INHALED GLUCOCORTICOIDS
IN ASTHMA

LUNG BIOLOGY IN HEALTH AND DISEASE

Executive Editor

Claude Lenfant
Director, National Heart, Lung and Blood Institute
National Institutes of Health
Bethesda, Maryland

Primary Pulmonary Hypertension, *edited by Lewis J. Rubin and Stuart Rich*

Parasitic Lung Diseases, *edited by Adel A. F. Mahmoud*

Pulmonary and Cardiac Imaging, *edited by Caroline Chiles and Charles E. Putman*

Lung Growth and Development, *edited by John A. McDonald*

Inhalation Delivery of Therapeutic Peptides and Proteins, *edited by Lex A. Adjei and P. K. Gupta*

Treatment of the Hospitalized Cystic Fibrosis Patient, *edited by David M. Orenstein and Robert C. Stern*

Dyspnea, *edited by Donald A. Mahler*

Lung Macrophages and Dendritic Cells, *edited by Mary F. Lipscomb and Stephen W. Russell*

Beta$_2$-Agonists in Asthma Treatment, *edited by Romain Pauwels and Paul M. O'Byrne*

The opinions expressed in these volumes do not necessarily represent the views of the National Institutes of Health.

INHALED GLUCOCORTICOIDS IN ASTHMA

MECHANISMS AND CLINICAL ACTIONS

Edited by

Robert P. Schleimer

*The Johns Hopkins University
School of Medicine
Baltimore, Maryland*

William W. Busse

*University of Wisconsin
Medical School
Madison, Wisconsin*

Paul M. O'Byrne

*McMaster University
Hamilton, Ontario, Canada*

Marcel Dekker, Inc.   **New York • Basel • Hong Kong**

Library of Congress Cataloging-in-Publication Data

Inhaled glucocorticoids in asthma : mechanisms and clinical actions /
    edited by Robert P. Schleimer, William W. Busse, Paul M. O'Byrne.
        p. cm. — (Lung biology in health and disease ; v. 97)
    Includes bibliographical references and index.
    ISBN 0–8247–9730–2 (hardcover : alk. paper)
    1. Asthma—Hormone therapy. 2. Glucocorticoids—Therapeutic use:
I. Schleimer, Robert P. II. Busse, W. W. (William W.)
III. O'Byrne, Paul M. IV. Series.
[DNLM: 1. Asthma—drug therapy. 2. Glucocorticoids—pharmacology.
W1 LU62 v.92 1997 / WF 553 I55 1997]
RC591.I536 1997
616.2'38061—dc20
DNLM/DLC
for Library of Congress

                                                                    96–32804
                                                                         CIP

The publisher offers discounts on this book when ordered in bulk quantities. For more information, write to Special Sales/Professional Marketing at the address below.

This book is printed on acid-free paper.

Marcel Dekker, Inc.
270 Madison Avenue, New York, New York 10016

Current printing (last digit):
10 9 8 7 6 5 4 3 2

PRINTED IN THE UNITED STATES OF AMERICA

INTRODUCTION

The history of asthma is a long one with which we associate names such as Maimonides, Hippocrates, Aretaeus the Cappodocian, and others whom we revere. One of the most striking descriptions of the disease is to be found in the writings of Thomas Willis in *Pharmaceutice Rationalis*, published in London in 1679:

> The organs of breathing, and the precordia themselves, which are the foundation and Pillars of Life, are shaken by this disease, as by an Earthquake, and so totter, that nothing less than the ruin of the whole animal Fabrick seems to be threatened; for breathing, whereby we chiefly live, is very much hindred by the assault of the disease, and in danger, or runs the risque of being quite taken away.

Early in the voyage of asthma understanding, the role of environmental allergens—"external causes," as Hippocrates said it—had been recognized. In contrast, the notion that asthma may be an inflammatory disease was not accepted until recently. Yet, long ago, descriptions of asthma evoked images of inflammation. for example, Thomas Willis referred to "extravasated blood" causing the "straitness of the Bronchia." It appears that William Osler must be credited for formally introducing the concept of inflammation; indeed, in the Principles and Practice of Medicine (1892) he stated that "in many cases it [asthma] is a special form of inflammation of the smaller bronchioles."

The quest for effective treatments for inflammation has engendered much research. As pointed out by the editors of this volume in their Preface, the 1949 description of Hench and his collaborators of the dramatic effect of cortisone and adrenocorticotropic hormone (ACTH) in patients with rheumatoid arthritis (1) was a landmark event in this search.

Later in the same year, two very important reports appeared simultaneously. One was based on "the prompt control of the chronic asthmatic state and the striking alterations in the tissues of the upper respiratory tract in five asthmatic patients (treated with ACTH)" (2). The other also reported "decided improvement" in one case of status asthmaticus, but, more important, it pointed out the following:

> 1) the fundamental process by which adrenalcortical steroids affect (asthma) is unknown . . . and
> 2) although the use of pituitary adrenocorticotrophic hormone and cortisone in human patients may result in dramatic remissions . . . , such use may also be attended with serious complications. (3)

It is fair to say that these two points have been with us ever since; they have led to considerable and brilliant research and have fueled endless debate.

This volume, edited by Drs. Schleimer, Busse, and O'Byrne, addresses these two points and reports the most up-to-date, if not definitive, answers. This was accomplished by bringing together a cadre of leading experts from several countries. Their discussion, disagreements, and agreements are reported in this unique and novel volume.

Ever since its beginning—only 20 years ago—the series of monographs Lung Biology in Health and Disease has had one goal: to assist the clinical and research communities by presenting ideas, and often solutions to problems. This volume has accomplished the goal superbly. The editors and authors are to be commended for such a major contribution.

As the Executive Editor of the series, I thank them for it and for the opportunity to share their wisdom with clinicians and investigators.

Claude Lenfant, M.D.
Bethesda, Maryland

References

1. Hench PS, Kendall EC, Slocumb CH, Palley HF. The effect of a hormone of the adrenal cortex and of pituitary adrenocorticotrophic hormone in rheumatoid arthritis; preliminary report. Proc Staff Meet Mayo Clin 1949; 24:181–187.
2. Bordley JE, Carey RA, McGehee HA, Howard JE, Kattus AA, Newman EV, Winkenwerder WL. Preliminary observations on the effect of adrenocorticotrophic hormone (ACTH) in allergic disease. Bull Johns Hopkins Hosp 1949; 85:396–398.
3. Elkinton JR, Hunt AD, Gadfrey L, McCrory WW, Rogerson AG, Stokes J. Effects of pituitary adrenocorticotrophic hormone (ACTH) therapy. JAMA 1949; 141:1273–1279.

PREFACE

Glucocorticoids are now widely recognized to be the most effective and potent drugs for the treatment of diseases of inflammation. Purified synthetic glucocorticoids first became available for clinical use around 1949. While Hench, Kendall, and Reichstein were rewarded for their efforts in glucocorticoid development with the Nobel Prize in Medicine shortly thereafter, sufferers of inflammatory diseases of the airways such as asthma were rewarded with medications that for the first time could effectively manage these debilitating diseases. In the period of enthusiasm following the introduction of these drugs into clinical use, the unrequited use of high doses for extended periods was found to result in a constellation of side effects that could be quite severe. As a result, the use of these drugs was gradually restricted to those patients with severe disease. The remarkable efficacy of steroids was hard to ignore, however, and the pharmaceutical industry expended a great deal of effort to improve these drugs.

A convenient feature of diseases of the airways, including hay fever (rhinitis) and asthma, is that the airways are accessible to medications that are applied locally. This fact has been exploited in an attempt to reduce undesirable side effects of steroids by the development of inhaled or intranasal steroids.

One problem with this approach is that a significant portion of the inhaled or sprayed dose of medication is swallowed. Since the swallowed steroid is absorbed into the circulation, it was necessary to develop steroids that would be rapidly metabolized by the liver following absorption. The fact that the circulatory system takes all blood from the gastrointestinal tract to the liver facilitated these efforts, and it was possible to design a number of steroids with structural features that render them quite susceptible to hepatic metabolism on the 16- and 17-carbon atoms of the steroid nucleus. A few of these steroids are now in clinical use. Their efficacy is uncontested and their side effects are usually minimal; as a result, these drugs have become exceedingly popular for clinical management of airway inflammatory diseases.

The purpose of this volume is to discuss in detail the general pharmacology of glucocorticoids as it applies to their use in airways disease, in the context of specific issues that apply to topically active glucocorticoids. Thus, it is our goal to initiate a dialogue on a wide range of issues from the molecular biology of glucocorticoid action to their clinical efficacy, side effects, and value for therapy of asthma and related diseases. While the prevailing view is that molecular studies can give new insights into cellular, systemic, and organismic effects of drugs, it is our firm belief that enhanced awareness of observations in the clinic can help guide the cellular and molecular studies that form the basis of our understanding of both drug action and the disease process. We have gathered an important group of investigators who have had a high impact in these various aspects of glucocorticoid actions.

It is our sincere hope that this volume will be of great value to clinicians, basic scientists, and clinical investigators. The interdisciplinary flavor of the volume was intentional, and the goal of this intermingling of disciplines is to stimulate new ideas, new concepts, new strategies, and, it is hoped, improvement of pharmacological management of asthma and other airways diseases. It is our firm belief that the value of glucocorticoids has not peaked and that new and still better glucocorticoid preparations will be developed. It is also our hope that advances in the understanding of glucocorticoid mechanisms of action will continue to be a wellspring for a new understanding of the mechanisms of allergic diseases as well as for the development of new strategies to combat these diseases.

We would like to express our gratitude to many individuals who helped make this project viable. The initial idea to have a meeting and volume such as this sprang from early conversations with Dr. Ralph Brattsand, the developer of budesonide, one of the most widely used inhaled glucocorticoids. We would like to thank Mr. Erik Lanner and Dr. Michael J. Fox for their generous support of this project. We would like to also acknowledge the invaluable assistance of Drs. Lisa Beck, Cristiana Stellato, and Lisa Schwiebert, as well as Ms. Bonnie Hebden, for their painstaking and attentive care in documenting the discussion sessions of the volume. Finally, we would like to thank the editor of this series, Dr. Claude Lenfant.

Robert P. Schleimer
William W. Busse
Paul M. O'Byrne

CONTRIBUTORS

Bengt I. Axelsson, Ph.D.   Assistant Director, Departments of Preclinical R&D and Pharmacology, Astra Draco AB, Lund, Sweden

Peter J. Barnes, D.M., D.Sc., F.R.C.P.   Professor and Chairman of Thoracic Medicine, National Heart and Lung Institute, Imperial School of Medicine, London, England

Lisa A. Beck, M.D.   Assistant Professor of Dermatology and Medicine, The Johns Hopkins Asthma and Allergy Center, The Johns Hopkins University School of Medicine, Baltimore, Maryland

John W. Bloom, M.D.   Associate Professor of Pharmacology and Medicine, Department of Pharmacology, University of Arizona College of Medicine, Tucson, Arizona

Bruce S. Bochner, M.D.   Associate Professor, Department of Medicine, Division of Clinical Immunology, The Johns Hopkins Asthma and Allergy Center, The Johns Hopkins University School of Medicine, Baltimore, Maryland

Ralph Brattsand, Ph.D.   Associate Professor of Experimental Pharmacology and Assistant Director, Departments of Preclinical R&D and Pharmacology, Astra Draco AB, Lund, Sweden

William W. Busse, M.D.   Professor of Medicine, and Head, Department of

Allergy and Immunology, Department of Medicine, University of Wisconsin Medical School, Madison, Wisconsin

Neil Clipstone, M.D. Department of Pathology, Howard Hughes Medical Institute, Stanford University School of Medicine, Stanford, California

Chris J. Corrigan, M.A., M.Sc., Ph.D., M.R.C.P. Clinical Senior Lecturer and Honorary Consultant Physician, Department of Allergy and Clinical Immunology, National Heart and Lung Institute, Imperial College, London, England

David J. Cousins, B.Sc. Research Associate, Department of Allergy and Respiratory Medicine, UMDS, Guy's and St. Thomas' Hospitals, London, England

Gerald R. Crabtree, M.D. Professor and Investigator, Department of Pathology and Developmental Biology, Howard Hughes Medical Institute, Stanford University School of Medicine, Stanford, California

Kelly Davenpeck, Ph.D. Fellow, Medicine, The Johns Hopkins Asthma and Allergy Center, The Johns Hopkins University School of Medicine, Baltimore, Maryland

Judah A. Denburg, M.D., F.R.C.P. Professor, Department of Medicine, McMaster University, Hamilton, Ontario, Canada

Jerry Dolovich, M.D. Professor, Department of Pediatrics, McMaster University and St. Joseph's Hospital, Hamilton, Ontario, Canada

Stephen R. Durham Reader and Honorary Consultant Physician, Department of Allergy and Clinical Immunology, National Heart and Lung Institute, Imperial College, London, England

Staffan Edsbäcker, Ph.D. Associate Director, Department of Human Pharmacology, Astra Draco AB, Lund, Sweden

Ann Efthimiadis, M.L.T. Registered Laboratory Technologist and Research Assistant, Department of Medicine, St. Joseph's Hospital and McMaster University, Hamilton, Ontario, Canada

Bradley Fletcher, M.D. Department of Biological Chemistry, University of California School of Medicine, Los Angeles, California

Jack Gauldie, Ph.D. Professor and Chairman, Department of Pathology, McMaster University, Hamilton, Ontario, Canada

Rebecca Gilbert, M.D. Department of Biological Chemistry, University of California School of Medicine, Los Angeles, California

Gerald J. Gleich, M.D. Professor of Immunology and Medicine, Department of Immunology, Mayo Clinic and Mayo Foundation, Rochester, Minnesota

Isabella Graef, M.D. Postdoctoral Fellow, Department of Pathology, Howard Hughes Medical Institute, Stanford University School of Medicine, Stanford, California

Qutayba Hamid, M.D. Associate Professor, Meakins-Christie Laboratories, McGill University, Montreal, Quebec, Canada

Frederick E. Hargreave, M.D. Professor, Department of Medicine, St. Joseph's Hospital and McMaster University, Hamilton, Ontario, Canada

Harvey Herschman, M.D. Professor, Department of Biological Chemistry, University of California School of Medicine, Los Angeles, California

Steffan N. Ho, M.D., Ph.D. Acting Assistant Professor, Department of Pathology, Stanford University School of Medicine, Stanford, California

Peter H. Howarth, M.D. Immunopharmacology Group, University Medicine, Southampton General Hospital, Southampton, England

Loren W. Hunt, M.D. Department of Immunology and Medicine, Allergic Disease Research Laboratory, Mayo Clinic and Mayo Foundation, Rochester, Minnesota

Manel Jordana, M.D., Ph.D. Associate Professor, Department of Pathology, McMaster University, Hamilton, Ontario, Canada

Michael Karin, Ph.D. Professor, Department of Pharmacology, University of California, San Diego, School of Medicine, La Jolla, California

A. B. Kay, F.R.C.P., Ph.D. Professor and Director, Department of Allergy and Clinical Immunology, National Heart and Lung Institute, Imperial College, London, England

Dean Klyber, M.D. University of California, Los Angeles, Los Angeles, California

Dean Kujubu, Ph. D. Department of Biological Chemistry, University of California School of Medicine, Los Angeles, California

Annika Laitinen, M.D. Assistant Professor, Department of Medicine, Institute of Biomedics, University of Helsinki, Helsinki, Finland

Lauri A. Laitinen, M.D. Professor and Head, Department of Medicine, University Central Hospital, Helsinki, Finland

Stephen J. Lane, M.D., Ph.D. Lecturer in Medicine, Department of Allergy and Respiratory Medicine, UMDS, Guy's and St. Thomas' Hospitals, London, England

Tak H. Lee, M.D., M.R.C.Path., F.R.C.P. Professor, Department of Allergy and Respiratory Medicine, UMDS, Guy's and St. Thomas' Hospitals, London, England

Donald Y. M. Leung, M.D., Ph.D. Professor and Head, Division of Pediatric Allergy-Immunology, National Jewish Center for Immunology and Respiratory Medicine, and University of Colorado Health Sciences Center, Denver, Colorado

E. R. McFadden, Jr., M.D. Director of Pulmonary and Critical Care Medicine and Argyle J. Beams Professor of Medicine, Department of Medicine, Case Western Reserve University School of Medicine, Cleveland, Ohio

Roger L. Miesfeld, Ph.D. Associate Professor, Department of Biochemistry, University of Arizona, Tucson, Arizona

Jeffrey Northrop, M.D. Department of Pathology, Howard Hughes Medical Institute, Stanford University School of Medicine, Stanford, California

Paul M. O'Byrne, M.D. Professor and Head, Division of Respirology, Department of Medicine, McMaster University, Hamilton, Ontario, Canada

Søren E. Pedersen, M.D. Professor and Consultant Pediatric Chest Physician, Department of Pediatrics, Kolding Hospital, University of Odense, Kolding, Denmark

Carl G. A. Persson, Ph.D. Professor, Department of Clinical Pharmacology, University Hospital, Lund, Sweden

Emilio Pizzichini, M.D. Visiting Professor, Department of Medicine, St. Joseph's Hospital and McMaster University, Hamilton, Ontario, Canada

Marcia Pizzichini, M.D. Visiting Professor, Department of Medicine, St. Joseph's Hospital and McMaster University, Hamilton, Ontario, Canada

Srinivasa Reddy, Ph.D. PGR IV, Department of Biological Chemistry, University of California School of Medicine, Los Angeles, California

Douglas S. Robinson, M.D. Senior Lecturer and Honorary Consultant, Department of Allergy and Clinical Immunology, National Heart and Lung Institute, Imperial College, London, England

Fahri Saatcioglu, Ph.D. Assistant Research Molecular Biologist, Department of Pharmacology, University of California, San Diego, School of Medicine, La Jolla, California

Bengt Sarnstrand   Astra Draco, Lund, Sweden

Robert P. Schleimer, Ph.D.   Professor of Medicine, The Johns Hopkins Asthma and Allergy Center, The Johns Hopkins University School of Medicine, Baltimore, Maryland

Lisa A. Schwiebert, Ph.D.   Instructor of Medicine, The Johns Hopkins Asthma and Allergy Center, The Johns Hopkins University School of Medicine, Baltimore, Maryland

Patricia J. Sime, M.B.Ch.B., M.R.C.P.   Department of Pathology, McMaster University, Hamilton, Ontario, Canada

Gerald C. Smaldone, M.D., Ph.D.   Associate Professor of Medicine, Physiology and Biophysics, Division of Pulmonary and Critical Care Medicine, Department of Medicine, State University of New York at Stony Brook, Stony Brook, New York

Jeffrey Smith, M.D.   Department of Biological Chemistry, University of California School of Medicine, Los Angeles, California

Ana R. Sousa, B.Sc.   Research Assistant, Department of Allergy and Respiratory Medicine, UMDS, Guy's and St. Thomas' Hospitals, London, England

Dontcho Z. Staynov, Ph.D.   Senior Lecturer, Department of Allergy and Respiratory Medicine, UMDS, Guy's and St. Thomas' Hospitals, London, England

Christiana Stellato, M.D.   Visiting Assistant Professor of Medicine, The Johns Hopkins Asthma and Allergy Center, The Johns Hopkins University School of Medicine, Baltimore, Maryland

Stanley J. Szefler, M.D.   Director of Clinical Pharmacology, Department of Pediatrics, National Jewish Center for Immunology and Respiratory Medicine, Denver, Colorado

E. Brad Thompson, M.D.   I. H. Kempner Professor and Chairman, Department of Human Biological Chemistry and Genetics, The University of Texas Medical Branch, Galveston, Texas

Luika A. Timmerman, M.S.   Graduate Student, Department of Pathology, Howard Hughes Medical Institute, Stanford University School of Medicine, Stanford, California

John H. Toogood, M.D., F.R.C.P.   Professor, Department of Medicine, Division of Clinical Immunology and Allergy, University of Western Ontario, London, Ontario, Canada

Diane Torry, M.Sc.   Graduate Student, Department of Pathology, McMaster University, Hamilton, Ontario, Canada

Guy M. Tremblay, Ph.D. MRC/CLA Postdoctoral Fellow, Department of Pathology, McMaster University, Hamilton, Ontario, Canada

Weilin Xie, Ph.D. Postdoctoral Fellow, Department of Biological Chemistry, University of California School of Medicine, Los Angeles, California

CONTENTS

**10. Inhibition of Inflammatory Cell Recruitment by Glucocorticoids:
Cytokines as Primary Targets** **203**

*Robert P. Schleimer, Lisa A. Beck, Lisa A. Schwiebert, Cristiana
Stellato, Kelly Davenpeck, and Bruce S. Bochner*

11. Airway Lymphocytes **239**

*Stephen R. Durham, Chris J. Corrigan, Douglas S. Robinson,
Qutayba Hamid, and A. B. Kay*

12. Effects of Corticosteroids on Basophils and Mast Cells **259**

Judah A. Denburg

INHALED GLUCOCORTICOIDS
IN ASTHMA

Part One

SUBCELLULAR ACTIONS OF GLUCOCORTICOIDS

1

Glucocorticoid Receptor Structure and Function

ROGER L. MIESFELD

University of Arizona
Tucson, Arizona

JOHN W. BLOOM

University of Arizona College of Medicine
Tucson, Arizona

I. Introduction

The glucocorticoid receptor (GR) is a ligand-regulated transcription factor that plays a critical role in modulating the expression of genes required for a variety of physiological processes. Biochemical and molecular biological analyses over the last decade have revealed that the mechanism of glucocorticoid action is due to ligand-dependent activation of GR transcriptional regulatory functions (1,2). The first part of this chapter summarizes key GR structure-function relationships known to be required for GR-mediated transcriptional control of gene expression as a consequence of sequence-specific GR DNA binding. The second part describes more recent data which demonstrates that the ligand-activated GR also inhibits gene expression by both direct and indirect mechanisms of transcriptional repression. This inhibitory function of the GR may be especially important for the action of inhaled glucocorticoids in the treatment of asthma (see refs., 3 and 4 and other chapters in this volume).

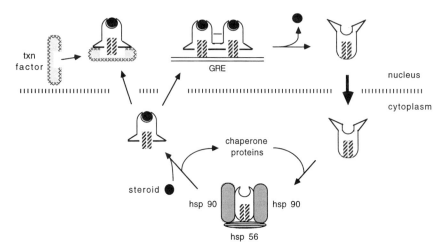

Figure 1 Glucocorticoid regulation of GR nuclear-cytoplasmic shuttling and GR transcriptional regulatory activities. GR exists in the unliganded form as a component of a large multisubunit protein complex in the cytoplasm. This complex contains a minimum of two subunits of hsp 90 and one subunit of hsp 56. Ligand binding results in activation and nuclear translocation of the receptor which is capable of both interacting with other transcription factors (txn factor) to cause transrepression and of binding to specific glucocorticoid response elements (GREs) on DNA leading to transcriptional transactivation. Dissociation of the steroid hormone from the receptor leads to a repartitioning of GR to the cytoplasm where it is then "refolded" by the hsp 90 and hsp 56 chaperone proteins into a conformation that is competent for ligand binding.

II. Biochemical Analyses of GR Functions

As shown in Figure 1, the unliganded and inactive GR exists primarily in the cytoplasm as part of a large multiprotein complex having an estimated molecular weight of ~330 kDa. This complex has been shown to contain a monomer of the ~90-kDa GR (5), two subunits of the heat shock protein (hsp) 90 (6,7), and one subunit of a ~56-kDa hsp referred to as hsp 56 (8). Initially, the GR-associated hsp 56 protein was identified as a 59-kDa immunofilin protein (9). There also appears to be one subunit of the hsp 70, and an acidic 23-kDa protein associated with the large unliganded GR complex (see ref. 10 for review). Ligand binding to the GR is thought to result in a conformational change in the receptor which leads to the disruption of the multisubunit complex and activation of GR functions. These activated receptors can either form homodimers and bind to specific DNA sequences called glucocorticoid response elements (GREs) located in GR target genes (2,11,12), or interact with other transcription factors and inhibit their activity (13–16).

When glucocorticoid levels in the cell decrease, the ligand dissociates from the receptor leading to a repartitioning of the GR from the nucleus to the cytoplasm. The mechanism of intracellular shuttling of the GR between the nucleus and the cytoplasm is not completely understood, but it has been suggested that hsp 90 and hsp 56 association with unliganded GR in the cytoplasm is required for the proper folding of the receptor into a conformation capable of ligand binding (10). This hormone-dependent activation and intracellular cycling of the GR is schematically shown in Figure 1.

The mechanistic basis of glucocorticoid signaling has been elucidated by combining classic biochemical analyses with structure-function studies of cloned GR cDNA sequences. The complete coding sequence of the GR from human (17), mouse (18), rat (19), and several other mammals (20,21) has been isolated and analyzed. A comparison of the GR amino acid sequences among various species has shown that the 66–amino acid DNA binding domain is highly conserved (100% identical between rats and humans) and there is only a ~5-10% amino acid difference in the rest of the protein (21). In humans, the GR gene is located on chromosome 5, and it has been mapped to chromosome bands 5q31-32 using in situ hybridization techniques (22,23).

Figure 2 shows a functional map of the GR as determined by a variety of experimental approaches. The three major protein domains are the carboxy-terminal hormone binding domain, the small DNA binding domain that comprises two repeats of a protein motif referred to as a zinc finger, and the amino-terminal (N-terminal) transcriptional transactivation domain. The evolutionary conservation of GR amino acid sequences between the various species characterized to date are also shown in Figure 2.

The following subsections summarize results from GR structure-function analyses which have led to the identification and characterization of numerous receptor activities. For organizational purposes, these functions will be presented in the context of the three major protein domains, which will be referred to as the hormone binding domain (HBD), the DNA binding domain (DBD), and the N-terminal domain (NTD).

A. GR Hormone Binding Domain

The ~250–amino acid carboxy-terminal GR HBD has so far eluded high-resolution protein structural analysis partly because of the difficulty in obtaining suitable material for x-ray crystallography. Nevertheless, much has been learned by investigating this region of the receptor using several strategies based on structure-function analyses. Figure 3 shows a linear map of the GR HBD, including the location of the minimal ligand binding region and the relative position of residues thought to be involved in ligand interactions. Note that many

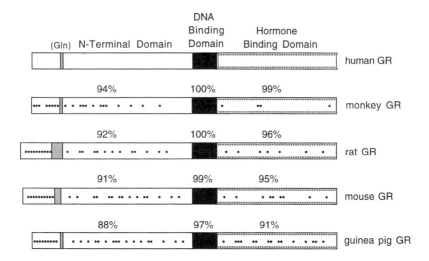

Figure 2   Functional map and evolutionary comparison of mammalian GR coding sequences. The linear map of the human GR coding sequence is shown at the top with the three major protein domains identified as the N-terminal domain, the DNA binding domain, and the hormone binding domain. The stippled box corresponds to the position of repeating glutamine residues (Gln), which vary from 2 in human GR to 19 in rat GR. The amino acid sequence homology of GR from four other mammalian species are shown for comparison. Dots indicate the position of amino acid substitutions in each mammalian receptor relative to human GR. The percentages refer to amino acid identity in each of the three domains relative to human GR.

of the GR HBD studies discussed below have been done with mouse or rat GR, but because of the high-sequence conservation between human, mouse, and rat GR (see Fig. 2), it is possible to extrapolate these data from rodents to humans.

The first approach used to study the GR HBD was based on obtaining purified native GR isolated from rat liver cells for covalent affinity labeling and partial proteolysis mapping to identify a minimum region required for hormone binding. These studies showed that ~ 135–amino acid GR subfragment fragment (amino acids 519–655 in human GR) was sufficient to bind hormone albeit with a 23-fold lower affinity than the intact domain (24). It has subsequently been shown using rat GR that the affinity label dexamethasone 21-mesylate covalently attaches to Cys 656 (25). In addition, it was found that the glucocorticoid triamcinolone acetonide can be cross linked by ultraviolet radiation to Met 622 and Cys 754 of purified rat GR (26). More recently, the thiol-blocking reagent methyl methanethiosulfonate was shown to interfere with glucocorticoid binding to rat GR by interacting with Cys 640, Cys 656, and Cys 661

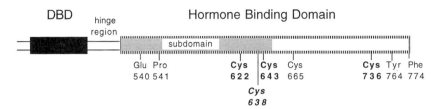

Figure 3 Functional map of the GR hormone binding domain (HBD). Schematic representation of the ~250–amino acid human GR HBD showing the relative position of the minimal ligand binding subdomain (stippled area) and the positions of amino acids shown to be important for high affinity ligand binding. The bolded amino acids were identified by ligand cross-linking studies and the plain text denotes amino acids which have been mutated and shown to decrease ligand affinities. Amino acid substitutions at the italicized amino acid Cys 638 were found to create "super" receptors. The amino acid numbering system is shown for human GR and was extrapolated from ligand binding studies using rat and mouse GR as described in the text.

(27). Together these ligand binding data implicate a number of cysteine residues in the GR HBD as potential interaction sites between the ligand and the receptor.

Chen and Stallcup (28) have recently used site-directed mutagenesis of cDNA encoding the mouse GR HBD to test the contribution of the cysteine residues to HBD function. Their results indicated that only mutations in Cys 742 and Cys 671 had substantial effects on ligand binding activity. It was found that by changing Cys 742 to serine or Cys 671 to serine or alanine, there was a 10- to 40-fold decrease in affinity for dexamethasone, whereas similar mutations in the other cysteines in the HBD had negligible effects. However, the deleterious effect of Cys 742 and Cys 671 mutations on GR functions could be overcome by using saturating levels of dexamethasone which resulted in normal levels of DNA binding and transcriptional transactivation.

The results of other studies examining the effect of point mutations in the GR HBD are also summarized in Figure 3. For example, alterations in mouse GR at Glu 546 completely eliminates ligand binding (18), whereas substitutions at Tyr 770 or Pro 547 only reduces binding affinities (29). Similarly, when Phe 780 in mouse GR was changed to an alanine, binding affinities for various hormones decreased from 25-fold for dexamethasone to 150-fold for hydrocortisone (30). Interestingly, when Cys 656 of rat GR was mutated to either a Gly or Ser residue, the ligand binding affinity of these receptors was actually increased, leading to the creation of "super" GRs (31). Point mutations in the human GR HBD have provided analogous results in that a Met to Arg replacement at residue 565 or a Ala to Gln conversion at residue 573 resulted in a

markedly higher ligand binding affinity and a sixfold increase in GR transactivation functions (32).

   Four other GR functions, in addition to ligand binding, have been mapped
to the HBD (see Fig. 3). These include residues required for hsp 90 interactions (33–35), receptor homodimerization (36–38), nuclear translocation
(39,40), and transcriptional transactivation (41,42). However, interpretations of
these data are not straightforward, since this region of the GR is likely to fold
into a complex structure that undergoes conformational changes in the presence
of ligand or when interacting with hsp 90 and hsp 56. Clearly, a better understanding of how these receptor functions are controlled by hormone interactions
awaits more definitive structural analyses of the GR HBD under a variety of
conditions.

B. GR DNA Binding Domain

Several comprehensive reviews have recently been written describing protein-
DNA interactions between the GR DBD and specific nucleotides within high-
affinity GR binding sites (43–45), and therefore these data will only be briefly
summarized here.

   The GR DBD is encoded within a 66–amino acid segment which forms
a structurally autonomous protein domain consisting of two zinc finger DNA
binding motifs. A schematic map of the GR DBD is shown in Figure 4. The
molecular structure of a GR DBD-DNA complex has been solved and shown

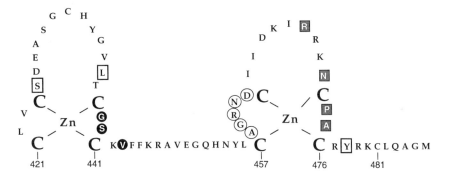

Figure 4   Functional map of the GR DNA binding domain (DBD). The two zinc finger DNA binding motifs are schematically shown as looped structures and the amino acid
sequence of the human GR DBD is written in single-letter code. Circles represent amino
acids identified to be important for GR-DNA interactions (filled circles) and GR-GR
homodimerization (open circles). Squares show amino acids found to be required for
transcriptional regulatory activities, independent of DNA binding, based on functional
analysis of GR transactivation (closed boxes) and GR transrepression (open boxes).

to consists of a GR DBD dimer interacting through alpha helices with the major groove in DNA (46). Each GR DBD monomer subunit contacts nucleotides specifying one half of a palindromic GRE binding site, and in addition, makes protein-protein contacts to form a second dimer interface within the DBD (the other dimerization interface is in the HBD). These structural data of the GR DBD were obtained by Luisi et al. (46) using multiple isomorphous replacement to solve the crystal structure of an 86–amino acid fragment of the rat GR (the extra 20 amino acids were on the carboxy end of the DBD). It was determined by this analysis that Lys 461, Val 462, and Arg 466 of the rat GR DBD are contained within an alpha helical region, and that all three of these residues make direct contact with multiple bases in the DNA.

Figure 4 summarizes the results from biochemical and molecular genetic studies which revealed that two additional amino acids contained within the first zinc finger also contribute to DNA binding specificity (47–51). These two residues, Gly 458 and Ser 459 in rat GR, coordinate with Val 462 to form a DNA sequence recognition motif referred to as the P box (52). This conserved GSckV sequence is found in the first zinc finger of the four GR subfamily steroid receptors which includes the androgen, progesterone, and mineralocorticoid receptors (53). DNA binding studies have shown that this GR subfamily of receptors all bind with high affinity to the DNA half-site sequence TGTTCT (54). In contrast, other steroid and nuclear receptors contain different P box sequences; for example, the estrogen receptor has the sequence EGckA in this region of the DBD specifying high-affinity binding to a DNA half-site sequence of TGACCT (52).

Other GR functions have also been mapped to the GR DBD suggesting that this small region of the receptor is important for making specific protein-protein contacts with other transcription factors. Using a yeast genetic screen to identify DBD mutants of rat GR, Schena et al. (48) found that two amino acids in the second zinc finger (Arg 488 and Asn 491) displayed defects in transcriptional regulatory activity in CV-1 cells without altering DNA binding affinities. Based on these results, they proposed that this region of the DBD may encode the previously identified enh 1 transcriptional transactivation function (55). Another rat GR DBD mutant called LS-7 has been described which has a similar phenotype in that this receptor is defective in transcriptional transactivation but not in DNA binding (56). The rat GR LS-7 mutations change Pro 493 and Ala 494 to Arg and Ser, respectively. Finally, with regard to transactivation functions that have been mapped to the GR DBD, it has been found that potentiation of GR-mediated transcriptional induction of SWI/SNF/BRM proteins in yeast (57) and human (58) cells requires amino acids in the DBD which may be distinct from those required for DNA binding.

Perhaps more relevant for understanding glucocorticoid action in asthma, it is known that transcriptional repression by the GR also requires sequences within the DBD. Functional mapping studies using various GR deletion mutants and GR fusion proteins have shown that the GR DBD is required for repression of gene activation by members of the AP-1 (13,14,59,60) and NF-κB (16,61) transcription factor families. In fact it has been shown that the rat GR LS-7 mutant is fully functional for AP-1 repression (62,63), suggesting that GR DBD-mediated transactivation and repression are separate functions and independent of DNA binding. In support of this conclusion, Heck et al. (64) have shown that Ser 425, Lys 436, and Tyr 478 in human GR are required for AP-1 repression but not for DNA binding, DBD dimerization, or transactivation. It has also been found that GR repression of NF-κB activity is mediated through the GR DBD (16). Figure 4 shows the relative location of these various GR DBD mutations and summarizes their effect on GR activity.

C. GR N-Terminal Domain

The largest of the three major GR protein domains is the NTD, which is defined as the N-terminal ~400 amino acids found within the first coding exon of the GR gene (this corresponds to the second exon [65]), as shown in Figure 5. Most notably, this portion of the receptor contains the transcriptional transactivation domain called tau 1 (66) or enh 2 (67). Transcriptional transactivation by NTD-encoded sequences is ligand independent in that tau 1–mediated transactivation can be observed using heterologous DNA binding

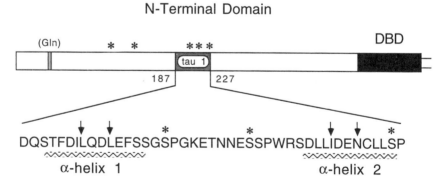

Figure 5 Functional map of the GR N-terminal domain (NTD). The relative position of the tau 1 core transactivation domain in human GR is shown as a stippled box (amino acids 187–227). The sequence of the 41–amino acid tau 1 core segment is also shown. The asterisks identify the corresponding position of serine residues in human GR, which were shown to be phosphorylated in mouse GR. The arrows identify amino acids in the tau 1 core which when replaced by proline residues, disrupted the structure of two predicted alphahelical regions (jagged lines).

domains derived from the *Escherichia coli* LexA (67) or yeast Gal 4 (68) proteins. The contribution of the NTD to GR function was first shown by the biochemical analysis of GR protein expressed in a class of glucocorticoid-resistant thymocyte mutant cell lines called nt^i for nuclear transfer increased (69). It was found that the nt^i GR could bind hormone and DNA but not mediate dexamethasone-induced apoptosis (70). Molecular characterization of the nt^i GR coding sequence revealed that this protein is truncated and translated from an aberrantly spliced mRNA lacking exon 2 and therefore the entire NTD (71). Genetic complementation experiments demonstrated that loss of the NTD-encoded tau 1 transactivation function was indeed responsible for the defect in GR-mediated thymocyte apoptosis (72). This particular alternate GR mRNA splicing pattern, however, may be rare in humans, since an examination of GR transcripts in thymocytes isolated from patients with steroid-resistant leukemia failed to identify any individuals with an nt^i GR defect (73).

To better understand the function of the NTD in GR-mediated transcriptional transactivation, Gustafsson and colleagues have characterized the tau 1 transactivation function by expressing portions of the human GR NTD in yeast cells. They initially found that high level expression of the human GR tau 1 region (amino acids 77–262) causes growth inhibition and inhibits expression of endogenous yeast genes (68). Based on the characteristics of this in vivo phenotype, and on results from in vitro transcription studies using a yeast cell free transcription system 74,75, they proposed that tau 1 residues interact with proteins required for basal transcription.

Dahlman-Wright et al. (76) have recently delineated a small "core" of 41 amino acids contained within the human GR tau 1 region which they show is responsible for transactivation function (see Fig. 5). To investigate the secondary structure of the tau 1 core polypeptide, they overproduced it in bacterial cells and used circular dichroism and nuclear magnetic resonance spectroscopy to characterize its biophysical properties in the presence and absence of trifluoroethanol (77). Their results indicate that the tau 1 core contains at least two segments with alpha helix propensity which can be disrupted by the insertion of proline residues leading to a loss of transactivation function. These results suggest that NTD-mediated transactivation is likely to be due to the function of a tau 1–encoded acidic activation domain based on the similarity of its biophysical properties with other known transcriptional activation domains (78).

The other important feature of the NTD is the presence of seven phosyphorylated residues which have been mapped to six serines and one threonine in the mouse GR (79) (this corresponds to five conserved serines in the human GR). The role of GR phosphorylation at these NTD phosphorylation sites was initially thought to be involved in GR transactivation. This model, however, appears not to be the case, since systematic site-directed mutagenesis of all seven of the phosphorylated residues was found to have little effect on trans-activation properties of the mouse GR (80). Another possibility is that GR phosphorylation at these sites may be important for receptor shuttling between the cytoplasm and the nucleus in response to hormone binding and cell cycle events. Several studies have shown that the GR is highly phosphorylated in the G_2/M phase of the cell cycle and unable to function efficiently as a ligand-activated transactivator (81,82). Based on the finding that four of the NTD phosphorylation sites are within consensus sequences for cell cycle–associated cyclin-dependent kinases and mitogen-activated protein kinases, a model as been proposed to account for basal and ligand-induced GR phosphorylation at different stages of the cell cycle (83). Because of these differences in GR activity during the cell cycle, it has been suggested that some forms of glucocorticoid resistance encountered during steroid therapy may be due to large numbers of steroid-nonresponsive G_2/M cells containing hyperphosphorylated GR (82).

III. GR-Mediated Control of Gene Expression

The molecular basis of glucocorticoid action is GR-mediated control of gene expression. This can either be due to transcriptional induction of specific GR target genes as a result of sequence-specific DNA binding and tau 1 trans-activation or GR-dependent transcriptional repression involving protein-protein interactions between the GR and other transcription factors. Although neither of these regulatory mechanisms is completely understood, it has become clear in the last several years that glucocorticoid signaling can lead to a variety of cellular responses depending on the physiological state of the cell (84). Since many of the beneficial effects of inhaled glucocorticoids in asthma treatment are likely to be the result of downregulation of cytokine gene expression (3,4), this section will summarize what is known about transcriptional repression in eukaryotes and then describe results from recent studies in which GR-mediated repression has been characterized.

A. Mechanisms of Transcriptional Repression in Eukaryotes

Complex transcriptional regulatory circuits in eukaryotes involve multiple levels of control and integration. Molecular characterization of numerous eukaryotic promoters and regulatory regions have shown that these DNA elements contain potential binding sites for large numbers of transcription factors (85). It is important to keep in mind that DNA-binding transcription factors are likely to represent only the first level of complexity, as it is now known that non-DNA binding accessory proteins, called adaptor molecules, are also required for transcriptional control (86). Moreover, chromatin structure (87) and DNA methylation at CpG residues (88) contribute to overall levels of transcription, perhaps by modulating transcription factor accessibility to regulatory sequences (85). Nevertheless, for the purposes of this chapter, transcriptional repression will be discussed only in the context of the protein-DNA and protein-protein interactions, as shown in Figure 6. Three basic mechanisms of transcriptional repression have been identified (see refs. 89 and 90 for reviews): activator competition, activator quenching, and direct inhibition.

Activator Competion

Activator competition describes the mechanism by which a repressor protein (R) is able to interfere with the ability of a transcriptional activator protein (A) to bind to its sequence-specific response element (RE) located within the regulatory region of a target gene (see Fig. 6A). This competition can be indepen-

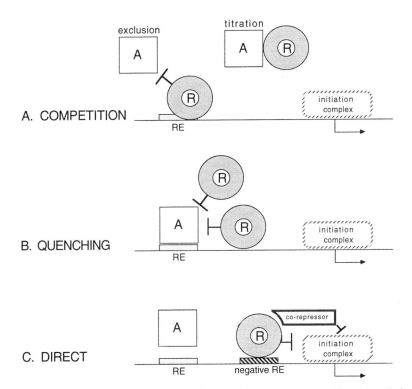

Figure 6 Mechanisms of transcriptional repression in eukaryotes. The three distinct mechanisms of transcriptional repression by activator competition, activator quenching, and direct inhibition are shown. R represents a repressor protein, A is an activator protein, and RE is a DNA binding site which functions as a response element. See text for details.

dent of DNA binding by either of the proteins, which is a form of repression by titration sometimes called "squelching" (91). Competitive titration has been suggested as a mechanism to explain the inhibitory function of a repressor protein called Id, which is a helix-loop-helix protein that inactivates basic helix-loop-helix proteins by forming nonfunctional heterodimers (92). A second type of activator competition is one that could be described as repression by exclusion. This mechanism is exemplified by the repressor protein GCF, which binds to a DNA sequence that overlaps an SP1 binding site in the epidermal growth factor promoter (93). When GCF is bound to these GC-rich sequences in the promoter, then SP1 is excluded and unable to bind an activate transcription. A similar competitive exclusion mechanism has been proposed to account for COUP-TF inhibition of estrogen receptor binding to overlapping sequences in the lactoferrin gene (94).

Activator Quenching

The second transcriptional repression mechanism, as shown in Figure 6B, is called activator quenching. As defined here, quenching is due to the repressor-mediated inhibition of transactivation function of a DNA bound activator protein. Repressor-mediated activator quenching does not require that the repressor be bound to DNA, although is often is (89,90). The distinction between activator competition (see, Fig. 6A) and activator quenching (see Fig. 6B) is whether or not the activator protein is bound to its response element as a prerequisite for repressor protein function. One of the best examples of activator quenching is the repressing effect of the *Drosophila* protein Snail on DNA-bound activators such as Dorsal (95). In this case, Snail only has repressing activity if Dorsal is functioning as an activator and when the Snail protein is bound to DNA. Importantly, Snail is not a dedicated transcriptional repressor, because it has no effect on basal transcription.

Direct Inhibition

Direct repression, as shown in Figure 6C, is characterized by repressor-mediated inhibition of transcription initiation complex assembly (89). Most importantly, direct repression can occur in the absence or presence of activator proteins. The *Drosophila* homeodomain protein Even-Skipped is an example of a eukaryotic repressor that inhibits transcription initiation complex formation (96). Some types of direct repression may be due to DNA-induced allosteric changes in the conformation of the repressor protein. For example, specific protein-DNA interactions at binding sites called negative response elements (NREs) may lead to the "unmasking" of repressor domains which only function under certain conditions (97). Such a mechanism of allosteric control of GR function has recently been proposed to explain the repressing activities of several DBD mutations in the rat GR (98). Figure 6C illustrates that adaptor proteins functioning as corepressors could mediate direct repression as a result of their association with DNA-bound regulatory proteins. Both allosteric control of repressing activity and interaction of regulatory proteins with corepressors could also be involved in mechanisms of activator quenching (see Fig. 6B).

B. GR-Mediated Transcriptional Repression

Based on studies in prokaryotic systems where transcriptional repression is most often the result of interference between a repressor protein and RNA polymerase (90), it was thought that GR-mediated repression would be due to competitive exclusion of activator proteins (53). However, this form of repression would not easily explain how the GR could be a repressor under some conditions, but an activator under others, if it were to be bound to the same GRE DNA sequence. One model to explain this apparent paradox was proposed by Sakai et al. (99) to account for GR-mediated repression of prolactin gene expression. According to this model, ligand-activated GR binds to "negative GRE" (nGRE) sequences (distinct from GRE sequences) in the prolactin promoter, which function as allosteric regulators of GR activity. Studies of the proopiomelanocortin gene promoter have suggested that GR-mediated repression of proopiomelanocortin expression could also be due to GR binding to such nGRE sequences (100). It is presently not known if GR-mediated repression of prolactin and proopiomelanocortin gene expression is the result of direct repression or if activator proteins are required for the GR effect.

Several other examples of DNA-dependent GR-mediated repression have now been reported as listed in Table 1. The best characterized of these is the composite GRE sequence in the proliferin gene which consists of a GR binding site that overlaps with a site for the AP-1 transcription factor (101). AP-1 is a heterodimeric transcription factor complex most often consisting of the two proteins c-*fos* and c-*jun* (102). Yamamoto and colleagues found that transcriptional repression of the proliferin gene required GR DNA binding, and their results have suggested that the GR might be quenching the transactivation function of the AP-1 complex (103). A similar GRE/AP-1 composite site has also been found in the herpes virus type 16 gene-regulatory region (104). The only other composite GRE characterized so far is in the promoter of the c-*fos* gene, and it contains overlapping GR and SRF (serum response factor) binding sites (105). It was shown in these studies that GR binds to SRF sites in the c-*fos* promoter, but it was not clear if GR-mediate repression of c-*fos* expression is due to activator competition or quenching.

Although there are several examples of DNA-dependent GR-mediated repression, as shown in Table 1, it may be that these represent the exception rather than the rule. In 1990, three groups of researchers simultaneously re-

Table 1 GR-Mediated Transcriptional Repression

Gene	GR DNA Binding?	Activator Protein	References
Prolactin	Yes	?	99
Proopiomelanocortin	Yes	?	100
Proliferin	Yes	AP-1	101
HPV 16	Yes	AP-1	104
c-*fos*	Yes	SRF	105
Collagenase	No	AP-1	62,106
IL-6	No	NF-κB	15
IL-8	No	NF-κB	108
MHC genes	No	NF-κB	16
ICAM-1	No	RelA	61
Ets-regulated genes	No	Spi-1/PU.1	110
Oct-regulated genes	No	Oct-2A, OTF-1	111,112
IL-2	No	NFIL-2B protein	113

ported that GR-mediated repression of AP-1 induction of the collagenase gene did not require GR DNA binding, but instead DNA-independent protein-protein interactions between GR and the AP-1 constituents c-*fos* and c-*jun* (62,106,107). These studies demonstrated that ligand-activated GR could inhibit phorbol ester activation of AP-1–regulated target genes, and moreover that AP-1 could repress glucocorticoid induction of GRE-containing reporter genes. A large number of studies have since confirmed that GR/AP-1 protein complexes are present in cells treated with both phorbol esters and glucocorticoids (see refs. 13 and 14 for reviews). This important finding helps to explain how glucocorticoids can have such a pronounced effect on cellular phenotypes, since GR-mediated "transrepression" would allow for the simultaneous induction and repression of both GR target genes and those controlled by AP-1.

Table 1 lists seven other genes which have recently been shown to be negatively regulated by GR transrepression. Two genes of particular relevance to glucocorticoid-suppressed inflammation are the interleukins IL-6 and IL-8 genes, both of which have been shown to be negatively regulated by GR-mediated repression of NF-κB function (15,108). NF-κB is a member of a multigene family of transcription factors whose activity is regulated at subcellular localization (109). Chemical cross linking has demonstrated that the GR interacts directly with the p65 subunit of NF-κB (15). It has also been shown that the GR interacts with RelA (61), another member of the NF-κB family (109), which leads to transcriptional repression of the intercellular adhesion molecule 1 (ICAM-1) gene promoter. Scheinman et al. (16) reported that p65 overexpression inhibits GR transactivation, and moreover that the GR DBD, but not GR DNA binding activity, was required for GR transrepression of NF-κB activity. Other transcription factors shown to be subject to GR transrepression include Spi-1/PU.1 (110), Oct-2A (111), OTF-1 (112), and the NFIL-2B binding protein (113) (see Table 1).

Most of the experiments done to date to characterize GR-mediated transrepression have relied on transient transfection assays and protein overexpression strategies, both of which could lead to an misinterpretation of the relevance of this phenomenon. However, there are at least two examples where GR/AP-1 cross signaling appears to be important physiologically. The best documented case is the developmental changes in GR activity during chick embryogenesis (114–116). Studies have shown that the level of GR protein in chick retinal glial cells is unchanged between days 6 and 10 even though the transactivation function of the GR rises significantly over this same period. To explain this observation, Vardimon and colleagues (115,117) examined the levels and activity of c-*jun* in day 6 and day 10 chicks and found that there was an inverse correlation between GR transactivation function and the amount of c-*jun* in these cells. A second example of where GR/AP-1 cross signaling may be playing role in vivo is in human T-cell apoptosis. Helmberg et al. (63) recently reported that the GR transactivation mutant LS-7 (56) is able to induce apoptosis in human Jurkat cells by a mechanism which is most consistent with GR transrepression of AP-1 functions. Moreover, studies in transgenic mice have suggested that thymocyte apoptosis may be similarly controlled by GR/AP-1 cross signaling (118,119).

IV. Summary and Perspectives

Understanding the molecular mechanisms of glucocorticoid action in asthma is an important next step in designing improved steroid and nonsteroidal therapies for the treatment of this prevalent disease (3,4). A working knowledge of the GR structure and function is now available, and it is clear from a large number of studies that GR-mediated transcriptional control is the basis of glucocorticoid action. Until recently, it was thought that most effects of glucocorticoids required direct DNA binding by the GR at either positive (GRE) or negative (nGRE) response elements located in the regulatory regions of GR target genes. There is now abundant evidence that the GR can also function in a DNA-independent manner to inhibit gene expression through a transrepression mechanism involving protein-protein interactions. Since AP-1 and NF-κB are known to be involved in the positive regulation of a number of genes that play a central role in inflammation, and GR transrepression mechanisms appear to be due to the formation of inactive GR/AP-1 and GR/NFκB complexes, it will be important to identify key AP-1– and NF-κB–regulated genes which are subject to GR-mediated transrepression.

As we extend our understanding of the molecular basis of anti-inflammatory action of glucocorticoids, it may be possible to develop more efficacious treatments of asthma based on combinatorial approaches. One avenue to pursue may be the development of glucocorticoid analogues that stimulate GR-transrepressing activities without inducing GR-transactivation functions. There are several new studies which suggest that this may be achievable. Heck et al. (64) found that three prototypical glucocorticoid antagonists, RU486, ZK98296, and ZK98299, are actually agonists in the context of GR/AP-1 transrepression. RU486 has also been shown to have the same effect on GR/NF-κB transrepression (16). This same type of ligand-selective effect has now been reported for several retinoic acid receptor agonist/antagonists which were shown to dissociate transactivation and AP-1 transrepression (120). These exciting findings suggest that ligand binding to the receptor causes subtle protein conformational changes in the GR DBD which can alter DNA binding but still allow for certain protein-protein interactions, such as those required for transrepression. Perhaps it may be possible to develop suitable inhaled steroids that could be used for the treatment of asthma which have this property of being selective agonist/antagonists of GR function.

Discussion

DR. HERSCHMAN: You estimate 10–100 genes are "regulated" by glucocorticoids. I presume you mean genes that are indirectly induced (or are constitutive genes that are suppressed) by glucocorticoids. However, there are many genes that are silent and not induced by glucocorticoids but whose induction by other agents is suppressed by glucocorticoids. This, I think, increases the number of "glucocorticoid regulated" genes substantially. (1) Many genes whose induction is blocked by glucocorticoids are not glucocorticoid suppressible when their promoters are used in transfection assays to drive reporter genes. Is this, as I am inclined to believe, a common phenomenon? (2) If so, does this imply that glucocorticoid suppression may be due to a DNA structure/chromatin context in many cases?

DR. MIESFELD: (1) From our interpretation of cDNA cloning data, and in limited cases three-dimensional protein gels, the number of rapidly regulated primary GR target genes (early-response genes) appears to be a defined subset of genes, I would guess about 10–100. Of course, when one includes cross-signaling pathways, the number is probably much greater because a potential nonoverlapping subset of genes is affected. Together then, a large number of genes may be potential targets depending on cell type, disease state, and compounding signals in addition to glucocorticoids. (2) Cross-talk interference by GR is not yet understood at the molecular level, but there is no reason to discount the role of DNA structure/chromatin.

DR. BARNES: You concentrated particularly on the interaction between GR and GRE, but many of the anti-inflammatory or immunomodulatory actions of glucocorticoids are likely to be due to repression of gene transcription. There are few instances of direct gene repression via nGREs and many examples of repression are secondary to interference with other transcription factors (such as AP-1 or NK-κB). Do you have information about the site of interaction between GR and these transcription factors?

DR. MIESFELD: There is clearly evidence that some mechanisms of GR-mediated transcriptional repression may involve direct protein-protein interactions. However, a caution must be taken because some of the studies were done under conditions of ectopic gene transfection and therefore protein levels may be greatly exaggerated compared to physiological conditions. The early AP-1–GR studies are an example of this. There is evidence from the study of rat prolactin gene repression by GR that this mechanism may involve a steric hindrance effect at what was termed a negative GRE. However, there was not a lot of examples as of yet of other "nGREs." It would follow that GR must not be functioning as a transcriptional activator under these conditions and, moreover, that GR can bind DNA at nonconsensus GRE sites.

DR. GLEICH: (1) Could you speculate regarding the possible mechanisms of the multiplicity of glucocorticoid actions? (2) Is there any evidence of glucocorticoid receptor heterogeneity? Is there one gene only and is there evidence of differential splicing of this gene product?

DR. MIESFELD: (1) Current models of glucocorticoids mechanisms at the molecular level have the common theme that multiple cell-specific and gene promoter-sensitive transcription factors interact with GR to result in a "jigsaw puzzle" of protein-protein interactions. Induction or repression of transcription is the observed outcome of these protein interactions. (2) Human GR maps to chromosome 5 and it is this genetic analysis which supports the existence of a single human GR gene.

DR. BARNES: There is recent evidence that there may be alternative splicing of the GR gene resulting in a form of GR (GRβ) that does not bind glucocorticoids and may have a blocking action by binding to GRE. It is possible that GRβ may be increased in glucocorticoid resistance.

DR. THOMPSON: Regarding the question as to whether three is one or many GRs, there seems to be a single gene for the GR, on chromosome 5. Indeed the GRβ form has been shown to be expressed in some cells. This form is a short C-terminal truncation of GRα and does not bind glucocorticoid. It may have some non-ligand-mediated functions. Pleiotropisms in the GR have been discovered-point mutations that do not seem to affect overall function. But as yet no one (to my knowledge) has demonstrated a subset of GRs responsible for specific gene effects. Based on spontaneous differential loss of glucocorticoid inducibility of genes in clones from the HTC cell line, I once proposed the formal possibility that there were gene-specific subsets of GRα. Based on the general data available today, it would seem that alterations in other transcription factors that interact with the GR is a likely explanation (Gehring U, Segnitz B, Foeller B, Francke U. Assignment of the human gene for the glucocorticoid receptor to chromosome 5. Proc Natl Acad Sci USA 1985; 82:3751–3755).

Dr. Miesfeld: One reason why it has been difficult to physically map gene-regulatory sequences that "specify" gene repression may be that transcriptional repression may in many cases involve DNA-independent mechanisms, i.e., indirect effects of activator protein inhibition. Transcriptional induction mechanisms appear to be more DNA-dependent working via specific DNA-binding sites.

References

1. Miesfeld RL, Okret S, Wikström A-C, Wrange Ö, Gustafsson JK, Yamamoto KR. Characterization of a steroid hormone receptor gene and mRNA in wild-type and mutant cells. Nature 1984; 312:779–781.
2. Miesfeld RL. Glucocorticoid action: Biochemistry. In: DeGroot LJ, ed. Endocrinology. 3rd ed. Philadelphia: Saunders, 1994:1656–1667.
3. Barnes PJ, Pedersen S. Efficacy and safety of inhaled corticosteroids in asthma. Am Rev Respir Dis 1993; 148(suppl.):S1–S26.
4. Barnes PJ, Adcock I. Anti-inflammatory actions of steroids: molecular mechanisms. Trends Pharmacol Sci 1993; 14:436–441.
5. Hutchison KA, Dittmar KD, Pratt WB. All of the factors required for assembly of the glucocorticoid receptor into a functional heterocomplex with heat shock protein 90 are preassociated in a self-sufficient protein folding structure, a "foldosome." J Biol Chem 1994; 269:27894–27899.
6. Bresnick EH, Dalman FC, Sanchez ER, Pratt WB. Evidence that the 90-kDa heat shock protein is necessary for the steroid binding conformation of the L cell glucocorticoid receptor. J Biol Chem 1989; 264:4992–4997.
7. Rexin M, Busch W, Gehring U. Protein components of the nonactivated glucocorticoid receptor. J Biol Chem 1991; 266:24601–24605.
8. Hutchison KA, Scherrer LC, Czar MJ, et al. FK506 binding to the 56-kilodalton immunophilin (Hsp56) in the glucocorticoid receptor heterocomplex has no effect on receptor folding or function. Biochemistry 1993; 32:3953–3957.

9. Tai P-KK, Albers MW, Chang H, Faber LE, Schrieber SL. Association of a 59-kilodalton immunophilin with the glucocorticoid receptor complex. Science 1992; 256:1315–1318.
10. Pratt WB. The role of heat shock proteins in regulating the function, folding, and trafficking of the glucocorticoid receptor. J Biol Chem 1993; 268:21455–21458.
11. Yamamoto KR. Steroid receptor regulated transcription of specific genes and gene networks. Annu Rev Genet 1985; 19:209–252.
12. Tsai M-J, O'Malley BW. Molecular mechanisms of action of steroid/thyroid receptor superfamily members. Annu Rev Biochem 1994; 63:451–486.
13. Ponta H, Cato ACB, Herrlich P. Interference of pathway specific transcription factors. Biochim Biophys Acta Gene Struct Expression 1992; 1129:255–261.
14. Schüle R, Evans RM. Functional antagonism between oncoprotein c-Jun and steroid hormone receptors. Cold Spring Harbor Symp Quant Biol 1991; 56:119–127.
15. Ray A, Prefontaine KE. Physical association and functional antagonism between the p65 subunit of transcription factor NF-kappaB and the glucocorticoid receptor. Proc Natl Acad Sci USA 1994; 91:752–756.
16. Scheinman RI, Gualberto A, Jewell CM, Cidlowski JA, Baldwin AS Jr. Characterization of mechanisms involved in transrepression of NF-kappaB by activated glucocorticoid receptors. Mol Cell Biol 1995; 15:943–953.
17. Hollenberg SM, Weinberger C, Ong ES, et al. Primary structure and expression of a functional human glucocorticoid receptor of cDNA. Nature 1985; 318:635–641.
18. Danielsen M, Northrop JP, Ringold GM. The mouse glucocorticoid receptor: mapping of functional domains by cloning, sequencing and expression of wild-type and mutant receptor proteins. EMBO J 1986; 5:2513–2522.
19. Miesfeld RL, Rusconi S, Godowski PJ, et al. Genetic complementation of a glucocorticoid receptor deficiency by expression of cloned receptor cDNA. Cell 1986; 46:389–399.
20. Brandon DD, Markwick AJ, Flores M, Dixon K, Albertson BD, Loriaux DL. Genetic variation of the glucocorticoid receptor from a steroid-resistant primate. J Mol Endocrinol 1991; 7:89–96.
21. Keightley M-C, Fuller PJ. Unique sequences in the guinea pig glucocorticoid receptor induce constitutive transactivation and decrease steroid sensitivity. Mol Endocrinol 1994; 8:431–439.
22. Francke U, Foellmer BE. The glucocorticoid receptor gene is in 5q31-q32. Genomics 1989; 4:610–612.
23. Theriault A, Boyd E, Harrap SB, Hollenberg SM, Connor JM. Regional chromosomal assignment of the human glucocorticoid receptor gene to 5q31. Hum Genet 1989; 83:289–291.
24. Simons SS Jr, Sistare FD, Chakraborti PK. Steroid binding activity is retained in a 16-kDa fragment of the steroid binding domain of rat glucocorticoid receptors. J Biol Chem 1989; 264:14493–14497.
25. Simons SSJr, Pumphrey JG, Rudikoff S, Eisen HJ. Identification of cysteine 656 as the amino acid of hepatoma tissue culture cell glucocorticoid receptors that is covalently labeled by dexamethasone 21-mesylate. J Biol Chem 1987; 262:9676–9680.

26. Carlstedt-Duke J, Strömstedt P-E, Persson B, Cederlund E, Gustafsson J-Å, Jörnvall H. Identification of hormone-interacting amino acid residues within the steroid-binding domain of the glucocorticoid receptor in relation to other steroid hormone receptors. J Biol Chem 1988; 263:6842–6846.

27. Chakraborti PK, Garabedian MJ, Yamamoto KR, Simons SS Jr. Role of cysteines 640, 656, and 661 in steroid binding to rat glucocorticoid receptors. J Biol Chem 1992; 267:11366–11373.

28. Chen D, Stallcup MR. The hormone-binding role of 2 cysteines near the C terminus of the mouse glucocorticoid receptor. J Biol Chem 1994; 269:7914–7918.

29. Byravan S, Milhon J, Rabindran SK, et al. Two point mutations in the hormone-binding domain of the mouse glucocorticoid receptor that dramatically reduce its function. Mol Endocrinol 1991; 5:752–758.

30. Chen D, Kohli K, Zhang S, Danielsen M, Stallcup MR. Phenylalanine-780 near the C-terminus of the mouse glucocorticoid receptor is important for ligand binding affinity and specificity. Mol Endocrinol 1994; 8:422–430.

31. Chakraborti PK, Garabedian MJ, Yamamoto KR, Simons SS Jr. Creation of "super" glucocorticoid receptors by point mutations in the steroid binding domain. J Biol Chem 1991; 266:22075–22078.

32. Warriar N, Yu C, Govindan MV. Hormone binding domain of human glucocorticoid receptor. Enhancement of transactivation function by substitution mutants M565R and A573Q. J Biol Chem 1994; 269:29010–29015.

33. Howard KJ, Holley SJ, Yamamoto KR, Distelhorst CW. Mapping the HSP90 binding region of the glucocorticoid receptor. J Biol Chem 1990; 265:11928–11935.

34. Housley PR, Sanchez ER, Danielsen M, Ringold GM, Pratt WB. Evidence that the conserved region in the steroid binding domain of the glucocorticoid receptor is required for both optimal binding of hsp90 and protection from proteolytic cleavage: a two-site model for hsp90 binding to the steroid binding domain. J Biol Chem 1990; 265:12778–12781.

35. Dalman FC, Scherrer LC, Taylor LP, Akil H, Pratt WB. Localization of the 90-kDa heat shock protein-binding site within the hormone-binding domain of the glucocorticoid receptor by peptide competition. J Biol Chem 1991; 266:3482–3490.

36. Wrange Ö, Eriksson P, Perlmann T. The purified activated glucocorticoid receptor is a homodimer. J Biol Chem 1989; 264:5253–5259.

37. Eriksson P, Wrange Ö. Protein-protein contacts in the glucocorticoid receptor homodimer influence its DNA binding properties. J Biol Chem 1990; 265:3535–3542.

38. Dahlman-Wright K, Wright A, Gustafsson J-Å, Carlstedt-Duke J. Interaction of the glucocorticoid receptor DNA-binding domain with DNA as a dimer is mediated by a short segment of five amino acids. J Biol Chem 1991; 266:3107–3112.

39. Picard D, Yamamoto KR. Two signals mediate hormone-dependent nuclear localization of the glucocorticoid receptor. EMBO J 1987; 6:3333–3340.

40. Cadepond F, Gasc J-M, Delahaye F, et al. Hormonal regulation of the nuclear localization signals of the human glucocorticosteroid receptor. Exp Cell Res 1992; 201:99–108.

41. Danielian PS, White R, Lees JA, Parker MG. Identification of a conserved region required for hormone dependent transcriptional activation by steroid hormone receptors. EMBO J 1992; 11:1025–1033.
42. Lanz RB, Rusconi S. A conserved carboxy-terminal subdomain is important for ligand interpretation and transactivation by nuclear receptors. Endocrinology 1994; 135:2183–2195.
43. Dahlman-Wright K, Wright A, Carlstedt-Duke J, Gustafsson J-Å. DNA-binding by the glucocorticoid receptor: a structural and functional analysis. J Steroid Biochem Mol Biol 1992; 41:249–272.
44. Freedman LP. Anatomy of the steroid receptor zinc finger region. Endocr Rev 1992; 13:129–145.
45. Freedman LP, Luisi BF. On the mechanism of DNA binding by nuclear hormone receptors: a structural and functional perspective. J Cell Biochem 1993; 51:140–150.
46. Luisi BF, Xu WX, Otwinowski Z, Freedman LP, Yamamoto KR, Sigler PB. Crystallographic analysis of the interaction of the glucocorticoid receptor with DNA. Nature 1991; 352:497–505.
47. Green S, Kumar V, Theulaz I, Wahli W, Chambon P. The N-terminal DNA-binding 'zinc finger' of the oestrogen and glucocorticoid receptors determines target gene specificity. EMBO J 1988; 7:3037–3044.
48. Schena M, Freedman LP, Yamamoto KR. Mutations in the glucocorticoid receptor zinc finger region that distinguish interdigitated DNA binding and transcriptional enhancement activities. Genes Dev 1989; 3:1590–1601.
49. Danielsen M, Hinck L, Ringold G. Two amino acids within the knuckle of the first zinc finger specify DNA response element activation by the glucocorticoid receptor. Cell 1988; 57:1131–1138.
50. Zilliacus J, Dahlman-Wright K, Wright A, Gustafsson J-Å, Carlstedt-Duke J. DNA binding specificity of mutant glucocorticoid receptor DNA-binding domains. J Biol Chem 1991; 266:3101–3106.
51. Alroy I, Freedman LP. DNA binding analysis of glucocorticoid receptor specificity mutants. Nucleic Acids Res 1992; 20:1045–1052.
52. Umesono K, Evans R. Determinants of target gene specificity for steroid/thyroid hormone receptors. Cell 1989; 57:1139–1146.
53. Miesfeld RL. The structure and function of steroid receptor proteins. CRC Crit Rev Biochem Mol Biol 1989; 24:101–117.
54. Beato M. Gene regulation by steroid hormones. Cell 1989; 56:335–344.
55. Miesfeld RL, Godowski PJ, Maler BA, Yamamoto KR. Glucocorticoid receptor mutants that define a small region sufficient for enhancer activation. Science 1987; 236:423–427.
56. Godowski P, Sakai D, Yamamoto K. Signal transduction and transcriptional regulation by the glucocorticoid receptor. In: Gralla JD, ed. DNA-Protein Interactions in Transcription. UCLA Symposium on Molecular and Cellular Biology, new series. New York: Liss, 1989; 95:197–210.
57. Yoshinaga SK, Peterson CL, Herskowitz I, Yamamoto KR. Roles of SWI1, SWI2, and SWI3 proteins for transcriptional enhancement by steroid receptors. Science 1992; 258:1598–1604.

58. Muchardt C, Yaniv M. A human homologue of *Saccharomyces cerevisiae SNF2/SWI2* and *Drosophila brm* genes potentiates transcriptional activation by the glucocorticoid receptor. EMBO J 1993; 12:4279–4290.
59. Kerppola TK, Luk D, Currant T. Fos is a preferential target of glucocorticoid receptor inhibition of AP-1 activity in vitro. Mol Cell Biol 1993; 13:3782–3791.
60. Liu W, Hillmann AG, Harmon JM. Hormone-independent repression of AP-1-inducible collagenase promoter activity by glucocorticoid receptors. Mol Cell Biol 1995; 15:1005–1013.
61. Caldenhoven E, Liden J, Wissink S, et al. Negative cross-talk between RelA and the glucocorticoid receptor: a possible mechanism for the antiinflammatory action of glucocorticoids. Mol Endocrinol 1995; 9:401–412.
62. Yang-Yen H-F, Chambard J-C, Sun Y-L, et al. Transcriptional interference between c-Jun and the glucocorticoid receptor: mutual inhibition of DNA binding due to direct protein-protein interaction. Cell 1990; 62:1205–1215.
63. Helmberg A, Auphan N, Caelles C, Karin M. Glucocorticoid-induced apoptosis of human leukemic cells is caused by the repressive function of the glucocorticoid receptor. EMBO J 1995; 14:452–460.
64. Heck S, Kullmann M, Gast A, et al. A distinct modulating domain in glucocorticoid receptor monomers in the repression of activity of the transcription factor AP-1. EMBO J 1994; 13:4087–4095.
65. Encío IJ, Detera-Wadleigh SD. The genomic structure of the human glucocorticoid receptor. J Biol Chem 1991; 266:7182–7188.
66. Giguère V, Hollenberg SM, Rosenfeld MG, Evans RM. Functional domains of the human glucocorticoid receptor. Cell 1986; 46:645–652.
67. Godowski PJ, Picard D, Yamamoto KR. Signal transduction and transcriptional regulation by glucocorticoid receptor-lexA fusion proteins. Science 1988; 241:812–816.
68. Wright APH, McEwan IJ, Dahlman-Wright K, Gustafsson J-Å. High level expression of the major transactivation domain of the human glucocorticoid receptor in yeast cells inhibits endogenous gene expression and cell growth. Mol Endocrinol 1991; 5:1366–1372.
69. Sibley CH, Tomkins GM. Mechanisms of steroid resistance. Cell 1974; 2:221–227.
70. Yamamoto KR, Gehring U, Stampfer MR, Sibley CH. Genetic approaches to steroid hormone action. Rec Prog Horm Res 1976; 32:3–32.
71. Dieken ES, Meese EU, Miesfeld RL. nt^i Glucocorticoid receptor transcripts lack sequences encoding the amino-terminal transcriptional modulatory domain. Mol Cell Biol 1990; 10:4574–4581.
72. Dieken ES, Miesfeld RL. Transcriptional transactivation functions localized to the glucocorticoid receptor N terminus are necessary for steroid induction of lymphocyte apoptosis. Mol Cell Biol 1992; 12:589–597.
73. Distelhorst CW, Miesfeld RL. Characterization of glucocorticoid receptors and glucocorticoid receptor mRNA in human leukemic cells: stabilization of the receptor by diisopropylfluorophosphate. Blood 1987; 69:750–756.
74. McEwan IJ, Wright APH, Dahlman-Wright K, Carlstedt-Duke J, Gustafsson J. Direct interaction of the t1 transactivation domain of the human glucocorticoid

receptor with the basal transcriptional machinery. Mol Cell Biol 1993; 13:399–407.

75. McEwan IJ, Almlöf T, Wikström A-C, Dahlman-Wright K, Wright APH, Gustafsson J. The glucocorticoid receptor functions at multiple steps during transcription initiation by RNA polymerase II. J Biol Chem 1994; 269:25629–25636.

76. Dahlman-Wright K, Almlöf T, McEwan IJ, Gustafsson J-Å, Wright APH. Delineation of a small region within the major transactivation domain of the human glucocorticoid receptor that mediates transactivation of gene expression. Proc Natl Acad Sci USA 1994; 91:1619–1623.

77. Dahlman-Wright K, Baumann H, McEwan IJ, et al. Structural characterization of a minimal functional transactivation domain from the human glucocorticoid receptor. Proc Natl Acad Sci USA 1995; 92:1699–1703.

78. O'Hare P, Williams G. Structural studies of the acidic transactivation domain of the Vmw65 protein of herpes simplex virus using ^{1}H NMR. Biochemistry 1992; 31:4140–4156.

79. Bodwell JE, Ortí E, Coull JM, Pappin DJC, Smith LI, Swift F. Identification of phosphorylated sites in the mouse glucocorticoid receptor. J Biol Chem 1991; 266:7549–7555.

80. Mason SA, Housley PR. Site-directed mutagenesis of the phosphorylation sites in the mouse glucocorticoid receptor. J Biol Chem 1993; 268:21501–21504.

81. Hsu S, Qi M, DeFranco DB. Cell cycle regulation of glucocorticoid receptor function. EMBO J 1992; 11:3457–3468.

82. Hu J-M, Bodwell JE, Munck A. Cell cycle-dependent glucocorticoid receptor phosphorylation and activity. Mol Endocrinol 1994; 8:1709–1713.

83. Bodwell JE, Hu L-M, Hu J-M, Ortí E, Munck A. Glucocorticoid receptors: ATP-dependent cycling and hormone-dependent hyperphosphorylation. J Steroid Biochem Mol Biol 1993; 47:31–38.

84. Bloom JW, Miesfeld RL. Molecular mechanisms of glucocorticoid action. In: Szefler S, Leung D, eds. Severe Asthma: Pathogenesis and Clinical Management. New York: Dekker, 1995:255–284.

85. Johnson PF, McKnight SL. Eukaryotic transcriptional regulatory proteins. Annu Rev Biochem 1989; 58:799–839.

86. Gill G, Tjian R. Eukaryotic coactivators associated with the TATA box binding protein. Curr Genet 1992; 2:236–242.

87. Clark D, Reitman M, Studitsky V, et al. Chromatin structure of transcriptionally active genes. Cold Spring Harbor Symp Quant Biol 1993; 58:1–6.

88. Bird AP. Functions for DNA methylation in vertebrates. Cold Spring Harbor Symp Quant Biol 1993; 58:281–285.

89. Cowell IG. Repression versus activation in the control of gene transcription. Trends Biochem Sci 1994; 1:38–42.

90. Herschbach BA, Johnson AD. Transcriptional repression in eukaryotes. Annu Rev Cell Biol 1993; 9:479–509.

91. Ptashne M. How gene activators work. Sci Am 1988; 260:40–47.

92. Benezra R, Davis RL, Lockshon D, Turner DL, Weintraub H. The protein Id: a negative regulator of helix-loop-helix DNA binding proteins. Cell 1990; 61:49–59.

93. Kageyama R, Pastan I. Molecular cloning and characterization of a human DNA binding factor that represses transcription. Cell 1989; 59:815–825.
94. Liu Y, Yang N, Teng CT. COUP-TF acts as a competitive repressor for estrogen receptor-mediated activation of the mouse lactoferrin gene. Mol Cell Biol 1993; 13:1836–1846.
95. Gray S, Szymanski P, Levine M. Short-range repression permits multiple enhancers to function autonomously within a complex promoter. Genes Dev 1994; 8:1829–1838.
96. Johnson FB, Krasnow MA. Differential regulation of transcription preinitiation complex assembly by activator and repressor homeo domain proteins. Genes Dev 1992; 6:2177–2189.
97. Saha S, Brickman JM, Lehming N, Ptashne M. New eukaryotic transcriptional repressors. Nature 1993; 363:648–652.
98. Lefstin JA, Thomas JR, Yamamoto KR. Influence of a steroid receptor DNA-binding domain on transcriptional regulatory functions. Genes Dev 1994; 8:2842–2856.
99. Sakai DD, Helms S, Carlstedt-Duke J, Gustafsson J-Å, Rottman FM, Yamamoto KR. Hormone-mediated repression: a negative glucocorticoid response element from the bovine prolactin gene. Genes Dev 1988; 2:1144–1154.
100. Drouin J, Sun YL, Chamberland M, et al. Novel glucocorticoid receptor complex with DNA element of the hormone-repressed POMC gene. EMBO J 1993; 12:145–156.
101. Diamond MI, Miner JN, Yoshinaga SK, Yamamoto KR. Transcription factor interactions: selectors of positive or negative regulation from a single DNA element. Science 1990; 249:1266–1272.
102. Curran T, Franza R Jr. Fos and Jun: the AP-1 connection. Cell 1988; 55:395–397.
103. Miner JN, Yamamoto KR. The basic region of AP-1 specifies glucocorticoid receptor activity at a composite response element. Genes Dev 1992; 6:2491–2501.
104. Mittal R, Kumar KU, Pater A, Pater MM. Differential regulation by c-*jun* and c-*fos* protooncogenes of hormone response from composite glucocorticoid response element in human papilloma virus type 16 regulatory region. Mol Endocrinol 1994; 8:1701–1708.
105. Karagianni N, Tsawdaroglou N. The c-*fos* serum response element (SRE) confers negative response to glucocorticoids. Oncogene 1994; 9:2327–2334.
106. Schüle R, Rangarajan P, Kliewer S, et al. Functional antagonism between oncoprotein c-Jun and the glucocorticoid receptor. Cell 1990; 62:1217–1226.
107. Jonat C, Rahmsdorf HJ, Park K-K, et al. Antitumor promotion and antiinflammation: down-modulation of AP-1 (Fos/Jun) activity by glucocorticoid hormone. Cell 1990; 62:1189–1204.
108. Mukaida N, Morita M. Ishikawa Y, et al. Novel mechanism of glucocorticoid-mediated gene repression. Nuclear factor-kappaB is target for glucocorticoid-mediated interleukin 8 gene repression. J Biol Chem 1994; 269:13289–13295.
109. Siebenlist U, Franzoso G, Brown K. Structure, regulation and function of NK-kB. Annu Rev Cell Biol 1994; 10:405–455.

110. Gauthier J-M, Bourachot B, Doucas V, Yaniv M, Moreau-Gachelin F. Functional interference between the Spi-1/PU.1 oncoprotein and steroid hormone or vitamin receptors. EMBO J 1993; 12:5089–5096.
111. Wieland S, Döbbeling U, Rusconi S. Interference and synergism of glucocorticoid receptor and octamer factors. EMBO J 1991; 10:2513–2521.
112. Kutoh E, Strömstedt P-E, Poellinger L. Functional interference between the ubiquitous and constitutive octamer transcription factor 1 (OTF-1) and the glucocorticoid receptor by direct protein-protein interaction involving the homeo subdomain of OTF-1. Mol Cell Biol 1992; 12:4960–4969.
113. Northrop JP, Crabtree GR, Mattila PS. Negative regulation of interleukin 2 transcription by the glucocorticoid receptor. J Exp Med 1992; 175:1235–1245.
114. Ben-Dror I, Havazelet N, Vardimon L. Developmental control of glucocorticoid receptor transcriptional activity in embryonic retina. Proc Natl Acad Sci USA 1993; 90:1117–1121.
115. Berko-Flint Y, Levkowitz G, Vardimon L. Involvement of c-Jun in the control of glucocorticoid receptor transcriptional activity during development of chicken retinal tissue. EMBO J 1994; 13:646–654.
116. Reisfeld S, Vardimon L. Cell to cell contacts control the transcription activity of the glucocorticoid receptor. Mol Endocrinol 1994; 8:1224–1233.
117. Dana SL, Hoener PA, Wheeler DA, Lawrence CB, McDonnell DP. Novel estrogen response elements identified by genetic selection in yeast are differentially responsive to estrogens and antiestrogens in mammalian cells. Mol Endocrinol 1994; 8:1193–1207.
118. Zacharchuk CM, Ashwell JD. Fruitful outcomes of intracellular cross-talk. Crosstalk between intracellular signalling pathways at the level of interacting transcription factors allows co-activation of two pathways to have a qualitatively different outcome from activation of either alone. Current Biol 1992; 2:246–248.
119. King LB, Vacchio MS, Ashwell JD. To be or not to be: mutually antagonistic death signals regulate thymocyte apoptosis. Int Arch Allergy Immunol 1994; 105:355–358.
120. Chen JY, Penco S, Ostrowski J, et al. RAR-specific agonist/antagonists which dissociate transactivation and AP1 transrepression inhibit anchorage-independent cell proliferation. EMBO J 1995; 14:1187–1197.

2

Negative Transcriptional Regulation by the Glucocorticoid Receptor Is Responsible for the Anti-inflammatory Activity of Glucocorticoids

MICHAEL KARIN and FAHRI SAATCIOGLU

University of California, San Diego
School of Medicine
La Jolla, California

I. Introduction

Steroid and thyroid hormones, as well as vitamins A and D and their metabolites, have pronounced effects on cellular physiology and differentiation. Although they are not absolutely required for cell survival, these substances are essential for the proper development and function of the entire organism. Most, if not all of their effects, are mediated through binding to their specific receptors, which belong to the nuclear receptor superfamily (1,2). Members of this family, which includes the glucocorticoid receptor (GR), are sequence specific DNA binding proteins that recognize *cis*-acting elements, known as hormone response elements (HREs), and act as ligand-activated transcription factors. Through binding to positively acting HREs (p-HREs), ligand-occupied receptors stimulate the transcription of hormone-inducible genes. This classic mode of gene regulation, which accounts for most cases of positive regulation by nuclear receptors, is fairly well characterized. However, nuclear receptors, and especially the GR, are also involved in negative regulation and can mediate repression of certain genes in response to ligand binding. The number of genes subjected to ligand-mediated repression approaches the number of genes which are ligand inducible (3). Despite recent advances, it has not been possible to formulate a simple, all-inclusive model accounting for negative gene regulation by nuclear receptors. One reason for this is that until now only a few genes have been studied in detail whose transcription is repressed by the liganded GR. Also, as more cases of negative regulation are studied, it has become apparent that DNA binding by the GR may not be sufficient or even required for ligand-dependent repression and an interplay with additional factors may be involved. The purpose of this chapter is to integrate these findings and describe two general mechanisms accounting for negative gene regulation by the GR. As shall be discussed, these mechanisms are likely to account for the potent anti-inflammatory and immunosuppressive activity of glucocorticoids.

II. Nuclear Receptor Superfamily

Sequence comparison of nuclear receptors indicates that they have a modular structure in which the centrally located DNA binding domain is the most highly conserved followed by the more variable C-terminal ligand binding domain (1,2) (Fig. 1). The DNA binding domain contains nine invariant cysteines involved in the formation of two "zinc fingers" (1,2). The N-terminal zinc finger dictates sequence specificity, whereas the C-terminal zinc finger contacts the sugar phosphate backbone to stabilize the DNA-receptor complex (see ref. 2 for review). Sequences present in the DNA binding domain facilitate dimerization after DNA binding even in the absence of the major dimerization surface, located in the ligand binding domain (4). The N-terminal domain is the least conserved region both in its sequence and size. This region is believed to modulate transcriptional activation by nuclear receptors and confer some specificity to their activity, probably through interaction with other transcription factors (5). The ligand binding domain, which is rich in hydrophobic amino acids, is relatively well conserved. In addition to ligand binding, this region contains the ligand-dependent activation function as well as the major dimerization surface (6). Like other family members, the GR binds DNA as a dimer (5,6). In addition, the unoccupied and probably unfolded ligand binding domain of the GR, like some of the other family members, binds heat shock proteins (hsps) (e.g., hsp 70 and hsp 90), an interaction that is thought to modulate receptor activity (7-9). As mentioned above, transcriptional activation by liganded nuclear receptors is mediated through two transcriptional activation functions (TAFs), known as TAF-1 and TAF-2, which are located at the N-terminal and C-terminal domains, respectively (5). Both TAF-1 and TAF-2 can be fused to heterologous DNA binding domains to generate chimeric activators that display their individual characteristics. Although activators containing TAF-1 are constitutively active, those containing TAF-2 are ligand dependent. However, in the intact molecule, the two functions may interact and modulate each other.

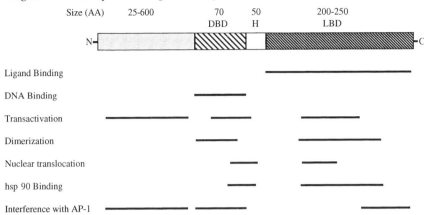

Figure 1 Domain structure of nuclear hormone receptors. The functional domains of nuclear receptors are schematically shown. Approximate sizes of domains in amino acids are indicated on the top. DBD, DNA binding domain, H, hinge region, LBD, ligand binding domain. Functions ascribed to the different domains are indicated by bars underneath.

A. Transcriptional Interference Between Nuclear Receptors and Other Transcription Factors

Repression by transcriptional interference results when a transcription factor is prevented from fruitfully interacting with the transcription initiation complex (TIC) through direct or indirect interactions with another transcription factor. Transcriptional interference may involve competition for binding to a common or overlapping *cis* active element, competition for a common mediator, a phenomenon also known as squelching, or formation of inactive complexes (see refs. 10 and 11 for reviews). Although nuclear receptors can interfere with transcriptional activation by several transcription factors, including CREB (12,13), Oct-1 (14), and bHLH proteins (15), interference with AP-1 activity has been most extensively studied and characterized, and is therefore discussed in detail here. Transcriptional interference between nuclear receptors and AP-1 was first demonstrated for the GR and falls in two categories depending on the type of response element involved: simple and composite. These will be discussed separately.

Transcriptional Interference at a Simple Response Element

Several laboratories have independently shown that AP-1 and some members of the nuclear receptor superfamily interfere with each others' transcriptional activity. Most of these studies concentrated on genes whose promoters contain

AP-1 binding sites and are known to be negatively regulated by glucocorticoids or retinoic acid (RA) in vivo, such as the genes coding for metalloproteases and interleukin-2 (IL-2). The collagenase and stromelysin genes encode the major matrix-degrading metalloproteases, which are capable of digesting collagen, fibronectin, and other structural components of connective tissue and basal lamina (16). Their deregulated expression in synoviocytes and macrophages is thought to be responsible for the destruction of bone and tendon in rheumatoid arthritis (RA) and other autoimmune disorders (16). Transcription of both collagenase and stromelysin is positively regulated by AP-1 which binds to a conserved site upstream to the TATA boxes in their promoters to mediate induction by growth factors and proinflammatory cytokines such as tumor necrosis factor alpha (TNF-α) and IL-1 (17). Interestingly, expression of both collagenase and stromelysin is dramatically repressed by glucocorticoids and retinoids (18–20). This repression most likely accounts for the therapeutic utility of glucocorticoids and RA as antiarthritic agents and is responsible for the downregulation of collagenase and stromelysin expression in inflamed synovia following glucocorticoid treatment (18–20). Analysis of the collagenase promoter indicated, that the element which mediates this repression is the AP-1 site (21–22). Furthermore, this AP-1 site can be inserted into other constitutively expressed promoters and confer on them growth factor and cytokine inducibility and repression by glucocorticoids and RA (21–23). Transient transfection experiments have shown that repression is mediated by the GR and RA receptor (RAR) and is strictly ligand dependent. Although the GR and RAR do not bind to the collagenase AP-1 site or any other site within the collagenase promoter, a functional DNA binding domain is required for repression (21,22,24). However, certain mutations within the DNA which severely attenuate the ability of the GR to activate promoters containing p-HREs (25) do not affect its ability to repress the collagenase promoter and interfere with AP-1 activity (22). In addition, the GR DNA binding domain can be replaced with a heterologous DNA binding domain, and the chimeric receptor retains its ability to interfere with AP-1 activity, although it can no longer interact with its cognate HRE (24). Deletion of the GR ligand binding domain, which converts it into a constitutive activator, renders it a ligand-independent repressor of AP-1 activity (21,22). Reciprocally, elevated expression of either the c-Jun or the c-Fos components of AP-1 prevents the activation of the MMTV promoter by GR (21,22,26). The repression of GR activity by c-Jun and c-Fos explains previous observations that growth factors, phorbol esters, and various activated oncogenes attenuate glucocorticoid-mediated gene transcription (26). The actual composition of the AP-1 complex interacting with the collagenase AP-1 site does not appear to be critical, as both c-Jun:c-Jun and c-Jun:c-Fos complexes can be repressed by activated the GR or RAR (22,23).

Like the GR and RARs, thyroid hormone (T3) receptors (T3Rs) are also capable of inhibiting AP-1 activity in response to ligand binding (27–29). Interestingly, v-ErbA, the oncogenic counterpart of the cellular T3Rα, has lost all of these activities owing to a deletion of nine amino acids at its extreme C-terminus (27,29). Single, double, or triple amino acid substitutions within this region completely abolished T3-dependent transcription, as well as interference with AP-1 activity (29). Decreased, but not abolished, T3 binding by these mutants does not fully account for the loss of transactivation and transcriptional interference activities. Furthermore, deletion of the homologous region in RAR resulted in similar loss of transcriptional activation and interference activities (29). The finding that v-ErbA had lost the ability to interfere with AP-1 (27,29) suggests that the inhibition of AP-1 activity could decrease the oncogenic potential of this mutant receptor. Indeed a large body of evidence indicates that elevated AP-1 activity is important for the proliferation of many (but not all) cell types (17). Therefore, the known antiproliferative effects of glucocorticoids and RA could be due to interference with AP-1 activity as originally suggested by Yang-Yen et al. (22,23). Indeed, it was recently demonstrated that glucocorticoids and RA block tetradecanoyl phorbol acetate (TPA)–induced anchorage independent growth at the same dose range required for interference with AP-1 activity (30).

Although both c-Jun and c-Fos were shown to interfere with activation by the liganded GR and RARs (22,23), there is limited data at present regarding other members of the AP-1 family. Among the Fos subfamily, Fos-B cannot repress transactivation by GR, whereas c-Fos is an efficient repressor (31). This functional difference between c-Fos and Fos-B has been traced to an N-terminal region in c-Fos which is absent in Fos-B (31). Information regarding the domains of Jun proteins that are required for interference with nuclear receptors is also limited. Although some investigators found that the c-Jun DNA binding domain is sufficient for repression of GR activity (24), other studies determined that the N-terminal activation domain is also required (J.-C. Chambard, unpublished results). Similar findings were reported regarding interference with estrogen receptor activity, which also requires the N-terminal activation domain of c-Jun (32).

Mixing of recombinant c-Jun and c-Fos proteins with partially purified or cell-free translated GR or RAR results in mutual inhibition of DNA binding activity (22,23). In vitro, the minimal DNA binding domain of c-Jun was sufficient for inhibition of GR and RAR binding to DNA (22,23). However, in vivo this part of c-Jun is not sufficient for inhibition of GR activity and the N-terminal activation domain is also required (J.-C. Chambard, unpublished results). In addition, no cross inhibition of DNA binding activity can be detected through the analysis of glucocorticoid- or TPA-treated cell extracts (22). Furthermore, genomic footprinting experiments on the collagenase promoter show that there is no change in the occupancy of the TPA response element (TRE) in the presence and absence of glucocorticoids in vivo (33). Thus, although confirmed and extensively studied by several different groups (22,23,24), mutual inhibition of DNA binding observed in vitro is unlikely to reflect accurately the in vivo interactions between AP-1 and nuclear receptors. These results suggest that a mechanism different from mutual inhibition of DNA binding is likely to operate in vivo. However, it is still possible that the activated receptor and AP-1 interact to block each other's ability to contact the TIC. Thus, if the GR sits on top of AP-1, it can block its interaction with the TIC or a mediator protein without affecting its contact with the collagenase promoter, which is consistent with genomic footprinting data (Fig. 2A). Since so far the in vitro interactions between purified AP-1 proteins and nuclear receptors are rather weak (21–23,35), other proteins may be required to stabilize these inhibitory interactions in vivo.

Alternatively, the receptor and AP-1 compete for an important cofactor required for efficient activation by both of them. The findings with T3R and RAR are most consistent with this mechanism. Single amino acid substitutions within the C-terminal of T3Rα abolished its ability to interfere with AP-1 and activate from a T3 response element but only partially interfered with T3 binding. This suggests that the C-terminal of T3R could be the site for interaction

---

Figure 2 A model illustrating the proposed mechanism of interference between the GCR and AP-1 from simple or composite response elements. (A) Interference at a simple response element. In the absence of ligand, AP-1 (dark hatched rectangle) binds to its cognate response element (TRE) and activates transcription by means of a cofactor (light shaded oval) which enables it to contact the transcriptional initiation complex (TIC). Upon binding ligand (small circle), the GCR (represented as in figure 2) gains the ability to interact with the cofactor, titrates it away from AP-1 and thereby inhibits AP-1 activated transcription (bottom left). Alternatively, liganded GCR binds to AP-1 which is already bound to the TRE causing a conformational change such that it can no longer contact the TIC (bottom right). Note that in this figure only the interference of AP-1 activity by GCR is shown, but a similar mechanism is likely to operate for the reverse situation where an activated AP-1 interferes with GCR activity. (B) Interference at a composite response element. In the absence of ligand, AP-1 (two small rectangles on DNA) binds to the composite response element (com-RE) either as a c-Jun:c-Jun homodimer (left) or a c-Jun:c-Fos heterodimer (right) giving rise to a low level of promoter activity. When ligand is added, the GR dimer binds to the com-RE and depending on the composition of the AP-1 complex, promoter activity is either activated or repressed. Since so far it has not been possible to detect a ternary complex involving AP-1, GR, and the com-RE, additional cellular factors may be necessary for this response as indicated (checkered oval with question mark).

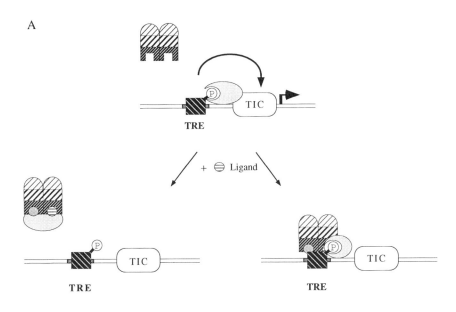

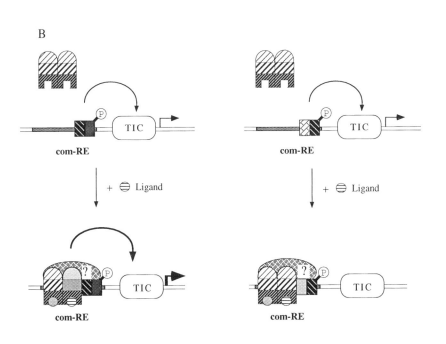

with a cofactor which is also required for efficient activation by AP-1 (see Fig. 2A). The finding that a mutant of RAR lacking the homologous region has also lost the ability to interfere with AP-1 (29) supports this hypothesis. In addition, the requirement for the N-terminal activation domain of c-Jun for effective interference with GR activity and the weaker interfering abilities of Jun-B and Jun-D are entirely consistent with this hypothesis. A definitive test of this hypothesis, however, relies on the isolation of the cofactor(s) required for efficient activation of transcription by AP-1 and nuclear receptors.

Transcriptional Interference at a Composite Response Element

Another gene that is repressible by glucocorticoids is the proliferin gene. Similar to collagenase and stromelysin, repression of proliferin expression is mediated through a *cis* element that is activated by TPA (36). However, unlike the collagenase promoter, footprinting of the proliferin promoter indicates that the *cis* element mediating repression is complex and contains both AP-1 and GR binding sites. A 25–base pair oligonucleotide, named plfG, corresponding to this element, bound both GR and AP-1 albeit with low efficiency, and when fused to a heterologous promoter, conferred both TPA induction and glucocorticoid repression (35).

Unlike the collagenase AP-1 site, repression through the plfG composite response element (com-RE) by the activated GR depends on the composition of the AP-1 complex. When the com-RE is occupied by c-Jun homodimers, the GR potentiates the activation produced by AP-1, but when the com-RE is bound by the c-Jun:c-Fos heterodimers, the activated GR represses the activation produced by AP-1. Simultaneous occupancy by both GR and AP-1 is a critical feature of the regulatory model presented for the com-RE (35). According to this model, transcriptional regulation through the com-RE involves both DNA-protein and protein-protein interactions in which the precise composition of the AP-1 bound to DNA determines the magnitude and direction of the hormonal response (35) (see Fig. 2B). Consistent with this view, and as pointed out in the previous section, it has been possible to detect direct protein-protein interactions between the GR and c-Jun and indirect interactions between the GR and c-Fos in the presence of c-Jun in vitro, but such interactions appear to be rather weak (21–23,35). It should also be noted that binding of GR to the com-RE has so far been demonstrated only with high concentrations of recombinant protein (35,36). This suggests that additional cellular factors may be involved, especially since so far no ternary complex, including the GR, AP-1, and the com-RE, was found. Recent in vitro binding studies suggest that some of the transcriptional properties of the GR at the com-RE may be explained by selective interference with DNA binding of different AP-1 components (34). However, no data are available at this time on the occupancy of com-RE in vivo. More detailed binding and mutagenesis studies of the proliferin com-RE is needed to assess mechanistic features of this putative co-occupancy model for cross talk between the GR and AP-1.

The mineralocorticoid receptor (MR), which binds to and activates from identical p-HREs as the GR, is unable to activate the com-RE (37). The analysis of GR/MR chimeras indicated that a segment within the GR amino-terminal is required for activity at the com-RE (37). So far, no other member of the nuclear receptor family has been shown to regulate transcription by binding to this com-RE. It is particularly important to examine whether the RARs and T3Rs which can interfere with AP-1 activity can affect the com-RE. A more detailed review of transcriptional interference from a composite response element has recently been published (38).

B. Inhibition of NF-κB Activation

Another transcription factor whose activity is inhibited by glucocorticoids is NF-κB. Unlike AP-1, which is constitutively nuclear, NF-κB is retained in the cytoplasm of nonstimulated cells through interaction with the IκB inhibitor (39,40,41). On cell stimulation with inflammatory mediators, such as TNF-α or IL-1, IκB is rapidly phosphorylated and proteolyzed (42,43), resulting in the liberation of NF-κB dimers which translocate to the nucleus. Once in the nucleus, NF-κB binds to target sites on responsive genes to activate their transcription (39,43). IκB synthesis itself is transcriptionally regulated by NF-κB, such that following NF-κB activation, IκB is resynthesized at a faster rate in negative feedback which restores NF-κB to the cytoplasm, thus terminating its activation (42–45).

It was reported that glucocorticoids also inhibit NF-κB transcriptional activity (46,47). In vitro, the GR was found to interact with p65, and this complex was precipitable by anti-GR antibodies (46,47). The p65 subunit of NF-κB, but not its p49 subunit, were found to repress activation of the MMTV-LTR by liganded GR (46). Correspondingly, p49 could not be cross linked or coprecipitated with the GR (46). These results suggested that the mechanism of NF-κB inhibition by the GR is similar to the mechanism of interference with AP-1 activity. The activated GR can interact with the p65 subunit of NF-κB and sequester it into a nonproductive complex. Since p65 harbors the major activation function of the NF-κB complex, its sequestration results in inhibition of NF-κB transcriptional activity. This model, however, predicts that glucocorticoids should not inhibit NF-κB DNA binding activity, as the NF-κB subunits p49 and p50 that have only minor activation functions (39,43) and do not interact with the GR (46) should still be able to dimerize and bind DNA.

We have recently confirmed that glucocorticoids are potent inhibitors of NF-κB activity and that inhibition together with the interference with AP-1 transcriptional activity could be a major contributor to the immunosuppressive activity of glucocorticoids (48). Contrary to the prediction that glucocorticoids should not inhibit the induction of NF-κB DNA binding activity, we found that treatment of several cell types with dexamethasone inhibited the appearance of NF-κB DNA binding activity following cell activation. This inhibition required expression of the functional GR and most importantly could be demonstrated in vivo. Administration of dexamethasone to mice blocked the induction of NF-κB activity by either lipopolysaccharide (LPS) or the potent T-cell activator anti-CD3 antibody (48). Close examination of the kinetics of NF-κB activation in cells incubated without or with glucocorticoids revealed that in the first 30 min, NF-κB binding activity is induced with similar kinetics, but after 30 min, this activity rapidly disappears in glucocorticoid-treated cells and persists in untreated cells. The inhibition of NF-κB activity by glucocorticoids was found to be dependent on new RNA and protein synthesis and was correlated with induction of a short-lived protein (48). Since IκB is a short-lived protein whose degradation is accelerated following cell activation (42,43), we examined the effect of glucocorticoids on its abundance. We found that cells expressing a functional GCR induce both IκB mRNA and protein synthesis and potentiate its postactivation induction in the presence of glucocorticoids (48). Therefore, glucocorticoid-treated cells reach higher levels of IκB faster than nontreated cells. As revealed by indirect immunofluorescence, this results in translocation of NF-κB from the nucleus to the cytoplasm in glucocorticoid-treated activated cells, whereas the GCR remains nuclear (48).

These findings reveal a much simpler mechanism that accounts for inhibition of NF-κB activity by glucocorticoids (Fig. 3). Instead of transcriptional interference between the activated GR and one or several components of NF-κB, the liganded GR binds and activates the IκB gene. This results in higher rates of IκB synthesis. Since any excess IκB that does not bind to NF-κB is rapidly degraded, IκB protein levels in glucocorticoid-treated nonactivated cells are not much higher than those in nontreated cells, although the levels of IκB mRNA are five- to sevenfold higher. Most importantly, however, following cell activation and the initial degradation of IκB, the levels of IκB reach the critical inhibitory concentration required for retention of NF-κB in the cytoplasm much faster than in nontreated cells. This results in relocation of activated NF-κB from the nucleus to the cytoplasm and termination of NF-κB–mediated gene induction. In activated cells not exposed to glucocorticoids, NF-κB remains in the nucleus for at least 4–5 hr resulting in efficient gene induction. As shall be discussed below, NF-κB has been implicated in the induction of many cytokines and other immunoregulatory molecules.

III. Physiological Implications

The ability of the GR to mediate both positive and negative effects on promoter activity in response to ligand binding indicates that the regulatory potential of

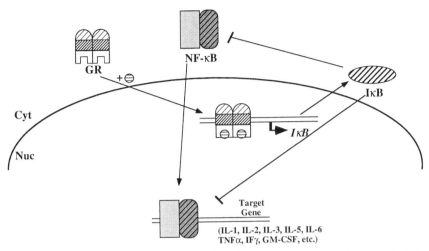

Figure 3 A model illustrating the proposed mechanism of interference between the GR and NF-κB. In the presence of ligand (small circle), GR binds and activates the IκB gene, which results in higher rates of IκB synthesis. Since any excess of NF-κB that does not bind to NF-κB is rapidly degraded, IκB levels in glucocorticoid-treated nonactivated cells are not much higher than those in nontreated cells, although the levels of IκB mRNA are five- to sevenfold higher. Following cell activation and initial degradation of IκB, the levels of IκB reach the critical inhibitory concentration required for retention of NF-κB in the cytoplasm much faster than in nontreated cells. This results in relocation of activated NF-κB from the nucleus (Nuc) to the cytoplasm (Cyt) and termination of NF-κB–mediated gene induction. In activated cells not exposed to glucocorticoids, NF-κB remains in the nucleus at least 4–5 hr resulting in efficient gene induction.

this transcription factor and most likely other members of its family is very broad. The ability of the GR to interfere with the activity of transcription factors whose activity is regulated in response to extracellular signals received at cell surface receptors, such as AP-1, CREB, and NF-κB, is extremely important, as it allows for a cross talk between glucocorticoids on the one hand and polypeptide hormone and cytokines on the other hand. This form of cross regulation is likely to be essential for the maintenance of cellular homeostasis and provide fine tuning to a variety of physiological processes, including cell proliferation and differentiation and inflammatory and immune responses. Some of the genes which are subject to this cross regulation include metalloproteases, such as collagenase and stromelysin, and many cytokine genes. The products of these genes, whose expression is activated by various growth factors, inflammatory mediators, and phorbol esters through AP-1 and NF-κB, play key roles in pathogenesis of various autoimmune disorders and regulation of immune and inflammatory responses (16,49). The inhibition of these genes by glucocorticoids is likely to contribute to the antiarthritic and immunosuppressive effects of these hormones (46,48).

Physiologically and clinically important glucocorticoid effects on lymphocytes include suppression of lymphokine production, inhibition of cell proliferation, and induction of apoptosis. Owing to this central role of IL-2 in the regulation of immune responses, suppression of its transcription by the activated GR is of particular interest. Activation of the IL-2 promoter is dependent on the cooperative action of at least four transactivating complexes binding to four different *cis* elements, designated as A, B, C, and E (50). The *cis* element closest to the TATA box, A, binds a complex of Oct-1 and AP-1 (51). Elements B and C bind AP-1 and the p50 homodimer form of NF-κB, respectively (52,53). Element E binds NF-AT, a complex of AP-1 and the cytoplasmic component NFATp (54–56). Deletion of any single *cis* element does not affect repression by glucocorticoids. However, constructs of multimerized single elements coupled to the minimal IL-2 promoter indicates that all of the activities containing AP-1 were repressed by glucocorticoids (57). In addition, NF-κB activity is also repressed by glucocorticoids (46–48), but NF-κB makes only a small contribution to IL-2 gene activation (48). Analysis of GR mutants indicates that the structural requirements needed for repression of IL-2 are the same as those required for interference with AP-1 activity (57). Importantly, dexamethasone effectively inhibited IL-2 transcription in a Jurkat cell line stably transfected with the activation-deficient glucocorticoid receptor mutant LS7 (25), which is still fully competent in interfering with AP-1 activity (58). Since this mutant is defective in gene activation, but not transcriptional interference (22), and the IL-2 promoter does not contain a GR binding site, it is quite clear that transcriptional interference is responsible for repression of this gene.

Transcriptional interference may also play a key role in glucocorticoid-induced apoptosis. Glucocorticoids kill immature thymocytes at rather low concentrations (59). At higher concentrations, they also kill certain subsets of mature T cells (60). Owing to their ability to induce apoptosis, glucocorticoids are an essential element in the chemotherapy of lymphomas and lymphocytic leukemias. In the human leukemic Jurkat cell line, the activation-defective but AP-1 repression-competent GR mutant LS7 proved as effective as the wild-type GR in mediating glucocorticoid-dependent apoptosis (58). Although the link between apoptosis and suppression of AP-1 activity may be a mere correlation, the repressive function of the GR, whose prototypic target is AP-1, seems to be sufficient for induction of apoptosis in lymphocytes. Although the putative "anti-apoptotic gene" or "survival gene" whose expression is inhibited by the activated GR remains to be identified, its gene product is expected to be involved in progression through the S phase in the cell cycle. When levels and/

or activity of this protein are decreased, it is possible that the S phase is not completed and an alternative abortive pathway is triggered resulting in activation of a nuclease responsible for nucleosomal cleavage and other events involved in programmed cell death.

AP-1 also plays critical roles in IL-2 gene activation and cell proliferation; however, it does not participate in the induction of all cytokine genes and other types of immunoregulatory genes. On the other hand, glucocorticoids inhibit the expression of many lymphokines, including IL-1, IL-3, IL-5, IL-6, γ-interferon, TNF-α, and granulocyte-macrophage colony-stimulating factor (GM-CSF) (61–68) in addition to IL-2. Furthermore, they also inhibit expression of class I and class II major histocompatibility complex (MHC) molecules and other adhesion molecules (68,69). It is hard to explain the repression of this rather impressive list of regulatory genes by the mere inhibition of AP-1 activity. On the other hand, many, if not all, of these genes are positively regulated by NF-κB (70,71). Thus, inhibition of NF-κB activation by glucocorticoids can easily account for much of their immunosuppressive and anti-inflammatory activity. NF-κB is induced in response to inflammatory stimuli, including LPS, and once induced it seems to be involved in activation of IL-1, IL-3, IL-6, IL-8, TNF-α, GM-CSF, class I and class II MHC genes, κ light chain genes, endothelial leukocyte adhesion molecule 1 (ELAM-1) and intercellular adhesion molecule 1 (ICAM-1) (72–81). Thus, the combined inhibition of AP-1 and NF-κB explains most of the anti-inflammatory activities of glucocorticoids. However, it should be pointed out that some of the NF-κB–inducible genes which may be involved in the inflammatory processes, such as ICAM-1 and vascular cell adhesion molecule 1 (VCAM-1), may not be downregulated by glucocorticoids (82) and require alternative explanations. Interestingly, the only positively regulated gene affected by glucocorticoids that is relevant for their anti-inflammatory activity is IκB, whose role is inhibition of NF-κB activation. Thus, it appears that the anti-inflammatory and immunosuppressive activity of glucocorticoids is based mostly on gene repression rather than gene activation.

Another example which underscores the physiological significance of interference between the GR and AP-1 is the involvement of c-Jun in the control of GR activity during development of retinal tissue (83). The expression of c-Jun is high in early embryonic retina and declines with age, and these changes in c-Jun expression are inversely correlated with GR transcriptional activity during development despite no significant change in GR protein levels. Elevation of c-Jun levels by TPA treatment or by overexpression of c-Jun caused a pronounced decline in GR-mediated transcription of various promoters which do not contain an AP-1 site, suggesting that this repression may be due to interference with GR activity from a single response element as discussed earlier.

Transcriptional interference between nuclear receptors and AP-1 is likely to play as major modulatory role in cell growth and differentiation. Glucocorticoids are inhibitory to the growth of various cell types and are used as antineoplastic agents (16,84). Beneficial effects of certain retinoids as antineoplastic agents have also been demonstrated (39,40,42,44,45,63,70,85–90). In addition, both glucocorticoids and retinoids have long been known to block tumor promotion by TPA in the mouse skin carcinogenesis model (88–90). These antiproliferative effects could be due to inhibition of AP-1 transcriptional activity by the liganded GR and RAR, since AP-1 is known to be stimulated by many different mitogens and tumor promoters (17). On the other hand, inhibition of GR and RAR activity by c-Jun and c-Fos can play an important role in relieving the inhibitory effect of glucocorticoids and retinoids on cell growth and thereby continue to cell proliferation and neoplastic transformation.

Taken together, it is possible that all of the therapeutic effects of glucocorticoids and retinoids which happen to be quite similar, despite the involvement of different nuclear receptors, are due to the inhibition of certain target genes by interference with other factors, such as AP-1. This raises the possibility that the side effects of the drugs used in many diseases, which happen to be quite distinct, are mediated by the classic gene induction mechanism involving the binding of receptors to cognate HREs. If correct, this assumption raises the interesting possibility that certain synthetic ligands may stimulate the transcriptional interference activities of nuclear receptors more efficiently than their ability to activate gene expression through their p-HREs. Such compounds may be more effective for treating diseases such as rheumatoid arthritis and other immune disorders, as their metabolic side effects are likely to be much milder than conventional receptor agonists. However, it is not clear whether such drugs would also be effective inhibitors of NF-κB, as its inhibition depends on induction of IκBα expression. Therefore, such compounds may not be as effective as immunosuppressive agent as glucocorticoids after all.

IV. Summary

Glucocorticoids, as do other steroid hormones, bind to nuclear receptors which act as ligand-modulated transcription factors. In many cases, ligand-activated nuclear receptors bind to p-HREs to induce gene transcription. However, ligand-activated receptors, especially the glucocorticoid receptor, also repress transcription of specific genes. Several mechanisms that account for negative regulation by glucocorticoids have recently emerged. One major form of negative regulation is based on transcriptional interference between the activated receptor and other transcription factors, such as AP-1. In this case, the liganded receptor prevents AP-1 or other positively acting transcription factors from fruitful interaction with the transcription initiation complex. A second mechanism accounting for negative regulation applies to repression of NF-κB activity by glucocorticoids. In this case, the activated receptor leads to induction of IκB, an inhibitor that associates with NF-κB and retains it in the cytoplasm. As AP-1 and NF-κB regulate the expression of many immunoregulatory genes, both of these mechanisms are likely to underlie the potent anti-inflammatory and immunosuppressive activity of glucocorticoids.

Acknowledgments

We would like to thank Arno Helmberg for helpful discussions. The work in the authors' laboratory was supported by a grant from the National Institutes of Health (CA50528) to M.K. F.S. was supported by postdoctoral fellowships from Tobacco Related Disease Research Program of California and American Heart Association, California Affiliate.

Discussion

DR. BRATTSAND: (1) Peter Herrlich et al. described in their reporter gene systems that inhibition of the AP-1-mediated pathway could be reached at a $10\times$ lower dexamethasone concentration than required for triggering GRE-mediated upregulation (Cell 1990; 62:1189). What do you know about the dose-response for inhibiting the NFκB pathway—does its threshold fit best with the AP-1 or the GRE findings above? (2) Is it possible to develop NFκB or AP-1 inhibitors that do not exert transactivation?

DR. SAATCIOGLU: (1) A 10-fold difference one might see for concentrations of ligand required for efficient transcriptional interference versus transactivation by the nuclear receptor in a transient transfection experiment may not be significant to translate into physiological effects. However, it is possible that the side effects of the drugs used are mediated by the classic gene induction mechanism by liganded receptors. (2) If this is correct, it should be possible to screen for and find synthetic ligands that activate the receptor for its transcriptional interference but not transactivation properties. Such ligands would be much more efficacious in treatment since they would have significantly decreased side effects. Indeed, such ligands have recently been discovered for the retinoic acid receptor but the biological efficacies remain to be determined.

DR. MIESFELD: The data showing that the LS7 GR mutant can still promote Jurkat cell apoptosis, without inducing MMTV transcription, need to be qualified by the finding that the MMTV GREs may be unusual and not potentially representative of all "GR inducible" cellular genes. We have found that the androgen receptor effectively induces mouse T-cell apoptosis without inducing MMTV transcription in the same cell.

DR. SAATCIOGLU: According to our current model, interactions between GR and AP-1 are not direct, but occur through a common cofactor. Our detailed mapping studies in T3R for anti-AP-1 activity clearly demonstrate that an essential part of the ligand-dependent transactivation domain may bind a cofactor that is absolutely required, reinforcing our model.

DR. THOMPSON: In the experiments showing that glucocorticoids induce IκB, did you measure its level of phosphorylation (since phosphorylation is required to release NF-κB, one could imagine a large increase in I-κB with a parallel change in phosphorylation)?

DR. SAATCIOGLU: Yes. With the reagents available to us at the moment, we did not see an effect on IκB phosphorylation by dexamethasone treatment. However, since phosphorylation of IκB is necessary but not sufficient for its degradation, one has to determine the effect of dexamethasone treatment, if any, on the whole process of IκB breakdown.

DR. GAULDIE: (1) Your data appear to imply that there are now at least three mechanisms for steroid suppression: induction of IκB, interference by protein interaction with NF-κB, and interference by protein interaction with AP-1. Is this your understanding? (2) How do you explain the data recently published by Ray et al. on the evidence for NF-κB interaction with GR dexamethasone in the suppression of IL-6 induction?

DR. SAATCIOGLU: (1) In the case of NF-κB, liganded GR activates the IκB gene through a putative GRE, which results in higher rates of IκB synthesis. This results in the retention of NF-κB in the cytoplasm, redistribution of activated NFkB from the nucleus to the cytoplasm, and NF-κB-mediated gene induction is terminated. In the case of AP-1, data from several laboratories suggest that there is competition for a common cofactor that is required for efficient transactivation by either protein. In this case, no GRE is involved, positive or negative. (2) See answer to Dr. Lane's question below.

DR. SEVERINSON: Is it known if the 5′-regulatory region of IκB contains a GRE site? Does the steroid receptor complex affect IκB director or indirectly?

DR. SAATCIOGLU: We did not find a GRE within -250 bp upstream of the MAD3 gene. We now have approximately 2.5 kb of the promoter and experiments are in progress to determine whether it contains a functional GRE.

DR. LANE: The effect of steroids is cell type- and stimulus-specific. Dexamethasone-mediated suppression of IL-8 in deletional mapping experiments and transient transfection studies in a glioblastoma cell line is by a NF-κB recognition site. Therefore, in this system, more than dexamethasone-mediated sequestration of NF-κB by IκB must be involved (Mukaida N, Morita M, Ishikawa Y, et al. Novel mechanism of glucocorticoid-mediated gene repression. NF-κB is target for glucocorticoid-mediated interleukin-8 gene repression. J Biol Chem 1994; 269:13289–13295).

DR. SAATCIOGLU: This study showed that inhibition of the IL-8 promoter activity by liganded glucocorticoid receptor is mediated through the NF-κB site. A physical interaction was demonstrated by coimmunoprecipitation experiments between p65 and GR, and p65 was shown to be retained in the nucleus after TPA-dexamethasone treatment by Western analysis. Although a direct interaction is possible between the two molecules, our immunofluorescence data clearly show that p65 translocates into the nucleus with TPA treatment and redistributes back to the cytoplasm upon addition of dexamethasone, in contrast to the in vitro findings of Mukaida et al. Since liganded GR is a nuclear protein, it is unlikely that direct binding of GR to p65 causes its redistribution and sequestration in the cytoplasm. I would like to suggest that our findings, which are obtained in situ, coupled with marked elevation of IκB mRNA and protein levels provide a more reliable and straightforward mechanism. However, we cannot rule out cell-type specific differences in the mechanism of anti-NF-κB activity by liganded GR.

DR. SCHLEIMER: If I understand your studies with the LS7 mutant correctly, one would expect that glucocorticoid would not inhibit the NFκB system and would not induce IκB. Have you tested this? Also, could you please tell us the importance of GR levels in determining responsiveness?

DR. SAATCIOGLU: This is a good experiment, but we have not done it.

DR. MIESFELD: GR protein levels can indeed be rate-limiting in cell-specific responses. It may be that natural variability in GR expression levels between patients could influence efficacy. Interestingly, heterozygous GR knockout mice (Schutz and co-workers) have GR-negative phenotypes in some cell types but are GR-normal in others, suggesting that the importance of GR levels may depend on the cell type being studied (Günther Schütz, German Cancer Research Center, Heidelberg, personal communication).

DR. GAULDIE: Is there anything to be learned from the fact that carrying out these transfections with reporter constructs in different cell types can lead to different answers; i.e., are different mechanisms involved in different cell types for the same gene?

DR. SAATCIOGLU: I think that the mechanism we have proposed to explain transcriptional interference between GR and AP-1, that they may be competing for a common cofactor, accommodates cell-type differences. For example, if the levels of this cofactor or any posttranslational modifications of it are different between the cell types, one would expect to find differences, both qualitative and quantitative.

DR. BRATTSAND: What is the role of dimerization of the receptor in interference with AP-1 activity?

DR. SAATCIOGLU: Our studies on anti-AP-1 activities of two other nuclear receptors, thyroid hormone receptor (T3R) and retinoic acid receptor (RAR), suggest that dimerization may have an effect since heterocomplexing of T3R and RAR with retinoid X receptors (RXRs) greatly increases their ability to inhibit AP-1. This also reinforces our model since the heterodimers are much more potent transactivators than the homodimers.

DR. BARNES: The interactions between glucocorticoids and other drugs need to be considered. There may be synergistic or inhibitory interactions that could be exploited, respectively. For example, we recently demonstrated a synergistic interaction between glucocorticoids and cyclosporin A in human T cells, which can be explained by the interaction between NF-AT or AP-1 and regulation of IL-2 gene expression. Other such interactions between GR and other tissue- or cell-specific transcription factors may be described in the future.

References

1. Evans R. The steroid and thyroid hormone receptor superfamily. Science 1988; 240:889–895.
2. Beato M. Gene regulation by steroid hormones. Cell 1989; 56:335–344.
3. Ivarie RD, Morris JA, Eberhardt NL. Hormonal domains of response: actions of glucocorticoid and thyroid hormones in regulating pleiotropic responses in cultured cells. Rec Prog Hormone Res 1980; 36:195–235.
4. Luisi BF, Xu WX, Otwinowski Z, Freedman LP, Yamamoto KR, Sigler PB. Crystallographic analysis of the interaction of the glucocorticoid receptor with DNA. Nature 1991; 352:497–505.
5. Gronemeyer H. Nuclear hormone receptors as transcriptional activators. In: Parker MG, ed. Steroid Hormone Action. New York: IRL Press, 1993:93–117.
6. Tsai M-J, O'Malley BW. Molecular Aspects of Cellular Regulation. In: Cohen P, Foulkes JG, eds. The Hormonal Control Regulation of Gene Transcription, London. Elsevier, 1991:101–116.
7. Catelli MG, Binart N, Jung-Testas I, Renoir JM, Bauleiu EE, Feramisco JR, Weich WJ. The common 80 kDa protein component of non-transformed 8S steroid receptor is a heat shock protein. EMBO J 1985; 4:3131–3135.
8. Howard KJ, Distelhorst CW. Evidence of the intracellular association of the glucocorticoid receptor with the 90-kDa heat shock protein. J Biol Chem 1985; 263:3471–3481.

9. Sanchez ER, Toft DO, Schlesinger MJ, Pratt WB. Evidence that the 90-kdalton phosphoprotein associated with the untransformed L-cell glucocorticoid receptor is a murine heat shock protein. J Biol Chem 1985; 260:12398–12401.

10. Levine M, Manley JL. Transcriptional repression of eukaryotic promoters. Cell 1989; 59:405–408.

11. Clark AR, Docherty K. Negative regulation of transcription in eukaryotes. Biochem J 1993; 296:521–541.

12. Akerblom IE, Slater EP, Beato M, Baxter, JD, Mellon PL. Negative regulation by glucocorticoids through interference with cAMP responsive enhancer. Science 1988; 241:350–353.

13. Stauber C, Altschimied J, Akerblom IE, Marron JL, Mellon PL. Mutual cross-interference between glucocorticoid receptor and CREB inhibits transactivation in placental cells. New Biologist 1992; 4:527–540.

14. Weiland S, Dobbeling U, Rusconi S. Interference and synergism of glucocorticoid receptor and octamer factors. EMBO J 1991; 10:2513–2521.

15. Lanigan, TM, Tverberg, LA, Russo, AF. Retinoic acid repression of cell-specific helix-loop-helix-octamer activation of the calcitonin/calcitonin gene-related peptide enhancer. Mol Cell Biol 1993; 13:6079–6088.

16. Werb, Z. Proteinases and matrix degradation. In: Kelley WN, Harris ED Jr, Ruddy S, Sledge CB, eds. Textbook of Rheumatology. Philadelphia: Saunders, 1989:300–321.

17. Angel P, Karin M. The role of Jun, Fos and the AP-1 complex in cell proliferation and transformation. Biochem Biophys Acta 1991; 1072:129–157.

18. Frisch SM, Ruley HE (1987) Transcription from the stromelysin promoter is induced by interleukin 1 and repressed by dexamethasone. J Biol Chem 262:3535–3542.

19. Offringa R, Smis AM, Houweling A, Bos JL, van der Eb AJ. Similar effects of adenovirus E1A and glucocorticoid hormones on the expression of the metalloprotease stromelysin. Nucl Acids Res 1988; 16:10974–10983.

20. Brinckerhoff CE, Plucinska IM, Sheldon LA, O'Connor GT. Half-life of synovial cell collagenase mRNA is modulated by phorbol myristate acetate but not by all-trans-retinoic acid or dexamethasone. Biochemistry 1986; 25:6378–84.

21. Jonat G, Rhamsdorf HF, Park KK, Cato ACB, Gebel S, Ponta H, Herrlich P. Antitumor promotion and inflammation: down regulation of AP-1 (Fos/Jun) activity by glucocorticoid hormone. Cell 1990; 62:1189–1204.

22. Yang-Yen HF, Chambard JC, Sun YL, Smeal T, Schmidt TJ, Drouin J, Karin M. Transcriptional interference between c-Jun and the glucocorticoid receptor: mutual inhibition of DNA binding due to direct protein-protein interaction. Cell 1990; 62:1205–1215.

23. Yang-Yen HF, Zhang XK, Graupner G, Pfahl M, Karin M. Antagonism between retinoic acid and AP-1: implications for tumor promotion and inflammation. New Biologist 1991; 3:1209–1219.

24. Schüle R, Rangarajan P, Kliewer S, Ransone LJ, Yang N, Verma IM, Evans RM. Functional antagonism between oncoprotein c-Jun and the glucocorticoid receptor. Cell 1990; 62:1217–1226.

25. Godowski PJ, Sakai DD, Yamamoto KR. Signal transduction and transcriptional regulation by the glucocorticoid receptor. In: Gralla JD, ed. DNA-Protein Interactions in Transcription. UCLA Symposia on Molecular and Cellular Biology, New Series. New York: Liss, 1989:197–210.

26. Vacca A, Screpanti I, Maroder M, Petrangeli E, Frati L, Gulino A. Tumor promoting phorbol ester and ras oncogene expression inhibit the glucocorticoid-dependent transcription from the mouse mammary tumor virus long terminal repeat. Mol Endocrinol 1989; 3:1659–1665.

27. Desbois C, Aubert D, Legrand C, Pain B, Samarut J. A novel mechanism of action for v-ErbA: Abrogation of the inactivation of transcription factor AP-1 by retinoic acid and thyroid hormone receptors. Cell 1991; 67:731–740.

28. Zhang XK, Wills KN, Husmann M, Hermann T, Pfahl M. Novel pathway for thyroid hormone receptor action through interaction with jun and fos oncogene activities. Mol Cell Biol 1991; 11:6016–6025.

29. Saatcioglu F, Bartunek P, Deng T, Zenke M, Karin M. A conserved C-terminal sequence that is deleted in v-ErbA is essential for the biological activities of c-ErbA. Mol Cell Biol 1993; 13:3675–3685.

30. Dong ZG, Birrer MJ, Watts RG, Matrisian LM, Colburn NH. Blocking of tumor promoter-induced AP-1 activity inhibits induced transformation in JB6 mouse epidermal cells. Proc Natl Acad Sci USA 1994; 91:609–613.

31. Lucibello FC, Slater EP, Jooss KU, Beato M, Muller R. Mutual transrepression of Fos and the glucocorticoid receptor: involvement of a functional domain in Fos which is absent in FosB. EMBO J 1990; 9:2827–2834.

32. Doucas V, Spyrou G, Yaniv, M. Unregulated expression of c-Jun or c-Fos proteins but not Jun D inhibits oestrogen receptor activity in human breast cancer derived cells. EMBO J 1991; 10:2237–2245.

33. König H, Ponta H, Rahmsdorf HJ, Herrlich P. Interference between pathway-specific transcription factors: glucocorticoids antagonize phorbol ester-induced AP-1 activity without altering AP-1 site occupation in vivo. EMBO J 1992; 11:2241–2246.

34. Kerppola TK, Luk D, Curran T. Fos is a preferential target of glucocorticoid receptor inhibition of AP-1 activity in vitro. Mol Cell Biol 1993; 13:3782–3791.

35. Diamond M, Miner JN, Yoshinaga SK, Yamamoto KR. Transcription factor interactions: selectors for positive or negative regulation from a single DNA element. Science 1990; 249:1266–1272.

36. Mordacq JD and Linzer DIH. Colocalization of elements required for phorbol ester stimulation and glucocorticoid repression of proliferin gene expression. Genes Dev 1989; 3:760–769.

37. Pearce D, Yamamoto KR. Mineralocorticoid and glucocorticoid receptor activities distinguished by nonreceptor factors at a composite response element. Science 1993; 259:1161–1165.

38. Miner JN, Yamamoto KR. Regulatory crosstalk at composite response elements. TIBS 1991; 16:423–426.

39. Baeuerle PA. The induction transcription activator NFκB: regulation by distinct protein subunits. Biochem. Biophys. Acta 1991; 1072:63–80.

40. Baeuerle PA, Baltimore D. IκB: A specific inhibitor of the NF-κB transcription factor. Science 1988; 242:540–546.
41. Haskill S, Beg AA, Tompkins SM, Morris JS, Yurochko AD, Sampson-Johannes A, Mondal K, Ralph P, Baldwin AS Jr. Characterization of an immediate-early gene induced in adherent monocytes that encodes IκB-like activity. Cell 1991; 65:1281–1289.
42. Sun SC, Ganchi PA, Ballard D, Greene WC. NF-κB controls expression of inhibitor IκBα: evidence for a inducible autoregulatory pathway. Science 1993; 259:1912–1915.
43. Beg AA, Baldwin AS, Jr. The IkB proteins: multifunctional regulators of Rel/NF-κB transcription factors. Genes Dev. 1993; 7:2064–2070.
44. Brown K, Park S, Kanno T, Franzoso G, Siebenlist U. Mutual regulation of the transcriptional activator NF-κB and its inhibitor, IκB-α. Proc Natl Acad Sci USA 1993; 90:2532–2536.
45. de Martin R, Vanhove B, Cheng Q, Hofer E, Csizmadia V, Winkler H, Bach FH. Cytokine-inducible expression in endothelial cells of an IkappaBα-like gene is regulated by NFkappaB. EMBO J 1993; 12:2773–2779.
46. Ray A & Prefontaine KE. Physical association and functional antagonism between the p65 subunit of transcription factor NF-κB and the glucocorticoid receptor. Proc Natl Acad Sci USA 1994; 91:752–756.
47. Mukaida N, Morita M, Ishikawa Y, Rice N, Okamoto S, Kawahara T, Matsushima K. Novel mechanism of glucocorticoid-mediated gene repression: NF-κB is target for glucocorticoid-mediated interleukin 8 gene repression. J. Biol. Chem. 1994; 269:13289-95.
48. Auphan N, DiDonato JA, Helmberg A, Rosette C, Karin M. Immunosuppression by glucocorticoids: inhibition of NF-κB activity through induction of IκB synthesis. Science 1995; 270:286–290.
49. Cantrell DA, Smith KA. The interleukin-2 T cell system: A new cell growth model. Science 1984; 224:1312–1316.
50. Durand DB, Shaw JP, Bush MR, Replogle RE, Belagaje R, Crabtree GR. Characterization of antigen receptor response elements within the interleukin 2 enhancer. Mol Cell Biol 1988; 8:1715–1724.
51. Ullman KS, Northrop JP, Admon A, Crabtree GR. Jun family members are controlled by calcium-regulated, cyclosporin A-sensitive signaling pathway in activated T lymphocytes Genes Dev 1993; 7:188–196.
52. Serfling E, Barthelmäs R, Pfeuffer I, Schenk B, Zarius S, Swoboda R, Mercurio F, Karin, M. Ubiquitous and lymphocyte-specific factors are involved in the induction of the mouse interleukin 2 gene in T lymphocytes. EMBO J 1989; 8:465–473.
53. Lenardo MJ, Baltimore D. A pleitropic mediator of inducible and tissue-specific gene control. Cell 1989; 58:227–229.
54. Shaw JP, Utz P, Durand DB, Toole JJ, Emmel EA, Crabtree GR. Identification of a putative regulator of early T cell activation genes, Science 1988; 241:202–205.
55. Jain J, McCaffrey PG, Valge-Archer VE, Rao A. Nuclear factors of activated T cells contains Fos and Jun. Nature 1992; 356:801–804.
56. McCaffrey PM, Luo C, Kerppola TK, Jain J, Badalian TM, Ho AM, Burgeon E,

Lane WS, Lambert JN, Curran T, Verdine GL, Rao A. Isolation of the cyclosporin-sensitive T cell transcription factor NFATp. Science 1993; 262:750–754.

57. Northrop JP, Crabtree GR, Mattila PS. Negative regulation of interleukin 2 transcription by the glucocorticoid receptor. J Exp Med 1992; 175:1235–1245.

58. Helmberg A, Auphan N, Caelles C, Karin M. Glucocorticoid-induced apoptosis of human leukemic cells is caused by the repressive function of the glucocorticoid receptor. EMBO J 1995; 14:452–460.

59. Wyllie A H. Glucocorticoid-induced thymocyte apoptosis is associated with endogenous endonuclease activation. Nature 1980; 284:555–556.

60. Galili U. Glucocorticoid-induced cytolysis of human normal and malignant lymphocytes. J Steroid Biochem 1983; 19:483–490.

61. Knudsen PJ, Dinarello CA, Strom TB. Glucocorticoids inhibit transcriptional and post-transcriptional expression of interleukin 1 in U937 cells. J Immunol 1987; 139:4129–4134.

62. Arya SK, Wong-Staal F, Gallo RC. Dexamethasone-mediated inhibition of human T cell growth factor and α-interferon messenger RNA. J Immunol 1984; 133:273–276.

63. Culpepper JA, Lee F. Regulation of IL-3 expression by glucocorticoids in cloned murine T lymphocytes. J Immunol 1985; 135:3191–3197.

64. Wang Y, Campbell HD, Young IG. Sex hormones and dexamethasone modulate interleukin-5 gene expression in T lymphocytes. J Steroid Biochem Mol Biol 1993; 44:203–210.

65. Zanker B, Walz G, Wieder KJ, Strom TB. Evidence that glucocorticosteroids block expression of the human interleukin-6 gene by accessing cells. Transplantation 1990; 49:183–185.

66. Collart MA, Belin D, Vassalli JD, Vassalli P. Modulations of functional activity in differentiated macrophages are accompanied by early and transient increase or decrease in c-*fos* gene transcription. J Immunol 1987; 139:949–955.

67. Beutler B, Krochin N, Milsark IW, Luedke C, Cerami A. Control of cachectin (tumor necrosis factor) synthesis: mechanisms of endotoxic resistance. Science 1986; 23:977–979.

68. Von Knebel Doeberitz M, Koch S, Drzonek H, Zur Hausen H. Glucocorticoid hormones reduce the expression of major histocompatibility class I antigens on human epithelial cells. Eur J Immunol 1990; 20:35–40.

69. Celada A, McKercher S, Maki RA. Repression of major histocompatibility complex IA expression by glucocorticoids: the glucocorticoid receptor inhibits the DNA binding of the X box DNA binding protein. J Exp Med 1993; 177:691–698.

70. Grilli M, Chiu JJS, Lenardo MJ. NF-kappaB and Rel: participants in a multiform transcriptional regulatory system. Int Rev. Cytol 1993; 143:1–62.

71. Baeuerle PA, Henkel T. Function and activation of NF-κB in the immune system. Annu. Rev. Immunol. 1994; 12:141–179.

72. Hiscott J, Marois J, Garoufalis J, D'Addario M, Roulston A, Kwan I, Pepin N, Lacoste J, Nguyen H, Bensi G, et al. Characterization of a functional NFκB site in the human interleukin-1 β-promoter: evidence for a positive autoregulatory loop. Mol Cell Biol 1993; 13:6231–6240.

73. Shakhov, AN, Collart MA, Vassalli, P, Nedospasov SA, Jongeneel. κB-type enhancers are involved in lipopolysaccharide-mediated transcriptional activation of the tumor necrosis factor α gene in primary macrophages. *J Exp Med* 171:35–47.

74. Lieberman TA, Lenardo M, Baltimore D. Involvement of a second lymphoid-specific enhancer element in the regulation of a immunoglobulin heavy-chain gene expression. *Mol Cell Biol* 1990; 10:3155–3162.

75. Mukaida N, Mahe Y, Matsushima K. Cooperative interaction of nuclear factor-κB- and cis-regulatory enhancer binding protein-like factor binding elements in activating the interleukin-8 gene by pro-inflammatory cytokines. *J Biol Chem* 1990; 265:21128–21133.

76. Schreck R, Baeuerle PA. NF-kB as inducible transcriptional activator of the granulocyte-macrophage colony-stimulating factor gene. *Mol Cell Biol* 1990; 10:1281–1286.

77. Voraberger G, Schafer R, Stratowa C. Cloning of the human gene for intercellular adhesion molecular 1 and analysis of its 5'-regulatory region: induction by cytokines and phorbol ester. *J Immunol* 1991; 147:2777–2786.

78. Whelan J, Ghersa P, Hooft van Huijsduijnen R, Gray J, Chandra G, Talabot F, DeLamarter JF. An NF-κB-like factor is essential but not sufficient for cytokine induction of endothelial leukocyte adhesion molecule 1 (ELAM-1) gene transcription. *Nucleic Acids Res* 1991; 19:2645–2653.

79. Mukaida N, Morita, M, Ishikawa, Y, Rice N, Okamoto S, Kasahara T, Matsushima K. Novel mechanism of glucocorticoid-mediated gene repression: nuclear factor-κB is target for glucocorticoid-mediated interleukin-8 gene repression. *J Biol Chem* 1994; 269:13289–13295.

80. Leung K, Nabel GJ. HTLV-1 transactivator induces interleukin-2 receptor expression through an NF-κB-like factor. *Nature* 1988; 333:776–778.

81. Ballard DW, Bohnlein E, Lowenthal JW, Wano Y, Franza BR Green WC. HTLV-I tax induces cellular proteins that activate the κB-element in the IL-2 receptor α gene. *Science* 1988; 241:1652–1655.

82. Kauer J, Bickel CA, Bochner BS, Schleimer RP. The effects of the potent glucocorticoid budesonide on adhesion of eosinophils to human vascular endothelial cells and on endothelin expression of adhesion molecules. J Pharmacol Exp. Ther 1993; 267:245–249.

83. Berko-Flint Y, Levkowitz G, Vardimon L. Involvement of c-Jun in the control of glucocorticoid receptor transcription activity during development of chicken retinal tissue. EMBO J 1994; 13:646–654.

84. Hackney JF, Gross SR, Aronow L, Pratt WB. Specific glucocorticoid binding macromolecules from mouse fibroblasts growing in vitro. Mol Pharmacol 1970; 6:500–512.

85. Hennekens CH. Vitamin A anologues in cancer chemoprevention. In: De Vita VT Jr, Hellman S, Rosenberg SA, eds. Important Advances in Oncology. Philadelphia: Lippincott, 1986:23–35.

86. Kraemer KH, DiGivanna JJ, Mushell AN, Tarone RE, Peck GL. Prevention of skin cancer in xeroderma pigmentosum with the oral use of isotretinoin. N Engl J Med 1988; 318:1633–1637.

87. Hong WK, Lippman SM, Itri LM, Karp DD, Lee JS, Byers RMSchantz SP,

Kramer AM, Lotan R, Peters LJ, Dimery IW, Brown BW, Goepfert H. Prevention of second primary tumors with isotretinoin in squamous cell carcinoma of the head and neck. N Engl J Med 1990; 323:795–804.

88. Verma AK. Inhibition of both stage I and stage II mouse skin tumor promotion by retinoic acid and the dependence of inhibition of tumor promotion on the duration of retinoic acid treatment. Cancer Res 1987; 47:5097–5101.

89. Belman S, Troll W. The inhibition of croton oil-promoted mouse skin tumorigenesis by steroid hormones. Cancer Res 32:450–454.

90. Scribner JD, Slaga TJ. Multiple effects of dexamethasone on protein synthesis and hyperplasia caused by a tumor promoter. Cancer Res 1973; 33:542–546.

3

Glucocorticoids Attenuate Induction of Two Primary Response/Immediate Early Genes, Prostaglandin Synthase 2 and Inducible Nitric Oxide Synthase, Whose Products Mediate Paracrine Cell Communication

HARVEY HERSCHMAN, REBECCA GILBERT, SRINIVASA REDDY,
BRADLEY FLETCHER, WEILIN XIE, JEFFREY SMITH,
and DEAN KUJUBU

University of California School of Medicine
Los Angeles, California

I. Primary Response/Immediate Early Genes

There exists a class of genes whose transcription is increased in response to cell stimulation as a result of activation of preexisting, latent transcription factors without requiring any intervening protein synthesis. These genes are referred to as primary response genes (PRGs) or immediate early genes (IEGs) (see ref. 1 for review). Transcriptional activation of IEGs occurs in response to cell stimulation in the presence of protein synthesis inhibitors. Transcription of IEGs can be induced by growth factors, hormones, neurotrophins, neurotransmitters, and many other ligands. The most well-studied IEGs encode transcription factors (c-*fos*, c-*jun*, *egr*-1/*zif*-268/TIS8, *nur*77/N10/TIS1). Induction of transcription factor IEGs is thought to be the first step in ligand-induced gene-expression cascades that result in changes in cellular phenotypes such as mitogenesis or differentiation. Other primary response/immediate early genes encode protein kinases (1), protein phosphatases (2), and cytokines (3).

Our laboratory has been interested in the immediate-early genes that are induced in response to mitogenic stimuli in quiescent, nondividing cells. To study mitogenesis, we used differential screening of a cDNA library prepared from Swiss 3T3 cells treated with tetradecanoyl phorbol acetate (TPA) in the presence of cycloheximide and identified cDNAs induced by this potent mitogen/tumor promoter (4). We refer to these IEGs as TIS genes (TPA-induced sequences). We assumed (1) expression of some TIS genes is unique to mitogenesis and (2) TIS gene-encoded proteins play causal roles in mitogenesis.

II. The TIS10 Gene Encodes a Second Prostaglandin Synthase/Cyclooxygenase

The prostanoids—prostaglandins, prostacyclins, and thromboxanes—modulate the immune response, wound healing, reproduction, bone development, hemostasis, thermoregulation, sleep, and other physiological functions. Aberrant prostanoid regulation is associated with arthritis, asthma, bone resorption, cardiovascular disease, nephrotoxicity, atherosclerosis, acute inflammation, immunosuppression, and cancer (5). Prostaglandin production in response to agents such as interleukin-1 (IL-1), serum, platelet-derived growth factor, TPA, and glycoprotein hormones has been characterized in fibroblasts and in endothelial, mesangial, and ovarian granulosa cells.

Prostaglandin synthase (PGS) produces PGH_2, the precursor for all the prostanoids, from arachidonic acid (arachidonic acid). Interdiction of prostaglandin production by nonsteroidal anti-inflammatory drugs (NSAIDs) such as aspirin occurs by inhibition of the PGS cyclooxygenase reaction and results in reduction of inflammation, pain, and fever, a lessening of risk for coronary occlusions, and a lowered incidence of colon cancer. Phospholipase A2 (PLA2) activation was thought to be the controlling step in ligand-induced prostanoid synthesis. PGS EC 1.14.99.1 (now termed PGS1) was assumed to be present in excess in cells and available to convert to PGH_2 the arachidonic acid released from membrane stores following ligand-induced PLA2 activation.

Sequencing of the TPA-induced TIS10 cDNA demonstrated that this gene encoded a protein with striking sequence similarity to PGS1 (6). We now refer to this gene as TIS10/PGS2, or simply as PGS2. PGS1 has a highly hydrophobic amino acid insertion located near the amino-terminal of the molecule (Fig. 1). In contrast, an 18–amino acid sequence is present in the TIS10/PGS2 molecule that is not found in PGS1. We subsequently demonstrated that PGS2 has cyclooxygenase and hydroperoxidase activities of a second, functional PGS (7). This gene was also cloned as a v-*src*–inducible cDNA from chicken fibroblasts by Xie et al. (8). Several other groups subsequently cloned the TIS10/PGS2 cDNA as a serum-inducible sequence from mouse fibroblast cell lines (9,10). Richards and her colleagues demonstrated the presence of a glycoprotein-hormone inducible PGS (rPGS*i*), distinct from PGS1, in rat ovarian granulosa cells (11) and subsequently demonstrated at the protein, serological, and

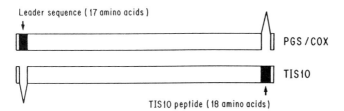

Figure 1 The PGS1 and TIS10/PGS2 proteins share regions of sequence identify and similarity. The unshaded areas indicate regions of sequence similarity or identity. The shaded area in the amino-terminal region of PGS1 (termed PGS/COX in the figure) indicates a 17–amino acid hydrophobic sequence present in PGS1 but absent in TIS10/PGS2. The shaded area in the caroboxyl-terminal region of TIS10/PGS2 indicates the 18–amino acid insertion present in TIS10/PGS2 but missing from PGS1.

message levels that rPGS*i* is the rat homologue of TIS10/PGS2 (11,12). TIS10/PGS2 message and protein are inducible in Swiss 3T3 cells and in ovarian granulosa cells in response to mitogen inducers (6,7) and glycoprotein hormones (11,12), respectively. Discovery of PGS2 has initiated both new drug discovery programs to identify NSAIDs that differentially inhibit PGS1 and PGS2 and studies designed to delineate the roles of the PGS1 and PGS2 enzymes in physiological processes and in pathophysiological conditions.

III. PGS2 Expression Is Induced in Fibroblasts by Mitogens and in Macrophages by Endotoxin/Lipopolysaccharide

We took advantage of the unique 18–amino acid insertion in PGS2 to prepare a PGS2-specific antipeptide antiserum. Treatment of 3T3 cells with TPA induces the accumulation of PGS2 antigen (Fig. 2). Subcellular fractionation experiments demonstrated that PGS2, like PGS1, is found in the microsomal fraction (7). As expected, induction of PGS2 antigen by TPA in 3T3 cells is blocked by inhibition of protein synthesis (Fig. 2). The specificity of the antipeptide PGS2 antiserum is demonstrated by the ability of the immunizing peptide to block the detection of PGS2 antigen.

Macrophages/monocytes play a major role in inflammatory and immune responses. Macrophages are activated by endogenous cytokines (e.g., tumor necrosis factor, γ-interferon) and by exogenous factors such as bacterial endotoxin/lipopolysaccharide (LPS). Activated macrophages secrete a variety of agents, including protein cytokines, oxygen free radicals such as O_2^-, H_2O_2, and NO, and lipid mediators such as prostaglandins, thromboxanes, and platelet-activating factor (PAF). Macrophage-produced prostaglandins are thought to play a major role in mediating inflammatory responses.

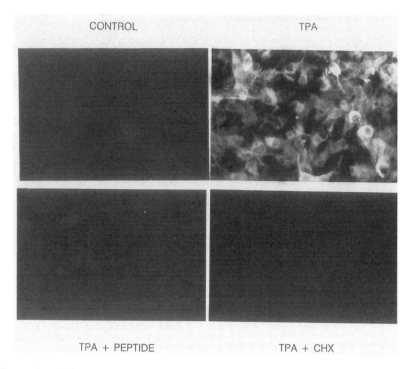

Figure 2 Antibody to the unique carboxyl-terminal region of TIS10/PGS2 can detect induced TIS10/PGS2 protein synthesis by immunofluorescence in phorbol-treated Swiss 3T3 cells. Indirect immunofluorescence of untreated Swiss 3T3 cells (upper left); cells treated with phorbol (50 ng/ml) for 6 hr (upper right); cells treated with phorbol (50 ng/ml) but incubated with 1 μM TIS10/PGS2–specific peptide 30 min prior to and during incubation with primary antibody (lower left); and cells treated with phorbol (50 ng/ml) and cycloheximide (10 μm/ml) for 6 hr (lower right). (Data reproduced from ref. 19.)

From previous studies with macrophages and monocytes, it seemed likely that LPS might similarly induce TIS10/PGS2 expression in macrophages. We used our antipeptide antiserum to characterize the LPS induction of TIS10/PGS2 protein in RAW 264.7 macrophage cells (Fig. 3). Untreated cells show no detectable TIS10/PGS2 antigen in Western analysis. Following treatment with LPS, TIS10/PGS2 antigen peaks between 6 and 14 hr. TIS10/PGS2 protein remains elevated for over 24 hr but eventually returns to near-basal levels despite the continued presence of LPS. Unstimulated RAW 264.7 cells showed essentially no reactivity with the antipeptide antiserum when analyzed by immunofluorescence (Fig. 4). In contrast, bright cytoplasmic fluorescence was

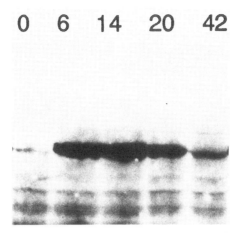

Figure 3 Western blot analysis of TIS10/PGS2 protein induction by LPS in RAW 264.7 cells. RAW 264.7 cells were treated with LPS (5 ng/ml) for the indicated times (in hours). Cell lysates were prepared and subjected to Western blot analysis using the TIS10/PGS2 antipeptide antiserum.

present 6 hr after cells were exposed to LPS. Little or no nuclear staining is present. We observe substantial perinuclear fluorescence, with additional diffuse staining of the surrounding cytoplasm. Peptide and cycloheximide inhibition again demonstrate the specificity of the antiserum and the requirement for protein synthesis for LPS-induced PGS2 protein accumulation.

IV. Glucocorticoids Inhibit Both the Production of Prostaglandins and the Induction of PGS2

Although induced prostaglandin synthesis in mitogen-stimulated fibroblasts and endotoxin-stimulated macrophages has been demonstrated previously, we repeated these experiments to be certain that, in our experimental systems, induction of PGS2 and prostaglandin production are correlated. TPA stimulates PGE_2 production in Swiss 3T3 cells (Fig. 5), and LPS stimulates PGE_2 production in RAW 264.7 cells (Fig. 6).

Stimulus-induced prostaglandin synthesis can be blocked by glucocorticoids in monocytes, macrophages, smooth muscle cells, and fibroblasts. We find that dexamethasone is able to prevent both mitogen-induced and endotoxin-induced PGE_2 production in 3T3 fibroblasts and RAW 264.7 macrophages (see Figs. 5 and 6).

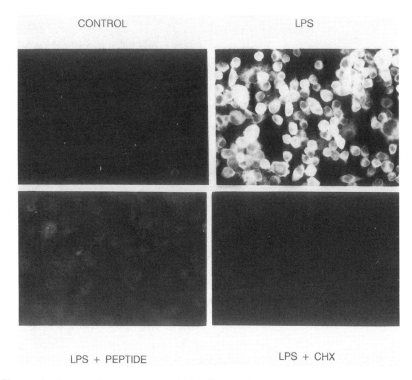

Figure 4 Immunofluorescence analysis of the TIS10/PGS2 protein induced in RAW 264.7 cells by LPS. Indirect immunofluorescence of untreated cells (upper left); cells treated with LPS (5 ng/ml) for 6 hr (upper right); cells treated with LPS (5 ng/ml) but antibody incubated with 1 μM TIS10/PGS2–specific peptide 30 min prior to and during incubation with primary antibody (lower left); and cells treated with LPS (5 ng/ml) and CHX (10 μg/ml) for 6 hr (lower right).

Several earlier studies reported that glucocorticoids inhibit the induction of prostaglandin synthase enzyme activity and/or PGS antigen synthesis (13). However, a concomitant change in the level of mRNA for the PGS EC 1.14.99.1 gene was not observed. The presence of two pools of PGS enzyme activity was suggested to explain these paradoxical results (14,15). One pool of PGS is thought to be constitutively expressed (unregulated), whereas the other PGS pool is proposed to be (1) inducible by various ligands and (2) sensitive to glucocorticoid inhibition. If Swiss 3T3 cells are first incubated with dexamethasone (DEX), then stimulated with TPA, DEX completely blocks the appearance of PGS2 protein (Fig. 7). Moreover, DEX blocks PGS2 antigen accumulation in response to other mitogenic stimuli in 3T3 cells (Fig. 8), sug-

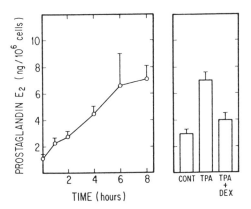

Figure 5 Dexamethasone inhibits TPA-induced PGE_2 synthesis and secretion in Swiss 3T3 cells. Left panel: Density-arrested 3T3 cells were treated with TPA (50 ng/ml) for the hours shown. Media were collected and prostaglandin concentrations were determined by radioimmunoassay. Right panel: Cells were either exposed to 2 μM dexamethasone for 4 hr or were left untreated and then exposed to TPA (50 ng/ml) for 4 hr. Media were collected and prostaglandin concentrations were determined. Data points are the the averages and standard deviations of three dishes. CONT, Control; DEX, dexamethasone. (Data reproduced from ref. 21.)

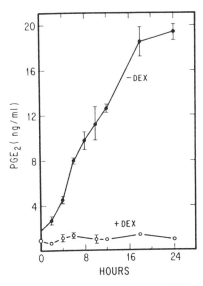

Figure 6 Dexamethasone inhibition of LPS-stimulated PGE_2 secretion in RAW 264.7 cells. RAW 264.7 cells were incubated in the presence or absence of DEX (2 μM) for 4 hr and then treated with LPS (5 ng/ml) for the times indicated. Media were collected, and prostaglandin E_2 concentrations were determined by radioimmunoassay.

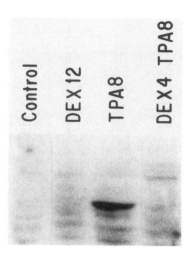

Figure 7 Dexamethasone pretreatment blocks accumulation by TIS10/PGS2 protein. Confluent cultures of 3T3 cells were either left untreated or exposed to TPA (50 ng/ml) dexamethasone (DEX) (2 μM) for 12 hr or dexamethasone followed by TPA for 8 hr. Extracts were prepared and subjected to electrophoresis and Western analysis with the PGS2 antipeptide antiserum. (Data reproduced from ref. 19.)

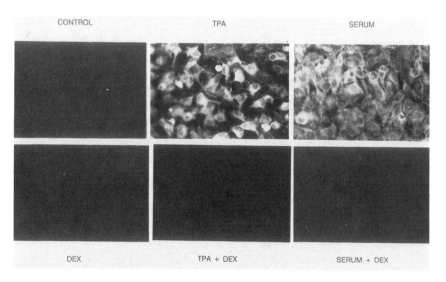

Figure 8 Dexamethasone inhibits phorbol- and serum-induced synthesis of TIS10/PGS2 protein. Control Swiss 3T3 cells (upper left); cells treated with phorbol (TPA, 50 ng/ml) for 6 hours (upper middle); cells treated with 20% serum for 6 hr (upper right); cells treated with dexamethasone (2 μm) for 10 hr (lower left); cells treated with dexamethasone for 4 hr followed by phorbol or 6 hr (lower middle); and cells treated with dexamethasone for 4 hr followed by serum for 6 hr (lower right) were fixed and subjected to indirect immunofluorescent analysis. (Data reproduced from ref. 19.)

gesting that the global inhibition of prostaglandin synthesis by steroid hormones may be mediated by inhibition of PGS2 expression.

V. Glucocorticoids Inhibit Mitogen-Stimulated Accumulation of PGS2 mRNA

The TIS10/PGS2 cDNA was initially cloned as a TPA-inducible cDNA. Expression of the PGS2 message in response to TPA is rapid and transient, peaking between 2 and 4 hr in 3T3 cells (Fig. 9). In addition, a number of inducers that act via several different signal transduction pathways to activate distinct transcription factors include TIS10/PGS2 mRNA accumulation (Fig. 9). Swiss 3T3 cells also express PGS1 (also known as cyclooxygenase I, and referred to as COX in Fig. 9). In contrast to PGS2, the PGS1 message is present in untreated cells and is not modulated by mitogenic stimulation. PGS2 and mRNA

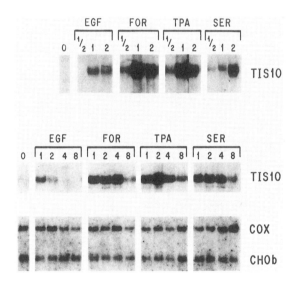

Figure 9 The TIS10/PGS2 gene is rapidly and transiently induced by a variety of ligands. Total RNA was prepared from density-arrested Swiss 3T3 cells treated with EGF (10 ng/ml), forskolin (FOR, 40 ng/ml), phorbol (TPA, 50 ng/ml), or 20% fetal bovine serum (SER) for 1, 2, 4, and 8 hr. RNA (10 μg/ml) was subjected to electrophoresis and transferred to nitrocellulose. Two separate electrophoretic analyses and blots were performed for the experiments shown here. One blot, the upper blot, showing times from 0 to 2 hr, was hybridized with a cDNA probe for TIS10/PGS2. The lower blot, showing times from 0 to 8 hr, was hybridized with cDNA probes for PGS2/COX2, PGS1/COX1, and CHOB. (Data reproduced from ref. 6.)

is also rapidly and strongly induced by LPS in RAW 264.7 cells, peaking between 4 and 8 hr after treatment (Fig. 10). The lower molecular weight band present in these autoradiographs is due to the presence of an alternative polyadenylic acid (polyA) addition site. The two PGS2 messages encode the same open reading frame (9).

If 3T3 cells are first preincubated with DEX and then exposed to TPA, accumulation of the TIS10/PGS2 message is completely suppressed (Fig. 11). In contrast, the PGS1 message (referred to as COX in Fig. 11) is neither elevated following TPA treatment nor reduced in the presence of DEX. The ability of DEX to attenuate TIS10/PGS2 mRNA accumulation in Swiss 3T3 cells is remarkably strong; a concentration of 2 nM DEX can completely prevent TIS10/PGS2 mRNA accumulation (Fig. 12). In contrast, TPA induction of *egr*-1/TIS8 mRNA accumulation (recall that this gene encodes a mitogen-induced IEG transcription factor) is not attenuated by DEX concentrations three orders of magnitude greater than the concentration required to attenuate TPA-induced PGS2 mRNA accumulation. Both cortisol (a physiological glucocorticoid) and the minearlocorticoid aldosterone inhibit TPA-induced TIS10/PGS2 mRNA accumulation at micromolar concentrations (Fig. 13). However, progesterone and testosterone, steroids that do not activate the glucocorticoid receptor, cannot inhibit PGS2 induction. These data suggest that glucocorticoid regulation of mitogen-induced TIS10/PGS2 mRNA accumulation occurs via the glucocorticoid receptor.

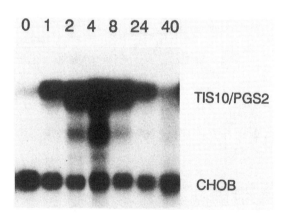

Figure 10   Induction of TIS10/PGS2 mRNA in RAW 264.7 cells. Cells were treated with LPS (5 ng/ml) for the times (in hours) indicated in the figure. Total RNA was isolated and used for Northern analysis. Ten micrograms of total cellular RNA was loaded in each lane. Filters were hybridized simultaneously with radiolabeled probes for TIS10/PGS2 and CHOB, a constitutive message used to normalize for mRNA loading.

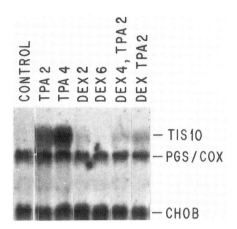

Figure 11 Dexamethasone inhibits phorbol-induced accumulation of TIS10/PGS2 mRNA. Swiss 3T3 cells were treated with phorbol (TPA, 50 ng/ml) or dexamethasone (DEX) (2 μM) for the times (in hours) indicated. DEX4, TPA2 cells were preincubated with DEX for 4 hr prior to exposure to phorbol for 2 hr. DEX TPA2 cells were incubated for 2 hr with phorbol and DEX with no preincubation. Total RNA was isolated, subjected to electrophoresis, and transferred to nitrocellulose; 10 μg of RNA was loaded in each lane. The blot was hybridized with cDNA probes for TIS10/PGS2, PGS1, and CHOB. (Data reproduced from ref. 21.)

Recall that the PGS2 gene can be induced in 3T3 cells by a number of distinct second-messenger–mediated pathways, activating a variety of transcription factors (see Fig. 9). Dexamethasone can also attenuate forskolin-mediated induction of the TIS10/PGS2 gene in Swiss 3T3 cells (Fig. 14). These data suggest that glucocorticoids modulate TIS10/PGS2 mRNA accumulation by a common molecular mechanism despite the wide variety of agents able to induce expression of this gene. Glucocorticoids block mitogen-induced accumulation of PGE_2 (see Fig. 1), TIS10/PGS2 protein (see Figs. 7 and 8), and TIS10/PGS2 message (see Figs. 11–14) in 3T3 cells. TIS10/PGS2 satisfies the proposed requirements for the long-sought, ligand-induced, glucocorticoid-inhibitable "second pool" (14,15) of prostaglandin synthase.

We utilized transcriptional run-on experiments to determine the level at which DEX inhibits mitogen-induced PGS2 mRNA accumulation in 3T3 cells (16). No transcription of the TIS10/PGS2, *egr*-1/TIS8, or TIS21 genes can be detected in unstimulated or DEX-treated 3T3 cells (Fig. 15). Treatment with TPA stimulates transcription of all three genes. In contrast, the transcription of the constitutive CHO-B gene is unaffected by mitogen or steroid exposure. The TPA-induced transcription of the TIS10/PGS2 gene is dramatically suppressed by DEX preincubation. In contrast, transcription of the TIS21 and *egr*-1/TIS8

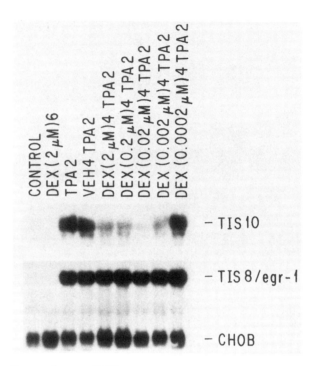

Figure 12 Dexamethasone (DEX) does not inhibit phorbol-induced accumulation of TIS8/*egr*-1 mRNA. Total RNA was prepared from Swiss 3T3 cells preincubated for 4 hr either vehicle (ethanol) or DEX at the concentrations shown and then treated with phorbol (50 ng/ml) for 2 hr. RNA was also prepared from DEX-treated, phorbol-treated, and untreated cells. The RNA preparations were subjected to Northern analysis. Each lane contains 10 μg of RNA. Blots were hybridized with TIS10/PGS2, TIS8/*egr*-1, and CHOB radioactive cDNA probes. (Data reproduced from ref. 21.)

genes is unaffected by DEX preincubation. The data suggest (1) that elevated transcription is a major mechanism for mitogen-induced PGS2 gene expression, and (2) that suppression of transcription is a major mechanism for steroid suppression of mitogen-induced PGS2 gene expression.

In the course of studying the structure of the TIS10/PGS2 gene (7), we cloned and sequenced 1 kilobase of the regulatory region 5' of the start site of transcription of the gene. We constructed a deletion series of this region fused to a luciferase reporter gene. A 371-bp fragment of the promoter is responsive to stimulation by serum, platelet-derived growth factor, or forskolin in transient transfection assays (Fig. 16). However, neither the 371-bp chimeric reporter construct nor longer reporter constructs carrying as much as 3 kb of sequence 5' of the PGS2 transcription start site are susceptible to glucocorticoid suppression (data not shown).

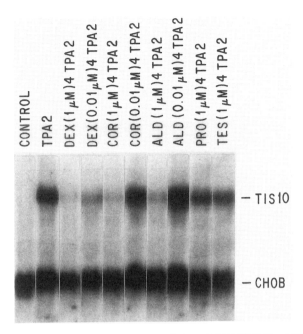

Figure 13 Glucocorticoid inhibition of TPA-induced TIS10/PGS2 mRNA accumulation. Cells were treated at the concentrations indicated with DEX, cortisol (*COR*), aldosterone (*ALD*), progesterone (*PRO*), or testosterone (*TES*) for 4 hr prior to exposure to TPA (50 ng/ml) for 2 hr G. Total RNA was prepared and subjected to northern analysis. Each lane contains 10 μg of RNA. (Data reproduced from ref. 21.)

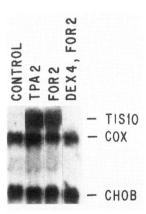

Figure 14 DEX inhibition of forskolin-induced TIS10/PGS2 and mRNA accumulation. Cells were treated with DEX (2 μM), TPA (50 ng/ml), or forskolin (*FOR*, 100 μM) for the times shown. Each lane contains 10 μg of RNA. (Data reproduced from ref. 21.)

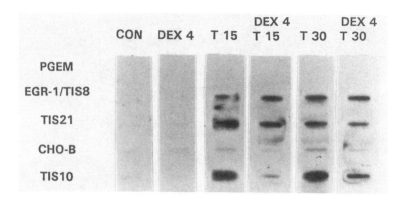

Figure 15 Dexamethasone (DEX) inhibits TPA-induced transcription of the TIS10/PGS2 gene. Swiss 3T3 cells were incubated with dexamethasone (2 μM) for 4 hr and then treated with TPA (T, 50 ng/ml) for 15 or 30 min. Control (CON) cells were treated either with DEX alone for 4 hr or with TPA for 15 and 30 min. Nuclei were prepared and allowed to incorporate radioactive nucleotides into RNA. RNA was isolated and hybridized to filters containing pGEM plasmid DNAs with inserts or with pGEM DNA (as a nonspecific control), TIS8/*egr-1*, TIS21, TIS10/PGS2, and CHOB. After washing, the filters were subjected to autoradiography. (Data reproduced from ref. 16.)

VI. Glucocorticoids Tonically Regulate PGS2 Expression In Vivo

Masferrer et al. (17) demonstrated that peritoneal macrophages from adrenalectomized mice have elevated prostaglandin synthase antigen and enzyme activity compared with sham-operated or hormone-supplemented animals. However, the antisera used in these experiments could not distinguish the two isoforms of COX/PGS. In a collaboration with the Searle group, we investigated whether adrenal glucocorticoids play a role in regulating prostaglandin production and both PGS1 and PGS2 expression in unchallenged animals (18). Peritoneal macrophages isolated from adrenalectomized mice produce substantially greater amounts of PGE_2 from exogenous arachidonic acid than do sham-operated animals (Fig. 17). DEX replacement therapy is able completely to block the adrenalectomy-induced elevation of PGE_2 synthesis.

We used antipeptide antisera that distinguish murine PGS1 and PGS2 to determine the effects of adrenalectomy on the expression of these two enzyme isoforms. PGS1/COX1 is present in peritoneal macrophages from sham-operated animals, and it is not modulated either by adrenalectomy or by DEX replacement therapy (Figs. 18 and 19). In contrast, no PGS2/COX2 antigen is present in peritoneal macrophages from sham animals (Figs. 19 and 20). However, adrenalectomy induces the accumulation of COX2/PGS2 antigen in peri-

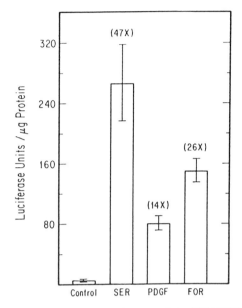

Figure 16 A fusion construct between 371 bp of the TIS10/PGS2 promoter and a luciferase reporter gene is responsive to serum, platelet-derived growth factor, and forskolin treatment. A construct in which the 371 bp of the TIS10/PGS2 promoter lying 5' of the start site of transcription was fused to the luciferase reporter gene was constructed (7). This fusion gene was transfected into NIH 3T3 cells. After stimulation with serum, platelet-derived growth factor or forskolin cell extracts were harvested and assayed for luciferase activity.

toneal macrophages examined 2 weeks after surgery. If peritoneal macrophages are examined from adrenalectomized animals following DEX injection, within 16 hr COX2/PGS2 antigen is no longer observable in the cells. Adrenalectomy also induces a substantial elevation in COX2/PGS2 mRNA accumulation; DEX-replacement therapy reverses the adrenalectomy-dependent accumulation of this message (Fig. 21). Neither adrenalectomy nor steroid administration modulate the level of COX1/PGS1 mRNA. We conclude that endogenous adrenal glucocorticoids play a tonic role in regulating COX2/PGS2 gene expression in macrophages in the intact animal.

VII. Ligand-Induced Prostaglandin Synthesis Requires PGS2 Gene Expression in Fibroblasts and Macrophages

Constitutive PGS1 and inducible PGS2 proteins are both found in the endoplasmic reticulum in 3T3 cells (19,20). Reiger et al. (20) suggest arachidonic acid

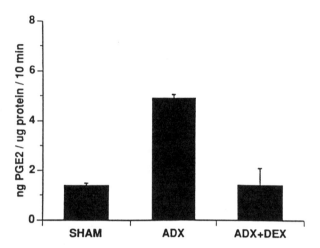

Figure 17 PGS enzyme activity in peritoneal macrophages from SHAM (sham-operated), ADX (adrenalectomized), and ADX+DEX–treated mice. After the in vivo treatments, peritoneal macrophages were collected, plated in cell culture dishes, and treated with arachidonic acid (30 μM) for 10 min at 37°C. The media were then analyzed by ELISA for PGE$_2$. The results are the mean±SEM of three separate experiments. (Data reproduced from ref. 18.)

will be equally accessible to both PGS enzymes. We found, however, that protein synthesis inhibition *blocks* TPA-induced PGE$_2$ accumulation in 3T3 cells (21) despite the presence of constitutive PGS1 (19,20). These data suggest that, at least in some cases, (1) PGS2 may play a required role in ligand-induced prostaglandin production and (2) arachidonic acid released in response to ligand activation may not be accessible to PGS1.

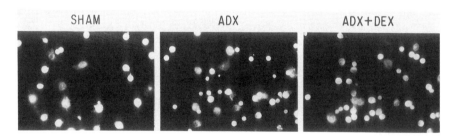

Figure 18 Immunostaining of PGS1 protein in peritoneal macrophages from SHAM, ADX, and ADX mice treated with 1 mg/kg of dexamethasone (ADX+DEX). Macrophages were collected by lavage, centrifuged, fixed, and stained for PGS1 immunofluorescence. (Data reproduced from ref. 18.)

SHAM   ADX   ADX + DEX

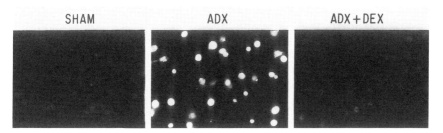

Figure 19 Western blot analysis of PGS1/COX1 and PGS2/COX2 proteins in peritoneal macrophages from SHAM, ADX, and ADX+DEX–treated mice. Macrophages were collected by lavage and centrifuged and Western blotting was carried out. Analysis with PGS1/COX1 antibody was performed on the samples in the left-hand panel; analysis with PGS2/COX2 antibody was carried out on the samples in the right-hand panel. (Data reproduced from ref. 18.)

We used antisense oligonucleotides (ASOs) to investigate the role of PGS2 expression in (1) mitogen-induced prostaglandin production in fibroblasts and (2) endotoxin/LPS-induced prostaglandin production in macrophages. Transfected PGS2 ASOs block TPA-induced PGS2 protein accumulation in 3T3 cells without interfering with PGS1 accumulation (22). Sense (SO) and random (RO) oligos have no effect. If 3T3 cells are first transfected with ASO, RO, or SO and then challenged with TPA, *murine PGS2 antisense oligonucleotides com-*

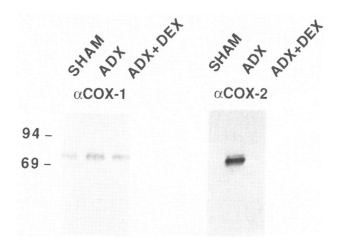

Figure 20 Immunostaining of PGS2 protein in peritoneal macrophages from SHAM, ADX, and ADX+DEX–treated mice. Macrophages were collected by lavage, centrifuged, fixed, and stained for PGS2. (Data reproduced from ref. 18.)

70

Herschman et al.

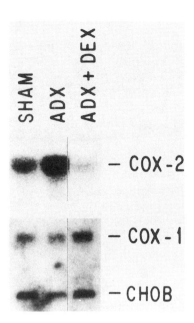

Figure 21 Expression of PGS1/COX1 and PGS2/COX2 mRNAs in peritoneal macrophages from SHAM, ADX, and ADX+DEX–treated mice. Macrophages were collected by lavage and cintrifugation. Total RNA was isolated, subjected to electrophoresis, transferred to nitrocellulose filters, and hybridized with PGS2/COX2 or PGS1/COX1 probes. The CHOB probe was used to normalize for differences in RNA loading. (Data reproduced from ref. 18.)

pletely block TPA-induced PGE$_2$ accumulation. SO and RO have no effect. To be certain that PGS2 ASO treatment did not inactivate PGS1, these same cell cultures were washed and then challenged with serum-free medium containing 10 µM exogenous arachidonic acid. All the cells, including those receiving ASOs, convert *exogenous* arachidonic acid to PGE$_2$, demonstrating that active PGS1 enzyme is present in these cells. PGS2 ASO also block prostaglandin production in serum and PDGF-treated 3T3 cells (22). To be certain that this result was not an artifact of using established cell lines, we demonstrated that PGS2 ASOs also block prostaglandin production in TPA-treated murine embryo fibroblast cultures (22). PGS2 ASOs also prevent PGE$_2$ production in LPS-treated RAW 264.7 macrophages and LPS-treated peritoneal macrophages (22).

To assess the possibility that PGS2 ASOs prevent mitogen-stimulated arachidonic acid release from membrane stores, we prelabeled 3T3 phospholipids with [^{3}H]arachidonic acid, transfected the cells with ASO, RO, or SO, challenged with TPA, and measured released radioactive arachidonic acid and radioactive PGE_2 by thin-layer chromatography and scintillation counting. PGS2 ASOs again block PGE_2 production (22) but do *not* prevent [³H]arachidonic acid release in cells treated with TPA. In fact, more [³H]arachidonic acid is released in the presence of ASO than with RO or SO, since the [³H]arachidonic acid released in the presence of PGS2 ASO cannot be converted to prostanoids. LPS-stimulated release of endogenous [³H]arachidonic acid also occurs in RAW 264.7 cells in the presence of PGS2 ASOs (22).

Our cycloheximide (21) and antisense (22) experiments demonstrate that ligand-induced PGS2 synthesis and enzyme activity is necessary for mitogen-induced prostaglandin production in murine fibroblasts and for endotoxin-induced prostaglandin production in murine macrophages. Constitutive PGS1 present in these cells cannot utilize as substrate endogenous arachidonic acid released from membrane phospholipids in response to mitogen or endotoxin. Induced PGS2 expression is likely to be (1) required for many prostaglandin-mediated cellular interactions and (2) an important target in the management of pathophysiological conditions involving prostanoids; for example, asthma, arthritis, acute inflammation, and colon cancer.

VIII. "Macrophage" Nitric Oxide Synthase Is Also a Glucocorticoid-Inhibited Primary Response/Immediate Early Gene

Like prostaglandins, nitric oxide is a major mediator of paracrine cellular communication, mediating vasodilation, neurotransmission, and macrophage defense. Nitric oxide is synthesized from L-arginine by the enzyme nitric oxide synthase (NOS). Like the prostaglandin synthases, there are several nitric oxide synthase genes that encode distinct proteins with similar enzymatic activities. One of the nitric oxide synthases is, like PGS2, induced in macrophages by endotoxin. This mac-NOS, also termed iNOS because it is inducible, has been cloned by three groups (23–25). Because (1) both iNOS and PGS2 are induced in macrophages and (2) both iNOS and PGS2 encode proteins whose products are mediate paracrine cell communication, we examined the inducibility of iNOS in murine fibroblasts and the modulation of iNOS expression by glucocorticoids.

TPA induces the expression of iNOS in 3T3 cells with kinetics similar to those observed for PGS2 (Fig. 22). Moreover, induction of iNOS occurs in the presence of cycloheximide; iNOS is a primary response/immediate early gene (26). Many of the inducers that stimulate PGS2 gene expression in 3T3 cells also stimulate iNOS message accumulation (Fig. 23). Like PGS2, the iNOS gene responses to a number of different stimuli, which activate distinct second-messenger pathways. Although the kinetics of induction of iNOS and

Herschman et al.

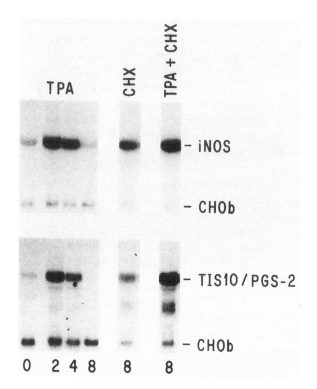

Figure 22 Induction of iNOS and TIS10/PGS2 mRNA by TPA in Swiss 3T3 cells.
Confluent, density-arrested Swiss 3T3 cells were treated for the times indicated (in hours)
with either TPA (50 ng/ml), CHX (10 µg/ml), or TPA plus CHX. Total RNA was isolated and analyzed by Northern analysis. Ten micrograms of total cellular RNA were
loaded per lane. Filters were hybridized with radiolabeled probes for iNOS, TIS10/PGS2,
or CHOB. (Data reproduced from ref. 26.)

PGS2 are similar, and these two genes respond to many of the same stimuli,
there *are* differences in the expression of the two genes. Expression of the v-
src oncogene is a potent inducer of PGS2 gene expression in 3T3 cells (27,28)
but does not stimulate expression of the iNOS gene (data not shown). In contrast, although LPS is unable to induce expression of PGS2 in 3T3 cells, LPS
is a potent inducer of iNOS (Fig. 24). Although glucocorticoids do not modulate the induced expression of most immediate early genes, DEX is able to block
iNOS induction by both mitogens and endotoxin in Swiss 3T3 cells (Fig. 25),
just as it does for PGS2.

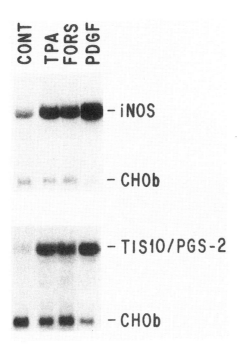

Figure 23 Induction of iNOS and TIS10/PGS2 mRNA in Swiss 3T3 cells by alternative ligands. Total cellular RNA was isolated from untreated, density-arrested Swiss 3T3 cells (CONT) and from cells treated for 2 hr with TPA (50 ng/ml), forskolin (100 μM), or PDGF (20 ng/ml). Ten micrograms of RNA were loaded per lane. (data reproduced from ref. 26.)

IX. Glucocorticoid Attenuation Defines a Subclass of Immediate Early Genes Whose Products Mediate Paracrine Cell Communication

We have demonstrated that glucorticoid hormones suppress ligand-induced expression of two primary response/immediate early genes, PGS2 and iNOS, whose products mediate paracrine cell communication. Glucocorticoids also inhibit the mitogen-induced expression of the JE and KC genes, two primary response/immediate early genes that encode cytokines that also mediate paracrine cell interactions (29–31). In contrast, mitogen-induction of c-*jun*, c-*fos*, *egr*-1/TIS8, and *nur*77/TIS1, which encode transcription factors, is not inhibited by DEX. Based on these observations, we propose that there exists a subclass of IEGs (1) whose induction is attenuated by glucocorticoids and (2) whose

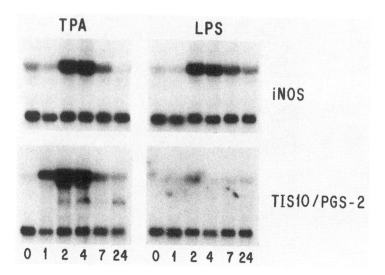

Figure 24 LPS induces iNOS, but not TIS10/PG-2, message in Swiss 3T3 cells. Density-arrested Swiss 3T3 cells were treated with TPA (50 ng/ml) or LPS (5 ng/ml) for the indicated times. Each lane contains 10 μg of RNA. (data reproduced from ref. 26.)

products, like PGS2 and iNOS, mediate paracrine communication following ligand stimulation.

To search for glucocorticoid attentuated–immediate early genes, or GA-IEGs, we used differential hybridization to screen a cDNA library prepared from Swiss 3T3 cells stimulated in the presence of cycloheximide. The "plus" probe was a ³²P-labeled cDNA prepared from RNA of cells treated with inducing ligands. The "minus" probe was prepared from cells treated similarly, with the exception that DEX was present. One hundred and twenty candidate clones were picked from 15,000 phages. Cross hybridization reduced the 40 phages with the highest differential hybridization scores to 10 groups. Northern analyses confirm that (1) each message is induced by ligand stimulation of 3T3 cells and (2) induction is attenuated by DEX. Part of our hypothesis has been confirmed; a subset of IEGs is subject to coordinate inhibition by glucocorticoids.

Five of the 10 GA-IEGs encode known paracrine modulators of cellular communication; (1) JE/MCP-1, (2) fic/MCP-3; (3) crg2/IP10, (4) thrombospondin 1, and (5) M-CSF. Readers should note that some of the relevant characteristics used to isolate these clones; for example fibroblast inducibility and DEX attenuation, were not previously known for these genes. Of the five previously unknown GA-IEG cDNAs, one has homology to a human interferon-induced protein, three partial sequences have no homology to known genes, and

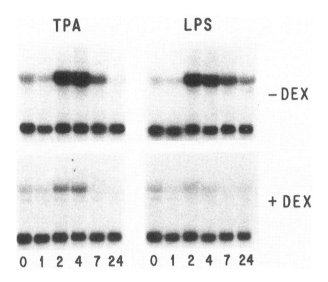

Figure 25 Dexamethasone inhibits TPA- and LPS-induced iNOS expression. Density-arrested Swiss 3T3 cells were preincubated for 4 hr in the absence or presence of DEX (2 μM) and then treated with TPA (50 ng/ml) or LPS (5 ng/ml) for the indicated times (in hours). Each lane contains 10 μg of RNA. (data are reproduced from ref. 26.)

one encodes a new member of the C-X-C chemokine family. This validates the second part of our hypothesis; many GA-IEGs encode proteins that mediate paracrine cell communication.

The results of our differential screen indicate the existence of a subset of primary response/immediate early genes whose induction by inflammatory stimuli is attenuated by glucocorticoids. Many of these GA-IEGs, such as PGS2, iNOS, and members of the C-C and C-X-C family of small cytokines, are now known to have important roles in inflammation. This suggests that the anti-inflammatory effects of glucocorticoids may be due in large part to the ability these steroid hormones have to attenuate the induction of this subset of IEGs. Understanding the mechanism(s) of the coordinate glucocorticoid attenuation of the induction of PGS2, iNOS, and other GA-IEGs that mediate paracrine cell communication will be critical for both our basic understanding of the regulation of gene expression and for the design of rational steroid therapeutic applications.

Acknowledgments

These studies were supported by grants GM24797 and AI34567 from the National Institutes of Health.

Discussion

DR. LIU: In the mast cell do you see free arachidonic acid released by stimulation?

DR. HERSCHMAN: We did not look in mast cells. However, in both mitogen-induced fibroblasts and endotoxin-stimulated macrophages, antisense oligonucleotides for TISIO/PGS-2 block ligand-induced PGE_2 production. As a result, cells in the presence of antisense oligonucleotides accumulate more free arachidonic acid in the medium, because the arachidonic acid has no place to go. This work was recently published (Reddy ST, Herschman HR. Ligand-induced prostaglandin synthesis requires expression of the TIS10/PGS-2 prostaglandin synthase gene in murine fibroblasts and macrophages. J Biol Chem 1994; 269:15473–15480).

DR. GLEICH: You showed the homologies between your novel chemokines and the IL-8 gene family. Is your new chemokine related to the known C-C or C-X-C families or possibly to the new family of cytokines exemplified by lymphotactin?

DR. HERSCHMAN: I am not familiar with lymphotactin. Our gene encodes a new member of the C-X-C chemokine family.

DR. BARNES: In the case of many immediate early genes, such as iNOS, COX-2, and IL-8, NF-κB appears to be an important transcription factor. Have you look at whether the inducible genes you have identified are driven by NF-κB?

DR. HERSCHMAN: PGS2 in fibroblasts can be induced by forskolin, PDGF, and serum. Each of these is thought to work through a distinct second-messenger pathway and activate different transcription factors. The PGS2 gene can be induced in neurons by depolarizatoin, in mast cells by aggregation of IgE receptors, and in macrophages by endotoxin. Each of these inductions can be blocked by glucocorticoids. If there is a common mechanism for glucocorticoid suppression of PGS2 induction, I doubt it will be via NFκB for these various inductions.

DR. PERRETTI: (1) Comment: In relation to the last question, I would like to say that we have been doing similar experiments with murine macrophages. LPS could stimulate both COX-2 and iNOS, and dexamethasone was able to inhibit the induction of these genes in this cell type. However, immunoneutralization of endogenous lipocortin-1 did not affect dexamethasone inhibition of COX-2 but abrogated the repression exerted by the steroid on iNOS induction. It is of interest that a GRE is present on the COX-2 promoter, whereas it is absent on the iNOS promoter. It is possible that lipocortin 1 selectively interferes with signaling, which leads to repression of iNOS and probably other genes. (2) If I may follow up with a question: MCP-1 and MCP-3 were, I believe, among the genes you have identified to be induced by LPS and represented by dexamethasone. Do these genes have a GRE in their promoter region?

DR. HERSCHMAN: I do not know.

DR. MIESFELD: If glucocorticoids can modulate cross-signaling pathways that are selectively activated by LPS or TPA or serum induction, then it is likely that more than one transcription factor mechanism is involved. It is difficult to see how NF-κB alone could explain all these effects.

DR. HERSCHMAN: In fact, our inducers in the establishment of the library were serum, TGFβ, and LPS. We find all combinations possible for LPS-induced dexamethasone-suppressed genes; some are inducible by serum but not TGFβ, and not inducible by either TGFβ or serum.

DR. SCHLEIMER: (1) Glucocorticoids affect many functional aspects of cells. I am therefore curious how you arrived at the hypothesis that genes involved in paracrine interactions would be selectively suppressed. (2) Would you please describe your studies with PGS2 knockout mice?

DR. HERSCHMAN: (1) The hypothesis was based on empirical observation. Mitogen induction of four immediate early genes, PGS2, iNOS, JE, and KC, is inhibited by dexamethasone. The products of these genes modulate paracrine cell communication. Induction of other immediate early genes that modulate transcription cascades to alter cellular phenotype (c-*fos*, c,*fos*, c-*jun*, *egr*-1/TISB/*zif*268, *nur*77/TIS1) is not inhibited by glucocorticoids. We proposed this might indicate a functional/regulatory subset of immediate early genes. (2) We have obtained germline transmission. Female heterozygotes are sterile. Male heterozygotes can father heterozygous pups with wide-type females.

DR. GAULDIE: For the genes you showed induced by LPS and suppressed by dexmethasone, you would not expect a GRE, if it were present, to be important since GRE is usually involved in *induction* and has no role to play in suppression. As an example, we and others have shown that the IL-6 gene induced by IL-1 in fibroblasts or LPS in macrophage and inhibited by steroid has four well-defined GRE elements in the 5'-region of the gene, but none are involved in either the stimulation or suppression mechanism.

DR. HERSCHMAN: Yes, I agree.

DR. MIESFELD: The first challenge is to choose a manageable model system using a specific cell type, GR-regulated gene, and realistic cross-talk signals. In asthma at this time, no one can agree on any of these three parameters (cell type, gene, and signal). In the future, it would be nice to develop a transgenic animal model of asthma.

DR. BRATTSAND: Glucocorticoid actions are often cell type-specific. How do you explain this?

DR. HERSCHMAN: In our hands, chimeric constructs with up to 5 kb of the PGS promoter are not inhibited by glucocorticoids. However, colleagues to whom we have sent these constructs tell us they can get 40–50% inhibition in an osteoblast cell line. We therefore think one may observe cell-specific modes of suppression by glucocorticoids for the same gene. Most workers believe stable transfectants more often reflect what is occurring in vivo than do transient transfectants. However, both assays are useful.

DR. MIESFELD: It is important not to discount the usefulness of transient transfection assays; there are as many examples of where it has been useful as there are cases where the reporter genes are inadequate. I agree that transcriptional repression mechanism may be more difficult to study by the standard transient assay. Moreover, it should be possible to use homologous recombination in cell lines to set up appropriate assay systems to study transcription repression at the normal gene locus.

DR. HERSCHMAN: I agree.

References

1. Simmons DL, Neel BG, Stevens R, Evett G, Erickson RL. Identification of an early-growth-response gene encoding a novel putative protein kinase. Mol Cell Biol 1992; 12:4164–4169.
2. Charles CH, Sun H, Lau LF, Tonks N. The growth factor-inducible immediate-early gene 3CH134 encodes a protein-tyrosine-phosphatase. Proc Natl Acad Sci USA 1993; 90:5292–5296.
3. Herschman HR. Primary response genes induced by growth factors and tumor promoters. Ann Rev Biochem 1991; 60:81–319.
4. Lim RW, Varnum BC, Herschman HR. Cloning of tetradecanoyl phorbol ester induced "primary response" sequences and their expression in density-arrested Swiss 3T3 cells and a TPA nonproliferative variant. Oncogene 1987; 1:263–270.
5. Smith WL, Marnett LJ. Prostaglandin endoperoxide synthase: structure and catalysis. Biochim Biophys Acta 1991; 1083:1–17.
6. Kujubu DA, Fletcher BS, Varnum BC, Lim RW, Herschman HR. TIS10, a phorbol ester tumor promoter-inducible mRNA from Swiss 3T3 cells, encodes a novel prostaglandin synthase/cyclooxygenase homologue. J Biol Chem 1991; 266:12866–12872.
7. Fletcher BS, Kujubu DA, Perrin DM, Herschman HR. Structure of the mitogen-inducible TIS10 gene and demonstration that the TIS10 encoded protein is a functional prostaglandin G/H synthase. J Biol Chem 1992; 267:4338–4344.

8. Xie W, Chipman JG, Robertson DL, Erikson RL, Simmons DL. Expression of a mitogen-responsive gene encoding prostaglandin synthase is regulated by mRNA splicing. Proc Natl Acad Sci USA 1991; 88:2692–2696.

9. O'Banion MK, Winn VD, Young DA. cDNA cloning and functional activity of a glucocorticoid-regulated inflammatory cyclooxygenase. Proc Natl Acad Sci USA 1992; 89:4888–4892.

10. Ryseck R-P, Raynoshek C, Macdonald-Bravo H, Dorfman K, Mattei M-G, Bravo R. Identification of an immediate early gene, pghs-B, whose protein product has prostaglandin synthase/cyclooxygenase activity. Cell Growth Diff 1992; 3:433–450.

11. Sirois J, Richards JS. Purification and characterization of a novel, distinct isoform of prostaglandin endoperoxide synthase induced by human chorionic gonadotropin in granulosa cells of rat preovulatory follicles. J Biol Chem 1992; 267:6383–6388.

12. Sirois J, Levy LO, Simmons DL, Richards JS. Characterization and hormonal regulation of the promoter of the rat prostaglandin endoperoxide synthase 2 gene in granulosa cells. J Biol Chem 1993; 268:12199–12206.

13. Seibert K, Masferrer JL, Jiyi F, Honda A, Raz A, Needleman P. The biochemical and pharmacological manipulation of cellular cyclooxygenase (COX) activity. Adv Prostaglandin Thromboxane Leukotriene Res 1990; 21:45–51.

14. Raz A, Wyche A, Siegel N, Needleman P. Regulation of fibroblast cyclooxygenase synthesis by interleukin-1. J Biol Chem 1988; 263:3022–3025.

15. Raz A, Wyche A, Needleman P. Temporal and pharmacological division of fibroblast cyclooxygenase expression into transcriptional and translational phases. Proc Natl Acad Sci USA 1989; 86:1657–1661 (1989).

16. Herschman HR, Kujubu DA, Fletcher BS, Ma Q-F, Varnum BC, Gilbert RS, Reddy ST. The TIS genes, primary response genes induced by growth factors and tumor promoters. Nucleic Acids Res Mol Biol 1994; 47:113–148.

17. Masferrer JL, Seibert K, Zweifel B, Needleman P. Endogenous glucocorticoids regulate an inducible cyclooxygenase enzyme. Proc Natl Acad Sci USA 1992; 89:3917–3921.

18. Masferrer J, Reddy ST, Zweifel B, Seibert K, Needleman P, Gilbert RS, Herschman HR. In vivo regulation of cyclooxygenase-2 by glucorticoids in peritoneal macrophages. J Pharm Exp Ther 1994; 270:1340–1344.

19. Kujubu DA, Reddy ST, Fletcher BS, Herschman HR. Expression of the protein product of the prostaglandin synthase-2/TIS10 gene in mitogen-stimulated Swiss 3T3 cells. J Biol Chem 1993; 268:5425–5331.

20. Reiger MK, DeWitt DL, Schindler MS, Smith WL. Subcellular localization of prostaglandin endoperoxide synthase-2 in murine 3T3 Cells. Arch Biochem Biophys 1993; 301:439–434.

21. Kujubu DA, Herschman HR. Dexamethasone inhibits mitogen induction of the TIS10 prostaglandin synthase/cyclooxygenase gene. J Biol Chem 1992; 267:7991–7994.

22. Reddy ST, Hershman HR. Ligand-induced prostaglandin synthesis requires expression of the TIS10/PGS2 prostaglandin synthase gene in murine fibroblasts and macrophages. J Biol Chem 1994; 269:15473–15480.

23. Lyons CR, Orloff GJ, Cunningham JM. Molecular cloning and functional expression of an inducible nitric oxide synthase from a murine macrophage cell line. J Biol Chem 1992; 267:6370–6374.

24. Xie Q-W, Cho JJ, Calaycay J, Mumford RA, Swiderek KM, Lee TD, Ding A, Troso T, Nathan C. Cloning and characterization of inducible nitric oxide synthase from mouse macrophages. Science 1992; 256:225-228.
25. Lowenstein CJ, Glatt CS, Bredt DS, Snyder SH. Cloned and expressed macrophage nitric oxide synthase contrasts with the brain enzyme. Proc Natl Acad Sci USA 1992; 89:6711-6715.
26. Gilbert RS, Herschman HR. Macrophage nitric oxide synthase is a glucocorticoid-inhibitable primary response gene in 3T3 Cells. J Cell Physiol 1993; 157:128-134.
27. Qureshi SA, Joseph CK, Rim M, Maroney A, Foster DA. v-Src activates both protein kinase C-dependent and independent signaling pathways in murine fibroblasts. Oncogene 1991; 6:995-999.
28. Xie W, Fletcher BS, Andersen RD, Herschman HR. v-src induction of the TIS10/PGS2 prostaglandin synthase gene is mediated by an ATF/CRE transcription response element. Mol Cell Biol 1994; 14:6531-6539.
29. Rameh LE, Armelin MC. Downregulation of JE and KC genes by glucocorticoids does not prevent the GO----G1 transition in BALB/3T3 cells. Mol Cell Biol 1992; 12:4612-4621.
30. Kamahara RS, Deng ZW, Deuel TF. Glucocorticoids inhibit the transcriptional induction of JE, a platelet-derived growth factor-inducible gene. J Biol Chem 1991; 226:13261-13266.
31. Deng ZW, Denkinger DJ, Peterson KE, Deuel TF, Kawahara RS. Glucocorticoids negatively regulate the transcription of KC, the mouse homologue of MGSA/GRO. Biochem Biophys Res Commun 1994; 203:1809-1814.

4

Glucocorticoids and Apoptosis of Hematopoietic Cells
Transcriptional and Posttranscriptional Control

E. BRAD THOMPSON

The University of Texas Medical Branch
Galveston, Texas

I. Introduction

Glucocorticoids have long been known to be profound regulators of cells of the allergic response system. The mechanisms by which this important regulation occurs are becoming clear. One mechanism regulating hematopoietic cells is apoptosis, a phenomenon in which intracellular systems are activated to cause a distinctive type of cell death (1). The concept of apoptosis began with histological observations of normal tissues showing stochastic death of cells that displayed morphology differing from the well-known necrotic process (2). In contrast to necrosis, apoptotic cells occurred randomly, displaying shrinkage and dissociation from surrounding tissues, a particular form of heterochromatization, and membrane blebbing. These were followed by condensation into dense apoptotic cells or fragmented apoptotic bodies which were subsequently taken up by surrounding parenchymal cells or macrophages, with little gross inflammatory reaction. All these features distinguish apoptosis from necrosis. At the time the concept of apoptosis was formulated, glucocorticoids had long been known to cause involution of the thymus and death of cortical thymocytes. Comparing the morphology of that process with that of spontaneous apoptosis showed great similarity. Since glucocorticoids regulate genes, the idea began that a gene-regulated process or processes was responsible for apoptosis. This has been solidified by finding that many specific ligands can set off morphological apoptosis in various cell types, and by the fact that systematic cell death during development often shows similar characteristics (3–5). In *Caenorhabditis elegans*, an increasingly well-known set of genes regulates such developmental loss of cells, and several of these genes are homologues to genes which are involved in mammalian cell apoptosis (6,7). A prolonged search for a single sequence of gene expression causing apoptosis has not yet yielded a universal mechanism. Increasingly, the conclusion is being reached that apoptosis is a common end point reached by the activation of a variety of specific paths. The task now is to define those specific paths using well controlled systems.

Glucocorticoids act in regulating the immune response system in two ways. First, they regulate cytokines and other growth factors which are important for the growth and viability of immune system cells. Second, glucocorticoids act directly upon individual cells in the immune system to alter genes involved in their immune functions or to directly affect their viability. The cytokine-directed and glucocorticoid-directed pathways seem to interact to control viability. In this paper I will discuss briefly the general concepts of these two types of control, with examples particularly pertinent to asthma. In the second portion of this paper, I will summarize the results of our studies on the mechanisms by which apoptosis takes place in a system of human lymphoid leukemic cells.

II. Mechanisms of Regulation of Gene Expression by Glucocorticoids, Transcriptional and Posttranscriptional

One consensus held about steroid hormones is that they regulate gene expression. That regulation may occur at several levels, from transcription through messenger RNA stability and even protein stability. This major paradigm has correctly shifted attention away from other possible actions of glucocorticoids that might affect immune responses; that is, allosteric regulation of proteins or alterations in membranes due to direct intercollation therein, which are hypotheses that prior to the 1960s were entertained as strong alternatives to the gene-regulation concept. As has been demonstrated repeatedly, glucocorticoids change the expressed levels of specific gene products at the transcriptional and posttranscriptional levels.

The direct cellular effects of glucocorticoids require the activation of the glucocorticoid receptor (GR) by the steroid. The intracellular steroid-receptor complex then functions as a transcription factor to alter the level of transcription of specific genes by several mechanisms. The ligand-activated GR has general DNA-binding capacity, with affinity for nonspecific DNA sequences yielding an apparent dissociation constant (Kd) of the order of magnitude of 10^{-6} M. Gene specificity is due to the thousandfold greater affinity of the steroid GR for specific sequences known as glucocorticoid response elements (GREs). A GRE_{PAL} is a 15-nucleotide sequence composed of a hexamer TGTYCT repeated as an imperfect palindrome separated by three nonspecific nucleotides. The precise sequence of the GRE_{PAL} varies from gene to gene, but a consensus sequence derived from several natural GREs is GGTACAnnnTGTYCT (8). GREs often occur in groups of two or three in the 5' promoter/regulatory regions of genes and the GRE can act with the properties of an enhancer; that is, it functions in either orientation and at varying distances from the initiation site of transcription. Indeed, some GREs have been found 3' of the transcription start site. Steroid-activated GR dimerizes cooperatively at each GRE_{PAL}. Acting from complete, palindromic GREs, the bound GR dimer acts to stimulate transcription, apparently by stabilizing the transcription preinitiation complex of RNA polymerase and its associated factors (9,10). In living cell systems, this action of the GR seems to require the constant presence of the ligand glucocorticoid. Studies of GR:GRE binding in chromatin on regulatory regions of the mouse mammary tumor virus and tyrosine aminotransferase genes suggest that the topological relationship of the GRE to specific nucleosomes also is critical for proper transcriptional control (11,12).

Alone the hexamers TGTYCT and GGTACA are referred to as GRE half-sites, and these are often found scattered through genes. The activated GR can bind as a monomer to these, with much greater affinity for the TGTYCT site, although still much less than for the full GRE_{PAL}. Alone GR interaction with GRE half-sites does not seem capable of regulating transcription. However, these sites may come into play as part of a second regulatory mechanism. This mechanism stems from the fact that the activated steroid GR can interact with other transcription factors to regulate genes through more complex sites. These may involve the binding sites for one or more factors; for example, an AP-1 site in proximity to a GRE half-site. At such combined sites (also termed complex or composite sites), functional interactions have been shown to occur between the GR and several important transcription factors, including Jun (of the Jun:Fos dimer AP-1), NF-κB, CREB, and C/EBP. The GR can bind directly to at least some of these factors, however, and as with the collagenase gene, AP-1:GR joint control of transcription appears to occur in the absence of a cognate GRE site (13). Even more complex, multifactor interactions have been described at a site controlling the transcription of the PEPCK gene (14). Recognition of these interactions between the GR and other transcription factors has led to the understanding that the balance of function between GR and the other factor(s) acting at a given site will determine the quantitative alteration in transcription. Thus, if a factor X acting alone at a site has a strong positive inductive effect and GR a weaker one, interaction with GR could cause a reduction in the rate of transcription, because the GR:factorX complex would be weaker in stimulating the transcription machinery than factor X by itself. If factor X levels are low or absent, basal transcription from the site would be very low, and then activated GR might be seen to stimulate from that site, because even its relatively weak action would cause an increase from the low basal state. In general, it can be seen that three sets of molecules are involved in such controls: the activated GR, its transcription factor "partners," and proteins in the large complex that makes up the "basal" transcription machinery, with which transcription factors interact. The complex and varying balance between these three components will determine the effect glucocorticoids have over many genes. Nonsteroidal influences on a cell that result in altered expression of any of these components can influence strongly how a particular gene responds to the addition of a glucocorticoid ligand. Such mechanisms allow for delicate and cell-specific, yet variable control by the steroid, since it is required to keep the GR in its active form as a transcription factor. Furthermore, glucocorticoidal gene control may alter the expression of other transcription factors and additional proteins important for gene expression. Depending on the half-lives of these other regulatory proteins, glucocorticoids can thus institute reverberating effects that may last for some time after the removal of the hormone. Many valuable reviews provide deeper access to the literature concerning the above general outline of glucocorticoid and related ligands, control over transcription and apoptosis (15–22).

In addition to transcriptional regulation, steroid hormones may regulate gene products posttranscriptionally. This was suggested early after the discovery that glucocorticoids induce expression of the products of specific genes. Indirect experiments on the induction of the tyrosine aminotransferase gene in liver and hepatoma cells were interpreted as indicative of posttranscriptional control (23). The methods available at the time did not allow clear resolution of the issue, and subsequently it was shown that the gene possesses several critical GREs and that acute induction is transcriptional (24). However, recent work has shown that, in cultured hepatoma cells, sustained induction of tyrosine aminotransferase by dexamethasone appears to result in loss of transcriptional stimulation and its replacement by message stabilization (25). Especially relevant to the control of the immune/inflammatory response is recent evidence suggesting that glucocorticoid control of interleukin-1 (IL-1) in human monocytes occurs posttranscriptionally. In this case, transcription is reduced and as well, the IL-1 mRNA appears to be destabilized by a GR-dependent action (26,27), so that by two mechanisms acting in concert, glucocorticoids are seen to downregulate IL-1 expression. A similar effect on mRNA has been observed for the downregulation of β-interferon (IFN-β) (28). Posttranscriptional effects of glucocorticoids on message stability have also been seen in the regulation of milk protein genes (29) and of HMGCoA reductase. Thus, glucocorticoids can provoke both stabilization and destabilization of specific mRNAs. Compared with the state of knowledge concerning regulation of transcription, less is known about the mechanisms by which these posttranscriptional effects occur. The GR seems to be required but is not necessarily involved directly in the effects on the RNA itself. In the case of IFN-β mRNA turnover, AU-rich sequences in the 3' untranslated region of the RNA were required for the stimulation of increased turnover by glucocorticoids. (Such sequences have been shown to be a signal for mRNA instability in a number of systems.) Regulation in the IFN-β and IL-1 systems appears to differ, since blocking protein synthesis with cycloheximide in the former did not block the effect of glucocorticoid, whereas in the latter, it did do so (27,28). How the GR works to alter mRNA synthesis without requiring protein synthesis is unknown, but it may be pertinent to recall that GR has been reported to bind RNA, although no specific confirmed binding sequence has been identified (30,31). Work on the mechanisms of posttranscriptional control has gone somewhat further in the case of estrogenic control over liver-specific mRNAs in *Xenopus*. In the frog, estrogen treatment causes a huge shift in the amounts of several liver mRNAs. Vitellogenin mRNA is stabilized, shifting in male frogs given estrogen from a half-life of about 16 hr to one of 500 hr. A 27-nucleotide region in the 3'-untranslated region of the vitellogenin mRNA has been identified to which an estrogen-induced stabilizing protein binds (32). At the same time, the mRNAs of the majority of secreted proteins are destabilized. Estrogens induce a ribonuclease found associated with the 80S ribosome on albumin mRNA; this nuclease is thought to play an important role in the increased turnover of mRNAs caused by estrogens (33). It is to be expected that similar mechanisms will be uncovered for glucocorticoidal regulation of mRNA stability.

In sum, through their receptor-activating action, glucocorticoids control the levels of gene expression by regulating both transcription and the stability of mRNAs. For any given gene, one or the other mechanism can predominate or be used exclusively, and the regulation can be up or down. Transcriptional regulation can involve direct binding of the GR to its cognate GRE site, resulting in gene activation; but in many genes, regulation comes about by the combined interactions of the GR and other transcription factors at sites different from the classic GRE_{PAL}. RNA stability can be regulated by glucocorticoids via their receptor, by as yet unknown mechanisms that do not require intervening macromolecular synthesis, or by the induction of proteins, perhaps mRNA-stabilizing proteins or destabilizing RNases as in the estrogenic control of frog liver gene expression. Through these mechanisms, glucocorticoids control gene expression of many regulatory molecules, ranging from proto-oncogenes and transcription factors to hormones and cytokines. Thus, the entry of a glucocorticoid signal into this pool of regulatory molecules can set off a ripple effect, as a relatively acute change in one factor brought about by the initial steroid:GR reverberates throughout the system. After the glucocorticoid:GR changes the level of expression of even a single transcription factor, the steroid's effect may become irreversible—not due to a primary effect on a particular downstream gene—but because of the primary effect of the initial signalling system. These principles are illustrated in Figure 1.

III. Glucocorticoids Cause Apoptosis of Cell Types Important in Asthma

A. Eosinophils

Lung infiltration by eosinophils is closely correlated with asthma. The occurrence of eosinophils in the lungs of asthmatics requires that these cells make their way from the circulation to the tissue, be activated, and in response to stimuli, release their mediators there. A significant part of the efficacy of glucocorticoids in the treatment of asthma is believed to come from their known ability to cause eosinopenia. In recent years, insight into the mechanisms involved has been achieved. Glucocorticoids—at least in the concentrations normally achieved therapeutically—do not seem to have much effect on the acute controls over eosinophil function. Thus, glucocorticoids were not found to inhibit eosinophil degranulation or IL-5-mediated activation (34). The synthetic glucocorticoid budesonide neither inhibited nor blocked expression of adhesion molecules by endothelial cells (35). Rather, there appears to be regulation of eosinophil number by glucocorticoids, and this seems to involve regulation of apoptosis in two ways. In cultured eosinophils, viability and shift to the hypodense state depends on the presence of any of several cytokines, IL-3, IL-5, granulocyte-macrophage colony-stimulating factor (GM-CSF), and IFN-γ. In their absence, the cells undergo apoptotic changes in 24–72 hr (36). Singly, or in combination, these cytokines will greatly prolong the survival of eosinophils in vitro. T lymphocytes produce each of these, and therefore the actions of glucocorticoids that reduce numbers of T lymphocytes or the production of these cytokines by T lymphocytes are secondarily antieosinophilic. GM-CSF is also produced by fibroblast and endothelial cells. Glucocorticoids in reasonable therapeutic concentrations, for example, 100 nM dexamethasone, partially inhibit basal GM-CSF production by cultured endothelial cells. But even 10-fold higher steroid had no effect on IL-1α–stimulated production of the cytokine (36). In short, glucocorticoids work to reduce the level of cytokines on which eosinophils depend for viability.

The second effect of glucocorticoids is directly on the eosinophils themselves. This appears to be a major point of impact of the steroids in this system. Eosinophils contain glucocorticoid receptors (37), and concentrations of

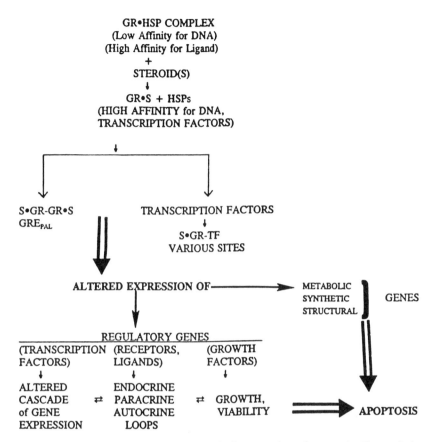

Figure 1 General pathways for glucocorticoid regulation of apoptosis. Transcription-ally inactive glucocorticoid receptor (GR) is complexed with a group of heat shock proteins (hsps). In this state, the GR binds its steroid ligand with high affinity. This results in release of the hsps and conversion of the GR with steroid bound (GR·S) to a transcriptionally active, DNA binding form, in which it can homodimerize at a classic palindromic GRE$_{PAL}$. Alternatively, the activated GR·S can interact with several other transcription factors to alter transcription from sites not containing the canonical GRE$_{PAL}$. This set of effects results in the alteration of expression of various genes, as shown. In some cases, the altered network of expressed genes results in apoptosis.

glucocorticoid which occupy these receptors cause accelerated apoptosis in vitro in the absence of cytokines, although the action of the steroids is more dramatic when minimal amounts of cytokine are used to support the vitality of eosino-phils (36). The addition of glucocorticoids then strongly produces apoptosis. Thus, glucocorticoids and cytokines are mutually antagonistic. Increasing the cytokine concentration can overcome the apoptotic effect of glucocorticoid (38–40). In other words, the glucocorticoid effect is to shift the viability dose-response curve for the cytokines to the right. That these glucocorticoid effects are receptor mediated is supported by appropriate dose-response curves, by the potency rank-order of glucocorticoids of known affinity for receptor, and by the absence of effect of sex steroids.

In sum, glucocorticoids may diminish the contribution of eosinophils to asthma by directly causing apoptosis of these cells while simultaneously acting to reduce the production of cytokines that enhance eosinophil growth and development. This latter effect can be occurring by regulation of cytokine production and by direct apoptotic reduction of some of the major cytokine-producing cells: for example, T-lymphoid cells. At the eosinophil, the balance between the actions of glucocorticoids and several cytokines determines whether apoptosis will occur. (For a valuable review of work prior to 1990 on the effects of glucocorticoids on allergic system cells, see ref. 41.) Figure 2 outlines some of the interactions by which glucocorticoids influence eosinophils: (1) by reducing the production of IL-2 and IL-1α on which T-lymphocytes and endothelial cells depend; (2) by inhibiting endothelial cell and T-lymphocyte production of cytokines on which eosinophils depend; and (3) by inhibiting T-lymphoid cell and eosinophil viability.

Among the direct effects of glucocorticoids on eosinophils, one of particular relevance for asthma is the inhibition of the expression of complement receptor type 3 (CR3). CR3 is necessary for many important functions of eosinophils. In cultured eosinophils, IL-3, IL-5, and GM-CSF all increased CR3 expression. Dexamethasone reduced basal CR3 expression and after 1 day blocked all or most of the increased receptor expression caused by the lymphokines (42). The lymphokine concentrations used and the timing of these experiments suggest that these dexamethasone effects occurred without a major contribution of dexamethasone-induced apoptosis. Thus, even under conditions where glucocorticoids do not kill eosinophils, the steroids can act to block critical eosinophil functions. Tomioka et al. found that although dexamethasone at 10^{-7} M reduced the level of CD11b in human eosinophils cultured for 2 or 3 days with 0.5 ng/ml of GM-CSF, the steroid did not prevent increased CD11b levels caused by combinations of GM-CSF and platelet-activating factor or GM-CSF and the chemotactic peptide FMLP (43). They concluded that the steroid did not inhibit a "priming function" of GM-CSF that rendered the cells sensitive to the additional factors.

B. Lymphocytes

As noted above, glucocorticoids are known to downregulate the production of cytokines by T cells. This is true of a considerable number of these regulatory

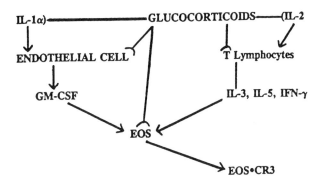

Figure 2 Interactions influencing apoptosis of T-lymphocytes and eosinophils. Glucocorticoids can cause apoptosis of activated or immature T cells and of eosinophils. This effect is antagonized by a variety of growth factors. Glucocorticoids also downregulate production of these factors in several cell types and thereby also reduce the growth of or cause the apoptosis of T cells and eosinophils. In the diagram, arrows indicate positive actions and curved symbols negative actions, discussed in the text.

molecules, including IL-1α, IL-2, IL-3, IL-4, IL-5, IL-6, IL-10, IFN-γ, and tumor necrosis factor (TNF) (44–47). Regulation of IL-2 reflects on the viability of T lymphocytes themselves, since IL-2 is the major lymphokine supporting their growth (48). IL-2 appears to be regulated by glucocorticoids at the transcriptional level (49) by a mechanism involving interactions with other factors (50). Some data indicate that in mitogen-stimulated human blood mononuclear cells, not IL-2 but a combination of IL-1, IL-6, and IFN-γ is required to prevent glucocorticoid inhibition of cell proliferation (51). Glucocorticoids also directly act to kill immature thymocytes or mitogen-stimulated T cells (52,53). Cells from patients with glucocorticoid-resistant asthma have been shown to be resistant to dexamethasone in vitro (54). Such patients may have a GR with reduced steroid affinity, and IL-2 plus IL-4 may be partly responsible for this effect (55). Other mechanisms may also be involved (56). Interestingly, although glucocorticoids decrease IL-2 production, they increase expression of the IL-2 receptor (47). The steroids also induce CD8 in rat and human acute lymphoblastic leukemia (ALL) CD4$^+$ cells (57,58).

B-lymphoid cells also can be sensitive to glucocorticoids, as evidenced by the apoptotic effects of these steroids on chronic lymphoblastic leukemia (CLL) (59) and myeloma (60) cells. In CLL, IL-2 is reported to antagonize the apoptotic effect of the steroid (59). In the myeloma system, induction of the GR itself and of transforming growth factor (TFG-β) may be involved in the apoptotic signal (60,61). For all types of lymphoid cells, resistance or sensitivity is dependent on the state of growth and differentiation of the cells. Fully mature, unstimulated cells are generally resistant. Immature cells vary depending on their status, and much is not understood about the determinant mechanisms. The recent work of Leung may be pertinent here (see Chapter 24).

In asthma, lymphoid cells probably contribute directly to the illness, and their apoptosis brought about by glucocorticoid treatment, along with the ability of glucocorticoids to decrease production of many of their cytokines by transcriptional and posttranscriptional mechanisms, are important explanations of the efficiency of steroid therapy.

C. Other Cell Types

Clear evidence of the direct apoptotic effects of glucocorticoids on basophils, mast cells, monocytes, and endothelial cells seems to be lacking. However, the production of several growth factors and lymphokines by these cells certainly is under steroidal control. Reduction of these proteins may therefore reduce the "support systems" for viability of cells such as eosinophils and lymphoid cells that clearly are susceptible to apoptosis, rendering them more sensitive to glucocorticoids.

Alveolar monocytes in vitro showed significantly reduced production of GM-CSF after treatment with budesonide, and a different pattern of inhibited expression of cytokines, as compared with monocytes obtained from the circulation (62). (It may be necessary to determine glucocorticoid effects on organ-specific cells in more than this case. Lymphoid and fibroblastic cells also behave in an organ-specific fashion.) As in other cell types, the balance between glucocorticoid and cytokine effects is seen in monocytes. Dexamethasone reduced IL-1β production in monocytes, and this reduction was prevented by simultaneous addition of IFN-γ (63,64).

Basophil migration but not outright viability is inhibited by glucocorticoids (65,66). These steroids also lower IgE-mediated release of histamine (67,68). As with certain other effects on various cells, glucocorticoidal inhibition of basophil histamine release was blocked by IL-3 (68).

According to Cohan et al., glucocorticoids do not seem able to inhibit the release of allergic reaction mediators from human alveolar mast cells, but reports seem to vary regarding their effect against these cells from other tissues (69,70). However, glucocorticoidal inhibition of cytokine production in T cells may lead to reduced numbers of mast cells. The possibility of a direct effect of glucocorticoids on normal mast cell proliferation is raised by the demonstration that dexamethasone reversibly diminished growth of mast cells transformed by the Kirsten sarcoma virus (71).

Even neutrophils, long thought resistant to glucocorticoid actions, have now been shown to modulate their cytokine systems after treatment with dexamethasone. The steroid acted synergistically with GM-CSF to increase IL-1 receptors on human neutrophils (72). Re et al. recently found that dexamethasone alone induced both type I and type II IL-1 receptors in neutrophils in vitro (73). The type II receptors were induced more quickly, were at higher levels, and were released from the cells. Owing to their structure, the ability of type II IL-1 receptors to transmit transmembrane signals is in doubt, and it is suggested that they serve as "decoys" to bind IL-1 in an inactive state. In monocytes, the production of a recently described "neutrophil priming activity" in a 3-kDa peptide was reduced by glucocorticoids. The reduction was seen in peripheral blood monocytes from steroid-sensitive but not steroid-insensitive asthmatic patients (74). IL-8 is a chemotactic cytokine produced by activated neutrophils as well as by monocytes. In both such cells, dexamethasone inhibits IL-8 production, as does IL-4 (75).

The general picture that emerges, therefore, is one of glucocorticoids regulating cytokine/growth factor production from many cell types, whereas also directly affecting the sensitivity of some cells, for example, eosinophils, to these factors. The combination of lowered production of cytokine/factors critical to viability and direct apoptosis-inducing effects of glucocorticoids results in cell death of the sensitive groups of cells. These include eosinophils and important sets of lymphoid cells. In addition, glucocorticoids may alter growth or inflammatory functions of some cells important in the pathobiology of asthma without killing them.

Pursuit of the detailed mechanisms of apoptosis is widespread. We have employed clones of a line of human CD4+ lymphoid cells derived from a child with ALL to study apoptosis. The next section briefly reviews our recent results.

IV. Apoptosis in CEM Cells

We have been studying the apoptosis evoked by application of glucocorticoids to a line of human ALL cells. From this CEM cell line we have isolated a number of clones which have proven extremely useful in studying the process. Clone CEM-C7 cells are sensitive to apoptosis by glucocorticoids, whereas clone CEM-C1 cells are resistant. Both have glucocorticoid receptors. These cells neither make nor depend on IL-2 (76) and can grow in completely defined medium (77). They therefore offer the opportunity to study apoptosis evoked by glucocorticoids in lymphoid cells without the complications of exogenous lymphokines. CEM-C1 cells express GR, and induction of the marker enzyme glutamine synthetase suggested that the receptor functioned normally (78). Also, somatic cell hybridizations showed that the CEM-C1 cells could complement receptor-deficient cells to restore glucocorticoid-induced apoptosis in the hybrids

(79). The glucocorticoid-sensitive clone CEM-C7 was shown to undergo spontaneous mutation to resistance at a haploid rate (80). Since the GR gene is autosomal, this suggested that they had become functionally haploid. This recently has been confirmed with the sequencing of their receptor genes (81,82). From CEM-C7 we have isolated a number of resistant cells, some of which have been characterized in detail. Clone ICR 27 is resistant owing to loss of the wild-type allele from CEM-C7. Properties of these three clones are illustrated in Table 1. As Table 1 shows, CEM-C7 cells contain one wild-type GR gene and one with a point mutation altering the *leu* at position 753 to *phe*. This renders the mutant receptor unable to bind and retain glucocorticoids correctly, whereas the normal GR continues to function properly. Clones C-1 and C-7 both have this heterozygous arrangement. The resistance of C-1 therefore depends on some other factor(s). Our recent data suggest that activation of the cAMP/protein kinase A pathway restores glucocorticoid sensitivity to these cells (83). The resistance of ICR-27 is due to the fact that the normal gene has been deleted, leaving only the mutant 753 *phe*. These experiments and similar work selecting for glucocorticoid resistance in mouse lymphoid lines (84) show unequivocally that the GR is necessary but not solely sufficient for glucocorticoids to cause apoptosis.

The successful cloning and complete sequencing of the human glucocorticoid receptor followed by domain analysis of its functions in regulating transcription produced our current knowledge of the domain structure of this transcription factor (21,85). Some of this structure is diagrammed in Figure 3. The human GR is a protein of 777 amino acids, and among its major functional regions are an amino-terminal transcription regulatory domain (amino acids 1–420), a middle DNA binding domain (DBD, amino acids 420–480), and a carboxyl-terminal steroid binding domain (SBD, 480–777). Within each of these are more specific sequences identified with specific functions. Nuclear localization signals are found in the DBD and SBD. Transcription regulation domains are found in both the N-terminal and SBDs. Three especially important subregions for transcription activation are tau 1, tau 2, and TAF, diagrammed as to approximate location in Figure 3. Other sites, such as those for specific protein/protein interactions, have also been mapped. The steroid binding domain contains regions important for binding of heat shock protein (hsp) 90, with which the glucocorticoid receptor complexes in its inactivated, high-affinity ligand binding form. Also bound to the GR are hsp 70 and several other protein factors (see ref. 21 for more details). The exact sites for these interactions have not been determined. When expressed in a recombinant cloning system, the DNA binding domain of the receptor is known to assume a specific tertiary structure which causes it to bind cooperatively with high affinity to the GRE_{PAL} (85). The DNA binding domain of the GR is structured such that two zinc atoms, each coordinately bound by four invariant cysteines, stabilize the three-

Table 1 Properties of CEM Cell Clones

Clone	Receptor				Glucocorticoid				Source
					Induction			Deinduction	
	Apoptosis	sites/cell	alleles[a]	expressed	GR[c]	GS[d]	c-*jun*	c-*myc*	
CEM-C7 "GR$^+$LY$^+$"[e]	Yes	~10,000	gr$^+$/gr^{mut}	GR$^+$/GR^{mut}	Yes	Yes	Yes	Yes	Cloned from CEM line without selection
ICR-27 "GR$^-$LY$^-$"[e]	No	≤1,000	gr$^-$/gr^{mut}	–[b]/GR^{mut}	No	No	No	No	Selected from mutagenized CEM-7 by dexamethasone
CEM-C1 "GR$^+$LY$^-$"[e]	No	~10,000	gr$^+$/gr^{mut}	GR$^+$/GR^{mut}	?	Yes	Yes	No	Cloned from CEM line without selection

[a]The GR point mutation in all three clones was leu753phe due to a single base change.
[b]Deletion.
[c]GR, glucocorticoid receptor.
[d]GS, glutamine synthetase.
[e]GR$^+$, functional GR; GR$^-$, nonfunctional GR; LY$^+$, cells lyse when exposed to glucocorticoid; LY$^-$, do not lyse.
Source: For original data, see refs. 78–82, 90, 91, and 95.

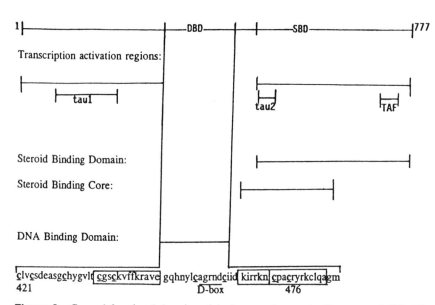

Figure 3   General functional domains of the human glucocorticoid receptor (hGR). The horizontal lines represent the primary amino acid sequence of the hGR, amino acids 1–777. *Approximate* locations of several major functional domains are shown. Lower line: amino acid sequence of the DNA Binding Domain (DBD). Cysteines that coordinate binding of two Zn atoms are underlined. These stabilize the helical structures shown in boxes. The DBD homodimerization contact region (D box) is also indicated by underlining. (For detailed reviews, see refs. 21 and 85.)

dimensional features of the molecule necessary for its interactions with the GRE. These in turn facilitate homodimerization of the peptide. Detailed knowledge of the forces and structures determining homodimerization of the holoGR at GREs is still lacking.

The importance of glucocorticoid-evoked apoptosis in biology and therapeutics mandated a study of the functional domains of the GR for apoptosis. For gene induction, the major tau 1 transactivation domain and the DNA binding domain had been shown to be essential. Removal of the steroid binding domain produced a receptor weakly constitutive for induction. However, deletion of tau 1 allowed the GR to still behave as a negative regulatory factor. We made use of the GR mutants created to study transcriptional regulation to examine apoptosis in our cell system. Conditions were determined that allowed electroporation and highly efficient transfection of the CEM cells with little loss of cell viability (86). This allowed demonstration that transfection of a plasmid expressing holoGR into the receptor-deficient, glucocorticoid-resistant ICR-27 cell line restored the lytic response to glucocorticoids. A chimeric receptor in which only the DNA binding domain was that of the GR, whereas the remainder of the molecule was an estrogen receptor, switched steroid sensitivity from glucocorticoids to estrogens (86). These data immediately suggested that the key region for induced cell death was the DNA binding domain of the GR. Subsequent detailed transfection experiments with a variety of mutants have repeatedly confirmed this fact (87–89). Deletion of the tau 1 region or almost all of the amino-terminal from the GR preserves glucocorticoid-induced cell death in the transfected cells. Deletion of the steroid binding domain on the other hand created a constitutively active receptor with potency as great as that of the holoreceptor. Even double deletions of both the amino- and carboxyl-terminals left a molecule that was highly potent in evoking the lytic response but no longer dependent on steroids. One particularly interesting mutant created a frame shift in the second "zinc finger" of the DNA binding domain. After isoleucine 465, the frame-shift alters the coding sequence so that the normal amino acids should be replaced by 21 amino acids unrelated to the GR normal sequence. This removes the two C-terminal cysteines, responsible for coordinate binding of zinc in the second zinc finger of the DNA binding domain, as well as the entire hinge region and steroid binding domain. We have overexpressed this mutant in the baculovirus system and find that it produces a shortened GR, which is consistent with the predicted size. Nevertheless, when expressed in transfected ICR-27 cells, this molecule too is lethal. It has been shown that it is the first zinc finger of the GR that is responsible for the primary specific recognition of the GRE, whereas the second finger is responsible for ancillary binding activity to phosphates in the DNA backbone as well as homodimerization. However, it was not known whether the mutant 465* was capable of binding a GRE. Using the truncated GR ("p465*") expressed from this mutant gene in the baculovirus system, we demonstrated by gel shift experiment that p465* can interact specifically with the glucocorticoid response element, albeit more weakly than GR. How is it that these molecules containing no steroid binding region and in some cases virtually only a DNA binding domain can be lethal? It is the focus of our research to find the detailed answer to that question, but several general concepts are clear. The strong lethal potency of the constitutive fragments, which contrasts so strikingly with their poor potency as transcription activators, suggests that activation of genes is not the key mechanism by which they kill these cells, unless there is very low level activation of some lethal gene whose product needs only to cross a minimal threshold in order to induce cell death. More likely, the small lethal fragments of the GR may be interfering with transcription machinery by meshing incorrectly with other transcription factors, causing a set of responses leading to cell death.

V. Gene Regulation by Glucocorticoids in Cloned CEM Cells: Downregulation of c-*myc* Appears to Be a Critical Step in Apoptosis

When glucocorticoids are given to CEM-C7 cells, a number of biochemical events take place, some beginning shortly after administration of the steroid, others appearing only after a considerable lapse of time. The early events include the onset of the induction of the GR itself, c-*jun* and glutamine synthetase, along with the onset of cell shrinkage and an abrupt reduction in c-*myc* mRNA and protein. The reduction of *myc* reaches a minimum by 12–24 hr (90,91). Beginning around 24 hr, one sees the start of accumulation of cells in G_0/G_1, and apoptosis follows over the next 1–2 days. As apoptosis begins, there is loss of key general macromolecular functions: breakdown of polysomes, reduction in thymidine kinase and in rRNA synthesis, and the appearance of low levels of lysed DNA of both small and large sizes. As we examined various clones of CEM cells for the striking downregulation of c-*myc*, one important fact stood out. In CEM-C1 cells (the clone which is resistant to apoptosis by steroids but which contains functional GR), c-*myc* was not downregulated (90). This was to offer a clue that *myc* regulation might be more than just a marker for the effect of a functional GR, and that downregulation of *myc* might have something to do with the lytic process. We hypothesized that negative *myc* regulation is an essential early step for apoptosis in CEM cells. Several tests of this hypothesis have been carried out. First, we transiently transfected into glucocorticoid sensitive clone CEM-C7 cells, plasmids containing genes that expressed c-*myc* under control of promoters that would not be downregulated by glucocorticoids. Three different constructs produced the same result. When c-*myc* levels were sustained, glucocorticoid-evoked apoptosis was significantly inhibited. Alternatively, the hypothesis would suggest that if *myc* were downregulated by an agent other than glucocorticoids, cell death should ensue as if glucocorticoids had been given. We carried out this test by the use of antisense oligonucleotides to c-*myc*. An oligonucleotide to the translation initiation site on the *myc* gene transcript abruptly downregulated c-*myc* levels, and this was followed by cell death a day or two later. Irrelevant oligonucleotides had no such effect (91). A third prediction of the hypothesis was that if cells could be rescued from the antiglucocorticoid effect, they should show a restoration of c-*myc* activity as a early event in the rescue. We carried out this test of the theory by use of the antiglucocorticoid RU38486. This glucocorticoid antagonist binds the GR with an affinity higher than that of dexamethasone, the standard synthetic glucocorticoid agonist used in our studies. Unlike dexamethasone, when bound to the receptor, RU486 cannot initiate the functional acts required to make the receptor alter gene expression. When RU486 was added together with glucocorticoids, it prevented cell death completely. RU486 alone had no

Table 2 Regulation of c-*myc* and Apoptosis in CEM-C7 Cells

Dex
↓

| | 6 | 12 | 24 | 48 | 72 | hr |

. . . . . . *myc* Reduced. . . . . Apoptosis→

Treatment	Interval (hr) 12–24	36–72
Dex	*myc* Reaches minimum	Apoptosis
Antisense c-*myc*	*myc* Reaches minimum	Apoptosis
RU38486	No change in *myc*	No apoptosis
Dex at t = 0 +RU at t = 0,6,12	*myc* Reduction blocked or rapidly reversed	Apoptosis blocked or stopped
Dex + c-*myc* expression vector	*myc* Reduction diminished	Apoptosis diminished

Source: From original data in refs. 87–89.

effect on cell growth and viability. Adding RU486 at various times after the addition of dexamethasone caused abrupt restoration of c-*myc* levels and either blocked completely the apoptotic process or at later times, such as 36 hr after dexamethasone, rescued the remaining viable cells (92). Outlined in Table 2, these results support our hypothesis. It seems that downregulation of c-*myc* by glucocorticoids in CEM cells is a critical early step in the apoptotic process. The downregulation of c-*myc* in CEM cells has been confirmed by independent groups (93,94), one of which also showed by blocking protein synthesis, that to kill the cells further protein synthesis is required beyond *myc* downregulation (93), which is consistent with our hypothesis as stated elsewhere (88). The c-*myc* protein is itself a transcription factor; therefore, we propose that a process occurs in which glucocorticoids remove from the pool of transcription factors a critical subset and that the removal leads to a sequence of transcription factor and gene expression events culminating in cell death.

Discussion

DR. BRATTSAND: Have the ribonucleases decomposing the mRNAs for IL-1β, IL-6, and GM-CSF been identified? Are there one or several species? If there were one ribonuclease species with a specificity for a group of central cytokines and growth factors, that might be a key anti-inflammatory mechanism of steroids.

DR. THOMPSON: While the process of their discovery is going on, no one can know how many RNases there eventually will be, so I really do not know the answer to your first question. A variety of substrate-specific RNases have certainly been described. Schoenberg's recent paper on an 80S ribosome-associated RNase induced by glucocorticoids in *Xenopus* with specific mRNAs suggests that there may be function-specific uses of RNases, and maybe such will be found in apoptosis (Pastori RL, Schoenberg DR. The nuclease that selectively degrades albumin mRNA in vitro associates with *Xenopus* liver polysomes through the 80S ribosome complex. Arch Biochem Biophys 1993; 305:313–319).

DR. BUSSE: (1) You indicated that there are different biochemical criteria for apoptosis. Would you comment on the association between the various biochemical markers for apoptosis and altered cell function? For example, is there a difference between DNA laddering and altered c-*myc* expression if one looks at one particular cell function? (2) When a cell undergoes apoptosis, does it contribute to tissue injury? For example, if an eosinophil undergoes apoptosis, is there still some tissue inflammation as its granular mediators are released?

DR. THOMPSON: (1) No. (2) I do not know specifically. Others may wish to comment. I could postulate that inactivation of the inflammatory substances occurs because tissue transglutaminase is activated, resulting in chemotactic factor inactivation by being crosslinked into apopotic bodies.

DR. GAULDIE: Since the normal mode of response to an apoptotic cell is engulfment by phagocytic (macrophage) cells without evidence of inflammation, this differs from necrosis, which is associated with inflammation. This suggests that lysis is not a normal mechanism for eosinophil killing by steroids.

DR. THOMPSON: Apoptosis is usually noninflammatory. The apoptotic bodies are engulfed by macrophages, or in some tissues by surrounding parenchymal cells (Kerr JFP, AH Wyllie, Currie AR. Apoptosis: a basic biological phenomenon with wide-ranging implications in tissue kinetics. Br J Cancer 1972; 26:239–257).

DR. GLEICH: Just a comment regarding the direct effect of glucocorticoids on the eosinophil and the question of whether glucocorticoids cause eosinophil lysis. Our laboratory has incubated eosinophils with glucocorticoids on numerous occasions and we have not shown any reduction in the numbers of viable eosinophils at 24 hr. On the contrary, we have found striking effects on the interaction between eosinophils and growth factors, such as IL-3, IL-5, and GM-CSF. Therefore, we believe that the effect of glucocorticoids is on the interaction between eosinophils and growth factors.

DR. HERSCHMAN: (1) Can the minimal construct of the GR that (i) binds DNA and (ii) induces apoptosis serve as a dominant negative in functional assays?

DR. THOMPSON: (1) The DBD does bind GREs specifically; in fact, that is how its structure was determined—as cocrystals with a GRE PAL. Our "minimal" DBD fragment that is lethal has reduced affinity compared with holo GR for a GRE PAL, but both have similar affinities for a composite AP-1,1/2 GRE site (by DNA gel-shift assay). We are investigating in detail the affinity and sequence specificity of binding of the "minimal" lethal DBD, but our data are not complete. I also strongly suspect that protein:protein interactions will be involved in its mechanism of action. (2) If by dominant negative you mean does it block the normal action of the holo GR, apparently not. For instance, addition of the 465 fragment as recombinant protein does not block holo GR stimulation of GRE-specific transcription in a cell-free system.

DR. BRATTSAND: What is the relationship between receptor occupancy and effect of GC?

DR THOMPSON: Gradations of GR concentration and/or of GR occupancy by glucocorticoid may differentially regulate various genes. As to GR concentration, as it varies in a specific cell type, so may response—though there can be large differences in GR between cell types, with some cells containing high GR levels being unresponsive. Experimentally, Yamamoto's laboratory varied GR levels over a fewfold by transfecting cells in tissue culture. There was increased sensitivity to dexamethasone causing enzyme induction, as GR content increased (Vanderbilt JN, Miesfeld R, Maler BA, Yamamoto KR. Intracellular receptor concentration limits glucocorticoid-dependent enhancer activity. Mol Endocrinol 1987; 1:68–74). It has also been noted that there is a regulatory region DNA sequence, unrelated to GREs or sites for common transcription factors, that, in conjunction with GRE-driven transcription, increases the sensitivity of the controlled gene to glucocorticoids (Oshima H, Simons SS. Jr. Modulation of transcription factor activity by a distant steroid modulatory element. Mol Endocrinol 1992; 6:416–428; Szapary D, Oshima H, Simons SS Jr. A new *cis*-acting element involved in tissue-selective glucocorticoid inducibility of tyrosine aminotransferase gene expression. Mol Endocrinol 1993; 7:941–952). For many genes under GR-GRE control, extent of induction corresponds to extent of occupancy of GR by ligand. When this additional sequence is in the regulatory domain, gene sensitivity to GR increases, so that full induction occurs well before saturation of GR by ligand. If such sequences are found in other genes, we can expect differential control at various glucocorticoid concentrations. Further, all the GR-transcription factor interactions becoming known surely will reveal varying degrees of regulation at various concentrations of steroid, due to differing protein:protein:DNA affinities and strength of regulation.

Dr. Brattsand: How rapidly can GRE be reused after it is vacated by glucocorticoid and GR? The nuclear form of the GR is hyperphosphorylated and must associate with hsp90. All these can affect the reutilization of the GR.

Dr. Thompson: GR is a relatively long-lived protein, with a $t_{1/2}$ of about 8–24 hr, as determined by various laboratories and in various cells. So probably the presence of ligand is limiting for GR function in most cases. There is a logical interpretation of several experiments suggesting that the GR cycles from cytoplasm to nucleus and back, and that it must be reprocessed somehow after reentering the cytoplasm before it can rebind ligand. It has been suggested by Alan Munck that alterations in GR phosphorylation level are required for proper cycling. Data from Pratt and Toft also suggest that hsp90 must bind GR to form a proper high-affinity site for glucocorticoid. Reformation of the hsp90 and GR complex therefore could also limit the content of active GR-steroid (Orti E, Mendel DB, Smith LI, Munck A. Agonist-dependent phosphorylation and nuclear dephosphorylation of glucocorticoid receptors. J Biol Chem 1989; 264:9724–9731; Orti E, Bodwell JE, Munck A. Phosphorylation of steroid hormone receptors. Endocr Rev 1992; 13:105–128).

Dr. Barnes: Is there any evidence that changes in hsp90 expression may alter GC responsiveness?

Dr. Thompson: Generally, cells contain a lot of hsp90; therefore, it does not seem to be limiting, unless of course there is a subtly specialized form of hsp90 responsible for binding GR. I am unaware of any evidence for such.

Dr. Herschman: Do you know of any precedent where glucocorticoids inhibit the production of an induced protein, but do not block mRNA accumulation?

Dr. Thompson: There are a few well-documented instances of estrogens causing allosteric changes in enzymes. Samuels showed that when GR binds glucocorticoid, its half-life is markedly reduced (McIntyre WR, Samuels HH. Triamcinolone acetonide regulates glucocorticoid-receptor levels by decreasing the half-life of the activated nuclear-receptor form. J Biol Chem 1985; 260:418–427). In their 1992 review, Pilkis and Granner refer to multiple levels of control by glucocorticoids (Pilkis SJ, Granner DK. Molecular physiology of the regulation of hepatic gluconeogenesis and glycolysis. Annu Rev Physiol 1992; 54:885–909).

References

1. Kerr JFR, Wyllie AH, Currie AR. Apoptosis: a basic biological phenomenon with wide-ranging implications in tissue kinetics. Br J Cancer 1972; 26:239–257.

2. Kerr JFR. Shrinkage necrosis: a distinct mode of cellular death. J Pathol 1971; 105:13–20.
3. Cohen JJ, Duke RC, Fadok VA, Sellins, KS. Apoptosis and programmed cell death in immunity. Ann Rev Immunol 1992; 10:267–293.
4. Raff MC. Cell death genes: drosophila enters the field. Science 1994; 264:558–669.
5. Bowen ID. Apoptosis or programmed cell death? Cell Biol Int 1993; 17:365–380.
6. Schwartz LM, Osborne, BA. Ced-3/ICE: evolutionarily conserved regulation of cell death. Bioessays 1994; 16:387–389.
7. Stewart BW. Mechanisms of apoptosis: integration of genetic, biochemical, and cellular indicators. J Natl Cancer Inst 1994; 86:1286–1296.
8. Truss M, Chalepakis G, Slater EP, Mader S, Beato M. Functional interaction of hybrid response elements with wild-type and mutant steroid hormone receptors. Mol Cell Biol 1991; 11:3247–3258.
9. Tsai SY, Srinivasan G, Allan GF, Thompson EB, O'Malley BW, Tsai M-J. Recombinant human glucocorticoid receptor induces transcription of hormone response genes in vitro. J Biol Chem 1990; 265:17055–17061.
10. Allan GF, Ing HN, Tsai SY, Srinivasan G, Weigel NL, Thompson EB, Tsai M-J, O'Malley BW. Synergism between steroid response and promoter elements during cell-free transcription. J Biol Chem 1991; 266:5905–5910.
11. Hager GL, Archer TK. The interaction of steroid receptors with chromatin. In: Nuclear Hormone Receptors. New York: Academic Press, 1991;217–234.
12. Truss M, Bartsch J, Hache RS, Beato M. Chromatin structure modulates transcription factor binding to the mouse mammary tumor virus (MMTV) promoter. J Steroid Biochem Mol Biol 1993; 47:1–10.
13. Konig H, Ponta H, Rahmsdorf HJ, Herrlich P. Interference between pathway-specific transcription factors: glucocorticoids antagonize phorbol ester-induced AP-1 activity without altering AP-1 site occupation in vivo. EMBO J 1992; 11:2241–2246.
14. Lucas PC, Granner DK. Hormone response domains in gene transcription. Annu Rev Biochem 1992; 61:1131–1173.
15. Thompson EB. Apoptosis and steroid hormones. Mol Endocrinol 1994; 8:665–673.
16. Thulasi R, Thompson EB. The role of glucocorticoids in cell growth, differentiation and programmed cell death. In: Khan S, Stancel GM, eds. Protooncogenes and Growth Factors in Steroid Hormone Induced Growth and Differentiation. Boca Raton, FL, CRC Press, 1993:221–240.
17. Beato M. Gene regulation by steroid hormones. Cell 1989; 56:335–344.
18. Schule R, Evans RM. Functional antagonism between oncoprotein c-jun and steroid hormone receptors. In: Antagonism Between c-jun and Steroid Hormone Receptors. Cold Spring Harbor, NY: Cold Spring Harbor Laboratory Press, 1991:119–127.
19. Tsai M-J, O'Malley BW. Molecular mechanisms of action of steroid/thyroid receptor superfamily members. Annu Rev Biochem 1994; 63:451–486.
20. Miner JN, Diamond MI, Yamamoto KR. Joints in the regulatory lattice: Composite regulation by steroid receptor-AP1 complexes. Cell Growth Diff 1991; 2:525–530.

21. Simons SS Jr. Function/activity of specific amino acids in glucocorticoid receptors. In: Vitamins and Hormones. New York: Academic Press, 1994:49:49-130.
22. Truss M, Beato M. Steroid hormone receptors: interaction with deoxyribonucleic acid and transcription factors. Endocr Rev 1993; 14:459-479.
23. Thompson EB, Granner DJ, Tomkins GM. Superinduction of tyrosine aminotransferase by actinomycin D in rat hepatoma (HTC) cells. J Mol Biol 1970; 54:159-175.
24. Schmid E, Schmid W, Jantzen M, Mayer D, Jastorff B. Transcription activation of the tyrosine aminotransferase gene by glucocorticoids and cAMP in primary hepatocytes. J Biochem 1987; 165:499-506.
25. Thompson EB, Gadson P, Wasner G, Simons SS Jr. Differential regulation of tyrosine amino-transferase by glucocorticoids: transcriptional and post-transcriptional control. In: Roy AK, Clark, JH, eds. Gene Regulation by Steroid Hormones IV. Rochester, NY: Springer-Verlag, 1988:63-77.
26. Hurme M. Siljander P, Anttila H. Regulation of interleukin-1β production by glucocorticoids in human monocytes: the mechanism of action depends on the activation signal. Biochem Biophys Res Commun 1991; 180:1383-1389.
27. Amano Y, Lee SW, Allison AC. Inhibition by glucocorticoids of the formation of interleukin-1α, interleukin-1β, and interleukin-6: mediation by decreased mRNA stability. Mol Pharm 1993; 43:176-182.
28. Peppel K, Vinci JM, Baglioni C. The AU-rich sequences in the 3′ untranslated region mediate the increased turnover of interfereon mRNA induced by glucocorticoids. J Exp Med 1991; 173:349-355.
29. Eisenstein RS, Rosen JM. Both cell substratum regulation and hormonal regulation of milk protein gene expression are exerted primarily at the posttranscriptional level. Mol Cell Biol 1988; 3183-3190.
30. Rossini GP, Masci G. Stabilization of glucocorticoid-receptor interactions in vitro by removal of RNA bound to receptor complexes in vivo. Life Sci 1990; 47:743-751.
31. Webb ML, Litwack G. Association of RNA with the glucocorticoid receptor and possible role in activation. In: Biochemical Actions of Hormones. New York: Academic Press, 1986; 13:379-402.
32. Dodson, RE, Shapiro DJ. An estrogen-inducible protein binds specifically to a sequence in the 3′ untranslated region of estrogen-stabilized vitellogenin mRNA. Mol Cell Biol 1994; 14:3130-3138.
33. Pastori RL, Schoenberg DR. The nuclease that selectively degrades albumin mRNA in vitro associates with xenopus liver polysomes through the 80S ribosome complex. Arch Biochem Biophys 1993; 305:313-319.
34. Kita H, Abu-Ghazaleh, R, Sanderson CJ, Gleich GJ. Effect of steroids on immunoglobulin-induced eosinophil degranulation. J Allergy Clin Immun 1991;87:70-77.
35. Kaiser J, Bickel CA, Bochner BS, Schleimer RP. The effects of the potent glucocorticoid budesonide on adhesion of eosinophils to human vascular endothelial cells and on endothelial expression of adhesion molecules. J Pharmacol Exp Ther 1993; 267:245-246.

36. Her E, Frazer J, Austen KF, Owen WF Jr. Eosinophil hematopoietins antagonize the programmed cell death of eosinophils. J Clin Invest 1991; 88:1982–1987.

37. Peterson AP, Altman LC, Hill JS, Gosney K, Kadin ME. Glucocorticoid receptors in normal human eosinophils: comparison with neutrophils. J Allergy Clin Immunol 1981; 68:212–217.

38. Wallen N, Kita H, Weiler D, Gleich GJ. Glucocorticoids inhibit cytokine-mediated eosinophil survival. Immunology 1991; 147:3490–3495.

39. Hallsworth MP, Litchfield TM, Lee TH. Glucocorticoids inhibit granulocyte-macrophage colony-stimulating factor-1 and interleukin-5 enhanced in vitro survival of human eosinophils. Immunology 1992; 75:382–385.

40. Lamas, AM, Leon OG, Schleimer RP. Glucocorticoids inhibit eosinophil responses to granulocyte-macrophage colony-stimulating factor. Immunology 1991; 147:254–259.

41. Schleimer RP. Effects of glucocorticosteroids on inflammatory cells relevant to their therapeutic applications in asthma. Am Rev Respir Dis 1990; 141:S59–S69.

42. Hartnell A, Kay AB, Wardlaw AJ. Interleukin-3–induced up-regulation of CR3 expression on human eosinophils is inhibited by dexamethasone. Immunology 1992; 77:488–493.

43. Tomioka, K, MacGlashan, DW, Jr, Lichtenstein, LM, Bochner, BS, Schleimer, RP. GM-CSF regulates human eosinophil responses to F-Met peptide and platelet activating factor. Immunology 1993; 151:4989–4997.

44. Ray A, Prefontaine KE. Physical association and functional antagonism between the p65 subunit of transcription factor NF-kB and the glucocorticoid receptor. Proc Natl Acad Sci USA 1994; 91:752–756.

45. Kunicka JE, Talle MA, Denhardt GH, Brown M, Prince LA, Goldstein G. Immunosuppression by glucocorticoids: inhibition of production of multiple lymphokines by in vivo administration of dexamethasone. Cell Immun 1993; 149(1):39–49.

46. Byron KA, Varigos G, Wootton A. Hydrocortisone inhibition of human interleukin-4. Immunology 1992; 77:624–626.

47. Rolfe FG, Hughes JM, Armour CL, Sewell WA. Inhibition of interleukin-5 gene expression by dexamethasone. Immunology 1992; 77:494–499.

48. Fernandez-Ruiz E, Rebollo A, Nieto MA, Sanz E, Somoza C, Ramirez F, Lopez-Rivas A, Silva A. IL-2 protects T cell hybrids from the cytolytic effect of glucocorticoids. Synergistic effect of IL-2 and dexamethasone in the induction of high-affinity IL-2 receptors. Immunology 1989; 143:4146–4151.

49. Northrop JP, Crabtree GR, Mattila PS. Negative regulation of interleukin 2 transcription by the glucocorticoid receptor. J Exp Med 1992; 175:1235–1245.

50. Vacca A, Felli MP, Farina AR, Martinotti S, Maroder M, Screpanti I, Meco D, Petrangeli E, Frati L, Gulino A. Glucocorticoid receptor-mediated suppression of the interleukin 2 gene expression through impairment of the cooperativity between nuclear factor of activated T cells and AP-1 enhancer elements. J Exp Med 1992; 175:637–646.

51. Almawi WY, Lipman ML, Stevens AC, Zanker B, Hadro ET, Strom TB. Abrogation of glucocorticoid-mediated inhibition of T cell proliferation by the synergistic action of IL-1, IL-6, and IFN-gamma. Immunology 1991; 146:3523–3527.

52. Neito MA, Lopez-Rivas A. Glucocorticoids activate a suicide program in mature T lymphocytes: protective action of interleukin-2. Ann NY Acad Sci 1992; 650:115–120.

53. Surh CD, Sprent J. T-cell apoptosis detected in situ during positive and negative selection in the thymus. Nature 1994; 372:100–103.

54. Haczku A, Alexander A, Brown P, Assoufi B, Li B, Kay AB, Corrigan C. The effect of dexamethasone, cyclosporine, and rapamycin on T-lymphocyte proliferation in vitro: comparison of cells from patients with glucocorticoid-sensitive and glucocorticoid-resistant chronic asthma. J Allergy Clin Immun 1994; 93:510–519.

55. Kam JC, Szefler SJ, Surs W, Sher ER, Leung DY. Combination IL-2 and IL-4 reduces glucocorticoid receptor-binding affinity and T cell response to glucocorticoids. Immunology 1993; 151:3460–3466.

56. Zubiaga AM, Munoz E, Huber BT. IL-4 and IL-2 selectively rescue Th cell subsets from glucocorticoid-induced apoptosis. Immunology 1992; 194:107–112.

57. Ramirez F, McKnight AJ, Silva A, Mason D. Glucocorticoids induce the expression of CD8 alpha chains on concanavalin A-activated rat CD4+ T cells: induction is inhibited by rat recombinant interleukin 4. J Exp Med 1992; 176:1551–1559.

58. Danel-Moore L, Kawa S, Kalmaz GD, Bessman D, Thompson EB. Induction of CD8 antigen and suppressor activity by glucocorticoids in a CEM human leukemic cell clone. Leuk Res 1993; 17:501–506.

59. Huang RW, Tsuda H, Takatsuki K. Interleukin-2 prevents programmed cell death in chronic lymphocytic leukemia cells. Int J Hematol 1993; 58:83–92.

60. Gomi M, Moriwaki J, Katagiri S, Kurata Y, Thompson EB. Glucocorticoid effects on myeloma cells in culture: correlation of growth inhibition with induction of glucocorticoid receptor mRNA. Cancer Res 1990; 50:1873–1878.

61. Johnson BH, Gomi M, Jakowlew SB, Moriwaki K, Thompson EB. Actions and interactions of glucocorticoids and transforming growth factor β on two related human myeloma cell lines. Cell Growth Diff 1993; 4:25–30.

62. Linden M, Brattsand R. Effects of a corticosteroid, budesonide, on alveolar macrophage and blood monocyte secretion of cytokines: differential sensitivity of GM-CSF, IL-1 beta, and IL-6. Pulm Pharmacol 1994; 7:43–47.

63. Linden M. The effects of beta 2-adrenoreceptor agonists and a corticosteroid, budesonide, on the secretion of inflammatory mediators from monocytes. Br J Pharmacol 1992; 107:156–160.

64. Geiger T, Arnold J, Rordorf C, Henn R, Vosbeck K. Interferon-gamma overcomes the glucocorticoid-mediated and the interleukin-4-mediated inhibition of interleukin-1 beta synthesis in human monocytes. Lymphokine Cytokine Res 1993; 12:271–278.

65. Yamaguchi M, Hirai K, Nakajima K, Ohtoshi T, Takaishi T, Ohta K, Morita Y, Ito K. Dexamethasone inhibits basophil migration. Allergy 1994; 49:371–375.

66. Charlesworth EN, Kagey-Sobotka A, Schleimer RP, Norman PS, Lichtenstein LM. Prednisone inhibits the appearance of inflammatory mediators and the influx of eosinophils and basophils associated with the cutaneous late-phase response to allergen. Immunology 1991; 146:671–676.

67. Marone G, Stellato C, Renda A, Genovese A. Anti-inflammatory effects of gluco-

corticoids and cyclosporin A on human basophils. Eur J Clin Pharmacol 1993; 45(Suppl 1):17–20.

68. Schleimer RP, Derse CP, Friedman B, Gillis S, Plaut M, Lichtenstein LM, MacGlashan DW Jr. Regulation of human basophil mediator release by cytokines. I. Interaction with antiinflammatory steroids. Immunology 1989; 143:1310–1317.

69. Cohan VL, Undem BJ, Fox CC, Adkinson NF Jr, Lichtenstein LM, Schleimer RP. Dexmethasone does not inhibit the release of mediators from human mast cells residing in airway, intestine, or skin. Am Rev Respir Dis 1989; 140:951–954.

70. Soda K, Kawabori S, Kanai N, Bienenstock J, Perdue MH. Steroid-induced depletion of mucosal mast cells and eosinophils in intestine of athymic nude rats. Int Arch Allergy Immunol 1993; 101:39–46.

71. Tchekneva E, Serafin WE. Kirsten sarcoma virus-immortalized mast cell lines. Reversible inhibition of growth by dexamethasone and evidence for the presence of an autocrine growth factor. Immunology 1994; 152:5912–5921.

72. Shieh JH, Peterson RH, Moore MA. Cytokines and dexamethasone modulation of IL-1 receptors on human neutrophils in vitro. Immunology 1993; 150:3515–3524.

73. Re F, Muzio M, DeRossi M, Polentarutti N, Giri JG, Mantovani A, Colotta F. The type II "receptor" as a decoy target for interleukin 1 in polymorphonuclear leukocytes: characterization of induction by dexamethasone and ligand binding properties of the released decoy receptor. J Exp Med 1994; 179:739–743.

74. Lane SJ, Wilkinson JR, Cochrane GM, Lee TH, Arm JP. Differential in vitro regulation by glucocorticoids of monocyte-derived cytokine generation in glucocorticoid-resistant bronchial asthma. Am Rev Respir Dis 1993; 147:690–696.

75. Wertheim WA, Kunkel SL. Standiford TJ, Burdick MD, Becker FS, Wilke CA, Gilbert AR, Strieter RM. Regulation of neutrophil-derived IL-8: the role of prostaglandin E2, dexamethasone, and IL-4. Immunology 1993; 151:2166–2175.

76. Johnson BH, Dean RR, Moran SM, Thompson EB. Glucocorticoid, interleukin-2 and prostaglandin interactions in a clonal human leukemic T-cell line. J Steroid Biochem Mol Biol 1992; 42:1–9.

77. Chilton DG, Johnson BH, Danel-Moore L, Kawa S, Kunapuli S, Thompson EB. Increased glucocorticoid responsiveness of CD4+ T-cell clonal lines grown in serum-free media. In Vitro Cell Dev Biol 1990; 26:561–570.

78. Zawydiwski R, Harmon JM, Thompson EB. Glucocorticoid-resistant human acute lymphoblastic leukemia cell line with functional receptor. Cancer Res 1983; 43:3865–3873.

79. Yuh YS, Thompson EB. Complementation between glucocorticoid receptor and lymphocytolysis in somatic cell hybrids of two glucocorticoid resistant human leukemic clonal cell lines. Somat Cell Mol Genet 1987; 13:33–34.

80. Harmon JM, Thompson EB. Isolation and characterization of dexamethasone-resistant mutants from human lymphoid cell line CEM-C7. Mol Cell Biol 1981; 1:512–521.

81. Ashraf J, Thompson EB. Identification of the activation-labile gene: a single point mutation in the human glucocorticoid receptor presents as two distinct receptor phenotypes. Mol Endocrinol 1993; 7:631–642.

82. Powers JH, Hillmann AG, Tang DC, Harmon JM. Cloning and expression of

mutant glucocorticoid receptors from glucocorticoid-sensitive and -resistant human leukemic cells. Cancer Res 1993; 53:4059–4065.

83. Saeed MF, Kawa S, Thompson EB. Synergistic interaction of the glucocorticoid and the PKA pathways in human lymphoblasts. Poster presentation at the 77th Annual Meeting of The Endocrine Society, Washington, DC, June 1995, Abstract #P2-426.

84. Dieken ES, Meese EU, Miesfeld RL. Anti glucocorticoid receptor transcripts lack sequences encoding the amino-terminal transcriptional modulatory domain. Mol Cell Biol 1990; 10:4574–4581.

85. Freedman LP. Anatomy of the steroid receptor zinc finger region. Endocr Rev 1992; 13:129–145.

86. Harbour DV, Chambon P, Thompson EB. Steroid mediated lysis of lymphoblasts requires the DNA binding region of the steroid hormone receptor. J Steroid Biochem 1990; 35:1–9.

87. Nazareth LV, Harbour DV, Thompson EB. Mapping the human glucocorticoid receptor for leukemic cell death. J Biol Chem 1991; 266:12976–12980.

88. Thompson EB, Nazareth LV, Thulasi R, Ashraf J, Harbour D, Johnson BH. Glucocorticoids in malignant lymphoid cells: gene regulation and the minimum receptor fragment for lysis. J Steroid Biochem Mol Biol 1992; 41:273–282.

89. Nazareth LV, Thompson EB. Leukemic cell apoptosis caused by constitutively active mutant glucocorticoid receptor fragments. Recent Prog Horm Res 1995; 50:417–421.

90. Yuh YS, Thompson EB. Glucocorticoid effect on oncogene/growth gene expression in human T-lymphoblastic leukemic cell line CCRF-CEM: specific c-myc mRNA suppression by dexamethasone. J Biol Chem 1989; 264:10904–10910.

91. Thulasi R, Harbour DV, Thompson EB. Suppression of c-myc is a critical step in glucocorticoid-induced human leukemic cell lysis. J Biol Chem 1993; 268:18306–18312.

92. Thompson EB, Thulasi R, Saeed MF, Johnson BH. Glucocorticoid antagonist RU486 reverses agonist-induced apoptosis and c-myc repression in human leukemic CEM-C7 cells. NY Acad Sci 1995; 761:261–275.

93. Wood AC, Waters CM, Garner A, Hickman JA. Changes in c-myc expression and the kinetics of dexamethasone-induced programmed cell death (apoptosis) in human lymphoid leukaemia cells. Br J Cancer 1994; 69:663–669.

94. Helmberg A, Auphan N, Caelles C, Karin M. Glucocorticoid-induced apoptosis of human leukemic cells is caused by the repressive function of the glucocorticoid receptor. EMBO J 1995; 14:452–460.

95. Harmon JM, Elsasser MS, Eisen LP, Urda LA, Ashraf J, Thompson EB. Glucocorticoid receptor expression in "receptorless" mutants isolated from the human leukemic cell line CEM-C7. Mol Endocrinol 1989; 3:734–743.

5

Lymphocyte Activation
The Interplay and Synergy of Immunosuppressants

ISABELLA GRAEF, NEIL CLIPSTONE, STEFFAN N. HO, LUIKA A. TIMMERMAN, JEFFREY NORTHROP, and GERALD R. CRABTREE
Stanford University School of Medicine
Stanford, California

I. Contingent Genetic Regulatory Events During T-Lymphocyte Activation

Presentation of antigen in the form of a MHC/peptide complex to T cells or the binding of soluble antigen to B cells initiates a sequence of events that activate these cells for immunological function. The term *activation* is a misnomer, since the sequence of events induced in T cells is more reminiscent of a developmental sequence or differentiation than a reversible activation. In all, well over 200 genes are activated or inactivated in T cells (Fig. 1), and studies in transgenic mice indicate that a considerable portion of the genome might be made transcriptionally active as T lymphocytes go from a resting dormant state to an immunologically active state. Although Figure 1 emphasizes the immunologically functional genes, a large number of genes are probably activated to handle the increased demand for protein synthesis, more rapid rates of metabolism, and the initiation of the cell cycle that requires that nearly all proteins be doubled prior to cell division.

The net effect of the process of T-cell activation is partly to coordinate the actions of many cells that do not express antigen receptors yet must respond

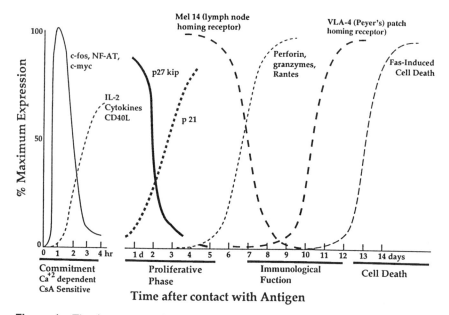

Figure 1 The time course of activation-induced changes in the expression of a number of illustrative gene products. The times indicated at the bottom are the time after activation of total peripheral blood T lymphocytes with a polyclonal activator and are probably correct for a specific antigen but most of the data are collected from examples obtained with human peripheral T cells activated with lectins. The lines indicate the level of the gene product for each of the indicated events and the dotted lines are used only for discrimination of the different time courses.

to specific antigen. This immune regulatory function is exerted through the secretion of cytokines and expression of cell surface molecules that mediate direct intercellular contact with other cell types. The spectrum of lymphokines secreted and thus the type of immune response initiated depends largely on the particular subset of T cells activated. Thus, cytokines like interleukin-3 (IL-3) and granulocyte macrophage colony-stimulating factor (GM-CSF) are involved in controlling the actions of macrophages and granulocytes, which do not themselves have antigen receptors. γ-Interferon, the exclusive product of activated T cells, induces high-affinity Fc-receptor and increased class II MHC expression on macrophages making them more effective agents in the fight against invading pathogens. The molecules that provide B-cell help are produced almost exclusively by activated T cells and are not present on resting T cells. These include IL-2, IL-4, IL-5, IL-6 and transforming growth factor β (TGFβ) as well as the CD40 ligand.

Signal transduction events leading to acquisition of differentiated function are not the result of a single wave of gene activation events but rather of a cascade of sequential gene activation events. The timing of events during activation very likely has a critical function in coordinating the actions of other cells. For example, certain molecules like the chemokine RANTES are produced late in the process of T-cell activation after entry into S phase and the completion of cell division (1). Whether RANTES has a stringent requirement for the completion of S phase is not known, and indeed whether a "completion mechanism" operates negatively on any of these late genes, similar to the requirement that S phase be complete before mitotic gene activation, is not known. The late action of RANTES and other chemokines may reflect a local requirement for chemotaxis late in the activation process after cells have lost their homing receptors and migrated to nonlymphoid tissues where an immune response is underway.

An interesting aspect of T-cell activation that mimics many developmental events is a change of homing receptors during the process. Naive postthymic T cells express a lymph node homing receptor, Mel 14 (LECAM-1), that directs their attachment to the high endothelial venules (HEV) of lymph nodes (LN) and enables them to pass between endothelial cells and gain entry to the paracortical regions of LNs. About 3 days after activation, which would commonly occur in a lymph node, they lose Mel 14 by a process that has not been elucidated (2). The loss of Mel 14 seems to coincide with the end of mitotic division, but the mechanism is unknown, other than that it depends on initial stimulation some 3 days early by antigen or pharmacological activators. Presumably this process would be blocked by drugs such as cyclosporin A and FK506 as well as glucocorticoids, infra vitam. The disappearance of Mel 14 is accompanied by the appearance of several very late activation antigens that seem to allow attachment of the lymphocyte to capillaries and small blood vessels at the site of inflammation. This sequential exchange of homing receptors may be critical to the final outcome of the battle against an infectious agent and represents a clear point of connection between the inflammatory side of the immune response; that is, the induction of stickiness in certain blood vessels by the products of an inflammatory reaction and the specific immune response by lymphocytes to foreign antigen. The coordinated loss and gain of cell surface molecules that direct localized attachment may serve as a convenient paradigm of similar developmental events such as neural crest migration.

The final act of T-lymphocyte activation appears to involve "suicide" leading to the physiological death of mature activated T cells to terminate an immune reaction. Mutations in either the fas ligand, as in *gld* mice, or in the tumor necrosis factor (TNF) receptor family molecule fas (CD95) itself, as in *lpr* mice, lead to a syndrome characterized by the accumulation of large numbers of CD4⁻CD8⁻, TCR⁺, B220⁺T lymphocytes, which appear to be deficient in activation-induced T-cell death (3). This accumulation seems to reflect a deficiency in activation-induced T-cell death at the end of an immune response, thereby implicating fas in the elimination of these cells. Fas is upregulated within 24 hr of T-cell receptor (TCR) stimulation, but the cells become sensitive to deletion via fas only several days later. Interestingly, both fas and bcl-2 are induced during the immune response suggesting that bcl-2 might be used to control and prevent cell death early in the process of T-cell activation before the cell has had as chance to carry out its normal functions. Here again, the sequential induction of genes initially set in motion by the antigen receptor leads to the sequential use of bcl-2 and fas to protect cells during the useful part of their life and to eliminate them later (4,5). Expression of fas is inhibited by cyclosporin A.

II. Signal Transduction and Transcriptional Pathways Initiating T-Lymphocyte Activation

The length of time that T lymphocytes must interact with antigen before becoming committed to the final response was initially defined from studies in which T lymphocytes were exposed to cultures of cells capable of presenting antigen derived from tumor cells and later the interaction terminated with a monoclonal antibody to the tumor antigen (6). These studies defined a period of about 1–2 hr for commitment to the process of T-cell activation. This period corresponds roughly to the time required for the induction of many of the early cytokines, about 40 min for IL-2 and 30–90 min for most of the others. Not surprisingly, most of the known immunosuppressants work within this time period. During the past 5 years, a detailed description of many molecules essential for the signal transduction pathways and early transcriptional events have emerged (see, e.g., reviews 7 and 8). Since the available immunosuppressants all function by inhibiting steps distal to the T-cell receptor, the costimulatory requirements, and the initial *src*-like tyrosine kinases, we will concentrate on the signaling and transcriptional mechanisms that are targets of the immunosuppressants; that is, those that occur long after the initial surface signaling mechanisms.

III. Calcineurin and *ras* as Essential Signaling Intermediates in T-Cell Activation

From the standpoint of understanding immunosuppressant action, one only needs to consider that antigen receptor signaling results in the activation of *ras* and the elevation of intracellular calcium concentrations, $[Ca^{2+}]_i$, since the critical steps affected by CsA, FK506, and glucocorticoids lie distal to these events. Although future efforts may find specific inhibitors of the *src*-like tyrosine kinases, *fyn* and *lck*, to date such molecules have not been detected despite extensive screening over the past 20–25 years for drugs that block the mixed lymphocyte reaction. Perhaps the *src*-like tyrosine kinase does not have enough specificity to serve as effective targets of immunosuppressant action. Signal transduction through the T-cell receptor induces an elevation of intracellular calcium and activation of *ras*. These intracellular second messengers then give rise to distinct, but connected, signaling pathways that culminate in the activation of a group of transcription factors such as NF-AT, Oct/Oap, Ap-1, and NF-κB (9,10). The net effect of this signaling pathway is to activate the cytokines, growth factors, and cell surface proteins that coordinate the immune response.

IV. The *ras*–AP-1 Pathway

T-cell receptor signaling activates *ras* by mechanisms that are as yet incompletely understood. The present evidence supports a cascade of signaling events that are initiated by oligomeriztion of antigen receptors due to binding of MHC bound antigen, with apparent activation of the *scr*-like tyrosine kinases *lck* and perhaps *fyn* as well as the *Syk* family tyrosine kinase ZAP-70 (see ref. 7 for review). PLCγ-1 becomes activated via tyrosine phosphorylation to yield the second messengers inositol 1,4,5-trisphosphate (IP3) and diacylglycerol (DAG). DAG regulates members of the PKC family of Ca^{2+}/phospholipid–dependent serine threonine kinases. PKC contributes to the activation of the *ras* pathway by phosphorylation of *ras*GAP (11). The means by which the early events of T-cell signal transduction activate *ras* via the PKC-independent pathway are debated, but three mechanisms have been proposed and are variously supported by current evidence. The phosphorylation of the *vav* rac/rho–like exchange factor suggests that it might have a role as a *ras* exchange factor (12). Second, the linker protein Shc has been suggested to directly couple T-cell receptor signaling to the *Sos ras* exchange protein via membrane recruitment of the *Grb-2/Sos* complex (13). Finally, a 36-tyrosine phosphorylated protein has been found to coprecipitate with *Sos*, *Grb-2*, and perhaps PLCγ in T cells, but apparently not in other cell types (14,15). The later findings are particularly enticing, since they suggest a cell type–specific coupling mechanism to *ras*.

The activation of *ras* is probably a site where the signaling pathways converge to a single necessary and sufficient step, which although subject to feedback controls through PKC is sufficient for activating several transcription factors such as AP-1. The mechanisms controlling *ras* have been extensively reviewed (16). Activation of *ras* appears to lead to several events in T cells, including (1) recruitment of c-*raf* to the cell membrane; (2) the activation of

PI3 kinase; (3) the activation of p70S6 kinase; (4) the activation of *jun* N-terminal kinase, JNK; and (5) the activation of the MAP kinase cascade. The sequence of signaling events that lead to the activation of the transcription factor AP-1 (see Chapter) involve either one or both kinase cascades activated by the MAP kinase family members. The well-studied MAP-kinase cascade initiated by *raf-ras* interactions leads from *ras* to *raf* to MAP kinase-kinase to MAP kinase to the serum response factor, which is essential for the activation of the c-*fos* gene. Alternatively, but not exclusively, ras activation can lead to the phosphorylation and activation of jun N-terminal kinase, JNK, through unknown intermediates. JNK phosphorylates and induces the transcriptional activity of the *jun* transcription protein. These two *ras*-induced events, that is, induction of *fos* protein and activation of the preexisting *jun* protein, lead to the assembly of the AP-1 transcription factor. At this point, glucocorticoids come to bear in the signal transduction and transcriptional control pathway (see below).

The background to understanding the site of action of cyclosporine and FK506 requires an explanation of the Ca^{2+} signaling pathway in T cells. The activation of PLCγ by mechanisms that involve the T-cell receptor and the tyrosine kinases results in the production of IP3 and DAG by the breakdown of the membrane phospholipid phosphatidylinositol 4,5-bisphosphate. The IP3 generated then interacts with the IP-3 receptor resulting in the leakage of Ca^{2+} out of intracellular compartments (17). At this point, the mechanisms that generate a sufficient raise in Ca^{2+} from basal levels of about 100 nM to a level greater than 1 μM to propagate the signaling pathway become unclear. Either Ca^{2+} leakage leads to the sensing of the loss and the induction of a rapid influx of Ca^{2+} from the external media by unknown mechanisms that most likely involve the intracellular CAML protein or Ca^{2+} released from internal stores is sufficient for activation (18). Most workers in this field favor the former hypothesis. Regardless of the mechanism by which $[CA^{2+}]_i$ is elevated, the next step in the signaling pathway seems very clear. The sustained rise in intracellular Ca^{2+} activates the calcium/calmodulin–dependent serine/threonine phosphatase calcineurin. Calcineurin is a three-component phosphatase made up of an A chain, which is the catalytic subunit, the B chain, which is a Ca^{2+} binding regulatory subunit, and finally the calmodulin protein, which is a Ca^{2+} binding regulatory subunit (19). The levels of intracellular Ca^{2+} achieved after T-cell activation are sufficient for activation of calcineurin (20). At this point, the pathway again becomes unclear. Calcineurin's best documented substrate is the phosphatase inhibitor, inhibitor I or DARP32 (21). Dephosphorylation of this protein leads to the activation of protein phosphatase 1, which is a broadly acting serine-threonine phosphatase.

The consequence of calcineurin activation is the nuclear translocation of the cytosolic components of NF-AT, NF-ATc, and NF-ATp (22,23). Although the simplest mechanism suggests that this occurs by dephosphorylation of NF-

AT by either calcineurin or protein phosphatase 1, this has not yet been documented and more convoluted explanation might apply, such as the dephosphorylation of an inhibitor such as a specialized IκB.

Once NF-AT has translocated to the nucleus, it combines with a nuclear component, NF-ATn, that can be replaced by *fos* or by *jun*; however, the identity of this subunit has never been elucidated. The nuclear subunit can be isolated from any tissue if the cells have been stimulated with PMA or activated *ras* (23). Production of the nuclear subunit requires both protein synthesis and RNA synthesis and hence must represent the activation of a new gene. AP-1 will replace this component both in transfection assays and in in vitro transcription. Additional studies will be required to determine their identity.

V. Mechanism of Action of the Major Immunosuppressants

The past 5 years have provided definitive identification of the sites of action of both the glucocorticoid and FK506/CsA classes of immunosuppressants. As noted by Karin and Saatcioglu, in Chapter 2, glucocorticoids form complexes with *jun* transcription factors resulting in the inactivation of the AP-1 complex. In some cases this requires an active glucocorticoid response element (GRE), whereas in other cases, such an element does not seem to be necessary. In the IL-2 gene there is only a very weak GRE next to a AP-1 site that appears to be essential for the induction of the IL-2 gene in transfection studies. However, glucocorticoid inhibition of IL-2 gene expression depends entirely on this site (24). Removal of this site reduces IL-2 gene expression by about 80–90%, and glucocorticoids inhibit about 80% of IL-2 gene transcription suggesting that this site is perhaps the only one that is responsive to glucocorticoids. Transcription directed by the NF-AT, the NF-κB, and the Oct/OAP sites are not sensitive to inhibition by glucocorticoids (24). The results with the NF-AT site seem curious, since if AP-1 were a component of NF-AT, one would expect it to be inhibited as well. The fact that it is not suggests that either NF-ATn is not AP-1 or that the mechanism is more complex than simple direct inhibition of AP-1.

CsA and FK506 are chemically very different immunosuppressants that bind to unrelated prolyl isomerases, cyclophilin and FKBP, forming inhibitory complexes that block the phosphatase activity of calcineurin, which is an essential component of the T-cell activation pathway (25–27). Neither drug nor receptor alone associate with or block calcineurin. The net effect of this block is a complete inhibition of the translocation of NF-ATc from the cytoplasm to the nucleus and hence a lack of T-cell activation and cytokine gene transcription. However, there are also other targets for calcineurin that are likely to play a a role in this process. For example, the transcriptional activity of NF-κB is inhibited by about twofold and certain AP-1 sites are inhibited by three- to fourfold (28). These effects are quite small compared with the several hundred- or thousandfold inhibition of properly initiated transcription at the NF-AT site.

Rapamycin has a structural similarity with FK506 but does not block cytokine transcription at the early stages of T-cell activation. Rapamycin inhibits proliferation of T cells in response to growth-promoting cytokines like IL-2 at the G_1 to S-phase progression via blocking the IL-2–mediated elimination of the cyclin-dependent kinase inhibitor p27^{Kip1} (29).

VI. Interplay and Possible Synergy Between Immunosuppressants

Glucocorticoids and CsA are often used together for suppression of transplant rejection and their independent mechanism of action supports this combined use. This is perhaps best illustrated for the control of the IL-2 gene. Here suppression by glucocorticoids and CsA maps to different sites with little or no crossover. As mentioned above, suppression of IL-2 promoter/enhancer function by CsA is related to the two NF-AT sites and the Oct/OAP site, with no detectable CsA inhibition at other sites. In contrast, inhibition by glucocorticoids requires the AP-1 site and the isolated AP-1 site is sufficient for inhibition by glucocorticoids (24). Thus, one would expect that each drug would make an independent contribution to the suppression of the promoter and thus IL-2 gene expression, hence mitigating drug toxicity while achieving a potent immunosupressive effect. These results suggest that these drugs might be used at reduced levels in certain treatments that allow independent modes of administration as will elaborated on in Chapter 25 by Barnes.

Discussion

Dr. Barnes: Cyclosporin A has inhibitory effects on mast cells and eosinophils. Presumably mechanisms other than activation of NF-AT are involved here?

Dr. Crabtree: It seems that both the toxicity and the therapeutic effects of CsA and FK506 are due to inhibition of calcineurin. This was shown using a panel of chemical analogues that bind to calcineurin to varying degrees. A perfect correlation was seen between the neutralization of calcineurin and renal toxicity. Thus, it is likely that the inhibitory effects on mast cells are mediated by calcineurin but the mechanism is not clear.

Dr. Leung: (1) What is the mechanism for loss of response to cyclosporin 1 hr after lymphocyte activation? (2) What is the mechanism for loss of response to glucocorticoids?

DR. CRABTREE: The localized time of sensitivity to CsA or dexamethasone appears to be related to the time during T-cell activation that calcineurin and AP-1 are used to activate transcription.

DR. LANE: Overexpression of calcineurin in cells can make them glucocorticoid-resistant. Is there any interaction between calcineurin and the glucocorticoid receptor? Is calcineurin found in other cells besides T cells (humans)? Are there increased levels of calcineurin in other diseases?

DR. CRABTREE: As far as we know, calcineurin is expressed in all tissues of all species from yeast to human. The sensitivity appears to be related to the low levels of calcineurin in T lymphocytes, meaning that cyclosporin will block the activation pathway at lower levels in T cells than other cells. We have not looked for an interaction between the glucocorticoid receptor and calcineurin.

DR. THOMPSON: Is there an INF-ATc analogous to IκB? Have you detected proteins involved in nuclear translocation?

DR. CRABTREE: We have done contransfection studies with the presently known IκBs and NF-ATc and find that none of them can oppose NF-AT-dependent transcription. Thus far, we do not know of any protein that interacts with NF-ATc other than AP-1, and even this occurs only at high concentrations.

DR. O'BYRNE: Why does it take so long for some of the delayed effects of T-cell activation, such as the production of RANTES, to occur?

DR. CRABTREE: RANTES expression and the expression of many genes that directly mediate the effects of T cells in the immune response (as opposed to those genes that coordinate the actions of other cells) such as granzyme are produced late, probably to carry out effects that are required late in the immune response. RANTES may be activated by a transcription factor induced by an early event.

DR. SEVERINSON: (1) What is the role of NF-AT in the regulation of other cytokine genes such as GM-CSF, IL-3, and IL-4? (2) NF-AT-like sequences have been identified in these cytokine genes, but there are conflicting results in the literature as to which factors bind to these NF-AT like sequences. NF-ATc, NF-ATp, ETs family members, and AP-1 family members have been identified. Could you please comment on this? (3) Are NF-AT cloned from human and murine sources functionally the same?

DR. CRABTREE: NF-ATc is necessary for production of a variety of cytokines, including IL-3, GM-CSF, IL-4, TNFα, and probably the CD40 ligand. However, it is difficult to know what precise NF-ATc family member is involved. The clones for murine and human NF-ATc family members are nearly identical, about 90% for human/murine NF-ATc. Furthermore, from transfection studies we find no difference.

DR. MIESFELD: Have you looked at Ca^{2+}-responsive elements? Possibly NF-AT binding sites?

DR. CRABTREE: We have looked at a limited number of other Ca^{2+}-responsive DNA elements and find that only some are responsive to NF-AT. Thus we think that NF-ATc family members are responsible for some of the Ca^{2+}-dependent gene activation responses but not all.

References

1. Schall TJ, Bacon K, Toy KJ, Goeddel DV. Selective attraction of monocytes and T lymphocytes of the memory phenotype by cytokine RANTES. Nature 1990; 347:669–671.
2. Jung TM, Gallatin WM, Weissman IL, Dailey MO. Down-regulation of homing receptors after T cell activation. J Immunol 1988; 141:4110–4117.
3. Watanabe-Fukunaga R, Brannan CI, Copeland NG, Jenkins NA, Nagata S. Lymphoproliferation disorder in mice explained by defects in Fas antigen that mediates apoptosis. Nature 1992; 356:314–317.
4. Itoh N, Tsujimoto Y, Nagata S. Effect of bcl-2 in Fas antigen-mediated cell death. J Immunol 1993; 151:621–627.
5. Ogasawara J, Watanabe-Fukunaga R, Adachi M, et al. Lethal effect of the anti-Fas antibody in mice. Nature 1993; 364:806–809.
6. Lowenthal JW, Tougne C, MacDonald R, Smith KA, Nabholz M. Antigen stimulation regulates the expression of IL-2 receptors in a cytolytic T lymphocyte clone. J Immunol 1985; 134:931–939.
7. Weiss A, Littman DR. Signal transduction by lymphocyte antigen receptors. Cell 1994; 76:263–274.
8. Crabtree GR, Clipstone NA. Signal transmission between the plasma membrane and nucleus of T lymphocytes. Annu Rev Biochem 1994; 63:1045–1083.
9. Durand DB, Bush MR, Morgan JG, Weiss A, Crabtree GR. A 275 bp fragment at the 5' end of the IL-2 gene enhances expression from a heterologous promoter in response to signals from the T cell antigen receptor. J Exp Med 1987; 165:395–407.
10. Shaw J-P, Utz PJ, Durand DB, Toole JJ, Emmel EA, Crabtree GR. Identification of a putative regulator of early T cell activation genes. Science 1988; 241:202–205.
11. Downward J, Graves JD, Warne PH, Rayter S, Cantrell DA. Stimulation of p21^{ras} upon T-cell activation. Nature 1990; 346:719–723.
12. Gulbins E, Coggeshall KM, Baier G, Katzav S, Burn P, Altman A. Tyrosine kinase-stimulated guanine nucleotide exchange activity of Vav in T cell activation. Science 1993; 260:822–825.
13. Ravichandran KS, Lee KK, Songyang Z, Cantley LC, Burn P, Burakoff SJ. Interaction of Shc with the ζ chain of the T cell receptor upon T cell activation. Science 1993; 262:902–905.
14. Sieh M, Batzer A, Schlessinger J, Weiss A. GRB2 and phospholipase C-gamma 1

associate with a 36- to 38-kilodalton phosphotyrosine protein after T-cell receptor stimulation. Mol Cell Biol 1994; 14:4435–4442.

15. Buday L, Egan SE, Rodriguez Viciana P, Cantrell DA, Downward J. A complex of Grb2 adaptor protein, Sos exchange factor, and a 36-kDa membrane-bound tyrosine phosphoprotein is implicated in ras activation in T cells. J Biol Chem 1994; 269:9019–9023.

16. McCormick F. How receptors turn Ras on. Nature 1993; 363:15–16.

17. Clapham DE. Calcium Signaling. Cell 1995; 80:259–268.

18. Bram RJ, Crabtree GR. Calcium signalling in T cells stimulated by a cyclophilin B-binding protein. Nature 1994; 371:355–358.

19. Hubbard MJ, Klee CB,. Functional domain structure of calcineurin A: Mapping by limited proteolysis. Biochemistry 1989; 28:1868–1874.

20. Fruman DA, Klee CB, Bierer BE, Burakoff SJ. Calcineurin phosphatase activity in T lymphocytes is inhibited by FK 506 and cyclosporin A. Proc Natl Acad Sci USA 1992; 89:3686–3690.

21. Cohen P. The structure and regulation of protein phosphatases. Annu Rev Biochem 1989; 58:453–508.

22. Clipstone NA, Crabtree GR. Identification of calcineurin as a key signalling enzyme in T cell activation. Nature 1992; 357:695–697.

23. Flanagan WF, Corthesy B, Bram RJ, Crabtree GR. Nuclear association of a T-cell transcription factor blocked by FK-506 and cyclosporin A. Nature 1991; 352:803–807.

24. Northrop JP, Crabtree GR, Mattila PS. Negative regulation of interleukin-2 transcription by glucocorticoid receptors. J Exp Med 1992; 175:1235–1245.

25. Liu J, Farmer JD, Lane WS, Friedman J, Weissman I, Schreiber SL. Calcineurin is a common target of cyclophilin-cyclosporin A and FKBP-FK506 complexes. Cell 1991; 66:807–815.

26. O'Keefe SJ, Tamura J, Kincaid RL, Tocci MJ, O'Neill EA. FK506 and CsA-sensitive activation of the interleukin-2 promoter by calcineurin. Nature 1992; 357:692–695.

27. Yang D, Rosen MK, Schreiber SL. A composite FKBP12-FK506 surface that contacts calcineurin. J Am Cancer Soc 1993; 115:819–820.

28. Emmel EA, Verweij CL, Durand DB, Higgins KM, Lacy E, Crabtree GR. Cyclosporin A specifically inhibits function of nuclear proteins involved in T cell activation. Science 1989; 246:1617–1620.

29. Nourse J, Firpo E, Flanagan WM, et al. Rapamycin prevents interleukin 2-mediated elimination of the cyclin-dependent kinase inhibitor, p27Kip1. Nature 1994;

Part Two

EFFECTS ON AIRWAY MUCOSA AND SUBMUCOSA

6

Airway Ultrastructure in Asthma

LAURI A. LAITINEN

University Central Hospital
Helsinki, Finland

ANNIKA LAITINEN

University of Helsinki
Helsinki, Finland

I. Introduction

Bronchial asthma has been identified as an inflammatory disease of the airways associated with epithelial cell injury and deposition of fibrous material in the subepithelial basement membrane (1–6) (Fig. 1.). It is not known if damage in the airway epithelium occurs prior to the inflammatory reaction or as a result of the action of released mediators from different types of inflammatory cells and mast cells (Fig. 2.). (2,5,7). The epithelium may have important functions in regulating the inflammatory processes (8). The interactions between the epithelial cytoskeleton and its transmembrane receptors with the epithelial basement membrane and stroma may play an important role in the pathogenesis of asthma.

II. Structural Epithelial Changes in Asthma

According to present understanding, reduced cell adhesion can lead to mechanical instability and apoptosis—programmed cell death. Epithelial cells maintain

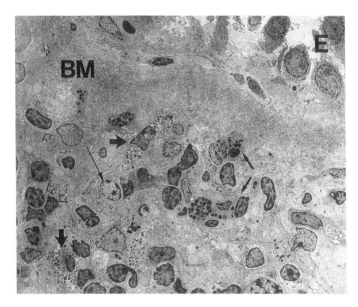

Figure 1 Transmission electron micrograph showing destroyed epithelium and an intense inflammatory reaction in the airway mucosa of a newly diagnosed asthmatic patient. The basement membrane (BM) beneath the epithelium (E) is seen to have a thick structure. Several types of cells are seen in the lamina propria. Open arrows, lymphocytes; short thick arrows, mast cells; long thin arrow, plasma cell; short thin arrows, eosinophils. Magnification ×2000.

contact with their underlying stroma by different types of junctions and cell adhesion molecules (8). The glycoproteins of the integrin family of receptors are the best characterized cell adhesion molecules. Various types of integrin receptors with different α and β subunits have been found in human airway epithelial cells (8). The distribution of integrins that bind primarily to laminin and collagen has been studied by immunocytochemistry. Normal bronchial epithelium expresses α_2 and α_6 strongly and less α_1 and α_3. The α_6 subunit was seen mainly at the basal surface, whereas the other subunits have a more even distribution through the epithelium. Integrin subunit α_v was readily visible in the epithelium, most prominently in the basolateral regions of epithelial cells. However, staining with the β_3 antibody was not found suggesting that in the epithelium the α_v subunit is associated with an alternate β subunit such as β_1 or β_5 (9). Recently an α_9 subunit has been described to be highly expressed in normal adult airway epithelium (10). The heterodimer form $\alpha_9\beta_1$ receptor has glycoprotein tenascin (Tn) as its known ligand. However, the other Tn bind-

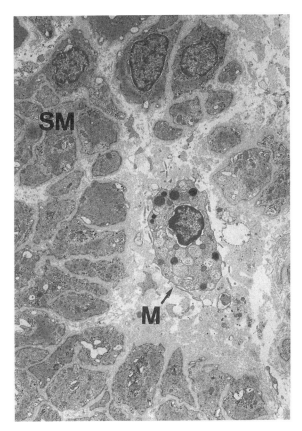

Figure 2 Micrograph showing airway smooth muscle (SM) in asthmatic airways. A highly degranulated mast cell (M) is seen between smooth muscle cells. Magnification ×7800.

ing integrin $\alpha_v\beta_6$ was not found in normal human airways (10). Shedding of the epithelial cells could be caused by weakened cellular attachment of adjacent columnar epithelial cells to each other or to the basal cells. A prominent feature described earlier, especially in severe asthma, was marked airway edema with shedding of airway columnar epithelial cells (11). So far, however, no changes at the cellular receptor site, which could explain shedding or fragility of the airway epithelium, have been reported in asthma.

In newly diagnosed asthmatics (7), a change in the structure of the epithelium from a predominantly ciliated epithelium to goblet cell hyperplasia (Fig. 3.) has been detected, possibly reflecting a reaction to irritation or a cell maturation defect (12).

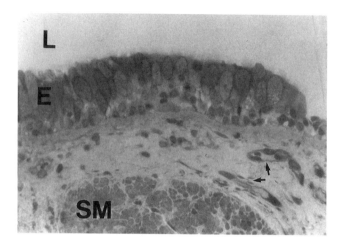

Figure 3 Micrograph of asthmatic airways showing goblet cell hyperplasia in the airway epithelium (E) at the light microscopical level. Arrows, blood vessels; SM, bronchial smooth muscle; L, lumen.

III. Extracellular Matrix and the Basement Membrane

The extracellular matrix (ECM) is composed of a mixture of macromolecules such as polysaccharide glycosaminoglycans, proteoglycans, and fibrous proteins of two functional types: structural (i.e., collagen and elastin) and adhesive (i.e., fibronectin and laminin). The glycosaminoglycan and proteoglycan molecules form a highly hydrated, gel-like "ground substance" in which the fibrous proteins are embedded.

The basement membrane is a thin layer of specialized extracellular matrix (13). Interactions of the bronchial epithelium with the extracellular matrix proteins are important during the development of the structural organization of the lung providing mechanical support and influencing cellular behavior (14). The cellular receptors mediate signals from the matrix to the cell, which in turn may alter the cell secretion. Many glycoproteins such as fibronectin and tenascin are involved during the development of airways. They are considered as transitional components of the basement membrane, because in adult lung, their expression is sparse or negative. Tenascin is reexpressed in the airway basement membrane in asthma (15), possibly reflecting increased turnover of the airway epithelium.

Thickening of epithelial basement membrane in asthma is partly due to increased expression of various collagens. This could be one reason for asthma to become more persistent. A thickened basement membrane has been described to be a characteristic of asthma (11,16,17).

IV. Effect of Treatment on Airway Structure in Asthma

After asthma has been revealed to be inflammatory disease in airways, there has been an increase in the use of anti-inflammatory drugs. Jeffery and co-workers (16) showed that treatment of atopic asthmatics with budesonide for 4 weeks reduced airway inflammation, but not even a longer treatment period could reduce the thickening of the basement membrane. Laitinen and co-workers (6) demonstrated that after 3 months of therapy with inhaled budesonide, the reduction of inflammatory cell numbers in the mucosa was associated with restoration of the normal epithelium.

Biopsy specimens taken during worsening of asthma are rare. In a case report, Laitinen et al. (18) showed that in addition to an intense infiltration of eosinophils in the mucosa during exacerbation of asthma, severe structural changes in the airway epithelium could be detected. The epithelium had lost both ciliated and goblet cells and it comprised only undifferentiated cells containing microvilli. When the patients' therapy consisting of a β_2-agonist was changed to an inhaled steroid, the lung function values rapidly improved. Biopsy specimens taken after 16 weeks of steroid therapy showed improvement in the epithelial structure. The epithelium consisted of predominantly ciliated cells and the inflammatory reaction had subsided. However, some changes could still be recognized in the epithelium such as intercellular edema and electron-dense cores in the mucous granules in goblet cells (Fig. 4.). Cells containing both cilia and mucus granules were seen (Fig. 5.). These types of cells are rarely described in the literature or seen in the human airway epithelium. They may reflect an intermediate stage of cellular differentiation in the airway epithelium.

In a recent study (15), the effect of inhaled budesonide treatment on airway subepithelial fibrosis in seasonal asthmatics was evaluated by immunohistochemistry. During 4 weeks of treatment with inhaled steroid, the glycoprotein tenascin content in the basement membrane area decreased in the inhaled steroid–treated group in comparison with the placebo group. No significant change in the thickness of the collagen band could be measured. This suggests that the inflammation, but not the fibrotic process, in the basement membrane is prevented by a short inhaled steroid treatment. Recently Trigg and co-workers (19) reported that 4 months of treatment with inhaled beclomethasone diprionate reduced both airway inflammation and subepithelial collagen III deposition in mildly asthmatic patients.

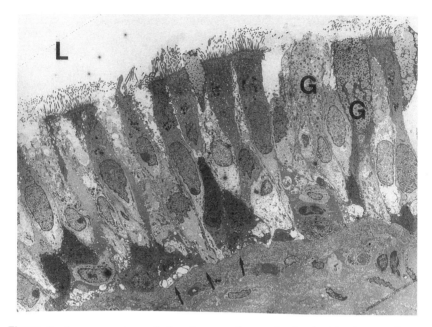

Figure 4 Low power transmission electron micrograph of asthmatic airways after 16 weeks of inhaled corticosteroid therapy. The epithelium has a predominance of ciliated cells. However, clear intercellular edema can still be seen and the mucous granules in the goblet cells (G) contain an electron-dense core. L, lumen; arrows, basement membrane. Magnification ×2000.

V. Conclusion

Biopsy studies performed at the electron microscopical level show severe structural changes in asthmatic airway epithelium, reflecting the importance of the epithelium which plays a dynamic role in asthma. The epithelium reacts to inhaled corticosteroid treatment. The epithelial damage and changes in its structural cell types may profoundly interact with the production of the extracellular matrix and the underlying basement membrane.

VI. Summary

At an early stage of the disease, the airways of asthmatics show morphological evidence of chronic inflammation. Both structural airway epithelial changes and the influx of inflammatory cells into the airway mucosa can be seen. Inhaled corticosteroid treatment has been shown to ameliorate allergic airway in-

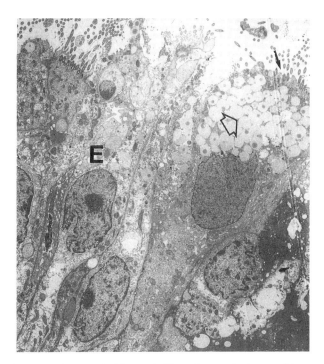

Figure 5 Same specimen as in Figure 4. The micrograph shows with greater magnification the airway epithelial (E) cells. On the right-hand side, there is one cell containing both atypical mucous granules (open arrow) and basal bodies and cilia (black arrow). Magnification ×5200.

flammation in asthma in several studies. At the electron microscopical level, normal epithelial structure, with ciliated epithelial cells outnumbering goblet cells, is restored during inhaled corticosteroid treatment. However, pathological changes which could cause asthma to become a more chronic disease have remained obscure. Recently many studies have been focused on the reversibility of collagen deposition in the airway epithelial basement membrane. Airway epithelial cell and stromal matrix interactions may be important to the chronicity of asthma and the development of permanent lung function abnormalities in asthma.

Acknowledgment

We acknowledge the financial support from the Finnish Lung and Health Association.

Discussion

DR. SMALDONE: (1) Were the biopsies from proximal or distal airways? (2) Because the cellular responses in chronic cough are similar in asthma, can some of the reported cellular observations in asthma be secondary to mechanical changes in the lung?

DR. LAITINEN: Our results are from biopsies taken from lobar bronchi: to first- and second-order segmental bronchi. We consider that mechanical factors are minor both in asthma and chronic cough.

DR. THOMPSON: The dose-response data of two proteoglycans to budesonide seems to show progressive effects from 10^{-9} to 10^{-5} M. Glucocorticoid receptors should be saturated at well below 10^{-5} M. It is difficult to interpret your results with respect to the GR theory of glucocorticoid action?

DR. HARGREAVE: What is the relationship between tenascin thickness and bronchial hyperreactivity.

DR. LAITINEN: We have done a study in Norwegian elite skiers of whom about half were hyperreactive to methacholine without asthma. Taking together these subjects and very hyperreactive asthmatics, we did not find a correlation between tenascin expression and bronchial hyperreactivity.

DR. DURHAM: You have shown a convincing reduction in the ratio of ciliated/ goblet cells in the bronchial epithelium in asthmatics and suggest this is due to an increase in goblet cells. Have you measured absolute goblet cell numbers? An alternative interpretation may be a reduction in ciliated cells as part of the epithelial disruption/damage in asthma.

DR. LAITINEN: The numbers correspond to absolute numbers of ciliated and goblet cells in biopsies where the epithelium is present.

DR. THOMPSON: What is tenascin? Do you know what cells produce it?

DR. LAITINEN: It is a glycoprotein discovered in the middle of the 1980s. It seems to be a crucial compound during the development of lung, but it should not be expressed in normal adult lung.

DR. LIU: Do allergic subjects with no asthma or airway hyperreactivity have inflammatory changes and airway eosinophils?

DR. LAITINEN: We are just studying the inflammatory cells, but we do not yet have the answer.

DR. LIU: Have you found inflammatory infiltrate in atopic patients with no sign of hyperreactivity?

DR. LAITINEN: We have not been able to study those patients.

DR. LEMANSKE: I would like to echo Mark Liu's comments by stating that the specificity of the histopathological changes in asthma need to be differentiated from those seen in other inflammatory lung disease characterized by cough, airway obstruction, etc., as well as those demonstrable in atopic individuals who do not have clinical asthma.

DR. HOWARTH: In response to Mark Liu's question regarding atopy and lower airway changes. We have previously found that in rhinitics who are atopic but have no lower airway symptoms and normal bronchial responsiveness, there is an increase in collagen deposition within the lamina reticularis and increased airway tissue eosinophil recruitment. These changes are less than those identified in clinical asthma but significantly greater than those identified in the normal airways. This may contribute to the difficulty in seeking relationships between duration of clinical asthma and bronchial hyperresponsiveness with collagen thickness, as subclinical changes are likely to precede the development of disease. I have a question for Dr. Laitinen relating to tenascin and epithelial disruption. The epithelial disruption appears to occur between the columnar ciliated epithelial cells and the basal epithelial cells. The basal epithelial cells remain firmly adhered to the true basement membrane (type IV collagen). As the tenascin is beneath the basement membrane, how do you perceive it induces a selective shedding/disruption of cell adhesion at this location?

DR. LAITINEN: Your assumption is correct. It is only our hypothesis. We do not know the mechanism yet.

DR. PERSSON: First, I would like to support the view that epithelial damage/repair processes initiated by mechanical trauma or otherwise may explain some of the features that are characteristic of the asthmatic airway mucosa, including plasma exudation and white cell traffic and activation. The other comment relates to the reduced frequency of epithelial nerves in asthma. Erjefalt et al. have demonstrated that epithelial peptidergic innervation (CGRP-positive nerves) appear in the new epithelium 15 hr after extensive denudation (Erjefalt JS, Erjefalt I, Sundler F, Persson CGA. In vivo restitution of airway epithelium. Cell Tissue Res, July 1995, in press). My question relates to the role of tenascin. Is it an important molecule in epithelial repair processes? I think particularly of the migration of flat poorly differentiated epithelial cells on a denuded basement membrane. (Erjefalt JS, Erjefalt I, Sundler F, Persson CGA. Microcirculation-derived factors in airway epithelial repair in vivo. Microvasc Res 1994; 148:161–178.)

DR. LAITINEN: Tenascin expression is located just under the basal lamina. Its effect on epithelial cell migration has not been studied.

DR. GAULDIE: Tenascin can be made by fibroblasts, and the location you have shown in the lamina reticularis suggests the fibroblast or myofibroblast is the cell responsible for synthesis in the asthmatics. It seems possible that the antiadhesion effects of tenascin could play a role in the desquamation of the epithelium from the basement membrane.

DR. BUSSE: Would you comment on the tissue distribution of fibronectin in the airway tissue of asthma?

DR. LAITINEN: We have studied fibronectin expression only in a small number of asthmatics. There is increased fibronectin expression in the areas of basement membrane where epithelium has been shed off.

DR. BARNES: Does the increase in collagen (types III, IV) correlate with severity or duration of asthma? There appears to be increased collagen deposition in the basement membrane of very mild asthmatics. That the extent of fibrosis is not greater in more severe asthma may reflect local antifibrotic mechanisms in the airway.

DR. LAITINEN: We have shown that in patients with more severe asthma there is increased expression of collagen types VII and IV in the airways basement membrane.

DR. BOCHNER: Despite the thickening within the basement membrane region of the airways and the increases seen in collagen and other matrix proteins, it is surprising that very few cells are actually seen within this region, since many infiltrating cells have β_1 integrin receptors for these matrix proteins and may be capable of tight adhesion to these molecules. Do you ever see accumulations of leukocytes in this region?

DR. LAITINEN: We see moving cells very seldom in the area of basement membrane. Whether these cells are binding by collagen receptors is impossible to know by electron microscopical method.

DR. GLEICH: Some persons have suggested that failure of a patient with asthma to achieve normal airflow after intensive treatment may be due to increased fibrosis in the basement membrane region. Do you have any impression whether this might be so? Do patients with persistent airway obstruction (after treatment with glucocorticoids) show greater degrees of airway fibrosis than normal glucocorticoid-responsive patients with asthma?

DR. LAITINEN: We have studied only expression of extracellular matrix proteins. When we compared that with pulmonary lung function of these patients, we did not find any correlation.

DR. LIU: Previous studies that have examined the relationship of clinical asthma severity, lung function, airway reactivity, or duration of disease to thickness at the basement membrane have not demonstrated a significant relationship.

Dr. Laitinen: We think that the reason for this lack of relationship is that methods for measuring the thickening of basement membrane are too crude. There are not clear borders for measuring the thickness of basement membrane, at stromal side in native specimens when antibodies that specifically stain a basement membrane-related component are not used.

Dr. O'Byrne: What is the relevance of the increase of smooth muscle cells as a marker?

Dr. Laitinen: Obstruction of airways is certainly caused more by an increase of smooth muscle than thickening of basement membrane.

References

1. Glynn AA, Michaels L. Bronchial biopsy in chronic bronchitis and asthma. Thorax 1960; 15:142-153.
2. Laitinen LA, Heino M, Laitinen A, Kava T, Haahtela T. Damage of the airway epithelium and bronchial reactivity in patients with asthma. Am Rev Respir Dis 1985; 131:599-606.
3. Beasley R, Roche WR, Roberts JA, Holgate ST. Cellular events in the bronchi in mild asthma and after bronchial provocation. Am Rev Respir Dis 1989; 139:806-817.
4. Jeffery PK, Wardlaw AJ, Nelson FC, Collins JV, Kay AB. Bronchial biopsies in asthma. An ultrastructural, quantitative study and correlation with hyperreactivity. Am Rev Respir Dis 1989; 140:1745-1753.
5. Bousquet J, Chanez P, Lacoste JY, Barneon G, Ghavanian N, Enander I, Venge P, Ahlstedt S, Simony-Lafontaine J, Godard P, Michel FB. Eisoniphilic inflammation in asthma. N Engl J Med 1990; 323:1033-1039.
6. Laitinen LA, Laitinen A, Haahtela T. A comparative study of the effects of an inhaled corticosteroid, budesonide, and a β_2-agonist, terbutaline, on airway inflammation in newly diagnosed asthma: a randomised double-blind, parrallel-group controlled trial. J Allergy Clin Immunol 1992; 90:32-42.
7. Laintinen LA, Laitinen A, Haahtela T. Airway mucosal inflammation even in patients with newly diagnosed asthma. Am Rev Respir Dis 1993; 147:697-704.
8. Albelda SM. Endothelial and epithelial cell adhesion molecules. Am J Respir Cell Mol Biol 1991; 4:195-203.
9. Damjanovich L, Albelda SM, Mette SA, Buck CA. Distribution of integrin cell adhesion receptors in normal and malignant lung tissue. Am J Cell Mol Biol 1992; 6:197-206.
10. Weinacker A, Ferrando R, Elliot M, Hogg J, Balmes J, Sheppard D. Distribution of integrins $\alpha v\beta 6$ and $\alpha 9\beta 1$ and their known ligands, fibronectin and tenascin, in human airways. Am J Respir Cell Mol Biol 1995; 12:547-557.
11. Dunnill MS, Massarella GR, Anderson JA. A comparison of the quantitative anatomy of the bronchi in normal subjects, in status asthmaticus, in chronic bronchitis, and in emphysema. Thorax 1969; 24:176-179.

12. Johnson NF, Hubbs AF. Epithelial progenitor cells in rat trachea. Am J Respir Cell Mol Biol 1990; 3:579–585.
13. Raghow R. The role of extracellular matrix in post inflammatory wound healing and fibrosis. FASEB J 1994; 8:823–831.
14. McGowan SE. Extracellular matrix and the regulation of lung development and repair. FASEB J 1992; 6:2895–2904.
15. Laitinen A, Altraja A, Linden M. Stållenheim G, Venge P, Håkansson L, Virtanen I, Laitinen LA. Treatment with inhaled budesonide and tenascin expression in bronchial mucosa of allergic asthmatics. Am J Crit Care Med 1994; 149:A942.
16. Jeffery PK, Godfrey RW, Ädelroth E, Nelson F, Rogers A, Johansson SÅ. Effects of treatment on airway inflammation and thickening of basement membrane reticular collagen in asthma. Am Rev Respir Dis 1992; 145:890–899.
17. Roche WR, Beasley R, Williams JH, Holgate ST. Subepithelial fibrosis in the bronchi of asthmatics. Lancet 1989; 1:520–524.
18. Laitinen LA, Laitinen A, Heino M, Haahtela T. Eosinophilic airway inflammation during exacerbation of asthma and its treatment with inhaled corticisteroid. Am rev Respir Dis 1991, 143:423–427.
19. Trigg CJ, Manolitsas ND, Wang J, Calderon MA, McAulay A, Jordan SE, Herdman MJ, Jhalli N, Duddle JM, Hamilton SA, Devalia JL, Davies RJ: Placebo-controlled immunopatholic study of four months of inhaled corticosteroids in asthma. Am J Respir Crit Care Med 1994; 150:17–22.

7

Sputum Indices of Inflammation in Asthma

FREDERICK E. HARGREAVE, EMILIO PIZZICHINI, MARCIA PIZZICHINI, ANN EFTHIMIADIS, and JERRY DOLOVICH

St. Joseph's Hospital
and McMaster University
Hamilton, Ontario, Canada

PAUL M. O'BYRNE

McMaster University
Hamilton, Ontario, Canada

I. Introduction

Lord Kelvin some time ago said, "When you can measure what you are speaking about, and express it in numbers, you know something about it; but when you cannot measure it, when you cannot express it in numbers, your knowledge is of a meagre and unsatisfactory kind. . . ."(1). Our knowledge of airway inflammation in asthma and other airway conditions is "meagre" and unsatisfactory because it has been investigated chiefly by invasive bronchoscopy, which is limited. The only noninvasive method to access directly airway inflammation is the examination of sputum. If this can be developed in a reliable way, it may be applied more widely to consecutive subjects, in severe as well as mild asthma, and repeatedly in the same person. This should greatly improve our understanding of the treatment, pathophysiology, and perhaps pathogenesis of these conditions. In this chapter, we will discuss sputum indices of airway inflammation in asthma and the effect of corticosteroid treatment on them. Initially, however, it is necessary to consider the methods of examination which are important for the accurate interpretation of results.

II. Methods of Examination of Sputum

A. Background

The introduction of reliable methods of sputum examination have been slow in coming. Over 100 years ago Gollasch (2) observed that eosinophils were increased in the sputum of asthmatics. This observation was used in the clinical evaluation of asthma in the 1950s to the 1970s (3–5). Cell counts were performed mainly on smears of sputum. During the 1970s and the 1980s there were sporadic measurements on the fluid phase of sputum histamine, leukotrienes, and eosinophil major basic protein (MBP) (6–10). In general, however, sputum examination was considered to be difficult and unreliable.

A resurgence of interest in sputum examination to measure indices of airway inflammation in research has occurred in the past 6 years. Cell counts in smears of sputum were found to be reproducible (11–13), responsive (14–15), and valid (11–13). The availability of sputum for examination can be increased by the inhalation of an aerosol of hypertonic saline (12,13,16). This was first introduced by Bickerman et al. (17) to induce sputum to diagnose lung cancer. In addition, the methods of processing sputum have improved from the examination of smears to the treatment of sputum with dithioethreitol or dithiothreitol (18,19) to disperse the cells, to study the cells on cytospins (16,20,21), or by flow cytometry (20,22) and to collect the cell supernatant for fluid phase measurements (16, 23–26). The methods are not difficult and give reproducible, responsive, and valid results. They are still evolving.

B. Sputum Induction

Two methods of inducing sputum by inhalation of an aerosol of hypertonic saline have been used. In one, the subject is premedicated with inhaled beta$_2$-agonist to inhibit any airway constriction caused by the hypertonic saline (12,16,27,28). An ultrasonic nebulizer is used to generate an aerosol of 3% hypertonic saline or 3% followed by 4% followed by 5%. The inhalations are given for 5- to 7-min periods, up to a total of about 20 min. In the other method, an aerosol of 4.5% hypertonic saline is generated by an ultrasonic nebulizer and inhaled for doubling times from 0.5 to 8 min, as in the method to measure airway responsiveness (13,29). In both methods, the mouth can be rinsed with water, the nose blown, and an FEV$_1$ performed before and after each inhalation to minimize contamination of the specimen by saliva and postnasal drip and to monitor the possibility of induced airway constriction, respectively. The inhalations are discontinued if the FEV$_1$ falls by 20% and an inhaled beta$_2$-agonist is given. After each inhalation, the subject is asked to try to cough sputum into a clear container.

In people who cannot produce sputum spontaneously, the induction of sputum is successful in 60–80% of procedures. There are a number of possible determinants of success which include various subject characteristics, technical factors concerned with the induction process, and aspects of the processing of the sputum (Table 1) (28). We have investigated the influence of the nebulizer, the concentration of saline, and the influence of pretreatment with a beta-agonist. Induction with an ultrasonic nebulizer is more successful than with a lower output jet nebulizer. Three percent saline or 3% followed by 4% followed by 5% is more successful than isotonic saline. Pretreatment does not influence the success of the procedure.

C. Sputum Processing and Examination

The method of examination of sputum that we use now is based on the evaluation by Popov et al. (21) and subsequent modification by Pizzichini et al. (30,31). The expectorated specimen is processed as soon as possible and within 2 hr. All portions of sputum that macroscopically appear to be free of salivary contamination are selected; occasionally, this is not possible macroscopically and selection is made with a phase contrast microscope to obtain a cellular sample with as small a number of squamous epithelial cells as possible. Dithiothreitol 10% (Sputolysin; Calbiochem Corp., San Diego, CA), diluted 1 to 10 with distilled water, is added. Dulbecco's phosphate-buffered saline (D-PBS) is added to stop the action of dithiothreitol. The mixture is then filtered, cell viability is measured by trypan blue, and a total cell count is obtained in a modified Neubauer hemocytometer. Cytospins can be made if only cells are to be examined. Alternatively, the cell suspension is spun at 790g and the supernatant collected and stored at -70°C for later fluid phase measurements. The cell pellet is resuspended in D-PBS and used either to prepare cytospins for differ-

Table 1 Possible Determinants of Success of Sputum Induction

Subject characteristics
   Cigarette smoking
   Healthy or disease
   Degree of inflammation
Induction
   Nebulizer output and particle size
   Saline concentration
   Duration of inhalation
   Beta-agonist pretreatment
   Details of encouragement
Processing of sputum
   Selection of sputum from saliva
   Effectiveness of dithiothreitol

ential cell counts (stained with Wright's), metachromatic cells (stained with toluidine blue), and immunocytochemistry or for flow cytometry. The quality of the cytospins is usually excellent (Fig. 1), the different cell types can be easily recognized, and 400 leucocytes can be counted in less than 5 min. Sometimes damaged cells and contamination by salivary squamous epithelial cells interfere with the counts. When the cell viability is <50% and/or squamous contamination is >20%, the accuracy of cell counts is less reproducible (32).

D. Evaluation of Sputum Examination

We have investigated the method of sputum assessment which involves selection of portions of induced sputum from saliva to see whether data are missed. We have compared the results of examination of the selected sample with the residual sample considered to be made up predominantly of saliva (Table 2) (30). Although the weight of the selected portion was only 6% of the whole sample, it contained the vast majority of viable nonsquamous cells. In addition, it only contained 1.2% salivary squamous cells, the viability of the nonsquamous cells was better, the quality of the slides were better, and the fluid phase eosinophil cationic protein (ECP) was five times higher. The median differential cell counts were similar. We conclude that the selection process employed

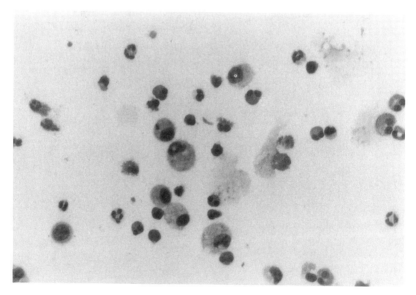

Figure 1 A cytospin of induced sputum showing eosinophils, neutrophils, macrophages, and debris.

Table 2 Differences Between a Selected Sample of Induced Sputum from the Residual Sample

	Wt (mg)	Total Cell Count (10^3/mg)	Squamous cells (%)	Viability (%)	Quality of slide (score)	ECP (μg/L)
Selected	437	5.9	1.2	86	7	768
Residual	6500	0.5	70	63	4	136

allowed examination of lower respiratory secretions only minimally contaminated with saliva and that data were not missed.

The repeatability of total and differential cell counts, various fluid-phase measurements, and lymphocytes in flow cytometry have been examined in stable subjects in specimens collected on 2 days within 7 days (Table 3, Fig. 2) (22,31). The repeatability was good as indicated by high intraclass correlation coefficients with the exception of total cell count (probably due to more variability between specimens), lymphocyte counts on cytospins (probably due to difficulty with accurate visual identification and the low percentage of these cells), and activated T-suppressor lymphocytes in flow cytometry (probably due to low numbers in the subjects studied).

III. Indices of Airway Inflammation in Asthma

In populations of asthmatics the sputum is characterized by an increase in the proportion of eosinophils and metachromatic cells and levels of eosinophil

Table 3 Repeatability (Expressed as Intraclass Correlation Coefficient) of Sputum Indices of Inflammation

Total cell count	0.35	Fluid-phase	
Differential cell counts		ECP	0.85
Eosinophils	0.94	MBP	0.80
Neutrophils	0.81	EDN	0.86
Macrophages	0.71	Albumin	0.94
Metachromatic cells	0.70	Fibrinogen	0.86
Lymphocytes	0.25	Tryptase	0.60
On flow cytometry		IL-5	0.69
T helper	0.94		
T suppressor	0.88		
Activated helper	0.77		
Activated suppressor	0.50		

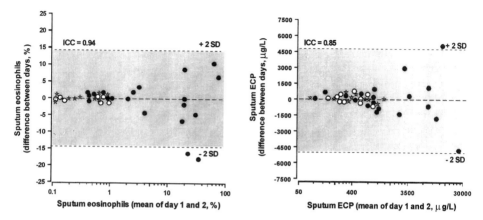

Figure 2 Repeatability of sputum differential eosinophil count and ECP levels (μg/L). Hatched area represents 2 SD around the mean of the difference. ICC is intraclass correlation coefficient.

cationic protein (ECP) compared with healthy subjects (Fig. 3) (11,12,16,31,33). There is also an increase in the proportion of neutrophils and levels of other eosinophil proteins (MBP and eosinophil-derived neurotoxin [EDN], tryptase, albumin, fibrinogen, and interleukin-5 (IL-5) (16,31). The increase in neutrophils was observed in cytospins prepared from dithiothreitol-treated sputum but not in the earlier used sputum smears, probably because of the better definition of cells in cytospins. The abnormalities observed, with the exception of the increase in neutrophils, albumin, and fibrinogen, also distinguish the asthmatic from smokers with nonobstructive bronchitis. Populations of asthmatics also differ from smokers with nonobstructive bronchitis in having a higher proportion of B(CD19+) lymphocytes and activated T-helper (CD4+, CD25+) cells in the sputum (22).

These observations are similar to those that have been observed in bronchoalveolar lavage (BAL) with the exception that the signal of abnormality is greater (34,35) and an increased proportion of neutrophils is evident. We believe that these differences are due to the fact that sputum samples the more proximal airways, whereas BAL samples the more distal respiratory areas and is diluted by saline lavage.

Various abnormalities in sputum in asthma correlate with one another (Table 4) (31). They can correlate with clinical parameters, although this varies between studies depending on the selection of subjects (12–15,22,27,31,36).

The extensive use of quantitative sputum examination has led to some unexpected findings. For example, it resulted in the recognition of the entity of eosinophilic bronchitis in which there is cough and sputum in the absence of any of the functional abnormalities of asthma; that is, in the absence of air-

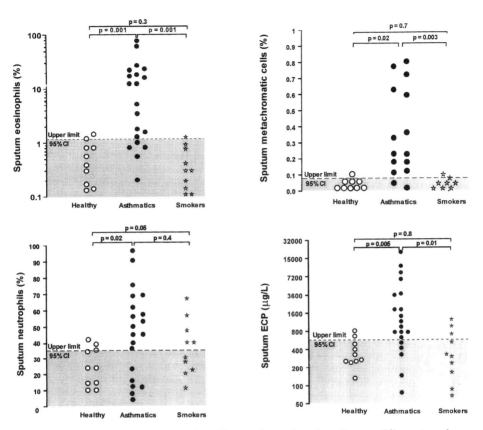

Figure 3 Sputum differential eosinophil, metachromatic cell, and neutrophil counts and ECP levels (μg/L) in healthy subjects, asthmatics, and smokers with little or no airflow obstruction.

Table 4 Correlation (rs)[a] Matrix for Sputum Differential Eosinophil Counts and Levels of Fluid-Phase Markers

	ECP	EDN	MBP	Albumin	Fibrinogen	IL-5[b]
Eosinophils	0.89	0.75	0.81	0.90	0.54	0.97
ECP		0.90	0.81	0.70	0.64	
EDN			0.89	0.70	0.62	
MBP				0.66	0.67	
Albumin					0.61	

[a]*P* values for all correlations < .001.
[b]Only in asthmatic subjects.

flow obstruction, variable airflow obstruction, or airway hyperresponsiveness (15,36). In addition, the measurements on sputum have demonstrated that acute exacerbations of asthma are not always associated with an increase in sputum eosinophils (26,37). This observation may well prove relevant to the investigation of the effects of anti-inflammatory medications which may show differential effectiveness depending on the type of inflammatory response. In addition, in studies of the antiinflammatory effects of drugs, the findings highlight the need to select subjects with defined inflammatory changes on which an effect of the anti-inflammatory treatment can be measured.

IV. The Effect of Corticosteroids on Inflammatory Indices

The use of sputum to study the effects of drugs on indices on airway inflammation promises to improve greatly our understanding of the treatment of airway diseases. So far, however, its use has only just begun and the results are sparse.

The anti-inflammatory effects of corticosteroids can be studied in three models. One model involves provocation inhalation tests to produce late asthmatic responses, increases in methacholine airway responsiveness, and airway inflammation (38). The protective effect of pretreatment can be examined. A second model consists of reducing inhaled corticosteroid in steroid-dependent asthmatic subjects to induce a mild and controlled exacerbation (39). This model can be used to investigate the protective effect of the drug if this is added before steroid reduction or to study the effect of reversing the inflammation which ensues after the corticosteroid has been reduced. Finally, there is the model of uncontrolled asthma or eosinophilic bronchitis (25,15) where active inflammation is present and reversal of the inflammation can be investigated by the addition of corticosteroid.

The effect of pretreatment with inhaled corticosteroid on allergen-induced asthmatic inflammation has been examined in three randomized, double-blind, placebo-controlled, crossover studies (40–42). In each of these studies, allergen inhalation preceded by placebo treatment caused early and late asthmatic responses and, at 24 hr, an increase from baseline in methacholine airway responsiveness and sputum differential eosinophil count. In the first two studies, pretreatment with inhaled beclomethasone, 250 μg and 500 μg, respectively, as a single dose just before allergen inhalation inhibited the late asthmatic response and the heightening of methacholine airway responsiveness but had no effect on the early response or the increase in proportion of eosinophils in the sputum. In the third study, budesonide, 400 μg daily, was given for 7 days before allergen inhalation. All of the effects of the inhaled allergen were inhibited, including the increase in sputum differential eosinophil count (Fig. 4).

We interpret these results to indicate that the earliest anti-inflammatory protective effects of inhaled corticosteroids does not affect the influx of eosinophils into the airways but the latter is inhibited by regular pretreatment. The nature of the earliest effects is unknown; a reduction of activation state and cytokine or mediator release by eosinophils or other cells are possibilities. Future studies to investigate the protective effect of drugs against airway inflammation should also utilize other sputum indices and, possibly, preceding regular treatment for a number of days.

Wong et al. (43) used the steroid reduction model to investigate whether the earliest indication of an exacerbation of symptoms in asthma was associated with an increase in sputum eosinophils and would benefit from treatment with increased inhaled steroid at that time. The question stemmed from the observation by Gibson et al. (39) that an exacerbation of symptoms often preceded deterioration of airway function. Thirty-two asthmatic adults, who needed inhaled corticosteroid to maintain control of the asthma, were enrolled in the study. The dose of inhaled steroid was reduced to produce an increase in symptoms detected by a daily diary with a sensitive scoring system. Then, when the symptoms had just increased, treatment with either budesonide, 800 µg, or placebo twice daily was added for 2 weeks in randomized double-blind paral-

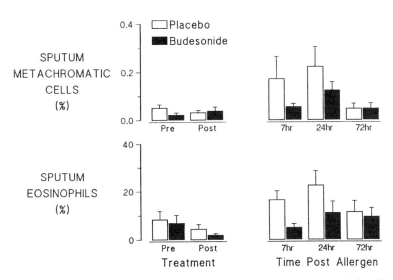

Figure 4 Sputum differential metachromatic and eosinophil counts pre and after 7 days, treatment with placebo and budesonide, 200 µg bid, and at 7, 24, and 48 hr after the same dose of inhaled allergen causing early and late asthmatic responses. Allergen inhalation increased the counts at 7 and 24 hr; this increase was inhibited by budesonide treatment.

lel group study. In the group that received budesonide, the exacerbation sputum differential eosinophil count was significantly heightened and the treatment improved symptoms and reduced the eosinophil count (Fig. 5). In the group that receive placebo, the exacerbation sputum eosinophil count showed a trend to be heightened and the treatment had no effect. However, individual subjects had increased symptoms without an increase in sputum eosinophils and improved symptoms without a decrease in eosinophils. The results of the group analysis therefore indicated that an increase in symptoms was an early indicator of asthmatic inflammation and that the addition of inhaled steroid at this point reversed this. However, the analysis in individual subjects also illustrated that symptoms on their own may not be specific for either an increase in sputum eosinophils or an improvement of these with treatment.

Claman et al. (25) investigated the effect of prednisone 0.5 mg/kg/day for 6 days, in asthmatic subjects on sputum eosinophils and ECP and on FEV_1 and peak expitatory flow (PEF) in a double-blind placebo-controlled parallel-group study. The prednisone treatment reduced eosinophil and ECP levels. However, there was only questionable improvement in the physiological parameters, presumably because the subjects for the study did not necessarily have uncontrolled asthma or abnormal inflammatory indices to begin with. In another study of

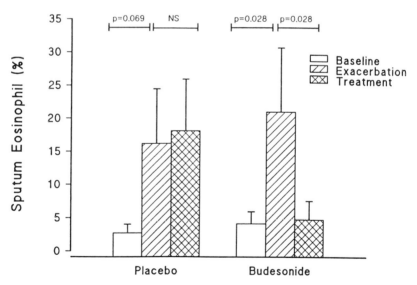

Figure 5   Sputum eosinophils (%) at baseline when inhaled corticosteroid was reduced to cause a symptomatic exacerbation and after treatment. There was an increase in eosinophils at the exacerbation which was significant in the group subsequently treated with budesonide. Budesonide treatment reversed the increase in eosinophils.

patients with eosinophilic bronchitis, Gibson (15) added inhaled beclomethasone, 400 μg twice daily, in an open uncontrolled study. The measurements on sputum, however, were made blind to the clinical characteristics. After 1 week of treatment, symptoms improved and sputum eosinophil counts fell in every subject (Fig. 6). The results of these two studies are consistent with those obtained by earlier workers using methods of examination of sputum which were not as well evaluated (4,44).

The effectiveness of steroid treatment on airway inflammation characterized by an increase in the proportion of eosinophils and level of ECP in sputum raises questions concerning the use of these measurements to predict a beneficial effect from steroid treatment (e.g., in smokers' bronchitis), to monitor optimal treatment and to investigate the antiinflammatory effects of different drugs.

V. Conclusions

Examination of spontaneous or induced sputum is the only noninvasive method to study directly airway inflammation. Methods of examination are evolving. The measurements are reproducible, responsive, and valid. They have been made in severe as well as mild disease and repeatedly in the same subject. They have begun to be used to investigate pathogenesis, pathophysiology, and treat-

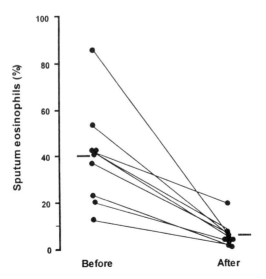

Figure 6 Sputum differential eosinophil count in patients with eosinophilic bronchitis before and one week after treatment with budesonide, 800 μg daily.

ment of asthma and other airway conditions. In populations of asthmatics there is an increase in the proportion of sputum eosinophils, metachromatic cells, neutrophils, eosinophil proteins, tryptase, IL-5, albumin, and fibrinogen. There appear to be increased proportions of B cells and activated helper T cells compared with smokers with nonobstructive bronchitis. Measurements are increased by allergen or isocyanate exposure in sensitized subjects and by reduction of steroid treatment. Treatment with corticosteroids can inhibit the allergen-induced increase in the proportion of eosinophils or metachromatic cells in sputum or can reverse the increased proportion of eosinophils or ECP levels in sputum during a natural exacerbation of asthma.

Acknowledgments

The original research in this article was supported by grants from Astra Pharma Inc., Boehringer Ingelheim (Canada) Ltd., and The Father Sean O'Sullivan Research Centre. We are grateful to Kabi Pharmacia Diagnostics for providing us with kits to measure ECP and tryptase and to Lori Burch for typing the manuscript.

Discussion

DR. LEMANSKE: Since many of the asthmatic patients you studied were atopic, I am curious to know if you have noted any differences between patients with allergic rhinitis and asthma versus nonatopic asthmatic individuals. I am concerned that postnasal drainage of cells and mediators in allergic rhinitis may confound your results.

DR. HARGREAVE: There is a possibility of contamination of the expectorate with postnasal drip. However, the procedure we used to collect induced sputum minimizes this possibility. We did not notice differences between atopic asthmatics and nonatopic asthmatics.

DR. BUSSE: In your studies of patients with chronic cough and high sputum eosinophilia, did the patients have airflow obstruction? If these patients did not have airflow obstruction, what role were the eosinophils playing? Furthermore, the number of eosinophils in the sputum were less, on average, than noted in the patients with eosinophilia and cough. What does this indicate for the role of eosinophils in the contribution to airway hyperresponsiveness and airflow obstruction?

DR. HARGREAVE: There was no airflow obstruction. The proportion of eosinophils in sputum can be as high in subjects with eosinophilic bronchitis without asthma as in those with asthma. One reason why the former group do not have airflow obstruction or hyperresponsiveness may be that the eosinophilic inflammation is occurring in proximal larger airways. Another possibility is that, although the eosinophilic inflammation is also occurring in smaller airways, the airway physiology is supernormal. Some evidence for this was seen in some subjects who had a heightening of methacholine airway responsiveness within the normal range which became evident when treatment with steroid was given and the responsiveness became less. (PG Gibson, FE Hargreave, A Girgis-Gabardo, et al. Chronic cough with eosinophilic bronchitis and examination for variable airflow obstruction and response to corticosteroid. Clin Exp Allergy 1995; 25:127–132.)

DR. MCFADDEN: Are there any data that demonstrate that differential inflammatory effects exist at different sites of the airways?

DR. HARGREAVE: Not that I am aware of. However, the work of Roland Ingram suggests that small airway involvement is needed to develop airway hyperresponsiveness. (LB Pliss, EP Ingenito, RH Ingram, Jr. Responsiveness, inflammation and effects of deep breaths on obstruction in mild asthma. J. Appl. Physiol. 1989; 66:2298–2304.)

DR. HOWARTH: Consistent with your suggestion that eosinophils may come from the large airways, Dr. Merrick in Southampton, investigating the distribution of inflammatory cells within different size airways in postmortem specimens from patients with asthma who died from an unrelated cause, found that eosinophils were rarely seen in small airways, whereas they are prominent in large airways. In contrast, mast cells are distributed throughout both large and small airways. This would suggest that if eosinophils are important to bronchial hyperresponsiveness small airway inflammation is not critical to this physiological measurement.

DR. MCFADDEN: What are the data that one must have eosinophils in the airway to have airway hyperreactivity? Eosinophils are undoubtedly important, but it is unlikely that they alone are the answer. I would make the plea that our postulates incorporate all of the available data, both positive and negative, otherwise we will continue to have difficulty focusing on what we do not know.

DR. DURHAM: First, a comment in response to Dr. McFadden: Eosinophils may be necessary but not sufficient for an allergen-induced late asthmatic response. The presence of eosinophils in BAL after challenge in the absence of a fall in FEV_1 is compatible with this. What would not be compatible would be a late response in the absence of eosinophilia, and this is not in generally seen. DeMonchy and Robinson found a good correlation between late fall in FEV_1 and BAL eosinophilia. (JGR DeMonchy, HK Kauffman, P Veng, et al.

Bronchoalveolar eosinophilia during allergen-induced late asthmatic reactions. Am. Rev. Respir. Dis. 1995; 131:373–376,; DS Robinson, DSQ Hamid, A Bentley, et al. Activation of CD1+ T cells, increased Th2-type cytokine mRNA expression, and eosinophil recruitment in bronchoalveolar lavage after allergen inhalation challenge in atopic asthmatics. J Allergy Clin Immunol 1993; 92:313–324, 1993.). Questions: (1) Does the baseline eosinophil count in sputum predict clinical response to corticosteroid in asthma? (2) Is sputum induction feasible in children where more invasive tests are not feasible?

Dr. Hargreave: It seems likely that an increase in the proportion of eosinophils in sputum will predict a beneficial effect from treatment with corticosteroid in asthma and other airway conditions. However, this still requires prospective investigation. Sputum induction has also been shown to be successful in children of 8 years and older. (I Pin, PG Gibson, R Kolendowicz, et al. Use of induced sputum cells counts to investigate airway inflammation in asthma. Thorax 1992; 47:25–29.). I am not aware of attempts at induction in younger children.

Dr. Barnes: In patients with COPD (chronic obstructive pulmonary disease), we find an increased population of neutrophils in induced sputum which is correlated with an increased concentration of IL-8. Glucocorticoid therapy does not reduce the neutrophil number or IL-8, suggesting that this is steroid resistant. In patients with asthma, you have demonstrated a relatively high proportion of neutrophils, but this population, in contrast to eosinophils, is not reduced by steroid treatment. Neutrophils might be important in acute exacerbations of asthma and may explain why glucocorticoids are not very effective in severe acute exacerbation of asthma. Have you studied neutrophils at earlier time points after allergen?

Dr. Hargreave: No.

Dr. Gleich: Note that endotoxin causes increases in lung neutrophils. One must be terribly careful to assure that patients with increased sputum neutrophils do not have endotoxin stimulation as a basis for the increased numbers of neutrophils. Such stimulation could be caused by bacterial infection or inhalation of endotoxin-containing materials.

Dr. A. Laitinen: Have you looked at the tryptase level in the sputum? Is there a difference between normal controls and asthmatics? What are the steroid treatment effects?

Dr. Hargreave: Tryptase can be increased in asthma but the effect of treatment has not been studied yet.

Dr. Denburg: After allergen challenge, we have observed that asthmatic sputum contains increased numbers of tryptase-positive cells by immunostaining.

The rise in tryptase-positive cells parallels, but is more modest than, the rise in toluidine blue–positive (i.e., metachromatic) cells.

DR. O'BYRNE: The subjects studied with allergen challenge in our laboratory are very mild, stable atopic asthmatic subjects. In the baseline state, they have very few EG2+ eosinophils in sputum.

DR. McFADDEN: In a segmental antigen challenge, eosinophils and other inflammatory cells increase in number and become activated, inflammatory cascades develop, mediators are released, and various cytokines are generated, yet there seems to be little overall adverse effects on the lung. Does airway reactivity rise? Do late reactions occur? In an antigen exposure in the wild, how much antigen is required to produce an asthma attack, an increase in reactivity, and where in the longitudinal distribution of the airways does it have its greatest impact? Is any of this known?

DR. HARGREAVE: In an antigen exposure in the wild, the amount of antigen required to produce an early asthmatic response depends on the concentration of IgE antibodies and the degree of airway responsiveness to bronchoconstrictor mediators like histamine or methacholine. The amount of antigen needed can be estimated from the skin sensitivity and PC_{20} histamine. (DW Cockcroft, KY Murdock, J Kirby, F Hargreave. Prediction of airway responsiveness to allergen from skin sensitivity to allergen and airway responsiveness to histamine. Am Rev Respir Dis 1987; 135:264–267.) The determinants of an allergen-induced increase in airway responsiveness are less clear. However, this seems to occur in association with the development of late asthmatic responses and the determinants of these include high IgE antibody levels. (PM O'Byrne, J Dolovich, FE Hargreave. Late asthmatic responses. Am Rev Respir Dis 1987; 136:740–751.) The inhaled dose of antigen required to elicit an early asthmatic response or an increase in airway responsiveness is not necessarily unnaturally large.

DR. PERSSON: I think that the hypertonic saline challenge in combination with forceful coughing to produce the sputum may cause some mechanical damage sufficient rapidly to cause accumulation of neutrophils (within 10 min). So my question is does spontaneously delivered sputum contain less neutrophils?

DR. HARGREAVE: No. (Pizzichini MMM, Popov TA, Efthimiadis A, Hussack P, Evans S, Pizzichini E, Polovich J, Hargreave FE. Spontaneous and induced sputum to measure indices of airway inflammation in asthma. Am J Respir Crit Care Med 1996. in press.)

References

1. Thomson Sir Wm. (Lord Kelvin). Electrical units of measurement. In: Popular Lectures and Addresses. London,: Macmillan, 1891:80–143.

2. Gollasch H. Zur kenntniss der asthmatischen sputums. Fortschritte der Medizin (Berlin) 1889; 7:361–365.
3. Hansel FK. Clinical Allergy. St. Louis: Mosby 1953.
4. Brown HM. Treatment of chronic asthma with prednisolone: significance of eosinophils in sputum. Lancet 1958; 2:1245–1247.
5. Chodosh S. Examination of sputum cells. N Engl J Med 1970; 282:854–858.
6. Thomas HV, Simmons E. Histamine content in sputum from allergic and nonallergic individuals. J Appl Physiol 1979; 26:793–797.
7. Turnbull LS, Turnbull LW, Leitch AG, Crofton JW, Kay AB. Mediators of immediate-type hypersensitivity in sputum from patients with chronic bronchitis and asthma. Lancet 1977; 2:526–529.
8. Bryant DH, Pui A. Histamine content in sputum from patients with asthma and chronic bronchitis. Clin Allergy 1982; 12:19–27.
9. O'Driscoll BRC, Cromwell O, Kay AB. Sputum leukotrienes in obstructive airways diseases. Clin Exp Immunol 1984; 55:397–404.
10. Frigas EO, Loegering DA, Solley GO, Farrow GM, Gleich GJ. Elevated levels of eosinophils granule major basic protein in the sputum of patients with bronchial asthma. Mayo Clin Proc 1981; 56:345–353.
11. Gibson PG, Girgis-Gabardo A, Morris MM, Mattoli S, Kay JM, Dolovich J, Denburg J, Hargreave FE. Cellular characteristics of sputum from patients with asthma and chronic bronchitis. Thorax 1989; 44:693–699.
12. Pin I, Gibson PG, Kolendowicz R, Girgis-Gabardo A, Denburg J, Hargreave FE, Dolovich J. Use of induced sputum cell counts to investigate airway inflammation in asthma. Thorax 1992; 47:25–29.
13. Iredale MJ, Wanklyn AR, Phillips IP, Krausz T, Ind PW. Non-invasive assessment of bronchial inflammation in asthma: no correlation between eosinophilia of induced sputum and bronchial responsiveness to inhaled hypertonic saline. Clin Exp Allergy 1994; 24:940–945.
14. Pin I, Freitag AP, O'Byrne PM, Girgis-Gabardo A, Watson RM, Dolovich J, Denburg JA, Hargreave FE. Changes in the cellular profile of induced sputum after allergen-induced asthmatic responses. Am Rev Respir Dis 1992; 145:1265–1269.
15. Gibson PG, Hargreave FE, Girgis-Gabardo A, Morris M, Denburg JA, Dolovich J. Chronic cough with eosinophilic bronchitis and examination for variable airflow obstruction and response to corticosteroid. Clin Exp Allergy 1995; 25:127–132.
16. Fahy JV, Liu J, Wong H, Boushey HA. Cellular and biochemical analysis of induced sputum from asthmatic and healthy individuals. Am Rev Respir Dis 1993; 147:1126–1131.
17. Bickerman HA, Sproul EE, Barach AL. An aerosol method of producing bronchial secretions in human subjects: a clinical technic for the detection of lung cancer. Dis Chest 1958; 33;347–362.
18. Cleland WW. Dithiothreitol, a new protective reagent for SH groups. Biochemistry 1964; 3:480–482.
19. Wooton OJ, Dulfano MJ. Improved homogenization techniques for sputum cytology counts. Ann Allergy 1978; 41:150–154.
20. Hansel TT, Braunstein C, Walker C, Blaser K, Bruijnzeel PLB, Virchow JC Jr,

Virchow C Sr. Sputum eosinophils from asthmatics express ICAM-1 and HLA-DR. Clin Exp Immunol 1991; 86:271–277.

21. Popov T, Gottschalk R, Kolendowicz R, Dolovich J, Powers P, Hargreave FE. The evaluation of a cell dispersion method of sputum examination. Clin Exp Allergy 1994; 24:778–783.

22. Kidney JC, Wong AG, Efthimiadis A, Morris MM, Sears MR, Dolovich J, Hargreave FE. Elevated B-cells in sputum of asthmatics: close correlation with eosinophils. Am J Repir Crit Care Med 1996; 153:540–544.

23. Fahy JV, Schuster A, Euki I, Boushey HA, Nadel JA. Mucus hypersecretion in bronchiectasis. The role of neutrophil proteases. Am Rev Respir Dis 1992; 146:1430–1433.

24. Fahy JV, Liu J, Wong H, Boushey HA. Analysis of cellular and biochemical constituents in induced sputum after allergen challenge: a method for studying allergic airway inflammation. J Allergy Clin Immunol 1994; 93:1031–1039.

25. Claman DM, Boushey HA, Liu J, Wong H, Fahy JV. Analysis of induced sputum to examine the effects of prednisone on airway inflammation in asthmatics subjects. J Allergy Clin Immunol 1994; 94:861–869.

26. Fahy JV, Kim KW, Liu J, Boushey HA. Prominent neutrophilic inflammation in sputum from subjects with asthma exacerbation. J Allergy Clin Immunol 1995; 95:843–852.

27. Maestrelli P, Calcagni PG, Saetta M, Di Stefano A, Hosselet JJ, Santoanastaso A, Fabbri LM, Mapp CE. Sputum eosinophilia after responses induced by isocyanates in sensitized subjects. Clin Exp Allergy 1994; 24:29–34.

28. Popov TA, Pizzichini MMM, Pizzichini E, Kolendowicz R, Punthakee Z, Dolovich J, Hargreave FE. Some technical factors influencing the induction of sputum for cell analysis. Eur Respir J 1995; 8:559–565.

29. Anderson SD, Smith CM, Rodwell LT, du Toit JI, Riedler J, Robertson CF. The use of nonisotonic aerosols for evaluating bronchial hyperresponsiveness. In: Spector SL, ed, Provocation Testing in Clinical Practice. New York: Dekker 1995:249–278.

30. Pizzichini E, Pizzichini MMM, Efthimiadis A, Hargreave FE, Dolovich J. Measurement of inflammatory indices in induced sputum: effects of selection of sputum to minimize salivary contamination. Eur Respir J 1996. In press.

31. Pizzichini E, Pizzichini MMM, Efthimiadis A, Evans S, Morris MM, Squillace D, Gleich G, Dolovich J, Hargreave FE. Indices of airway inflammation in induced sputum: reproducibility and validity of cell and fluid-phase measurements. Am J Respir Crit Care Med 1996. In press.

32. Efthimiadis A, Pizzichini MMM, Pizzichini E, Kolendowicz R, Weston S, Dolovich J, Hargreave FE. The influence of cell viability and squamous cell contamination on the reliability of sputum differential cell counts. Am J Respir Crit Care Med 1995; 151:A384.

33. Virchow JC Jr, Holscher U, Virchow C Sr. Sputum ECP levels correlate with parameters of airflow obstruction. Am Rev Respir Dis 1992; 146:604–606.

34. Fahy JV, Wong H, Liu J, Boushey HA. Comparison of samples collected by spu-

tum induction and bronchoscopy from asthmatic and healthy subjects. Am J Respir Crit Care Med 1995; 152:53–58.

35. Kidney J, Pizzichini E, Ädelroth E, Popov T, Hussack P, Efthimiadis A, O'Byrne P, Dolovich J, Hargreave FE. Comparison of sputum, bronchoalveolar lavage (BAL) and blood inflammatory cells in asthma. Am J Respir Crit Care Med 1995; 151:A384.

36. Gibson PG, Dolovich J, Denburg J, Ramsdale EH, Hargreave FE. Chronic cough: eosinophilic bronchitis without asthma. Lancet 1989; 1:1346–1348.

37. Turner MO, Hussack P, Sears MR, Dolovich J, Hargreave FE. Exacerbations of asthma without sputum eosinophilia. Thorax 1995; 50:

38. O'Byrne PM, Dolovich J, Hargreave FE. Late asthmatic responses. Am Rev Respir Dis 1987; 136:740–751.

39. Gibson PG, Wong BJO, Hepperle MJE, Kline P, Girgis-Gabardo A, Guyatt G, Dolovich J, Denburg JA, Ramsdale EH, Hargreave FE. A research method to induce and examine a mild exacerbation of asthma by withdrawal of inhaled corticosteroid. Clin Exp Allergy 1992; 22:525–532.

40. Wong BJO, Dolovich J, Ramsdale EH, O'Byrne P, Gontovnick L, Denburg JA, Hargreave FE. Formoterol compared to beclomethasone and placebo on allergen-induced asthmatic responses. Am Rev Respir Dis 1992; 146:1156–1160.

41. Pizzichini MMM, Kidney JC, Wong BJO, Morris MM, Efthimiadis A, Dolovich J, Hargreave FE. Effect of salmeterol compared with beclomethasone on allergen-induced asthmatic and inflammatory responses. Eur Respir J 1996. In press.

42. Gauvreau GM, Doctor J, Watson RM, Jordana M, O'Byrne PM. Effect of inhaled budesonide on allergen induced airway and inflammatory responses. Am J Respir Crit Care Med 1995; 151:A41.

43. Wong BJO, Gibson PG, Hussack P, Girgis-Gabardo A, Ramsdale EH, Dolovich J, Hargreave FE. Early asthma exacerbations by steroid reduction—examination of inflammation and treatment with inhaled budesonide. Am Rev Respir Dis 1993; 147:A291.

44. Baigelman W, Chodosh S, Pizzuto D, Cuples AL. Sputum and blood eosinophils during corticosteroid treatment of acute exacerbations of asthma. Am J Med 1903; 75:929–936.

8

Tissue Remodeling and Fibroblast Heterogeneity in Asthma and Other Chronic Airways Inflammatory Diseases

JACK GAULDIE, PATRICIA J. SIME, GUY M. TREMBLAY, DIANE TORRY, and MANEL JORDANA

McMaster University
Hamilton, Ontario, Canada

BENGT SARNSTRAND

Astra Draco
Lund, Sweden

I. Introduction

Examination of biopsy material from patients with asthma and other chronic inflammatory diseases of the airways, well-recognized and prominent features are thickening of the bronchial epithelial basement membrane, deposition of a subepithelial collagen band in the lamina reticularis, and the presence of myofibroblasts, cells not normally found in the subepithelial tissue (1–4). Whether these features are typical of a "fibrotic" reaction or represent a unique stromal cell response, the fibroblast in the subepithelial compartment in asthma is likely to contribute to the pathology and physiology of the tissue, with impact that needs to be considered when delineating the pathobiology of this disorder.

There are numerous other examples of fibrotic components of chronic airways diseases, and many of these share common features of excess collagen deposition and the presence of myofibroblasts. In this regard, three issues need consideration when examining the effects of steroid treatment on the airways of asthmatic subjects. The first issue involves the different types of matrix proteins made by stromal cells and how corticosteroids influence their expression and thereby the integrity of the tissue. The second issue involves the stromal cells as effectors with release of important growth and inflammatory cytokines and how corticosteroids affect the expression of these molecules. The third issue involves the fact that chronic inflamed tissue contains stromal cells with an altered phenotype which may or may not be affected by such treatment.

II. Matrix Metabolism

The matrix plays a profound role in providing the mechanical support for tissue, and in particular during reorganization and repair of damaged tissues. Moreover, the extracellular components of this matrix can influence cell distribution, differentiation, and tissue organization. Such components are involved in the reorganized asthmatic tissue, and their expression is influenced by treatment with corticosteroids (the extracellular matrix [ECM] in asthma was recently reviewed by Roche [3]). Although expression of these many extracellular and intracellular matrix components is modulated by various growth factors and cytokines, corticosteroids are also potent regulators of both extracellular and intracellular matrix molecules.

The most prominent component of the ECM are the various collagen molecules that are both fibrillar, such as types I, III, and V, deposited within the interstitium in increased amounts in fibrous tissue, and those classed as nonfibrillar, such as types IV and VII, which make up a major portion of the basement membrane in the lung. The report by Roche et al. (1) showed the presence of an abnormal subepithelial band of fibrillar collagen made up of types III and V. These studies and others (4–8) demonstrate the presence of increased collagen and fibroblasts within the interstitial tissue. Despite this evidence of "fibrotic" pathology, little attention is paid to the resolution or enhancement of these abnormalities on treatment. Although inflammatory cell infiltration is readily altered by steroid treatment (4,5,7,9), similar decreases in collagen deposits or numbers and types of fibroblasts are not so apparent. In one study (5), an increased number of fibroblasts was noted on budesonide treatment lasting 3 months, whereas another study (4) found no decrease in the thickness of the collagen deposition after short- or long-term treatment with inhaled steroid. On further examination, Altraja et al. (8) found that a 3-month exposure to inhaled steroid had no effect on the distribution of either type III or VII collagens in the basement membrane zone in bronchial biopsies from asthmatic patients.These studies contrast with that of Trigg et al. (7), who examined biopsies from asthmatic patients exposed to inhaled steroid for 4 months. They found that the thickness of the type III collagen deposit in the bronchial reticularis was reduced, implying that prolonged exposure to steroid could alter the tissue integrity and return the bronchial structure toward normal. Which of these findings has validity in the general patient population requires a further number of independent studies examining both the thickness and subtype distribution of collagen with longer term steroid exposure. Complexing the issue is a series of in vitro studies on pulmonary vascular smooth muscle cells that show steroid stimulates collagen secretion in rapidly proliferating cells (10,11). In vivo while corticosteroid ameliorates the pulmonary hypertension in rats caused by exposure to 10% O_2 for 3 days, this results in an increase in the proportion of collagen in the vessel wall (12). Recognising differences in skin and lung fibroblasts, nonetheless, steroid treatment also reduced the content of elastin in skin fibroblasts through inhibition of gene transcription (13), and similar responses would be expected from lung and airways fibroblasts albeit at different levels of sensitivity. Taken together these studies indicate that treatment with inhaled steroid may result in a beneficial decrease in the inflammation seen in asthmatic tissue but may not be beneficial and possibly be deleterious to the restructured components of the airways.

In addition to collagen, steroids have effects on other components of the matrix. Sarnstrand et al. (14) showed that fibroblasts derived from human lung tissue were more sensitive to steroid mediated inhibition of hyaluronic acid synthesis. Similar inhibition of proteoglycan synthesis would be expected in vivo, and this would result in an altered milieu in the basement membrane with differences in electrical charge of the membrane, cross linking of the ECM components and cell adhesion and signal transduction (3). A decrease in the content of the proteoglycans might also affect the hydration and permeability of the basement membrane.

Tenascin and laminin are other glycoproteins derived from the mesenchyme that play a role in the integrity of the interstitium and basement membrane of the lung. In a study using bone marrow stromal cells and fibroblasts, Ekblom et al. (15) showed marked downregulation of both tenascin and laminin expression by exposure to corticosteroids, and recently Laitinen et al. (16) extended these findings to asthma showing that treatment with inhaled budesonide for 4–6 weeks drastically reduced the content of tenascin in the bronchial epithelial basement membrane zone. The fact that others have shown that further components of ECM and basement membrane, including fibronectin, which plays a prominent role in cell adhesion and chemotaxis, are upregulated by exposure to steroids (17) indicates that treatment of patients with long-term inhaled corticosteroid is likely to have a profound effect on the content and distribution of the numerous components of ECM with differential regulation causing distortion of the normal distribution and an alteration in the integrity and function of the basement membrane.

III. Effector Function of Airways Fibroblasts

In addition to their role in the synthesis of ECM components, recent studies demonstrate that tissue structural cells such as the fibroblast are important effector cells secreting a broad spectrum of growth factors and immune- and inflammation-regulating cytokines (recently reviewed in refs. 18–20). The fibroblast response in inflammation derives from being stimulated by the presence of primary stimulating cytokines, including interleukin-1 (IL-1) and tumor necrosis factor (TNF). As a result, chemokines and growth factors (e.g. IL-8, monocyte chemotactic peptide [MCP-1], granulocyte-macrophage colony-stimulating factor [GM-CSF], and transforming growth factor [TGFβ]) are secreted (Table 1), and since structural cells represent a greater contingent within the tissue than inflammatory cells, this suggests a major contribution to the inflammatory milieu within the asthmatic tissue. There are two basic mechanisms involving regulation of fibroblast effector function by steroid treatment. The first is a direct effect with inhibition of cytokine gene expression. In most cases, fibroblasts and other structural cells require stimulation to express cytokines. In this regard, steroid treatment interferes with the normal upregulation seen after stimulation with factors such as IL-1 and TNF (21–23). Although several possible mechanisms have been suggested, the most likely involves interference by the steroid/steroid receptor complex with nuclear factors such as AP-1 (24) and NF-κB (25,26) preventing binding to suitable promoter sequences and thereby directly inhibiting gene transcription. This has been suggested for IL-6 production by fibroblasts (26), but in addition, there appears to be evidence for posttranscriptional regulation by steroid in lung fibroblasts (27). A further important example is seen in Figure 1 in which human pulmonary fibroblasts

Table 1 Cytokines Made by Fibroblasts

Cytokine	Possible effects in asthma	Inhibited by corticosteroid
IL-8		+
MIP-1	Chemotaxins of inflammatory cells	+
MCP-1		+
RANTES		+
IL-6	Immune regulation	+
IL-1	Inflammation	+
CSFs		
GM⁻	Eosinophil viability	+
G⁻	Neutrophil viability	+
M⁻	Monocyte viability	-
TGF-β	Myofibroblast differentiation	+
	Collagen syntheses	
bFGF	Fibroblast proliferation	?
PDGF	Proliferation and chemotaxis of structural cells	+
SCF	Mast cell proliferation	?
HGF	Epithelial cell growth and differentiation	+

MIP-1, macrophage inflammatory peptide 1; RANTES, monocyte chemokine; bFGF, basic fibroblast growth factor; PDGF, platelet derived growth factor; SCF, stem cell factor; HGF, hepatocyte growth factor or scatter factor.

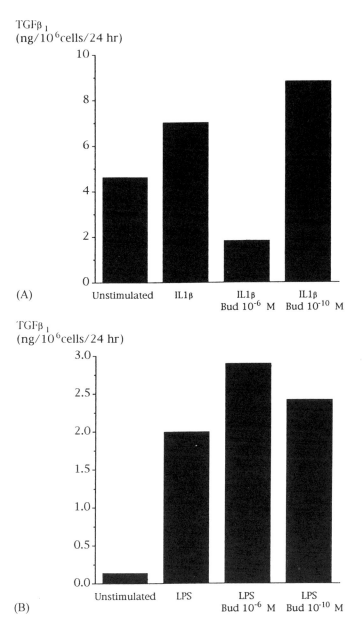

Figure 1 Effect of corticosteroid on production of TGF-β_1. (A) IL-1β (10 ng) was used to stimulate human pulmonary fibroblasts to produce TGF-β_1. Budesonide (10^{-6} and 10^{-10} M) was added to inhibit the production of cytokine. (B) LPS (10 μg) was used to stimulate human peripheral blood monocytes to produce TGF-β_1. Budesonide (10^{-6} and 10^{-10} M) was not able to inhibit cytokine production.

stimulated by IL-1 release significant levels of TGF-β (7–9 ng/10^6 cells/24 hr) and this production is profoundly inhibited by treatment with 10^{-6} M budesonide. This sensitivity for inhibition of TGF-β expression by steroid is not general, as peripheral blood monocytes are not affected by steroid treatment, and recently Khalil et al. (28) showed a similar lack of response to steroid by rat alveolar macrophage in a model of pulmonary fibrosis.

A second and indirect interaction with fibroblasts can be expected in steroid-exposed tissue. As seen above, steroid decreases the expression of proteoglycans such as a transmembrane β-glycan (29) and small extracelluar proteoglycans, including biglycan and decorin, from structural cells. These molecules are able to bind and inhibit the biological activity of TGF-β and preserve the integrity and activity of other growth factors such as the heparin binding family of fibroblast growth factors (FGFs) within the interstitium (30–33). Steroid treatment should result in downregulation of both cytokine and proteoglycan expression from the fibroblast, yet in the presence of activated macrophage or monocytes, TGF-β release could still occur with vastly decreased binding and inhibitory capacity in the tissue resulting in abnormal tissue matrix formation through unchecked stimulation of matrix gene expression. The result is a decrease in the effector function of fibroblasts concomitant with alteration in matrix formation by these same cells.

IV. Fibroblast Heterogeneity

The most notable cellular aspect of structural changes in asthmatic biopsy tissue is the presence of myofibroblast-like cells beneath the bronchial epithelium (6). Myofibroblasts possess fibroblast morphology and contain contractile elements (intracellular matrix) which are best seen on examination by electron microscopy. In some cases, the contractile elements may contain an actin filament that is normally found in smooth muscle cells (smooth muscle actin, SMC) (34,35). Although myofibroblasts are found in both normal and asthmatic subjects, they were increased in atopic asthma and found to correlate positively with the depth of collagen layer under the bronchial epithelium (recently reviewed in ref. 2). These cells may be very important in defining the nature of cellular responses in the airways, as the anatomical site they occupy, just below the epithelial layer, can allow them exposure to leukocyte-derived mediators and, in turn, can influence the behavior of inflammatory cells, such as eosinophils, that migrate through the layer and accumulate in the bronchial epithelium (Fig. 2). The presence of these cells and their potential role in airways responses is reminiscent of the findings of similar cells in granulation or healing tissue and

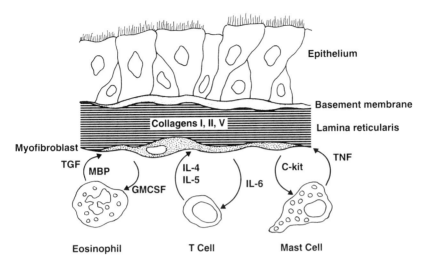

Figure 2 Scheme showing the relationship of the myofibroblast, collagen layer, and inflammatory cells with cytokine interactions. GM-CSF, granulocyte-macrophage colony-stimulating factor; TNF, tumor necrosis factor. (Adapted from ref. 4.)

in experimental tissue with evidence of developing fibrosis (36; see ref. 37 for review).

We have previously shown that chronically inflamed lung tissue, as found in fibrosis, contains phenotypically altered fibroblasts, sometimes expressing smooth muscle actin. Similar heterogeneity is seen in upper airways with fibroblast lines derived from nasal polyp tissue demonstrating phenotypic differences from normal cells (18–20,38–40). Differences include rates of proliferation, intrinsic activation, and enhanced expression of growth factors, such as GM-CSF, and recently extend to differences in production of hyaluronic acid and proteoglycans (41; Westergren-Thorsson G., et al., unpublished data). We have also shown differences in the ability to form colonies in soft agar, a condition similar to anchorage-independent growth seen with "transformed" cells (42,43). Such characteristics might account for the apparent "aggressive" nature of fibrosis. More notable is the finding that corticosteroids in vitro enhance the colony-forming activity of both fibrotic lung fibroblasts and a transformed fibrosarcoma cell line, HT1080 (Fig. 3). Whether this extends to effects of steroid in vivo needs to be examined.

The relationship of fibroblast phenotype, especially myofibroblast, and cytokine modulation is best seen through the induction of smooth muscle ac-

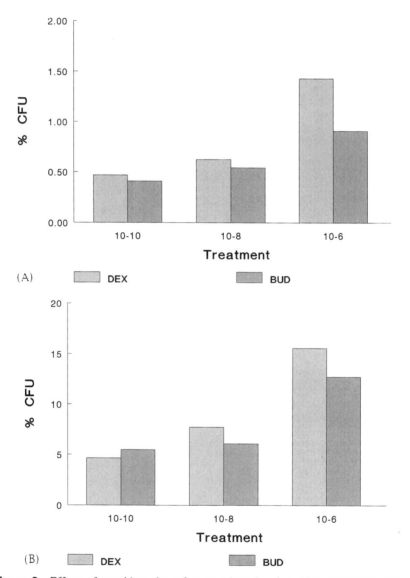

Figure 3 Effects of steroid on the soft agar colony-forming ability (% CFU) of human fibroblasts. (A) Line established from fibrotic lung tissue, passage 5. (B) HT-1080 fibrosarcoma transformed line. DEX, dexamethasone; BUD, budesonide.

tin in these cells. Recently, cytokines such as GM-CSF and TGF-β have been shown to be capable of inducing fibroblast differentiation to myofibroblasts with expression of smooth muscle action (SMA) in vitro and to some extent in vivo in experimental animals (37,44–46) and in human cells (47). We have previously shown the presence of both cytokines in nasal polyp tissue (48,49), and we thus examined fibroblast lines isolated from nasal polyps and lung tissue and skin for SMA expression. Basal expression of SMA was very evident in nasal derived lines (normal and polyp) but was not detectable in lines derived from lung tissue or skin. However, when these lines were exposed to TGF-β, 1 ng/ ml for 6 days, there was a marked induction of SMA expression, and this induction was not inhibited by the presence of budesonide at 10^{-8} or 10^{-6} M (Fig. 4A). In the case of nasal cell lines, incubation with budesonide alone caused a diminution in the basal expression of SMA (Fig. 4B), indicating that SMA expression in these cells was likely derived from autostimulation by a factor derived from the nasal cells whose release was inhibitable by steroid (40). These data are consistent with the finding that the number of SMA-positive cells seen in nasal polyp biopsies can be reduced by topical and systemic treatment with steroid (50).

As an extension to these studies, we have examined fibroblast lines derived from asthmatic tissue. These cells, identified as myofibroblasts (6), are negative for SMA expression under basal culture conditions, but on exposure to TGF-β, there is remarkable expression of SMA, much more so than similarly treated normal lung or skin cell lines (40). These findings are similar to those seen with SMA-negative cells found in keloid, a further example of chronically inflamed or repairing tissue (37). Whether expression, induced or endogenous, of smooth muscle actin by these myofibroblasts in asthma tissue contributes to the altered contractile or reactive nature of the bronchial tissue needs to be investigated. In addition, whether steroid functions directly on these cells or interferes with the development of the phenotype in an indirect manner, their presence must be considered in examining the tissue changes while on a long-term treatment with inhaled steroid.

V. Summary

Structural cells within the bronchial tree in asthmatic subjects are likely to be important contributors to the pathological and physiological abnormalities characteristic of this disease. Steroid treatment can regulate synthesis of a number of effector mediators from these cells, as well as produce changes in their matrix protein metabolism. Whether steroids can influence the phenotype of the myofibroblast present in the tissue remains to be determined, as do the effects

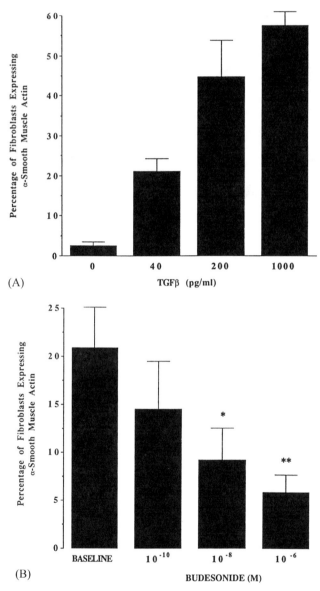

(A)

(B)

Figure 4 In vitro effect of budesonide on α-smooth muscle actin expression. (A) Four nasal polyp fibroblast cell lines. *Significantly different than baseline. **Significantly different than baseline and budesonide 10^{-10} M. ANOVA followed by Scheffe test ($P < .05$) (B) Two normal lung fibroblast cell lines. This induced expression cannot be prevented by incubation with budesonide 10^{-6} M.

of longer term steroid exposure on the overall function of structural cells in the bronchial tree.

Discussion

Dr. Brattsand: Why do we not see bronchial atrophy as we do when using topical steroid on the skin?

Dr. Gauldie: There are differences in response of the lung fibroblast and the skin fibroblast to challenge with inflammatory mediators. This may explain the differences, but I don't have another reasonable explanation.

Dr. Brattsand: One reason for the lack of atrophy in the lung seems to be that its fibroblasts have a lower intrinsic sensitivity to glucocorticoid than those of skin. We raised fibroblast lines from skin and lung samples of the same patients and compared their sensitivity for steroids regarding blocking hyaluronan and glycosaminoglycan synthesis. For inducing the same block, the lung fibroblasts needed about 100 times higher steroid concentration. One reason may be that these fibroblasts produce partly different glycosaminoglycans—lung fibroblasts make a lot of heparin sulfate, the synthesis of which seems less sensitive to steroids. (B Särnstrand, A Jeppson, A Malmstrom, R Brattsand. Effect of glucocorticosteroids on hyaluronic acid synthesis in vitro in human fibroblast-like cells from lung and skin. In: JC Hogg, R Ellul-Micallef, R Brattsand, eds. Glucocorticoids, Inflammation, and Bronchial Hyperreactivity. Amsterdam, Excerpta Medica 1985:157–166.)

Dr. Persson: I think the exceedingly profuse mucosal microcirculation may be an important factor potentially explaining why steroids do not produce the local side effects in the airways as are seen after topical application on the skin.

Dr. Leung: Do you have any data on the basis for altered structural cells in asthma or patients with idiopathic pulmonary fibrosis (IPF)? Is this an acquired phenotype or is there a genetic basis to this defect?

Dr. Gauldie: The phenotype in culture remains quite stable, but we are early in our studies on the cells isolated from bronchial biopsies of asthmatics. We need to study these cells in the similar way as our lung and nasal polyp cell lines.

Dr. Barnes: In the clones of fibroblasts from IPF that show increased proliferation, is there evidence that the cells are more responsive to growth factors or less responsive to growth inhibitors?

Dr. Gauldie: The chronic inflammation-derived cell lines are more sensitive to growth factors in vitro and some are able to undergo autocrine growth in vitro. They can provide suitable levels of their own growth factors. They are not transformed or immortal. They are normal cells with a different phenotype of behavior.

DR. O'BYRNE: (1) Do myofibroblasts contract in response to agonists? (2) Are there other functional differences between fibroblasts and myofibroblasts?

DR. GAULDIE: These are interesting questions, but as yet no functional measurements have been made.

DR. BRATTSAND: This comment pertains to Dr. Leung's statement that there is a lower risk of provoking skin atrophy in atopic dermatitis (that in other skin diseases), and that the atopic state in some way protects against connective tissue atrophy. If that protection from atrophy is relevant also in airways, does it mean that there is a higher risk of atrophic changes on long-term treatment in nonatopic asthmatics?

DR. LEUNG: The clinical observation in atopic dermatitis is that uninvolved noninflamed skin is much more susceptible to topical steroid–induced dermal atrophy than lesional inflamed skin. Perhaps the reason that bronchial atrophy doesn't occur in asthma is that inflammation alters steroid responsiveness. A word of caution must therefore be considered in the treatment of early childhood asthma or mild asthma in adults with topical steroids as a first-line therapy.

DR. GAULDIE: I think it is very important to recognize that (1) we show positive (stimulatory) effects on colony formation by steroid. (2) Dr. Lauri Laitinen showed an increase in bronchial fibroblast counts in steroid-treated patients. These data raise an issue regarding the effect on the tissue integrity on long-term steroid treatment of the airway. This is not a caution, but the issue should be recognized and studied.

DR. MCFADDEN: Why is tissue repair different in asthma as compared with other airway diseases such as chronic bronchitis, cystic fibrosis, and/or bronchiestasis. In these illnesses, airway destruction, occlusion of the lumen, and thickening of the walls occur. These are not features of asthma. Would you care to speculate as to why these differences exist?

DR. GAULDIE: It is not clear what events are necessary to induce a chronic response versus an acute repair response. We believe that it is crucial that genes such as TGF-β are switched on at some point in the response in order for the chronic change such as fibrosis to occur. We know that acute/repair responses do not show TGF-β expression in the tissue, but chronic responses do. As to what cells are involved and/or the cascade of cytokines necessary, that is not clear and is only now being investigated in asthmatic tissue.

DR. A. LAITINEN: Is there any difference in the productive capacity between these different types of fibroblasts especially concerning collagen synthesis?

DR. GAULDIE: We have not tested this, but I think it should be feasible with the techniques now available.

DR. BARNES: The relative lack of fibrosis in asthma is striking in comparison with other inflammatory diseases of the airways which involve neutrophils. This may suggest that eosinophils may protect against fibrosis. It would be of interest to study the interaction between eosinophil and neutrophil products with fibroblasts?

References

1. Roche WR, Williams JH, Beasley R, et al. Subepithelial fibrosis in the bronchi of asthmatics. Lancet 1989; 1:520-523.
2. Roche WR. Fibroblasts and asthma. Clin Exp Allergy 1991; 21:545-548.
3. Roche WR. Fibroblasts and extracellular matrix in bronchial asthma. In: Busse WW, Holgate ST, eds. Asthma and Rhinitis, Boston: Blackwell Scientific, 1995:554-562.
4. Jeffery PK, Godfrey RW, Ädelroth E, et al. Effects of treatment on airway inflammation and thickening of basement membrane reticular collagen in asthma. A quantitative light and electron microscope study. Am Rev Respir Dis 1992; 145:890-899.
5. Laitinen LA, Laitinen A, Haahtela T, et al. A comparative study of the effects of an inhaled corticosteroid, budesonide, and a β_2-agonist, terbutaline, on airway inflammation in newly diagnosed asthma: A randomized, double-blind, parallel-group controlled trial. J Allergy Clin Immunol 1992; 90:32-42.
6. Brewster CE, Howart PH, Djukarovic R, et al. Myofibroblasts and subepithelial fibrosis in bronchial asthma. Am J Respir Cell Mol Biol 1990; 3:507-511.
7. Trigg CJ, Manolitsas ND, Wang J, et al. Placebo-controlled immunopathologic study of four months of inhaled corticosteroids in asthma. Am J Respir Crit Care Med 1994; 150:17-22.
8. Altraja A, Laitinen A, Kämpe M, et al. Inhaled budesonide has no effect on the distribution of collagen types III and VII in bronchial epithelial basement membrane in allergic asthmatics (abstr). Am J Respir Crit Car Med 1994; 149:A632.
9. Laitinen LA, Laitinen A, Heino M, et al. Eosinophilic airway inflammation during exacerbation of asthma and its treatment with inhaled corticosteroid. Am Rev Respir Dis 1991; 143:423-427.
10. Leitman DC, Benson SC, Johnson LK, et al. Glucocorticoids stimulate collagen and noncollagen protein synthesis in cultured vascular smooth muscle cells. J Cell Biol 1984; 98:541-549.
11. Järveläinen H, Halme T, Ronnemaa T, et al. Effect of cortisol on the proliferation

and protein synthesis of human aortic smooth muscle cells in culture. Acta Med Scand 1982; 660(Suppl):114–122.

12. Poiani GJ, Tozzi CA, Thakker-Varia S, et al. Effect of glucocorticoids on collagen accumulation in pulmonary vascular remodelling in the rat. Am J Respir Crit Care Med 1994; 149:994–999.

13. Kāhāri V-M. Dexamethasone suppresses elastin gene expression in human skin fibroblasts in culture. Biochem Biophys Res Commun 1994; 201:1189–1196.

14. Sārnstrand B, Jeppsson A, Malmstróm A, et al. Effect of glucocorticoids on hyaluronic acid synthesis in vitro in human fibroblast-like cells from lung and skin. In: Hogg JC, Ellul-Micallef R, Brattsand R, eds. Glucocorticosteroids, Inflammation and Bronchial Hyperreactivity. Amsterdam: Excerpta Medica, 1985:157–166.

15. Ekblom M, Fässler R, Tomasisni-Johansson B, et al. Downregulation of tenascin expression by glucocorticoids in bone marrow stromal cells and in fibroblasts. J Cell Biol 1993; 123:1037–1045.

16. Laitinen A, Altraja A, Kämpe M, et al. Treatment with inhaled budesonide and tenascin expression in bronchial mucosa of allergic asthmatics (abstr). Am J Respir Crit Care Med 1994; 149:A942.

17. Oliver N, Newby RT, Furche LT, et al. Regulation of fibronectin biosynthesis by glucocorticoids in human fibrosarcoma and normal fibroblasts. Cell 1983; 33:287–296.

18. Gauldie J, Torry D, Cox G, et al. Effector function of tissue structural cells in inflammation. In: Holgate ST, Austen KF, Lichtenstein LM, Kay AB, eds. Asthma: Physiology, Immunopharmacology, and Treatment. London: Academic Press, 1993:211–225.

19. Tremblay GM, Jordana M, Gauldie J, et al. Fibroblasts as effector cells in fibrosis. In: Phan SH, Thrall RS, eds. Pulmonary Fibrosis. New York: Marcel Dekker, 1994: 541–577.

20. Kirpalani H, Gauldie J. Differentiation and effector function of pulmonary fibroblasts. In Busse WW, Holgate ST, eds. Asthma and Rhinitis, Boston: Blackwell Scientific, 1995:539–553.

21. Tobler A, Meier R, Seitz M, et al. Glucocorticoids downregulate gene expression of GM-CSF, NAP-1/IL-8, and IL-6, but not of M-CSF in human fibroblasts. Blood 1992; 79:45–51.

22. Cox G, Ohtoshi T, Vancheri C, et al. Promotion of eosinophil survival by human bronchial epithelial cells and its modulation by steroids. Am J Respir Cell Mol Biol 1991; 4:525–531.

23. Mukaida N, Zachariae CC, Gusella GL, et al. Dexamethasone inhibits the induction of monocyte chemotactic-activating factor production by IL-1 or tumor necrosis factor. J Immunol 1991; 146:1212–1215.

24. Ponta H, Cato AC, Herrlich P, et al. Interference of pathway specific transcription factors. Biochim Biophys Acta 1992; 1129:255–261.

25. Ray A, LaForge KS, Sehgal PB, et al. On the mechanisms for efficient repression of the IL-6 promoter by glucocorticoids: Enhancement of TATA box, and RNA start site (Inr motif) occlusion. Mol Cell Biol 1990; 10:5736–5746.

26. Ray A, Prefontaine KE. Physical association and functional antagonism between the p65 subunit of transcription factor Nf-κB and the glucocorticoid receptor. Proc Natl Acad Sci USA 1994; 91:752–756.

27. Zitnik RJ, Whiting NL, Elias JA, et al. Glucocorticoid inhibition of interleukin-1-induced interleukin 6 production by human lung fibroblasts: Evidence for transcriptional and post-transcriptional regulatory mechanisms. Am J Respir Cell Mol Biol 1994; 10:643–650.

28. Khalil N, Whitman C, Zuo LI, et al. Regulation of alveolar macrophage transforming growth factor-β secretion by corticosteroids in bleomycin-induced pulmonary inflammation in the rat. J Clin Invest 1993; 92:1812–1818.

29. Andres JL, Ronnstrand L, Cheifetz S, et al. Purification of the transforming growth factor-β (TGF-β) binding proteoglycan β-glycan. J Biol Chem 1991; 266:23282–23287.

30. Border WA, Noble NA, Yamamoto T, et al. Natural inhibitor of transforming growth factor-β protects against scarring in experimental kidney disease. Nature 1992; 360:361–364.

31. Folkman J, Klagsburn M, Sasse J, et al. A heparin-binding angiogenic protein—basic fibroblastic growth factor—is stored within basement membrane. Am J Pathol 1988; 130:393–400.

32. Saksela O, Moscatelli D, Sommer A, et al. Endothelial cell-derived heparin sulfate binds basic fibroblast growth factor and protects it from proteolytic degradation. J Cell Biol 1988; 107:743–751.

33. Yamaguchi Y, Mann DM, Ruoslahti E, et al. Negative regulation of transforming growth factor-β by the proteoglycan decorin. Nature 1990; 346:281–284.

34. Skalli O, Schurch W, Seemayer T, et al. Myofibroblasts from diverse pathologic settings are heterogeneous in their content of actin isoforms and intermediate filament proteins. Lab Invest 1989; 60:275–285.

35. Sappino AP, Schurch W, Gabbiani G. Differentiation repertoire of fibroblastic cells: Expression of cytoskeletal proteins as a marker of phenotypic modulation. Lab Invest 1990; 63:144–161.

36. Zhang K, Rekhter MD, Gordon D, et al. Myofibroblasts and their role in lung collagen gene expression during pulmonary fibrosis. A combined immunohistochemical and in situ hybridization study. Am J Pathol 1994; 145:114–125.

37. Schmitt-Gräff A, Desmoulière A, Gabbiani G. Heterogeneity of myofibroblast phenotypic features: An example of fibroblastic cell plasticity. Virchows Archiv 1994; 425:3–24.

38. Jordana M, Schulman J, McSharry C, et al. Heterogeneous proliferative characteristics of human adult lung fibroblast lines and clonally-derived fibroblasts from control and fibrotic tissue. Am Rev Respir Dis 1988; 137:579–584.

39. Gauldie J, Jordana M, Cox G, et al. Fibroblasts and other structural cells in airway inflammation. Am Rev Respir Dis 1992; 145:S14–S17.

40. Tremblay GM, Chakir J, Dubé J, et al. Smooth muscle actin expression by myofibroblasts from bronchial tissue of asthmatic subjects (abstr). Am J Respir Crit Care Med 1995; 151:A541.

41. Särnstrand B, Westergren-Thorsson G, Sime PJ, et al. Fibroblast clones differs in

proliferation rates and proteoglycan production. Am J Respir Crit Care Med 1995; 151:A560.

42. Torry DJ, Richards CD, Podor TJ, et al. Anchorage-independent colony growth of pulmonary fibroblasts derived from fibrotic human lung tissue. J Clin Invest 1994; 93:1525–1532.
43. Torry DJ, Richards CD, Podor TJ, et al. Modulation of the anchorage-independent phenotype of human lung fibroblasts derived from fibrotic tissue following culture with retinoid and corticosteroid. Exp Lung Res. In press.
44. Vyalov SL, Gabbiani G, Kapanci Y, et al. Rat alveolar myofibroblasts acquire α-smooth muscle actin expression during bleomycin-induced pulmonary fibrosis. Am J Pathol 1993; 143:1754–1765.
45. Rubbia-Brandt L, Sappino A-P, Gabbiani G, et al. Locally applied GM-CSF induces the accumulation of a smooth actin containing myofibroblasts. Virchows Arch B Cell Pathol 1991; 60:73–82.
46. Mitchell JJ, Woodcock-Mitchell JL, Perry L, et al. In vitro expression of the α-smooth muscle actin isoform by rat lung mesenchymal cells: Regulation by culture condition and transforming growth factor-β. Am J Respir Cell Mol Biol 1993; 9:10–18.
47. Verbeek MM, Otto-Hölles J, Wesseling P, et al. Induction of α-smooth muscle actin expression in cultured human brain pericytes by transforming growth factor-β1. Am J Pathol 1994; 144:372–382.
48. Ohno I, Lea R, Finotto S, et al. Granulocyte/macrophage colony-stimulating factor (GM-CSF) gene expression by eosinophils in nasal polyposis. Am J Respir Cell Mol Biol 1991; 5:505–510.
49. Ohno I, Lea RG, Flanders KC, et al. Eosinophils in chronically inflamed human upper airway tissues express transforming growth factor β1 gene (TGFβ1). J Clin Invest 1992; 89:1662–1668.
50. Tremblay GM, Nonaka M, Sarnstrand B, et al. Myofibroblast differentiation in nasal polyposis: Downregulation by topical steroids (abstr). Am J Respir Crit Care Med 1994; 149:A632.

9

Airway Microcirculation, Epithelium, and Glucocorticoids

CARL G. A. PERSSON

University Hospital
Lund, Sweden

I. Introduction

At the turn of the 19th century, detailed histological studies and direct in vivo observations had demonstrated a profuse superficial microcirculation in the nose and the bronchi, specifically including the asthmatic airways (reviewed in ref. 1). It was also a vascular hypothesis of asthma that already then prompted the first successful trial of a steroid drug in this disease (2). This original work was carried out by Solis-Cohen (3) (Fig. 1).

The mucosal output in inflammatory airway diseases consists of cells, secretions, and material emanating directly from the subepithelial microcirculation. The latter involves microvascular-epithelial exudation of "bulk" plasma. Luminal entry of plasma now emerges as a specific physiological response that potentially may show the distribution, the intensity, and the time course of significant inflammatory processes in the airways. Mucosal exudation of plasma occurs in allergic, occupational, and infectious airway diseases as well as in airways subjected to challenge with inflammatory agents (4–9). As might be expected, glucocorticoid treatment of asthma and rhinitis is associated with markedly reduced microvascular-epithelial exudation of plasma. The anti-

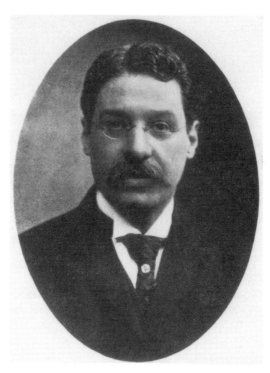

Figure 1 Solomon Solis-Cohen, M.D. (1857–1948). A Lecturer on Medicine and Therapeutics (Jefferson Medical College, Philadelphia, Pennsylvania) and Professor of Clinical Medicine, Solis-Cohen designed and delivered a course entitled "Therapeutic measures other than drugs" (1887–1890). He edited 11 volumes of *A System of Physiologic Therapeutics* (1901–1905). In between he published an intriguing report on the antiasthma effects of the oral intake of desiccated adrenals. Although not previously recognized as such, this report may well have been the original demonstration of the particular efficacy of steroid drugs in asthma (see text). (Kindly provided by F.B. Wagner, M.D. University Historian of the Thomas Jefferson University, Philadelphia, Pennsylvania.)

exudative effect alone may be a significant anti-inflammatory action, because the extravasated plasma harbors a richness in peptide mediators, cytokines, adhesive proteins, proteases, and immunoglobulins (Fig. 2). Plasma-derived effector solutes may, in fact, decide much of the molecular disease milieu in vivo.

This chapter first pays a tribute to Solomon Solis-Cohen. Then it deals with mechanisms and roles of microvascular-epithelial exudation of plasma in upper and lower airways. One consideration is whether the antiexudative effect of topical airway glucocorticoids reflects a direct microvascular antipermeability

Proteins	Adhesive Molecules (fibrinogen, fibronectin, etc.)
	Proteases - Antiproteases
	Cytokine Modulating Proteins
	Immunoglobulins
	Other
Cytokines	Growth factors (PDGF, IGF, TGF-β, etc.)
	Interleukins
	Several cytokines bound, carried, and targeted by
	α_2-macroglobulin and other plasma proteins
Peptides	Complement Fragments
	Bradykinins
	Fibrinolysis Peptides
	Other

Figure 2 Components of extravasated plasma.

action or whether the antiexudative efficacy of glucocorticoids is exclusively an indication of how effectively these drugs can inhibit the cellularly driven inflammatory process in the airways. This chapter also deals with the mucosal absorption ability, which may be abnormally low in airway disease despite the occurrence of epithelial shedding. Finally, recent experimental observations on the restitution of airway epithelium in the presence and absence of topical steroid drugs are reviewed. The focus throughout this chapter is on exploratory work carried out in vivo.

II. Treatment of Asthma by Oral Intake of Desiccated Adrenals

In an erudite essay, Solis-Cohen reported on the effects of the oral intake of "adrenal substance" in asthma (3). His account was based on long-term treatment involving at least 12 patients (another patient may well have been Solis-Cohen himself, because he suffered from both hay-fever and asthma). In an interesting piece of introduction, Solis-Cohen underscores that, "the balanced action of contending forces producing mobile or stable equilibrium, and the motion that takes place in the direction of an inferior force, are not merely problems of physics, but also of biology, and of that special branch of biology which deals with the disturbances we call disease."

Solis-Cohen soon reveals his focus: "We have not yet learned to realize the large part that the activities of the blood-vessels may take in determining symptomatology and lesions." Then we are being briefed about the complex pathology of asthma: "the immediate mechanism of the paroxysm is bronchial spasm" or "is dependent on irregular turgescence of the bronchial mucosa." He further houses "no doubt that in some cases turgescence of the bronchial mucosa is preceded, accompanied or succeeded by inflammatory or subinflammatory conditions, associated with exudation." Solis-Cohen lists a versatile range of associations with asthma including "nasal abnormalities" and "patients who are subject to urticaria". . . . "or who exhibit particular idiosyncrasies". . . . and concludes that, although the ultimate nature of the involved mechanisms remain unknown, "Clinically, however, the fault is found in the vascular taxis." Evidently Solis-Cohen was an astute clinical observer. He was also much influenced by the European school of thought represented by Stoerck, Cohnheim, Weber, and Curschman (see refs. 1 and 10), who saw asthma as a vascular disease with exudative inflammation. Solis-Cohen was most likely impressed by the good effect on the nasal passages that was produced by topical vasoconstrictor agents, with one of these agents being the then just available adrenal extract. No one, neither Solis-Cohen nor any of his colleagues, seems to have appreciated the possibility of a distinction between the active drug of a hydrophilic extract (adrenaline) and the drug that would be contained in the desiccated adrenal glands and that would be absorbed well after oral intake (steroids). Although unfortunate, this apparent mistake cannot diminish the original value of the clinical observations made and reported by Solis-Cohen.

Solis-Cohen states clearly that the adrenal substance cannot serve acutely "to cut short a paroxysm." "It has, however, been useful in averting the recurrence of paroxysms and in finally bringing about a state of freedom from fear of their recurrence." Solis-Cohen thus distinguishes this treatment that "provides control the the underlying condition" from "hyoscine" (an inhaled anticholinergic) that is "given for immediate control of paroxysms." He includes narrations on the effect of adrenal substance which agree so well with the current experience with the antiasthma steroid drugs: "The constant dyspnea first disappeared, the the paroxysmal nocturnal attacks became less frequent and less severe. Recovery was not rapid but was continuous." Solis-Cohen commendably finishes his essay with the following paragraph:

> What the active agent is and how much or how little of that active agent is absorbed, I must leave to laboratory students to determine. Clinically, I have watched closely and critically enough to satisfy myself that neither the susceptibility of patients to suggestion, nor the activity of the observer's imagination are sufficient in themselves to account for the whole of the results.

Owing to the confusion with adrenal extract by researchers, physicians, and, eventually, also by medical historians, Solis-Cohen's explicit challenge was to be unmet for several decades. It took 50 years before the good effect of purified steroids could be demonstrated in asthma (2). By then and for many additional years, Solis-Cohen's original work was forgotten, or it was interpreted to be one of the first demonstrations of the effect of adrenaline in asthma (2).

My tribute to Solis-Cohen in this chapter is prompted by three factors. Not only would he have carried out the original drug discovery work on the most important treatment principle in asthma (steroids). He also focused on the vascular aspects of this disease, and his work illustrates the importance of making innovative observations under complex in vivo conditions.

III. Focus on In Vivo Functions

The bulk of novel information on airway epithelium and vascular endothelium now emanates from studies employing reductive biological sciences approaches and cell culture techniques. However exciting and important, the novel molecular and cellular approaches may not always be applied with complete success unless the gross physiology and pathophysiology of the airway mucosa have first been well assessed. This caution may not be less in studies dealing with the actions of glucocorticoids, a class of compounds with exceedingly rich and complex pharmacological mechanisms. Somewhat conservatively the present chapter will, therefore, adhere to the experimental strategy of having the proper in vivo function established first. The point may be illustrated by several examples: After exploring, for almost 10 years, the structure-activity relationships of novel xanthine derivatives, including enprofylline, in various complex biosystems eventually including asthmatic subjects, it could be pragmatically demonstrated that antagonism of the physiological actions of adenosine should probably be avoided in asthma therapy, because it brought no good results but several side effects to xanthine drug therapy (cf. theophylline) (11,12). As a corollary, the role of adenosine as a mediator of asthma was also questioned (11–14). The in vivo data on enprofylline and other xanthines were disseminated at a time when isolated cell and receptor binding approaches had just produced a widely accepted paradigm maintaining that adenosine antagonism was the mechanism of action of theophylline, and further that adenosine was a major mediator of asthma (see ref. 14). The exploratory in vivo approach involving chemical structure-pharmacological activity observations thus clashed with concepts and language developed largely on the basis of more reductive biomedical research findings. Another example concerns a current paradigm stating that the airway barrier is abnormally pervious to inhaled molecules in asthma and rhinitis. In accord, reductive science approaches now provide mechanisms explaining how the perviousness is produced and also how glucocorticoids may act to prevent this result. At the same time, however, functional in vivo studies employing increasingly improved physiological methods (15) demonstrate that the absorption rate across the mucosa, if it is at all altered, may actually be decreased in allergic rhinitis and asthma (16–18). The present focus on "in vivo functions first" does not reduce the need for critical comparisons between animal and human findings. Recent concept testing has thus demonstrated that neurogenic inflammation (exudation), which is a major mechanism in guinea pig and rat airways, may not at all be present in human airways (19–21). Such observations may currently limit the interest in neurogenic exudation mechanisms. Equally, data emanating from studies of the interaction between glucocorticoids and the biology of neurogenic regulation of microvascular permeability may now be difficult to translate into human airway relevance.

It is difficult to discuss inflammation and anti-inflammatory actions without paying attention to the microcirculation-dependent milieu that characterizes the various tissue compartments in inflammation, defense, and repair. In airways subjected to inflammatory provocations and in airways where an inflammatory process is going on, extravasation of plasma, without molecular size restriction, may dramatically alter the composition of proteins, cytokines, and peptide mediators in the lamina propria, in the epithelial basement membrane, in the epithelium, and on the mucosal surface (see Fig.2). This microcirculation-plasma–derived molecular milieu would affect cellular and other inflammatory activities in ways which may be difficult to reproduce in vitro. (See also Section XI). The exuded plasma lays down important adhesive proteins such as fibronectin and fibrin(ogen). It provides proteases-antiproteases, binding proteins, and immunoglobulins. The extravasated bulk plasma contains many cytokines, including growth factors. Moreover, some of the plasma proteins, notably α_2-macroglobulin, are known to bind, carry, and target a wide variety of cytokines (22). The plasma-derived peptide mediators are not confined to the bradykinins. Fibrinolysis peptides, complement fragments, and numerous other biologically active molecules are dynamically produced by the extravasated protein systems in contact with airway tissue and surface components (see Fig. 2). In studies of the pharmacology of inflammatory processes and, equally, in studies of the pharmacology of defense and repair mechanisms, the complex as yet only partly understood contributions from the microcirculation need to be considered.

IV. Exudation of Plasma as an Airway End–Organ Response

The classic signs of inflammation, rubor, dolor, calor, tumor, and functio laesa seem of limited help in identifying the active inflammatory process in the airways. Rubor may simply characterize an airway embarrassed by irritants; that is, such factors that increase blood flow but do not produce inflammation (Fig. 3). It is notable that the airway mucosal blood flow is already so rich under

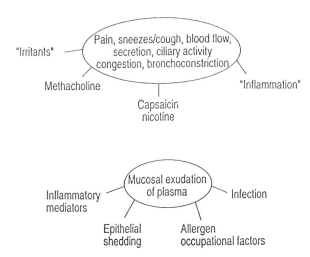

Figure 3 Several airway end-organ responses can be associated with inflammation. However, most of these responses are nonspecific and, as indicated above, are also readily induced by simple irritants, which merely evoke transient neural activity. These nonspecific responses may indirectly be inhibited by topical airway steroids as a consequence of the anti-inflammatory effects of these drugs. (Below) Mucosal exudation of plasma is singled out as a response that is a specific inflammatory response. In human airways, neither irritants nor methacholine-like challenges will produce the exudation response. Allergen, occupational agents, viral infection, epithelial shedding, select inflammatory mediators, proteases, and cytokines are required to produce airway mucosal exudation of plasma. Airway steroids inhibit release of the vasoactive agents, and, in addition, may reduce the exudative responsiveness of the mucosal microcirculation.

baseline conditions that moderate changes in flow may not be critical to airway end-organ functions in inflammation. This possibility is supported by the observation that a potent vasoconstrictor, such as oximetazoline, was completely devoid on inhibitory effects of inflammatory stimulus-induced plasma exudation in human nasal airways (23). Although glucocorticoids are known to produce vasoconstriction in the poorly blood-perfused skin, studies in human nasal airways suggest that glucocorticoids may not significantly reduce mucosal blood flow (24).

Dolor and calor, that is, pain and heat, may not be characteristic features of the inflammatory condition in asthma and rhinitis. "Tumor", in contrast, is clearly important. However, what is behind the visible swelling? The airway mucosa may be swollen owing to intravascular pooling of blood as in the venous sinuses of the nose. This kind of thickening is abrogated by sympathomimetic α-receptor agonists. Long-term treatment with topical steroids also inhibits the congestion-induced nasal blockade (25), but whether this result to any extent reflects a direct vasoconstrictor action of the drugs now remains highly speculative. The "swelling" that is observed through a bronchoscope may be composed of several factors. Congestion may contribute, but its importance is not known. Structural changes with increased numbers of vessels and cells and the increased presence of extracellular matrix molecules, exuded from the microcirculation and secreted by cells, may well contribute. Once established, airway structural changes may not readily be affected by drugs. Early institution of steroid therapy in childhood and adult asthma has been demonstrated to improve the disease significantly more than if steroid therapy starts at later stages of the asthmatic disease process (26,27). This important information has been interpreted to suggest that steroids may stop ongoing remodeling mechanisms but may not reverse a chronically altered airway back to normal.

A common bronchial mechanism, which may be difficult to distinguish from tumefaction, is simple bronchoconstriction that moves a normal or thickened mucosa, regularly or irregularly, inward to reduce the patency of the airway lumen. The bronchoconstriction may not be directly affected by steroid treatment. At least it was observed in a rat study that 3 weeks' continuous treatment with budesonide changed neither the sensitivity nor the reactivity of airway smooth muscle to constrictor or relaxant agents (28). The most common interpretation of the cause of airway swelling is edema, which simply means that the extravascular tissue holds abnormaly large amounts of fluid. Edema is also a widely accepted basic characteristic of asthmatic airways, although its presence in asthma is more based on histological pictures than on irrefutable quantitative research. Considerable or sustained extravasation of plasma is normally expected to produce tissue edema. This may occur in chronic inflammation, but the acute mucosal challenge-induced increase in vascular permeability, causing extravasation of plasma from the superficial microcirculation, may not produce mucosal edema but may rather result in luminal entry of bulk plasma (see Section V). As discussed in more detail below, glucocorticoids inhibit chronic plasma exudation in asthma and rhinitis.

Julius Cohnheim once stated that inflammation is exclusively an in vivo phenomenon occurring in tissues with an active microcirculation (see ref. 5). In airway disease, this would primarily mean involvement of the profuse capillary-venular plexus that resides in the lamina propria sometimes going as superficially as to penetrate part of the epithelial basement membrane. This mucosal end-organ supplies not only inflammatory cells, it also extravasates bulk plasma with its protein-peptide effector systems. Cohnheim clearly saw that extravasation of cells and plasma can occur independently of each other, although both utilize paraendothelial routes in postcapillary venules when leaving the circulation (29,30) (Fig. 4). The notion that plasma extravasation in living tissues is a sine qua non to inflammation was championed by Spector,

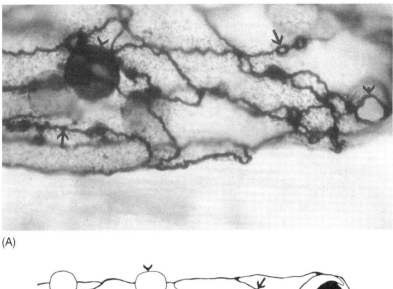

(A)

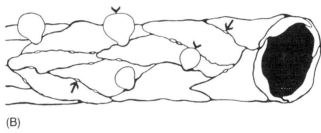

(B)

Figure 4 (A) Light micrograph of a tracheal whole-mount preparation where endothelial cell borders in the mucosal microcirculation (venules) have been visualized by a silver staining technique. These venules are actively involved in extravasation of plasma and leukocytes, respectively. (B) The morphological correlates to the increased vascular permeability are distinct sites of endothelial cell separation represented by small silver dots (arrow). At separate interendothelial sites, leukocytes are adhering and moving across the venular wall (these sites emerge as silver rings; arrowhead). (The graph and the drawing were provided by Jonas Erjefält; see also refs 29 and 30.)

Willoughby, and others in the 1950s and the 1960s (see ref. 5). Even today plasma extravasation and, in the airways, mucosal exudation of plasma may deserve attention as a breaking point demonstrating that cellular and other mechanisms of inflammation have reached the activity level where tissue end-organs become significantly affected (31). Plasma exudation also differs from many other airway end-organ responses by being rather specific to inflammation (31) (see Fig. 3). Bronchial tone, dilatation of venous sinuses, airway secretion, and blood flow are all increased both by inflammation and by simple irritant type of provocations, which also evoke neural reflex activity. Among the most powerful airway reflexes are coughs and sneezes, which both may be reduced by effective anti-inflammatory therapy (25,32). But, again, these reflexes are not exclusive to inflammation, nor are they always induced by inflammation.

The final classic sign of inflammation, "functio laesa," is true in the general sense that asthmatic airway inflammation may be a major cause of breathing difficulties. However, in more specific terms, this sign may be difficult to reconcile with most cases of asthma and rhinitis where hyperfunction rather than hypofunction may be prevalent and contribute to the phenomenon of nonspecific airway hyperresponsiveness. In addition, specific hyperresponsiveness of individual mucosal end-organs such as the secretory apparatus, the sensory innervation, and, particularly, the microcirculation itself may develop in inflammatory airway diseases (31). Nonspecific airway hyperresponsiveness in asthma and rhinitis is attenuated by glucocorticoid treatment (25,32). However, little is so far known about the effects of these drugs on the increased responsiveness that is expressed by individual mucosal end-organs of the airways (31).

V. Exudation Pathways

The acute plasma exudation response to airway mucosal challenges involves a series of events all occurring within minutes after challenge (1,5,29,31). By indirect, cellular release mechanisms, the inflammatory challenge results in increased mucosal tissue levels of vasoactive agents. Such an agent itself may constitute a directly acting challenge. The vascular permeability-increasing agents act on the venular wall endothelium that is equipped with cell surface receptors for various mediators. Through stimulation, the cell to cell contact is lost at distinct points in the walls of the postcapillary venules (29). The mechanism of interendothelial gap formation has been widely accepted as a contractile event, but the gaps might also be produced by reduced adhesion along tiny stretches of the endothelial cell-cell contact lines (29) (see Fig. 4). Through these gaps or holes in the venular wall, nonsieved plasma is moved by the hydrostatic pressure gradient (about 20 cm H_2O) that exists between the venules and the extravascular tissue. The extravasation is a dramatic event that locally abolishes the colloid osmotic pressure gradient between the microvessels and the tissue. It seems clear that the venular endothelial cell is an important target for experimental compounds and drugs that produce antiexudative effects by direct antipermeability mechanisms. In animal studies, acute steroid treatment may very markedly produce such antipermeability effects (32), whereas in human airways, longer term treatment appears to be required to reduce the exudative responsiveness of the subepithelial microcirculation (see later).

During the first 10–20 seconds after challenge the airway, the lamina propria is flooded with the plasma exudate. Apparently unhindered, the exudate then passes through the epithelial basement membrane and further up between epithelial cells that normally are separated at the base. At the apical pole circumference, the epithelial cells are tightly connected. However, not even the tight junctions of an intact epithelial lining are significant obstacles to the further flux of exudate into the airway lumen (reviewed in refs. 1, 31, and 33). The luminal entry of plasma may be described as a self-sustained process occurring as long as sufficient amounts of plasma press on the basolateral aspects of epithelial cells (see below). This mechanism appears to exclude the epithelial barrier function as an important direct target for the antiexudative effect of glucocorticoids (Fig. 5) or other drugs. The bulk plasma that is moved to the mucosal surface is not identical to circulating plasma. Promptly after extravasation, several protein systems of the blood plasma will be activated generating a great variety of peptides and oligoproteins. Enzymes and other factors involved in the local production of plasma-derived mediators may in theory be affected by glucocorticoids. However, in a study demonstrating the inhibition of bradykinin levels in allergic rhinitis (6), this action could be fully explained by a global antiexudative effect of the glucocorticoid drug. By preventing the

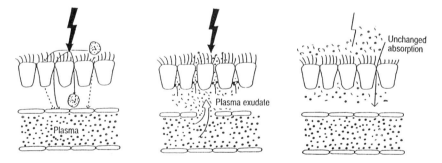

Figure 5 Challenge with allergen, leukotriene-type mediators, and several other proinflammatory factors produces dose-dependent extravasation, lamina propria distribution, and luminal entry of "bulk" plasma. This process may occur without disrupting the epithelial lining and without increasing the absorption ability of the airway mucosa. Thus, in defense and inflammation, all plasma protein systems, irrespective of molecular size, may appear on the surface of the intact airway mucosa. In inflamed airways, topical steroids inhibit the plasma exudation process through inhibition of inflammatory cells. Steroids may also reduce the microvascular exudative responsiveness through direct effects on the venular endothelium (see text).

extravasation of all plasma proteins, including kininogens (substrates for kinin formation), glucocorticoid treatment would inhibit the formation of plasma-derived active agents in the airways.

The extravasated plasma will also have excellent opportunities to interact with interesting molecules that are present in the lamina propria. For example, several plasma proteins, from the 70,000-Da albumin to the 700,000-Da α_2-macroglobulin (22), may be avid binders of different molecules such as mediators, cytokines, and drugs. The tissue flooding is, therefore, not merely a passive lamina propria lavage. The extravasated plasma may offer specific piggy-back riding to the airway surface (1). In airway disease conditions, simple histamine challenges, which produce graded exudations of bulk plasma, may, through this action, also increase dose dependently airway lavage fluid levels of select cytokines, such as interleukin (IL-6) (34), that are known to be bound by α_2-macroglobulin and other plasma proteins. A potential lamina propria lavage (1) induced by the plasma exudation process may have to be considered when bronchial and nasal lavage fluids, or biopsies, are examined in studies of disease mechanisms and anti-inflammatory drug effects.

Erjefält et al. (35), employing colloidal gold (5 nm in diameter) as plasma tracer, have recently observed that the plasma exudate is moved between all epithelial cells in the area and all around each cell. Hence, the burden on each unit length of cell junction would also be minute at pronounced rates of exudation of bulk plasma. This finding tallies with previous observations demonstrating a noninjurious nature of the mucosal exudation process (reviewed in refs. 1 and 36). Based on these data generated in animal and human airways, luminal entry of plasma was forwarded as a first-line mucosal defense mechanism of major importance (36). A novel mechanism has also been found and suggested to explain how the extravasated bulk plasma may pass through epithelial tight junctions (37,38). Using intact airway tube preparations mounted in organ baths that allow separate regulation of mucosal and serosal bathing fluids, it has thus been demonstrated that a slightly increased hydrostatic pressure load (<5 cm H_2O) on the basolateral aspects of the epithelial lining cells is sufficient for moving macromolecular solutes to the mucosal surface. Indeed, this process is reversible and repeatable much in the same way as in vivo exudation evoked by challenge with histamine-type mediators. The epithelial junctions evidently yield and close so that luminal entry of macromolecules occurs without being associated with or followed by increased mucosal absorption of polar solutes (reviewed in ref. 33). It is perhaps surprising that this noninjurious epithelial mechanism of passage of bulk plasma has remained undetected by physiologists, who rather have seen luminal entry of plasma as a mechanism of epithelial damage (se ref. 33). The hydraulic epithelial mechanism for transmission of large solutes into the airway lumen is not affected by the presence of exudative agents or antiexudative drugs in the organ bath (38). It thus appears that the plasma exudate itself, by its distribution and by its localized hydrostatic pressure influence, opens valve-like paracellular pathways for its luminal entry (see Fig. 5). The ease by which extravasated plasma enters the airway lumen is underscored by the observation that inflammatory stimulus-induced exudation of plasma in the guinea-pig tracheal mucosa occurred without any detectible increase in the regional lymph protein transport (39).

Taken together the experimental data indicate that the active physiological and pharmacological regulation of mucosal exudation of plasma takes place at the level of the microvascular wall. This is the site where inflammatory agents produce the interendothelial holes that govern the whole airways exudation process. It seems functional that mediators and drugs shall not act on the epithelial lining cells to regulate selectively the epithelial passage of plasma into the lumen. A tightening effect on the epithelium in this respect would, in fact, not be a desirable drug action, because it would increase the tendency of edema formation in the airway mucosa.

VI. Acute Challenge–Induced Exudation

A nonspecific contractile and secretory mediator such as acetylcholine and its analogues (e.g., methacholine, carbachol) are without exudative effects in the airways (1,5,7). Furthermore, irritants such as nicotine and capsaicin, which evoke strong neurogenic responses, are without exudative effects in human nasal airways (19–21). This latter observation is in sharp contrast to findings in guinea pig airways, where agents such as capsaicin produce pronounced mucosal exudation of plasma (40). An important inference is that plasma exudation in human airways is more specific to inflammation than in rodent airways, because simple neural reflex mechanisms may not produce this response. Mediators such as histamine, bradykinin, and leukotriene D_4 produce graded exudative responses over a wide range of concentrations in both guinea pig and human airways (see refs. 31 and 36). Select cytokines, proteases, fibrinolysis, peptides, and other agents may also induce plasma exudation. The exudative response is not only dose dependent, it is also fully reversible and reproducible within short periods of time (31). These characteristics of histamine-type mediators have been utilized to assess the vascular antipermeability effects of drugs such as glucocorticoids given prior to challenge with the mediator. Animal experiments have thus demonstrated that glucocorticoids significantly inhibit extravasation within 30–60 min after drug application (see ref. 32). These data have received attention, particularly since the antipermeability action is sustained for several hours irrespective of whether the glucocorticoid drug has been washed away or not. Indeed, the latter observation has quickened the intriguing hypothesis of a hit and run mode of action of inhaled airway steroids.

The human nasal mucosa lends itself to airway-specific, well-controlled challenge and lavage studies in situ. To take advantage of these possibilities, a nasal pool technique has been developed (15). Using a compressible nasal pool device, it is possible fill the entire ipsilateral nasal cavity with fluid and solutes. A large airway mucosal surface area can thus be exposed to defined concentrations of agents and tracers. After a selected mucosal exposure time, the pool fluid may, almost quantitatively, be recovered into the device. Thus, the exposed mucosal surface is also gently lavaged by the nasal pool fluid, providing the opportunity to sample mucosal indices selectively from the area of interest. This gentle lavage procedure can be carried out numerous times in sequence without causing undue changes in mucosal function. The technique also allows exposure of the same airway mucosal surface area at repeated provocations. It has not been possible to attain similarly controlled experimental conditions in human tracheobronchial airways. However, many mechanisms of the airway mucosa in health and disease can be examined in the nose and the findings may be extrapolated to the lower airways (31).

Using the nasal pool device, Greiff et al. (15) have demonstrated graded exudative effects of different mucosal surface concentrations of histamine. Between 20 µg/ml and 2000 µg/ml this amine produces 5-fold to more than 100-fold increases in lavage fluid levels of plasma proteins (albumin to α_2-macroglobulin). After a clinical dose of budesonide or placebo had been administered to the ipsilateral nasal cavity, a low exudative concentration of histamine (40 µg/ml) was employed as challenge at hourly intervals. It was thought that the threshold stimulus level that was thus employed would provide sensitive conditions under which any vascular antipermeability action of applied glucocorticoids should be readily revealed. However, in these experiments, topical steroid treatment completely lacked antiexudative effects (41), suggesting that the previous findings in animal airways, demonstrating acute inhibition by steroids of mediator-induced vascular permeability, cannot easily be translated to human airways. If confirmed in studies involving patients with asthma, these novel human airway data question the therapeutic relevance of the acute antipermeability effect of steroids. They also remove part of the experimental basis for the hypothesis of a hit and run action of topical airway steroids.

In a study involving 42 healthy subjects, Greiff et al. (42) examined the effects of prolonged steroid treatment on histamine-induced mucosal exudation of plasma. Placebo and budesonide (100 µg per nasal cavity twice daily) were given to parallel groups for 3 weeks in a double-blind design. Nasal challenges with isotonic saline and histamine (40 and 400 µg/ml) were carried out, using the nasal-pool technique, before and late into the treatment periods. Lavage fluids levels of α_2-macroglobulin were measured as an index of mucosal exudation of bulk plasma. Histamine produced concentration-dependent exudation before as well as after treatment with either placebo or budesonide. However, the responsiveness to histamine was somewhat reduced by the steroid. In contrast to acute treatment, these data indicate that sustained budesonide treatment reduces the microvascular exudative responsiveness to histamine in human airways. Since maintenance therapy with topical airway steroids attenuates the microvascular permeability response to inflammatory mediators, inhibition of plasma exudation in airway diseases by these drugs may reflect both a direct microvascular antipermeability effect and inhibitory effects on inflammatory cells that, if not inhibited, release vasoactive factors into the airway tissue. Luminal entry of bulk plasma may be a major mucosal defence mechanism that neutralizes offending agents on the airway surface even before they penetrate into the tissue (36). It is important, therefore, that the ability of the airway microcirculation to respond with exudation of plasma will not be lost in steroid-treated airways. Although the exudative responsiveness was reduced (42), the 3 weeks' treatment with a large topical dose of budesonide did not completely prevent the plasma exudation response, not even that produced by a low concentration of histamine (42).

VII. Microvascular-Epithelial Exudation of Plasma in Late-Phase Responses

Allergen challenge in subjects with allergic airway disease may produce both immediate and late-phase plasma exudation responses (5). Similarly, in sensitized guinea pigs, allergen challenge produces dual plasma exudation responses (43). (Neurogenic exudation is not involved in the allergic response even of the guinea pig airways.) If the allergen challenge is given to the whole guinea pig lung, involving also the peripheral parenchymal tissue, the late-phase exudation appears to be sustained for about 20 hr (44). If only the large tracheobronchial airway is challenged, the immediate, airway-specific exudation phase is over in about an hour. Then follows a late airway exudation phase that peaks about 5 hr after challenge and then fades off (43). Single-dose glucocorticoid treatment prevents the late-phase exudation responses in guinea pigs (43,45) and humans (5,46). Inhibition of the late-phase response may be associated with glucocorticoid-induced inhibition of eosinophil accumulation in the airways, but any causal interrelationship between these two events has not been demonstrated. Effects on the late-phase exudation in guinea pig large airways may potentially predict the clinical efficacy of glucocorticoid compounds. Thus, a clinically effective drug such as budesonide is effective in this model. In contrast, tipredane, although a potent steroid receptor binder, seems to be without significant effects both clinically and in the guinea pig tracheobronchial late-phase exudation system (45). By prolonged treatment with topical steroids also, the immediate exudation and obstruction response to allergen challenge is blunted (44). A contributory mechanism may be the reduced microvascular responsiveness that is produced by repeated administration of airway glucocorticoids over several weeks (42).

Differing from allergens, the occupational small molecular weight chemical toluenediisocyanate (TDI) also produces a strong and sustained plasma exudation response in airways that have not previously been exposed to TDI and thus have not been sensitized to this reactive agent. Within a wide dose range, 3 nl to 30 μl, TDI produces dose-dependent plasma exudation into guinea pig tracheobronchial airways of previously unexposed guinea pigs (47). These doses applied restrictedly on the large tracheobronchial airways of guinea pigs may be compared with the accepted exposure level which corresponds to a daily human body burden of about 15 μl TDI. The acute TDI-induced sustained plasma exudation response in nonsensitized guinea pigs peaks 5 hrs after challenge and continues for about 15 additional hours. In sharp contrast to the allergen challenge-induced late-phase exudation, the acute and sustained TDI-induced response is completely insensitive to pretreatment with glucocorticoids irrespective of whether these drugs are given topically or systemically. This does not mean that TDI produces such toxic and injurious effects that would be far beyond pharmacological modulation. On the contrary, the plasma exudation response to the first TDI exposure in guinea pig large airways is readily preventable by pretreatment with select experimental compounds (48). These novel molecules thus exhibit anti-inflammatory properties that are additional to the range of pharmacological actions produced by glucocorticoids. It is not yet known whether "anti-TDI-inflammation" compounds have a therapeutic utility in the treatment of occupational asthma or other inflammatory airway diseases.

Guinea pigs that receive repeated challenges with 3 nl of TDI, applied restrictedly on the large tracheobronchial airways, develop an increased inflammatory responsiveness to TDI (49). Thus, challenge with exceedingly low doses of TDI (0.3 nl) in the sensitized animals is associated with pronounced eosinophilia (45) and a marked and sustained exudative response. This TDI-induced plasma exudation response, in contrast to that observed in nonsensitized animals, is inhibited by glucocorticoid pretreatment (45,49). It has also been demonstrated that exposure to TDI in patients with occupational asthma produces a late-phase response that encompasses a plasma exudation process (46). The TDI challenge-induced plasma exudation in these patients is inhibited by pretreatment with inhaled glucocorticoids, whereas chromones are without effect (46).

VIII. Plasma Exudation in Disease

Plasma exudation in inflammatory airway diseases was first demonstrated through determination of plasma proteins in sputum samples obtained in asthma and chronic bronchitis. Almost equally early it was observed that steroid treatment significantly reduces the sputum level of different plasma indices (5). Interestingly, the inhibition of exudation seems to occur without concomitant reduction of sputum levels of secretory indices. Indeed, the latter may increase along with reduced sputum volume (5). The relatively poor antisecretory effect of glucocorticosteroids adds to a long list of significant qualitative differences between airway secretory and exudative processes (reviewed in refs. 33 and 50) and support the notion that the plasma exudation response may reflect airway inflammation better than other physiological end-organ responses in the airways. A further aspect is the possibility that the presence of luminal plasma exudate is subject to circadian rhythmicity. In coronavirus inoculation-induced common cold, the plasma-derived proteins on the nasal surface was about 20-fold greater during late night and early morning hours than during daytime and evening hours (51). It is not known to what extent the increase in plasma exudates on the airway surface is due to decreased removal or to an increased exudation rate. Irrespective of the cause, it may be particularly important to reduce plasma exudation during the night to prevent the accumulation of adverse amounts of exudate and its derived agents in both upper and lower airways.

Albumin is usually the only plasma protein that has been analyzed in the numerous bronchoalveolar lavage fluids (BALFs) obtained from asthmatic lungs. However, BALF levels of albumin alone may not always be a useful indicator of the plasma exudation process (50). Indeed, it has now been demonstrated in studies of the acute response to allergen challenge that BALF albumin may be unchanged, whereas large plasma proteins, such as fibrinogen and α_2-macroglobulin, are significantly increased (9,52). Such a result could even be expected: The inflammatory stimulus-induced luminal entry of plasma is almost a bulk flux of proteins with little size restriction (1,31,50) and, differing from albumin, the much larger plasma proteins are normally present in low concentrations. Additional confounding aspects include the fact that BALF contains material that has accumulated on the surface for variable and unknown periods of time, and the fact that BALF variably samples both airway and alveolar lining surface material. This latter aspect may pose a general problem in as much as asthma is an airway and not a pulmonary disease. Nevertheless, in analyzing several proteins in BALF, Van de Graaf et al. (8) have demonstrated that 6 weeks' treatment with inhaled budesonide significantly reduces plasma exudation in chronic asthma. By determination of a large plasma protein (fibrinogen) and a plasma-derived mediator (bradykinin) in nasal lavage fluids, Svensson et al. (6) have also demonstrated inhibition of plasma exudation by budesonide in seasonal allergic rhinitis during several weeks of natural pollen exposure.

Airway glucocorticoids may combine a potent anti-inflammatory pharmacology with little effects on airway mucosal defense (53). A complex treatment regimen involving topical and systemic steroid treatment thus did not seem to affect the plasma exudation indices of airways in patients with rhinovirus inoculation–induced common cold (54). A lack of antiexudative effects in acute common cold as well as the lack of effect at the first exposure to TDI (49) can be interpreted as an inability of steroids to prevent plasma exudation when it is expressed as a defense mechanism at acute events (36). Similarly, steroids may not reduce the accumulation and activation of neutrophils and eosinophils in airway defense and repair (55), and even in vitro steroids may have little effects on the neutrophils (56). The pharmacology of airway steroid drugs may thus involve a balance between the potent effects on inflammation on one hand and little interference with defense and repair on the other hand. Long-term treatment with airway steroids in asthma and rhinitis is also reported to be associated with an unchanged or a reduced frequency of airway infections (32). Indeed, it is common clinical practice to advise patients with asthma to continue steroid treatment and even increase the daily dose of inhaled steroids during periods of airway infection.

Common cold–induced inflammation has been demonstrated to be associated with increased microvascular exudative responsiveness in the human nose (57). Piedimonte et al. (58), studying the rat trachea have further demonstrated that the elevated baseline vascular permeability and the elevated vascular responsiveness that were present after Sendai virus inoculation–produced infection were inhibited by systemic dexamethasone treatment. Svensson et al. (59) and Greiff et al. (60) have demonstrated that seasonal allergic rhinitis may be characterized by an increased exudative responsiveness. Histamine challenges carried out during daytime or night hours thus produced much larger plasma exudation responses, measured as the luminal entry of α_2-macroglobulin, late into the season as compared with outside the allergic disease period. In view of the possibility that exudative hyperresponsiveness is a general feature of allergic and inflammatory airway diseases, the ability of topical steroids, to reduce the exudative responsiveness by prolonged treatment (42) may assume particular clinical importance.

IX. Roles of Exuded Plasma

The recent observations on mucosal exudation mechanisms in animal and human airways may call for a revision of the generally acknowledged roles of plasma exudation in airway diseases. Because of the swift luminal entry of bulk plasma, increased microvascular permeability in the airways may no longer, without further qualification, be equated with airway edema. Also, the presence of plasma proteins in the airway lumen may no longer be interpreted as a convincing sign of epithelial damage. More specifically, just because plasma is exuded into the airway lumen, this may not tell us anything at all about the perviousness of the airway mucosa to inhaled molecules. It may further be difficult to conclude about the occurrence of tracheobronchial plasma exudation merely from measurements of BALF levels of albumin; and it may be a mistake to conclude that a protein that did increase in BALF must come from a cellular source just because the level of albumin did not exhibit a simultaneous increase. In addition, we probably need to know whether plasma exudation has occurred or not to interpret properly the appearance of many cellularly derived indices, including cytokines on the mucosal surface; particularly we may have to define those conditions in which the indices merely have been carried from the lamina propria to the surface by the plasma exudate (1).

Even if plasma extravasation in the airways does not always produce mucosal edema, there are several other sequelae to be considered. Extravasated plasma may deposit its targeting and carrier proteins as well as its fibrinous macromolecules in the lamina propria, in the basement membrane, and both in and on the epithelial lining. Plasma may thus be an important source providing adhesive protein components to the mucosal extracellular matrix. For example, plasma-derived fibrin, fibronectin, and other proteins in the epithelium and on the mucosal surface may govern the traffic and the activity of leukocytes in airway inflammation. By continuously supplying these proteins, together with plasma-derived growth factors, and complement fragments, kinins, fibrinolysis molecules, and numerous other peptides (Fig. 2), the extravasation process in the airways may be a crucial component of airway inflammation. As reviewed elsewhere (4,5), plasma proteins may further produce a range of physical effects in the airways. They may impede the hydration of mucins and form complexes with mucins to increase the viscosity of the airway surface material that thus may stick to the mucosa also at sites where the airway already is narrow and where ordinary secretions would not have stayed. This effect and the volume of the exudate (that increasingly may attract fluid) would severely affect the mucociliary transport apparatus. Plasma-derived proteases have many potential effects, one of which is to destroy surfactant material to compromise the patency of small airways. Against a background of stagnated exudate-mucus material in the lumen, an additional exudation response together with a moderate contraction of the bronchial smooth muscle may cause extremely severe obstruction (4).

This discussion can only be a very incomplete sketch of the potential roles of exuded plasma in the pathology of airways diseases. However, it should provide a sufficient basis for forwarding the view that inhibition of the plasma exudation of airways by glucocorticoid drugs is not merely a sign of the antiinflammatory efficacy of this treatment. Rather, the antiexudative effect alone will have to be considered an important anti-inflammatory drug action in its own right.

X. The Importance of Reducing Airway Mucosal Perviousness in Asthma

Fraenkel (1), who examined the airways of patients who had died of asthma around 1900, suggested that epithelial shedding and a denuded basement membrane is a common, distinguishing characteristic of asthmatic bronchi. In recent decades, renewed proposals carrying a similar message have received much attention. The additional evidence includes the observation of denuded airways in biopsy specimens obtained from patients with less than severe asthma (61). The denudation hypothesis of asthma thus seems strongly rooted 90 years before Fraenkel and, as a consequence, work involving denuded airways in vitro proliferate. The airway denudation hypothesis is coupled with an increased "permeability" hypothesis (33), simply because the tightest membrane barrier of the airways is no longer present. The notion of an increased mucosal permeability is also popular, because it explains easily the nonspecific airway hyperresponsiveness that is present in most cases of asthma and that is attenuated by glucocorticoid treatment (32). The culprit causing the denudation is thought to be well identified. The eosinophil leukocyte is guilty not only by association; this cell also harbors toxic proteins with demonstrated epithelium-damaging properties (62). A further potential support for the role of the eosinophil in denudation is the fact that it is inhibited by steroids that are known to normalize many structural derangements of asthmatic epithelial lining cells (63). Before the role of mucosal eosinophils came into focus, Dunnill (64) and other pathologists believed that extravasated plasma could lift off sheets of epithelial cells on its way into the airway lumen. Again, by inhibition of plasma exudation, glucocorticoids would reduce such epithelial damage. However, there are now other findings to be considered, including the demonstration that the acute plasma exudation process does not cause epithelial damage, nor does it cause increased mucosal absorption of hydrophilic solutes (reviewed in refs. 1 and 33). Moreover, it has recently been demonstrated that epithelial restitution occurs speedily and unimpeded by topical glucocorticoid treatment (55) in the presence of activated neutrophils and eosinophils (30). Although clearly attractive hypotheses exist, it may now have to be concluded that the actual cause and the mechanisms involved in epithelial shedding in asthma remain to be assessed.

It is the tight junctions at the apical pole of epithelial lining cells that constitute the main barrier to mucosal penetration of inhaled molecules. A disruption and even more so a shedding of epithelial cells would, therefore, be expected to produce clear increases in the mucosal absorption of a large variety of solutes, including polar molecules, that normally pass through paracellular routes. Different laboratories have also made efforts to demonstrate an increased airway absorption permeability (reviewed in refs. 1, 33, and 36). Although it has been reported that the absorption permeability is increased in asthma, and that it correlates with the degree of abnormal responsiveness in these patients, most published data have in reality produced evidence against the paradigm (33). Halpin et al. (17), realizing that mucociliary clearance rates may vary greatly between subjects and between different study days, administered absorption tracer and mucociliary transport tracer (technetium albumin) at the same time. Based on their findings, including the correction for mucociliary transport, Halpin et al (17) reported that the absorption permeability in asthma may be significantly reduced. Findings in allergic rhinitis (33) preempt this observation.

Also in allergic rhinitis the idea of a hyperpermeability is widely entertained in various reviews and reports (33). Ultrastructural pictures show widened paracellular epithelial pathways in the allergic mucosa exactly as predicted by the champions of the hyperpermeability paradigm, and published reports purportedly show increased nasal airway absorption. Although frequently quoted, these paradigm-supporting reports have generally not been confirmed. In contrast, the opposite has been demonstrated in many cases (33). Greiff et al. (16), employing the nasal pool technique that noninvasively provides control of important variables such as exposed airway surface area, mucosal concentration of absorption tracer, and time of exposure (15), demonstrated that the nasal absorption ability was significantly reduced late into the allergic rhinitis season compared with outside the season. Hence, several weeks of exudative eosinophilic airway inflammation had somehow produced an abnormally tight function of the airway mucosa. A reduced absorption of peptide molecules has now been demonstrated under similar disease conditions and employing the same nasal pool technique (18). If the absorption barrier of the airway mucosa is more effective in inflammatory airway diseases than in health, a therapeutic action may, logically, involve a reduction of that mucosal barrier. Hence, it now seems important to ask what is the mechanism of increased barrier tightness and also to examine whether anti-inflammatory drug intervention may increase the perviousness of the barrier function in asthma and rhinitis.

XI. Airway Epithelial Restitution In Vivo

Epithelial repair or restitution occurs in healthy airways and may be extensive in inflammatory airway diseases. Early experimental studies have shown that traumatic removal of the tracheal epithelium with mucosal damage and bleeding eventually is followed by a process whereby remaining epithelial cells in the margin of the damage flatten and move medially to cover the wounded area (65). During the last 2 years, a novel in vivo method of shedding-like denudation has been developed and utilized in a series of experiments, including a study of the effects of topical steroid treatment on the epithelial restitution process. The technique involves the insertion of an oral steel probe into the guinea pig trachea and a gentle stroke with the probe along the mucosal surface in a noncartilaginous area of the airway. Without surgery and without causing damage to the basement membrane or, indeed, without causing any bleeding, an 800-μm wide denuded zone with distinct margins is thus created along the mucosal surface above the trachealis muscle (66). Immediately after epithelial removal in this model, both ciliated and secretory cells from the intact, remaining epithelium dedifferentiate (cilia being "internalized" and secretory granules being released), flatten out, and migrate over the basement membrane. It seems very important that migration can start promptly. The migration rate is also very fast, particularly during the first minutes after the "shedding" (2–3 μm/min) (66,67). The new aspects on epithelial restitution are reviewed elsewhere (68).

An instantaneous response to the denudation is plasma exudation (67). This latter result was expected, because the epithelium seems to hold a nitric oxide–generation mechanism that tonically suppresses the permeability of the subepithelial microcirculation (69). The exuded plasma creates a gel that soon attracts numerous neutrophils. The gel is a dynamic structure that continuously is supplied by exuded plasma. It covers the basement membrane until a new, flat, and tight epithelium has been established. The speedy migration thus occurs in close association with plasma-derived adhesive proteins such as fibronectin and fibrin as well as other plasma- and leukocyte-derived factors that may promote repair. The gel provides both a provisional cover and a proper supramembranal milieu for a speedy and efficient restitution process (Figs. 6, 7). Unfortunately, this in vivo milieu may not easily be reproduced in vitro. When exactly the same denudation technique that had been used in vivo was applied in experiments with guinea pig isolated, intact tracheae immersed in culture medium, no reepithelialization occurred. Or exceedingly slow and sporadic repair-like phenomena were observed. Zahm et al. (70), who used epithelial cell cultures grown on a collagen matrix, reported on the "rapid" repair occurring after removal of circular sheets of 25–75 epithelial culture cells. However, despite the fact that they had included several repair-promoting agents in their culture medium, including growth factors, the rate of early culture cell migration after a patchy damage was less than one-twentieth of that observed in the in vivo studies discussed above (66,67).

The current in vivo observations suggest that shedding, even of clusters of epithelial cells, may not cause prolonged states of denudation because epithelial restitution would occur promptly. It may further be inferred that those airway biopsy specimens that exhibit sharp edges between a denuded basement membrane and the columnar epithelium may frequently be artefacts unless there

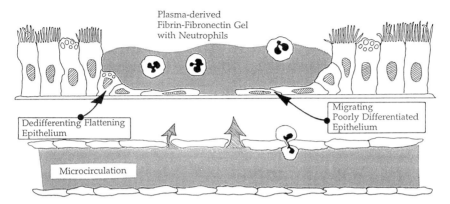

Plasma-derived
Fibrin-Fibronectin Gel
with Neutrophils

Dedifferentiating Flattening
Epithelium

Migrating
Poorly Differentiated
Epithelium

Microcirculation

Figure 6 After denudation, epithelial restitution occurs speedily under the provisional cover of a plasma-derived and leukocyte-rich gel. This important repair process may not be impeded by topical airway steroids. (Drawing by Jonas Erjefält.)

are also clear signs of dedifferentiation of the columnar cells and migration of poorly differentiated, flat cells. Since a provisional plasma-derived barrier may be created promptly, and since epithelial restitution by migration may occur fast in vivo, it is hypothesized that abnormal degrees of epithelial shedding may well occur in airways which exhibit maintained barrier functions that efficiently impede mucosal penetration if inhaled molecules. Furthermore, if only columnar cells are being shed, the remaining cobblestone appearing surface of basal cells will promptly change into flattened basal cells that establish cell to cell contact (68,71). Accordingly, this milder form of shedding may not result in grossly impeded airway barrier functions. The flattened repair cells occurring after

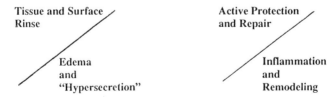

Tissue and Surface Rinse

Edema and "Hypersecretion"

Active Protection and Repair

Inflammation and Remodeling

Figure 7 The physical aspects (left) and the physiological-biological aspects of the plasma exudation of airways (right) are both important in defense (including repair) and in disease. Antiexudative drugs should, therefore, not be overly and indiscriminately effective. Glucocorticoids may prevent plasma exudation in disease and disease-like conditions but may not generally impede this process, so that active defenses and repair can be well maintained by the airway mucosa.

shedding-denudation events would provide reduced junctional lengths per unit mucosal surface area. This is offered as one potential tightening mechanism explaining observations of reduced airway absorption in disease (33).

Epithelial lining cells and the profuse subepithelial microcirculation are the first targets to be reached by inhaled molecules whether these are drugs such as glucocorticoids or inflammatory factors such as allergens and occupational chemicals that may damage the epithelium. The highest concentration of active solutes will also be present in these superficial parts of the airways; at least initially after the inhaled material has ben deposited on the mucosa. Since shedding-like removal of epithelium activates a range of humoral and cellular mechanisms (66,67) that are potentially sensitive to the actions of glucocorticoids, a number of questions present themselves. What is the steroid action on the microvascular responses, including extravasation of plasma and leukocytes and their activation? What is the effect of these drugs on epithelial cells dedifferentiation, migration, and sealing? And what is the effect on the ensuing proliferation phase involving the new and the old epithelium and also involving increased mitogenic activity in subepithelial fibroblasts and smooth muscle (66)? The controlled experimental conditions established in the recently developed guinea pig model has made it possible to examine the effects of topical steroid treatment on epithelial restitution.

A dose of budesonide that produces a full antiallergic effect (also when given to the whole lung) was given topically on the very site for epithelium removal (55). The drug was administered three times: 1 day before the removal, seconds after the removal (directly on the naked strip of basement membrane just prior to the appearance of exuded plasma), and 1 day after the removal. Budesonide promptly enters the airway tissue where it has a considerable retention time allowing a dosing interval of 24 hr as used in these experiments (32). After topical administration, budesonide produced no detectable effect of epithelial dedifferentiation, migration, sealing, or proliferation. Nor did budesonide affect the establishment over the denuded area of a plasma-derived gel containing numerous leukocytes. Most leukocytes were neutrophils, but eosinophils were also present and partly "degranulated" equally in control and budesonide-treated airways (55). Hence, epithelial repair in healthy airways was not impeded by budesonide. In inflammatory airway disease, several additional possibilities need consideration. An important effect of airway steroids may then be the prevention of epithelial damage in addition to allowing for proper repair. Since epithelial shedding-restitution may be causing part of the pathophysiology and cellular pathology of inflamed airways (30,68), it may even be hypothesized that the well-known anti-inflammatory effects of steroids in asthma and rhinitis may in part reflect simple prevention of epithelial cell damage. The plasma exudation response, the leukocyte response, and the restitution of a tight epithelium must together be considered major defense reactions in the airways. Although further studies are now warranted, the data obtained so far (55) suggest that topical airway steroids may not interfere with epithelial repair mechanisms of the airway mucosa. The lack of detrimental effect in this respect agrees with the clinical experience in asthma where treatment with inhaled glucocorticoids is seen to promote the development of a normal, intact epithelial lining (61,63).

XII. Summary

The profuse airway mucosal microcirculation has several important functions in asthma and rhinitis. One of its major roles lies in the process of extravasation of bulk plasma. This response is nonspecific in the sense that any kind of inflammatory insult will cause it. Thus, allergic reactions, infectious processes, occupational diseases, and challenge with any of a large number of inflammatory agents are associated with extravasation of plasma from the subepithelial microcirculation. However, the response is specific to inflammation, since it may not be produced by simple irritants which merely evoke various neurogenic responses in the human airways, nor may it be produced by contractile and secretory agents such as metacholine. The extravasated plasma is distributed in the lamina propria and the epithelium, including its basement membrane, and it moves to the mucosal surface. The latter passage, mucosal exudation, results from plasma moving up between epithelial cells gently forcing its way through the vast stretches of apical epithelial cell to cell junctions. The obligatory luminal entry of plasma makes it possible to examine the macromolecular permeability of the mucosal microcirculation simply by determining plasma indices in samples obtained from the airway surface.

Glucocorticoids inhibit plasma exudation in asthma and allergic rhinitis, but these drugs may not inhibit the plasma exudation response that occurs in acute infection or in other acute provocation conditions. The antiexudative effect of glucocorticoids in disease and in late phase reactions may thus not severely impede the plasma exudation response that is required to maintain a proper airway defense capacity.

Prolonged treatment of the airways with glucocorticoid drugs reduces the plasma exudation response by two mechanisms. The major effect may be the inhibition by glucocorticoids of various cellular activities that in turn lowers the levels of vasopermeability factors in the mucosa. The less well-explored action is a direct microvascular antipermeability effect that has been recorded in human airways only after repeated treatment with a topical airway steroid. The total action, seen as an effectively reduced airways plasma exudation process, is therapeutically important in proportion to the actual role played by exuded plasma in driving and perpetuating the inflammatory process and equally in causing sequelae such as increased airway responsiveness, structural changes, and luminal plugs.

The contributions to airway inflammation of the plasma-derived protein systems and their activation products may now receive relatively little attention, perhaps reflecting the greater popularity of in vitro over in vivo experiments in exploratory research. However, it is likely that in active inflammatory conditions, the lamina propria, the epithelial basement membrane, the epithelium, and the airway surface are endowed with exuded plasma products such as adhesive proteins, proteases, immunoglobulins, and cytokines and cytokine-modulating proteins. There is also a wide range of biologically active plasma-derived peptides.

The plasma exudation that occurs in airways after acute challenge with allergen or histamine-type mediators may not cause any epithelial damage, nor may it be associated with any change in the absorption capacity of the airway mucosa. Furthermore, it has now been demonstrated that exudative, eosinophilic airway diseases (allergic rhinitis and asthma) may be associated with an abnormally low absorption permeability of the airway mucosa. These recent findings seriously challenge the current paradigm of a generally increased perviousness of the airway mucosa in inflammatory airway diseases. Studies are now warranted to assess the effects of anti-inflammatory drug intervention on a reduced airway absorption ability in rhinitis and asthma.

The junctions of the epithelial lining cells are the rate-limiting structures in airway mucosal absorption of hydrophilic molecules. Hence, the question arises, How can epithelial shedding be extensive in inflamed airways without being associated with an increase in the absorption permeability? One piece in this puzzle is the increasing awareness that denuded epithelial basement membranes may not be overly characteristic of asthmatic airway. Indeed, some typical pictures of denuded asthmatic bronchi may be artefacts. It further seems likely that epithelial restitution, after shedding, is an exceedingly fast process, which is not reduced by airway steroids. Since flattened and migrating epithelial cells may cover small denuded areas within a few minutes, absorption may not increase; owing to the large size of the repair cells, paracellular absorption may even decrease.

Shedding-repair processes produce a series of physiological and cellular responses in the airways. In health, these are functionally important and lead to repair and homeostasis. However, in disease, the epithelial shedding-restitution process may assume major importance as a cause of some of the pathophysiology, the cellular pathology, and the structural changes that we now regard as characteristics of asthmatic bronchi. It seems to be an increasingly important target, for glucocorticoids and for novel antiasthma drugs, to protect the airway epithelium from damage so that shedding/restitution–evoked processes can be reduced to a minimum in asthma.

It has been concluded that topical airway steroids may combine a potent anti-inflammatory pharmacology, involving airway microcirculation and epithelium, with little effects on several of those "inflammation-like" responses that are vital to airway defense and repair.

Acknowledgments

I am indebted to F.B. Wagner, M.D., University Historian of The Thomas Jefferson University, Philadelphia, Pennsylvania, who kindly supplied the photograph and biographical details of Dr. Solomon Solis-Cohen, M.D., and I am indebted to D.J. Bucceri, P. Giroux, and M. Fox, M.D., at Astra USA Inc., for generous assistance in this matter. I acknowledge the expert secretarial help that I have received from Mai Broman in producing this chapter. Finally, I thank the "Airway Research Group" in Lund, that carried out the research upon which this chapter is built.

Discussion

DR. O'BYRNE: Are neutrophils required for epithelial reconstitution?

DR. PERSSON: This question requires consideration of two potential roles of neutrophils. It appears that the presence of neutrophils in the plasma-derived gel that covers the denuded basement membrane is important in bacterial and other defense reactions required during the healing period. Both the basement membrane and the migrating, poorly differentiated, flat epithelial cells are particularly vulnerable and presumably need the protection against bacteria, etc., provided by the neutrophils. The other possible role would be that neutrophils could release factors which are important for the epithelial restitution process. Indeed, we have observed that where the migration front moves particularly fast, neutrophils are particularly abundant on the basement membrane.

DR. PERRETTI: In the hamster cheek pouch study you mentioned, I believe that the steroid was given systemically. How do you think this relates to your study with the topically applied steroid? Have you looked at the effect of systemic budesonide on the histamine-induce plasma extravasation you have measured?

DR. PERSSON: This study employed topical budesonide treatment. So the same type of drug application was effective in animals but lacked effect in human airways.

DR. DENBURG: (1) In your epithelial regeneration model, do you see nerve regeneration? (2) How are you sure that cells regenerating are epithelial cells rather than blood-derived progenitors?

DR. PERSSON: (1) CGRP (calcitonin gene-related peptide)–positive nerve fibers (tachykininergic nerves) appear in the new epithelium about 15 hr after denudation. (2) By continuously observing by scanning electron microscopy how the remaining intact epithelial cells dedifferentiate, flatten, and migrate to cover the denuded basement membrane.

DR. GAULDIE: How do you explain the rapid functions of glucocorticoids?

DR. PERSSON: Since we did not find a rapidly induced antipermeability effect in human airway microcirculation, we have not given this question much thought. Obviously the acute vascular antipermeability effect has to be delineated in animal studies, but it now seems of little relevance for human airway function. However, there is one condition in which topical airway steroids (budesonide) have proved to be acutely very effective. Pedersen has thus observed that in children with croup, budesonide has marked effects within 2 hr after drug administration. To explain this clinical efficacy seems an important challenge. (S Husby, L Agertoft, S Mortensen, S Pedersen. Treatment of croup with nebulized steroid (budesonide): a double blind, placebo controlled study. Arch. Dis. Child. 1993; 68:253–255.)

DR. SMALDONE: Future studies need to reconcile the following: rapid healing of epithelium (your model), easily damaged epithelium, abnormal biopsies in patients with mild asthma, and normal mucociliary function in mild asthma.

DR. PERSSON: I think our data on rapid restitution of epithelium after shedding are well compatible with and perhaps can explain the observation that the absorption barrier is not compromised in asthma and rhinitis despite the occurrence of increased epithelial shedding in these diseases. Also, I think that some of the typical histological pictures of asthmatic airways where the basement membrane is denuded without extensive repair going on may be artifacts.

DR. LIU: Could you speculate on the reason that one application of steroids does not affect histamine-induced permeability, whereas prolonged steroid treatment inhibits the response to histamine?

DR. PERSSON: We interpret the effect as a change in the venular endothelial cell responsiveness that is not induced acutely but may require days to weeks of steroid exposure to be fully expressed.

DR. DURHAM: Are the inhibitory effects of corticosteroids on increases in mucosal vascular permeability stimulus specific?

DR. PERSSON: The reduced exudative response to histamine in human nasal airways treated for 3 weeks with topical budesonide may be a nonspecific effect of the steroid on venular endothelial cells.

DR. HOWARTH: You demonstrated that regular therapy with budesonide decreased acute histamine-induced plasma protein leakage. What was the effect of therapy on baseline nasal lavage levels, as this is relevant to chronic disease, and how do you think your findings fit with the identification that oral steroid therapy has no effect on allergen-induced skin wheal generation.

DR. PERSSON: In airways diseases including asthma and allergic rhinitis, steroids significantly inhibit baseline levels of plasma indices on the mucosal surface. The low and normal levels of plasma proteins in healthy airways may not be much affected by steroid treatment, although this aspect needs to be examined in greater detail, including studies of nocturnal exudation of plasma that may be slightly elevated compared with daytime exudation also in health. (L Greiff, A Akerlund, M Andersson, et al. Day-night differences in mucosal plasma proteins in common cold. Acta Otolaryngol 1995; in press.) With regard to your second question, my only comment is that the pharmacology of airway mucosal microcirculation may be quite different from that of the skin, because the skin lacks a reactive epithelium and a profuse superficial bed.

DR. GLEICH: Do you find evidence of fibrosis after epithelial stripping and regeneration after one or repeated procedures?

DR. PERSSON: After a single denudation episode, the repair process goes toward complete healing with a normal mucosa established within a few days. At this stage, the epithelium is fully differentiated with normal numbers of ciliated and secretory cells. There is no fibrosis although a transient increase in mitosis ([^{3}H]thymidine incorporation, bromdeoxyuridine staining) had occurred in subepithelial fibroblast–smooth muscle cells.

DR. BARNES: Is there any evidence for an increased proportion of goblet cells in the epithelial cells repopulating denuded areas of the airway? Have you looked at differences between acute and chronic epithelial denudation in this respect?

DR. PERSSON: The immediate response to denudation is release of PAS-positive material from secretory cells in the vicinity of the lesions. PAS-positive cells are normal in number and distribution in both the old and the new epithelium when restitution and differentiation are completed (4–5 days after denudation). This is after a single denudation maneuver in noninflamed airways. What will happen after repeated denudations is now being examined. Other means of acutely damaging the epithelium than mechanical denudation (such as with topical challenge with toluenediisocyanate [TDI]) may produce different effects on the goblet cell population. We have demonstrated that after a single exposure to TDI, the guinea pig airway mucosa is acutely inflamed for 24 hr and then follows a phase of markedly increased secretory cell numbers that lasts for several weeks.

DR. McFADDEN: (1) Do you have any data on how vascular permeability changes with chronic inflammatory states? (2) Are there any data regarding the existence of abnormal autonomic control of the airway microcirculation in inflammatory states like asthma?

DR. PERSSON: (1)We have observed in both seasonal rhinitis and virus inoculation–induced common cold that the airway microcirculation develops a significantly increased responsiveness so that the plasma exudation response to topical challenge (e.g., with histamine) is abnormally great. (2) Cholinergic transmitters (acetylcholine and analogues) are completely devoid of effects on vascular permeability. Circulating adrenaline (epinephrine), particularly in animals, may attenuate plasma exudation responses through stimulation of venular endothelial β_2 receptors. Finally, the reputed neurogenic exudation of plasma (neurogenic inflammation) that is so readily evoked in guinea pigs may not occur at all in human airways. At least we have demonstrated that when nicotine and capsaicin are applied on healthy nasal airways or on airways with long established allergic inflammation, marked secretory and painful effects are produced, but we have not been able to record the slightest tendency to a plasma exudation response.

DR. O'BYRNE: Is there any evidence that epithelial cells from asthmatic airways are functionally different ex vivo compared with normal airways?

DR. PERSSON: I think the epithelial cells change as soon as you remove them from their proper in vivo milieu.

DR. JORDANA: I think that nasal polyps are probably the best scenario to study chronic airway inflammation. Here you see closely intertwined both epithelial denudation and hyperplasia. I wonder if you had a chance to study nasal polyp tissue? A second comment is that another very interesting scenario to study is nasal polyps from patients with cystic fibrosis, because they have two distinctive features. One, they are heavily infiltrated with neutrophils but not eosinophils. Second, in spite of a fairly massive neutrophilic inflammation, the epithelium looks remarkably well preserved.

DR. PERSSON: I agree that nasal polyp tissue may provide good models for studies of inflammatory mechanisms. I think that currently we know too little about the occurrence of plasma-derived extracellular matrix and other plasma-derived proteins—cytokines and peptides—in polyps. The epithelium that has survived the surgical artifacts may be in different stages of inflammatory changes, and we see many poorly differentiated flat cells suggesting that repair migration may be extensive in this tissue. We have not examined nasal polyps in cystic fibrosis.

References

1. Persson CGA. Airway epithelium and microcirculation. Eur Respir Rev 1994; 4;23, 352–362.
2. Persson CGA. Glucocorticoids for asthma—early contributions. Pulm Pharmacol 1989; 2:163–166.
3. Solis-Cohen S. The use of adrenal substance in the treatment of asthma. JAMA 1900; 1164–1166.
4. Persson CGA. Role of plasma exudate in asthmatic airways. Lancet 1986; 2:1126–1129.
5. Persson CGA. Plasma exudation and asthma. Lung 1988; 166:1–23.
6. Svensson C, Klementsson H, Andersson M, Pipkorn U, Alkner U, Persson CGA. Glucocorticoid-reduced attenuation of mucosal exudation of bradykinins and fibrinogen in seasonal allergic rhinitis. Allergy 1994; 49:177–183.
7. Prescott T, Kaliner MA. Vascular mechanisms in rhinitis In: Busse WW, Holgate ST, eds. Asthma and Rhinitis. Oxford, UK: Blackwell, 1995; 777–790.
8. Van de Graaf EA, Out TA, Roos CM, Jansen HM. Respiratory membrane permeability and bronchial hyperreactivity in patients with stable asthma. Effects of therapy with inhaled steroids. Am Rev Respir Dis 1991; 143:362–368.
9. Svensson C, Grönneberg R, Andersson M, Alkner U, Andersson O, Billing B, Giljam H, Greiff L, Persson CGA. Allergen challenge-induced entry of alpha-2-macroglobulin and tryptase into human nasal and bronchial airways, J Allergy Clin Immunol 1995; 96:239–246.
10. Persson CGA. On the medical history of asthma and rhinitis. In: Mygind N, Pipkorn U, Dahl R, eds. Rhinitis and Asthma. Similarities and Differences. Copenhagen: Munksgaard, 1990:9–20.
11. Persson CGA. Overview of the effects of theophylline. J Allergy Clin Immunol 1986; 78:780–787.
12. Persson CGA. Development of safer xanthine drugs for treatment of obstructive airway disease. J Allergy Clin Immunol 1986; 78:817–824.
13. Persson CGA. Use of enprofylline to delineate endogenous actions of adenosine. In: Paton DM, ed. Adenosine and Adenine Nucleotides. London, Taylor and Francis, 1988: 217–224.
14. Persson CGA, Pauwels R. Pharmacology of anti-asthma xanthines. In: Page CP, Barnes PJ, eds. Handbook for Experimental Pharmacology. Vol 98. Pharmacology of Asthma, Berlin: Springer-Verlag, 1991:207–225.
15. Greiff L, Alkner U, Pipkorn U, Persson CGA. The 'nasal pool' device applies

controlled concentrations of solutes on human nasal airway mucosa and samples its
surface exudations/secretions. Clin Exp Allergy 1990; 20:253–259.

16. Greiff L, Wollmer P, Svensson C, Andersson M, Persson CGA. Effect of seasonal
allergic rhinitis on airway mucosal absorption of chromium-51-labelled EDTA.
Thorax 1993; 48:648–650.

17. Halpin DMG, Currie D, Jones B, Leigh TR, Evans TW. Permeability of bronchial
mucosa to [113m]In-DTPA in asthma and the effects of salmeterol. Eur Respir J 1993;
6:512s.

18. Greiff L, Lundin S, Svensson C, Andersson M, Erjefält JS, Wollmer P, Persson
CGA. peptide absorption in human allergic airways (abstr.). Eur Respir J 1995;
8:124s.

19. Greiff L, Svensson C, Andersson M, Persson CGA. Effects of topical capsaicin in
seasonal allergic rhinitis. Thorax 1995; 50:225–229.

20. Bascom R, Kagey-Sobotka A, Proud D. Effect of intranasal capsaicin on symptoms
and mediator release. J Pharmacol Exp Ther 1991; 259:1323–1327.

21. Greiff L, Erjefält I, Wollmer P, Andersson M, Pipkorn U, Alkner U, Persson
CGA. Effects of nicotine on the human nasal airway mucosa. Thorax 1993;
48:651–655.

22. James K. Interactions between cytokines and α_2-macroglobulin. Immunol Today
1990; 11:163–166.

23. Svensson C, Baumgarten CR, Alkner U, Pipkorn U, Persson CGA. Topical vasoconstrictor oxymetazoline does not affect histamine-induced mucosal exudation of
plasma in human and nasal airways. Clin Exp Allergy 1992; 22:411–416.

24. Bende M, Lindqvist N, Pipkorn U. Effect of a topical glucocorticoid, budesonide,
on nasal mucosal blood flow as measured with 133Xe wash-out technique. Allergy
1983; 38:461–464.

25. Mygind N, Naclerio RM. Allergic and Non-allergic Rhinitis. Clinical Aspects.
Copenhagen: Munksgaard, 1993:1–199.

26. Haahtela T, Jarvinen M, Kava T, Laitinen LA. Comparison of a β_2-agonist
terbutaline with an inhaled steroid in newly detected asthma. N Engl J Med 1991;
325:388–392.

27. Barnes PF, Pedersen S. Efficacy and safety of inhaled corticosteroids in asthma.
Am Rev Respir Dis 1993; 148:S1–S26.

28. Gustafsson B, Persson CGA. Effect of three weeks' treatment with budesonide on
in vitro contractile and relaxant airway effects in the rat. Thorax 1989; 44:24–27.

29. McDonald DM. Endothelial gaps and permeability of venules in rat tracheas exposed to inflammatory stimuli. Am J Physiol 1994; 266:L61–83.

30. Erjefält JS, Sundler F, Persson CGA. Eosinophils, neutrophils and venular gaps in
the airway mucosa at epithelial removal-restitution. Am J Respir Crit Care Med
1995; in press.

31. Persson CGA, Svensson C, Greiff L, Andersson M, Wollmer P, Alkner U, Erjefält
I. The use of the nose to study the inflammatory response of the respiratory tract
(editorial). Thorax 1992; 47:993–1000.

32. Brattsand R, Selroos O. Current drugs for respiratory diseases. Glucocorticoids.
Drugs and the Lung 1994; 101–220

33. Persson CGA, Andersson M, Greiff L, Svensson C, Erjefält JS, Sundler F, Wollmer P, Alkner U, Erjefält I, Gustafsson B, Linden M, Nilsson M. Airway permeability. Clin Exp Allergy 1995; 23:807–814.
34. Persson CGA, Alkner U, Andersson M, Greiff L, Linden M, Svensson C. Histamine-challenge-induced "lamina propria lavage" and mucosal out-put of IL-6 in human airways (abstr.). Eur Respir J 1995; 8:125s.
35. Erjefält JS, Erjefält I, Sundler F, Persson CGA. Epithelial pathway for luminal entry of bulk plasma. Clin Exp Allergy 1995; 25:187–195.
36. Persson CGA, Erjefält I, Alkner U, Baumgarten C, Greiff L, Gustafsson B, Luts B, Pipkorn U, Sundler F, Svensson C, Wollmer P. Plasma exudation as a first line respiratory mucosal defence. Clin Exp Allergy 1991; 21:17–24.
37. Persson CGA, Erjefält I, Gustafsson B, Luts A. Subepithelial hydrostatic pressure may regulate plasma exudation across the mucosa. Int Arch Allergy Appl Immunol 1990; 92:148–153.
38. Gustafsson BG, Persson CGA. Asymmetrical effects of increases in hydrostatic pressure on macromolecular movement across the airway mucosa. A study in guinea-pig tracheal tube preparation. Clin Exp Allergy 1991; 21:121–126.
39. Erjefält I, Luts A, Persson CGA. Appearance of airway absorption and exudation tracers in guinea-pig tracheobronchial lymph nodes. J Appl Physiol 1993; 74:817–824.
40. Persson CGA, Erjefält I. Inflammatory leakage of macromolecules from the vascular compartment into the tracheal lumen. Acta Physiol Scan 1986; 126:615–616.
41. Greiff L, Andersson M, Svensson C, Alkner U, Persson CGA. Glucocorticoids may not inhibit plasma exudation by direct vascular antipermeability effects in human airways. Eur Respir J 1994; 7:1120–1124.
42. Greiff L, Alkner U, Andersson M, Svensson C, Persson CGA. Three weeks' treatment with topical budeosnide reduces microvascular exudative responsiveness to histamine. Am J Respir Crit Care Med 1995; 151:A39.
43. Erjefält I, Greiff L, Alkner U, Persson CGA. Allergen-induced biphasic plasma exudation responses in guinea-pig large airways. Am Rev Respir Dis 1993; 148:695–701.
44. Andersson PT, Persson CGA. Developments in antiasthma glucocorticoids. In: O'Donnell Sr, Persson CGA, eds. Directions for New Antiasthma Drugs. Basel, Birkhäuser, 1988:239–260.
45. Erjefält I, Persson CGA. Effect of budesonide on allergen- and toluenediisocyanate (TDI)–induced late phase airway exudation of bulk plasma. Am J Respir Crit Care Med 1995; 151:A223.
46. Fabbri LM, Mapp C. Bronchial hyperresponsiveness, airway inflammation and occupational asthma induced by toluene diisocyanate. Clin Exp Allergy 1991; 21:42–47.
47. Persson CGA, Gustafsson B, Luts A, Sundler F, Erjefält I. Toluene diisocyanate produces and increase in airway tone that outlasts the inflammatory exudation phase. Clin Exp Allergy 1991; 21:715–724.
48. Persson CGA, Erjefält I. Xanthines and xanthine-like drugs for asthma. In:

Costello, JF, Piper PJ, eds. Methylxanthines and Phosphodiesterase Inhibitors in the Treatment of Airways Disease. London: Parthenon Publishing Group, 1994; pp 11–26.

49. Erjefält I, Persson CGA. Increased sensitivity to toluene diisocyanate (TDI) in airways previously exposed to low doses of TDI. Clin Exp Allergy 1992; 22:854–862.

50. Persson CGA. Plasma exudation in the airways: mechanisms and function. Eur Respir J 1991; 4:1268–1274.

51. Greiff L, Åkerlund A, Andersson M, Svensson C, Alkner U, Persson CGA. Day-night differences in mucosal plasma proteins in common cold. Acta Otolaryngol 1995; in press.

52. Salomonsson P, Grönneberg R, Gilljam H, Andersson O, Billing B, Enander I, Alkner U, Persson CGA. Bronchial exudation of bulk plasma at allergen challenge in allergic asthma. Am Rev Respir Dis 1992; 146:1535–1542.

53. Persson CGA, Pipkorn U. Glucocorticoids. In: Waksman BH, ed. Fifty Years Progress in Allergy. Chem Immunol 1990; 49:264–277.

54. Farr BM, Gwaltney JM Jr, Hendley JO. A randomized controlled trial of glucocorticoid prophylaxis against experimental rhinovirus infection. J Infect Dis 1990; 162:1173–1177.

55. Erjefält JS, Erjefält I, Sundler F, Persson CGA. Effects of topical budesonide on epithelial restitution in vivo in guinea-pig trachea. Thorax 1995; 50:785–792.

56. Schleimer RP, Freeland HS, Peters SP, Brown KE, Derse CP. An assessment of the effects of glucocorticoids on degranulation, cheomtaxis, binding to vascular endothelium and formation of leukotriene B4 by purified human neutrophils. J Pharmacol Exp Ther 1989; 250:598–605.

57. Greiff L, Andersson M, Åkerlund A, Wollmer P, Svensson C, Alkner U, Persson CGA. Microvascular exudative hyperresponsiveness in human coronavirus-induced common cold. Thorax 1994; 49:121–127.

58. Piedimonte G, McDonald DM, Nadel JA. Glucocorticoids inhibit neurogenic plasma extravasation and prevent virus-potentiated extravasation in the rat trachea. J Clin Invest 1990; 86:14090–1415.

59. Svensson C, Andersson M, Greiff L, Alkner U, Persson CGA. Exudative hyperresponsiveness to histamine in seasonal allergic rhinitis. Clin Exp Allergy 1995; 25:942–950.

60. Greiff L, Alkner U, Andersson M, Svensson C, Persson CGA. Day and night exudative hyperresponsiveness of airway microcirculation in seasonal allergic rhinitis. Am J Respir Crit Care Med 1995; 151:A586.

61. Laitinen LA, Laitinen A, Persson CGA. Role of epithelium. In: Weiss EB, Segal MS, eds. Bronchial Asthma. Boston: Little Brown, 1990:296–308.

62. Venge P, Håkansson L. The eosinophil and asthma. In: Kaliner MA, Barnes PJ, Persson CGA eds. Asthma its Pathology and Treatment. New York: Dekker, 1991:477–502.

63. Lundgren R, Söderberg M, Hörstedt P, Stenling R. Morphological studies of bronchial mucosal biopsies from asthmatics before and after ten years of treatment with inhaled steroids. Eur Respir J 1988; 1:883–889.

64. Dunnill MS. The pathology of asthma with special reference to the change in the bronchial mucosa. J Clin Pathol 1960; 13:27-33.
65. Wilhelm DL. Regeneration of tracheal epithelium. J Pathol Bacteriol 1953; 65:543-550.
66. Erjefält JS, Erjefält I, Sundler F, Persson CGA. In vivo restitution of airway epithelium. Cell Tissue Res 1995; 281:305-316.
67. Erjefält JS, Erjefält I, Sundler F, Persson CGA. Microcirculation-derived factors in airway epithelial repair in vivo. Microvase Res 1994; 48:161-178.
68. Persson CGA, Erjefält JS. Airway epithelial restitution following shedding and denudation. In: Crystal RG, West JB, Weibel ER, Barnes PJ, eds. The Lung: Scientific Foundations, 2nd ed. New York; Raven, 1996, Chapter 200.
69. Erjefält JS, Erjefält I, Sundler F, Persson CGA. Mucosal nitric oxide may tonically suppress airways plasma exudation. Am J Respir Crit Care Med 1994; 150:227-232.
70. Zahm JM, Chevillard M, Puchelle E. Wound repair of human surface respiratory epithelium. Am J Respir Cell Mol Biol 1991; 5:242-248.
71. Erjefält JS, Greiff L, Sundler F, Persson CGA. Basal cells promptly flatten out at detachment of the columnar epithelium in human and guinea-pig airways [abstract]. Eur Respir J 1995.

10

Inhibition of Inflammatory Cell Recruitment by Glucocorticoids

Cytokines as Primary Targets

ROBERT P. SCHLEIMER, LISA A. BECK, LISA A. SCHWIEBERT, CRISTIANA STELLATO, KELLY DAVENPECK, and BRUCE S. BOCHNER

The Johns Hopkins Asthma and Allergy Center
The Johns Hopkins University School of Medicine
Baltimore, Maryland

I. Introduction

The tremendous growth in the use of glucocorticoids for asthma in the last decade stems largely from the development of potent inhaled glucocorticoids which have substantially reduced systemic side effects by virtue of their high-lipid solubility, high affinity for the receptor, prolonged contact time in the lung, and relatively rapid metabolism once absorbed from the gastrointestinal tract (1–3). The remarkable efficacy of glucocorticoids in general, and in asthma in particular, results from the fact that these drugs are analogues of the endogenous hormones which homeostatically regulate overexpressed inflammatory responses (4). It is now appreciated that the ubiquitously expressed inflammatory cytokines interleukin-1 (IL-1) and tumor necrosis factor (TNF), which stimulate the liver to produce acute-phase proteins and stimulate the brain to induce fever during severe inflammatory responses, can activate the hypothalamic-pituitary-adrenal axis and induce cortisol release from the adrenals completing a feedback loop to dampen inflammation (5). That endogenous glucocorticoids regulate inflammation is suggested by numerous studies showing that removal of the adrenal gland can exacerbate inflammatory responses, sometimes with disastrous consequences. The purpose of this chapter is to consider the mechanisms that may be involved in the ability of glucocorticoids to inhibit inflammatory responses in the lung in particular. Perhaps as a result of the fact that glucocorticoids are endogenous regulators of inflammatory responses, they interfere with a multitude of target cells and molecules in the inflammatory cascade. Although the molecular targets include genes involved in the release and/or expression of inflammatory enzymes, chemical mediators, and components of plasma and the extracellular matrix, the main focus of this chapter is how glucocorticoid suppression of cytokine gene expression leads to diminished leukocyte infiltration at sites of inflammation.

The beneficial effects of glucocorticoids in asthma are now felt to result largely from their ability to reduce airways inflammation. This effect on inflammation in turn results in an improvement of airways function, a diminution in airways secretions, a decrease in airways reactivity, and a restoration of airways integrity. The effects of glucocorticoids on airways secretion, although well accepted, are at present only partially understood. Another chapter in this volume discusses their effects on plasma exudation into the airways (6; see Chapter 9). A relatively unexplored area of glucocorticoid action is their effect on the activation and function of secretory cells in the airways; namely, goblet cells and serous cells in mucous glands. Many of the effects of glucocorticoids on both the vasculature and the mucus-secreting cells are likely to be secondary to a reduction in inflammatory mediators that activate vascular and secretory cells. One mechanism by which glucocorticoids reduce mediators is by suppressing the influx of circulating cells, including eosinophils, lymphocytes, monocytes, and basophils. Thus, although the topic at hand (the effects of glucocorticoids on leukocyte infiltration) is narrow, the impact of this effect on tissues affected by these infiltrating cells can be profound.

II.   Inhibition of the Activation of Genes of Inflammation: A Major Mechanism of Glucocorticoid Action

For decades it was believed that glucocorticoids worked by stabilization of lysosomes. This concept, which was based on the ability of millimolar concentrations of steroids to prevent degranulation of leukocytes and dissolution of lysosomes, has been rejected; the concentrations of glucocorticoids required for these effects are too high and the selectivity for glucocorticoids, compared with nonglucocorticoid steroids, is not observed. Starting in the 1960s, it was recognized that gene induction by glucocorticoids occurs through a receptor-mediated mechanism, and a search for glucocorticoid second messengers began in earnest (7). Great interest was focused on lipocortin, a glucocorticoid-induced product, which was reported to inhibit phospholipase A_2, the enzyme responsible for generating arachidonic acid feeding both the cyclooxygenase and lipoxygenase pathways (8,9). Although subsequent studies have questioned whether glucocorticoids (or lipocortin itself) inhibit arachidonic acid metabolite release through this mechanism (10), lipocortin has numerous anti-inflammatory effects in vivo and in vitro (11,12).

In the last two decades, the ability of glucocorticoids to inhibit the production of various inflammatory enzymes and cytokines has been recognized (13–17). Recently, several molecular mechanisms underlying this action have been described: (1) the binding of the glucocorticoid receptor complex to transcription factors such as AP-1 and others, thereby squelching their transcriptional regulatory actions (18,19); (2) the binding of the glucocorticoid receptor complex to negative glucocorticoid regulatory elements (nGREs) (20,21)); (3) the ability of glucocorticoids to negatively regulate mRNA stability, as for IL-1β and IL-6 mRNAs, by an as yet unidentified mechanism (22,23); and (4) the glucocorticoid-mediated induction of IκB, an inhibitor of the transcription factor NFκB (see Chapter 2). Inflammatory enzymes whose induction is inhibited by glucocorticoids include collagenase, elastase, stromelysin, plasminogen activator, phospholipase, and the inducible forms of cyclooxygenase and nitric oxide synthase (13–16) (also see Chapter 3). Other chapters in this volume describe the ability of glucocorticoids to modulate the expression of these inflammatory proteins in detail. The focus of this chapter is the relevance of cytokines as important glucocorticoid targets.

III. Effects of Glucocorticoids on Leukocyte Accumulation in Allergic Diseases and Experimental Allergen Challenge Model Systems

The pathology of asthma is characterized by infiltration of the airways with eosinophils and mononuclear cells, especially lymphocytes (24–27). The ability of glucocorticoids to suppress infiltration of the airways by these cell types has only been recognized in the last decade or so, largely owing to the fact that studies with bronchoscopy and biopsy or bronchoalveolar lavage (BAL) were not previously routinely performed. Biopsy studies in asthmatic subjects have established that glucocorticoid treatment can reduce infiltration of the airways with eosinophils and lymphocytes as well as reduce the number of mucosal mast cells in the airways (28,29; see Table 1). Studies in BAL have confirmed that glucocorticoids reduce the number of eosinophils as well as the amount of eosinophil proteins [major basic protein (MBP), eosinophil cationic protein (ECP)] in BAL fluids of asthmatic individuals (30). Similar results to those in asthma have been obtained in the nose in studies of seasonal rhinitis in which glucocorticoids reduce the increase of eosinophils and their products during the

Table 1 Inhibition by Glucocorticoids of Leukocyte Accumulation in Asthma and Experimental
Antigen Challenge Models in Humans[a]

Asthma	
Lundgren et al.	(28)
Laitinen et al.	(29)
Adelroth et al.	(30)
Burke et al.	(31)
Djukanovic et al.	(215)
Montefort et al.	(74)
Robinson et al.	(128)
Experimental antigen challenge	
Lungs	
Liu et al.	(69)
Nose	
Pipkorn et al.	(204)
Pipkorn et al.	(205)
Bascom et al.	(206)
Bascom et al.	(207)
Jacobson et al.	(208)
Masuyama et al.	(129)
Lee et al.	(111)
Skin	
Slott et al.	(209)
Massey et al.	(210)
Rebuck et al.	(211)
Rebuck et al.	(212)
Mancini et al.	(213)
Charlesworth et al.	(214)

[a]Reference numbers are in parentheses.

natural allergen season (see Table 1). The primary cell in the BAL fluid is the macrophage; it has been difficult to detect any effects of glucocorticoids on macrophage number, although Burke et al. found a decrease in activated (HLA-DR+) macrophages (or dendritic cells) in a biopsy study of steroid-treated asthmatics (31).

The effect of glucocorticoids on cellular infiltration is much more readily demonstrable in allergen challenge systems, since antigen doses utilized are often quite large and the extent of the cellular infiltrate can be great. Responses to experimental allergen challenges are often biphasic; the first phase has generally been attributed to the immediate consequences of mast cell activation and the pursuant release of chemical mediators (32–34). This early phase includes airways constriction, wheal and flare in the skin, and sneezing and nasal congestion at the respective target challenge sites. Glucocorticoid treatment, especially prolonged administration of inhaled glucocorticoids, can dampen the acute-phase response, probably as a result of a decrease in the number of mucosal mast cells (35,36; see Chapter 12). The late-phase allergic reaction probably has several components which are distinguished by the nature of the cell infiltrate. During the initial period of the late-phase response, there is a relatively nonspecific infiltration of antigen challenge sites with virtually all white blood cell types, including eosinophils, lymphocytes, monocytes, and neutrophils (37). The neutrophil influx appears to be relatively transient compared with that of the other cell types and by the later stages of the experimental allergen challenge-induced late phase, the cellular infiltrate appears to be primarily composed of eosinophils, monocytes, and lymphocytes (38,39). Studies in the nose, skin, and airways, by both lavage and biopsy after antigen challenge, have shown repeatedly that glucocorticoids are quite effective in damping, or in some cases almost completely inhibiting, the influx of cells in these three sites (see Table 1). The following sections consider the role of cytokines in allergic cell infiltration and as a target of glucocorticoid action.

A. Cytokines and Allergic Inflammation

The focus of this section is confined to oligopeptide mediators, cytokines, and chemokines in allergic cell infiltration and as a target of glucocorticoid action. We have divided these cytokines into four main groups: The first is nonspecific endothelial activators, which includes IL-1 and TNF; the second is specific endothelial activators, which includes IL-4 and IL-13; the third is eosinophil-priming cytokines, which includes IL-3, IL-5, granulocyte-macrophage colony-stimulating factor (GM-CSF), and γ-interferon (IFN-γ), and the fourth is chemokines, a family of small oligopeptide inducers of cell movement and activation.

Nonspecific Endothelial Activators

Numerous cell types are capable of producing IL-1 and TNF. In fact, these cytokines appear to act as ubiquitous alarm molecules for local inflammatory responses (40–42). It is therefore quite difficult to analyze with absolute certainty what cell types generate these cytokines during allergic reactions and what their overall role in allergic inflammation is (Fig. 1). We hypothesize that nonspecific endothelial activation is partly responsible for the nonselective recruitment of leukocytes in the early stages of the antigen challenge-induced late phase (43,44). Nonspecific endothelial activation is well known to induce neutrophil binding and transendothelial migration (45); injection of IL-1 or TNF

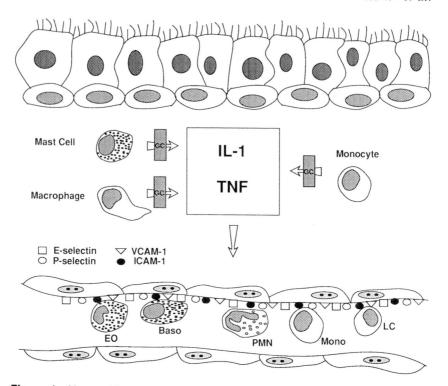

Figure 1 Nonspecific endothelial activation in allergic reactions. Resident cells are shown on the left and recruited cells on the right in this and Figures 2, 3, and 4. IL-1 and TNF activate expression of adhesion molecules on the endothelial surface. Documented effects of glucocorticoids to inhibit cytokine generation are indicated by the shaded box with GC in it. See text for discussion.

induces rich neutrophil infiltrates in animals (46,47) and humans (48,49). It is well established that experimental allergen challenge results in rapid activation of endothelial cells to express adhesion molecules, including E-selectin and intercellular adhesion molecule 1 (ICAM-1), which serve to indicate that nonspecific endothelial activation has occurred (and therefore that nonspecific endothelial activators have been released; see Fig. 1) (50–56). When antigen challenge occurs in a quiescent tissue (as in an out-of-season challenge of an allergic individual), it seems probable that these cytokines are produced by resident cells; the most likely candidates are mast cells and macrophages. Mast cells have been shown to store TNF and release it through an IgE-mediated mechanism in both rodents and humans (53,54,57,58). Macrophages in the airways have been shown to bear low-affinity IgE receptors and can be activated to produce IL-1 via exposure to antigen (59,60). Other tissue resident cells, including epidermal Langerhans cells, bear high-affinity IgE receptors (61). Kay et al. recently reported FcεRI on CD68-positive macrophage-like cells in airway biopsies of both nonatopic and atopic asthmatics (61a).

Glucocorticoids are extremely good inhibitors of the production of IL-1 and TNF-α in most cell types and tissues that have been studied (3). In fact, the inhibitory effects of glucocorticoids on IL-1 production were among the first recognized anti-cytokine effects of these drugs (62–65). Administration of glucocorticoids in vivo in humans has been shown to lead to an inhibition of production of IL-1 by lung macrophages (60). Studies by Wershil et al. have shown that glucocorticoids can inhibit TNF-α release and synthesis in murine mast cells (66). Although glucocorticoids do not inhibit the release of preformed or newly synthesized mediators from human mast cells from lung or other tissues, their effects on mast cell cytokine release in humans are unknown and must be determined (67). Relatively few studies have assessed the effects of glucocorticoid treatment in vivo on the production of these cytokines in allergic reactions. Although glucocorticoids inhibit IL-1 and TNF-α production in vivo in other types of reactions in mice (64,68), only the study by Borish et al. (60), and a study by Lane (see Chapter 14) have shown that glucocorticoids inhibit IL-1 production in human allergic reactions. Whether glucocorticoids inhibit nonspecific endothelial activation in vivo in humans has not received adequate study. Antigen challenge in the lung is associated with the elevation of E-selectin in BAL fluids (55); this increase in E-selectin is dramatically inhibited by pretreatment of allergic subjects with 3 days of prednisone administration prior to segmental antigen challenge (69). As to the effect of glucocorticoids on adhesion molecule expression in allergic reactions, recent studies by Bachert et al., using antigen challenge of explanted nasal mucosa from allergic individuals, have shown inhibition of endothelial activation by in vitro treatment with glucocorticoids (70). Similarly, Albelda's group has found that glucocorticoids inhibit endothelial activation in a model in which human skin is transplanted to SCID mice (AAAAI '95). In either case, whether glucocorticoids inhibit endothelial activation by inhibiting local release of cytokines was not directly established. This issue is critical, since in vitro studies with cultured endothelial cells have established that endothelial activation per se is not inhibited by glucocorticoids when the endothelial-activating cytokine is added to the experiment (71,72). Studies by Lane et al. failed to find an inhibitory effect of steroids on E-selectin expression at sites of tuberculin challenge (73). Montefort et al. found no effect of BDP treatment on mucosal expression of ICAM-1 or endothelial leukocyte adhesion molecule 1 (E-selectin) in asthmatic subjects using immunohistochemistry and a simple grading system (74).

Putting the above observations together, there appears to be an early component of the allergic late-phase reaction in which nonspecific endothelial activation occurs. It is necessary to assess the effects of glucocorticoids on this early component. Two main possibilities exist in our view. The first is that this nonspecific activation of endothelium results from mast cell degranulation and release of stored TNF. In this case, we would predict that the early endothelial activation would not be inhibited by steroids in humans and that the early wave of neutrophil influx itself would not be prevented. It is possible, of course, that steroids are effective on human mast cells in vivo (unlike their effects in vitro). The second possibility is that the cytokines which are responsible for the early endothelial activation are derived from other cells or are transcriptionally induced in mast cells. In such cases, we would expect that steroids are more likely to inhibit the early nonspecific endothelial activation. Careful studies are clearly needed to determine the effects of glucocorticoids on both the early cellular infiltration, the early activation of endothelium, and the early production of endothelium-activating cytokines.

P-selectin and Allergic Inflammation

The adhesion molecule, P-selectin, was first identified as an adhesive glycoprotein redistributed from alpha granules to the plasma membrane of platelets following their activation (75,76). P-selectin shares a similar basic chemical structure with the other selectins consisting of a lectin domain, an epidermal growth factor domain, nine complement regulatory-like protein repeats, and small transmembrane and cytoplasmic domains (77). Using monoclonal antibodies to survey other tissues, P-selectin was also found to be present on the surface of vascular endothelial cells in many organs, with the greatest expression on small veins and venules (76). As with platelets, unstimulated endothelial cells do not have significant quantities of P-selectin present on their surface, but activation of endothelial cells results in very rapid (i.e., within 1–3 min) expression of the molecule on the cell surface (76,78). P-selectin is stored in the Weibel-Palade bodies of endothelial cells (76), and it is translocated to the endothelial surface on stimulation with histamine, thrombin, phorbol 12-myristate 13-acetate (PMA), calcium ionophore A23187, and oxygen-derived free radicals (79–82). Expression of P-selectin on the endothelial surface is transient, with P-selectin being rapidly reinternalized. Like E-selectin, P-selectin mediates the earliest interaction between leukocytes and the endothelium (i.e., leukocyte rolling) (78,79,81), interacting with leukocyte-expressed carbohydrate ligands.

The role of P-selectin in allergic inflammation has not been fully investigated despite recent evidence which suggests that P-selectin does interact with leukocyte ligands on T cells (83) and eosinophils (84,85) as well as neutrophils and monocytes (85,86). P-selectin has been demonstrated to mediate acute mast cell–mediated leukocyte rolling and adherence in vivo (87,88). Utilizing a model

of rat intravital microscopy, Gaboury et al. demonstrated that mast cell activation resulted in a significant increase in leukocyte rolling and adherence which
could be blocked with a P-selectin–neutralizing monoclonal antibody (88). The
mechanism underlying this mast cell–induced change in leukocyte-endothelium
interaction appears to be mediated by mast cell–released histamine, as
diphenhydramine effectively attenuated the response. In this connection, others (89,90) have demonstrated that direct application of histamine can induce
P-selectin–mediated leukocyte rolling and adherence which is blocked by H1
receptor antagonists. Since P-selectin is not capable of mediating firm adherence of leukocytes to the endothelium, the mechanism by which P-
selectin–neutralizing monoclonal antibodies and histamine receptor antagonists
block leukocyte adherence is most likely due to disruption of the role of P-
selectin in mediating leukocyte activation. As demonstrated by Lorrant et al.
(79,91), P-selectin can tether the unstimulated leukocyte to the endothelial cell
surface, positioning it for exposure to endothelium-expressed mediators, such
as platelet-activating factor (PAF), which can fully activate the leukocyte and
result in firm adherence. These investigators demonstrated coexpression of P-
selectin and PAF on the surface of stimulated human umbilical vein endothelial
cells, and they also demonstrated a cooperativity of P-selectin with PAF in
bringing leukocytes in contact with the stimulated endothelium and in facilitating
the processes necessary for firm adherence and activation of the expression of
inflammatory genes such as MCP-1 (79,91,92).

In addition to activation of P-selectin expression by small molecules, there
is also evidence that the cytokines involved in allergic inflammation may affect endothelial expression of P-selectin. Gotsch et al. demonstrated the ability of TNF-α to regulate P-selectin at the transcriptional level in mouse endo-
thelioma cells. TNF-α resulted in maximal cell expression of P-selectin at 3–4
hr following stimulation (93). As Wershil et al. found dexamethasone to attenuate TNF-α release from mast cells, steroids may influence the expression of P-
selectin as well as E-selectin. Similarly, recent studies by Suzuki et al. demonstrate that high levels of circulating glucocorticoids in spontaneously
hypertensive rats decreased histamine-mediated leukocyte adherence, an effect
they attributed to decreased P-selectin expression (94). Thus, although it is
tempting to speculate that P-selectin expression may be disrupted by glucocorticoids, as with other endothelial adhesion molecules, the effect of glucocorticoids on P-selectin expression in vivo remains unknown.

Specific Endothelial Activation in Allergic Reactions

Investigators in several laboratories realized at about the same time that the
endothelial adhesion molecule vascular cell adhesion molecule 1 (VCAM-1)
(95), which binds to the leukocyte counterligand VLA-4, may participate in

binding of eosinophils and other cells which participate in allergic reactions (basophils, lymphocytes, monocytes) by inducing rolling, adhesion, and perhaps transendothelial migration of these cells into tissue sites (96–101). Of particular interest is the fact that VCAM-1 does not bind to neutrophils, which lack the counterreceptor, and the finding that the allergic disease–associated cytokine, IL-4, can induce the expression of VCAM-1 on endothelium without inducing either E-selectin of ICAM-1 (Fig. 2) (102–104). IL-4 in turn has been found to induce eosinophil, basophil, and lymphocyte adhesion, but not adhesion of neutrophils, to endothelial cells (104). These observations and others have led to the concept that specific endothelial activation by IL-4, and/or the related cytokine IL-13, leads to VCAM-1 expression and allergic cell re-

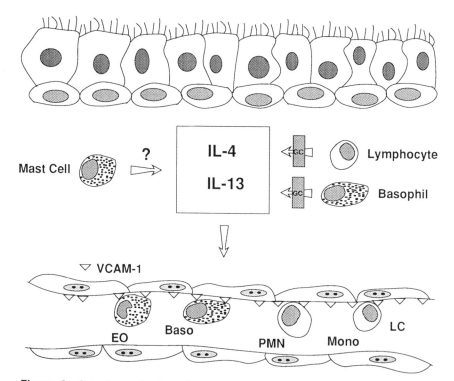

Figure 2 Selective activation of endothelial VCAM-1 expression. IL-4 and IL-13 activate endothelial VCAM-1 expression. Glucocorticoids inhibit production of IL-4 and IL-13. It is not known whether glucocorticoids inhibit mast cell IL-4 production. See legend for Figure 1 and text.

cruitment (104,105). Numerous studies in animals and humans have shown correlations among IL-4 levels, VCAM-1 expression, and eosinophils (50,56,106–113). Disruption of the VCAM-1/VLA-4 adhesion system inhibits allergic cell recruitment in several animal species (114–117). Elegant in situ hybridization studies on allergic reactions as well as in allergic diseases have firmly established that IL-4 (and IL-13) is generated during allergic inflammation (118,119, and Huang et al in press). The relative importance of various cellular source(s) of IL-4 and IL-13 in allergic reactions and allergic diseases is not completely known (120). However, numerous studies have shown that in challenge reactions lymphocytes are the primary mRNA-expressing cell type in both biopsies and BAL (120,121). Immunohistochemical studies have revealed, however, that mast cells may be an additional source of IL-4 (121–123). Recent studies have shown that eosinophils and basophils can also express IL-4 mRNA and/or protein (124,125, and Jordana et al, Moqbel et al., AAAAI 1995). In our view, based on the quantitative data in vitro and the fact that $CD4^+$ lymphocytes appear to be required for allergic late-phase reactions, the cell type of primary importance for IL-4 generation is likely to be the lymphocyte (126,127). The effects of glucocorticoids on specific endothelial activation can be subjected to a similar analysis to that which was presented for nonspecific endothelial activation (see Fig. 2). Glucocorticoids have been shown to be effective inhibitors of IL-4 production by lymphocytes in vitro (128–131). No published studies are yet available on the effects of glucocorticoids on IL-4 production or release from basophils, eosinophils, or mast cells. However, that portion of expression by these cell types which is inducible (as opposed to what may be stored and released) is expected to be inhibited by glucocorticoids. In vitro studies have shown that activation of endothelial adhesion molecule expression by IL-4 or IL-13 is not inhibited by glucocorticoids (72,105). Any inhibitory effect of glucocorticoids on endothelial activation to express VCAM-1 would therefore occur indirectly by reducing the release of IL-4 (and presumably IL-13). Glucocorticoids clearly do inhibit IL-4 production in allergic reactions and allergic diseases. In situ hybridization studies have shown a marked reduction of IL-4–positive cells after glucocorticoid treatment in asthma as well as following experimental antigen challenge in both the nose and the lungs (128–131). Although no studies are available to our knowledge on the effects of steroids on levels of IL-4 protein in BAL fluids, one study has shown that the quantity of IL-4 mRNA in BAL lysates 18 hr after antigen challenge is reduced by at least 90% following treatment with prednisone (130). Thus far, no studies on the effects of glucocorticoids on VCAM-1 expression following antigen challenge or in steroid-treated asthma have been reported.

Eosinophil-Priming Cytokines and Glucocorticoid Action

Cytokines play several important roles in the development, movement, and activation of human eosinophils. The primary cytokine in eosinophil generation appears to be IL-5, although IL-3 and GM-CSF can also induce eosinophil generation (132–135). All three of these cytokines, which act through distinct receptor α chains that share a common β chain, can dramatically prolong eosinophil survival, can increase eosinophil adhesion molecule expression and adhesion to endothelium and other surfaces, can profoundly potentiate eosinophil movement across an endothelial barrier and in simple Boyden chamber systems, and potentiate degranulation (136–142). These actions, often referred to as "priming," are now appreciated to be important in allergic diseases.

The source of eosinophil-priming cytokines in allergic reactions or allergic diseases is difficult to assess (Fig. 3). Studies of BAL fluid indicate that both IL-5 and GM-CSF are present at levels high enough to induce eosinophil survival and/or for detection in ELISA or bioassays. Antigen challenge increases the level of both of these cytokines (143–146). The cellular source of GM-CSF is most difficult to assess, since numerous resident cells, including epithelium, endothelium, macrophages, and even fibroblasts can potentially produce it. Several infiltrating cells, including lymphocytes and monocytes, can produce GM-CSF as well (147,148). In the case of IL-3 lymphocytes are likely to be the primary source, although in rodents, mast cells have been shown to make it (57,149,150). For IL-5, lymphocytes also are expected to be the primary source, although it has been detected in other cells, including mast cells and eosinophils themselves (149,151). Lymphocyte production of IL-5 and IL-3 in vitro is profoundly inhibited by glucocorticoids (152,153); effects of glucocorticoids on mast cell IL-5 release have not been documented. GM-CSF production is suppressed in vitro by glucocorticoids in most of the cell types listed above, including epithelium, monocytes, macrophages, and lymphocytes (23,154,155). Interestingly, the production of GM-CSF by human umbilical vein endothelial cells in vitro is not inhibited by glucocorticoid treatment (unpublished observations). In vivo, glucocorticoids have been found to reduce the number of cells expressing mRNA for GM-CSF, IL-3, and IL-5 in both allergic late-phase reactions as well as in asthma, as determined by in situ hybridization (128, and see Chapter 11). In BAL, IL-5 mRNA was found to be reduced by 90% in glucocorticoid-treated individuals 20 hr after segmental allergen challenge when compared with matched placebo-treated controls (130). Interestingly, in the same study, levels of GM-CSF in the BAL fluid were unaffected, suggesting that this cytokine may have been produced by a glucocorticoid-resistant cell type (possibly endothelial cells) (69).

Effects of glucocorticoids on eosinophil activation and priming by cytokines varies among in vitro test systems. Studies of GM-CSF–induced in-

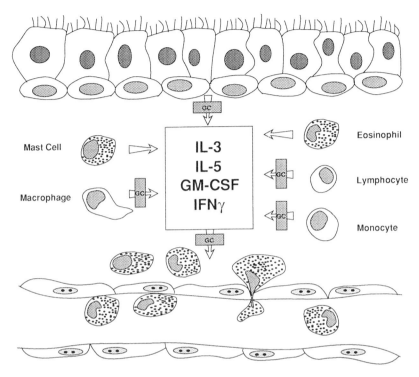

Figure 3 Eosinophil-priming cytokines and allergic disease. Cytokines prolong eosinophil survival and activate eosinophil functional responses. Glucocorticoids inhibit generation of cytokines and block the prolongation of survival. See legend for Figure 1 and text.

creases in eosinophil adhesion and CD11b expression failed to find an inhibitory effect of glucocorticoids (141), although IL-3–induced CD11b expression was inhibited by glucocorticoids (156). Studies by Kita et al. have shown that glucocorticoid treatment in vitro does not inhibit the potentiation of eosinophil degranulation caused by IL-5 or other eosinophil-priming cytokines (157), although Fujisawa et al. recently reported that dexamethasone inhibits IL-5–induced eosinophil degranulation (158). That eosinophil-priming cytokines are operative in vivo in antigen challenge models in the lungs seems clear from the finding that eosinophils isolated from BAL during a late-phase reaction display increased adhesive properties, increased superoxide generation, and increased transendothelial migration (55,142,159,160). Whether glucocorticoids have direct effects on these responses in vivo is almost impossible to determine, since they are so effective in reducing eosinophil numbers, making these studies impractical.

Lamas et al. and others have shown that the prolongation of eosinophil survival by IL-3, IL-5 and GM-CSF is dramatically inhibited by glucocorticoids (161–166). Interestingly, the effect of glucocorticoids depends on the concentration of the cytokine present: if cytokine levels are high enough, the glucocorticoid effect is lost. The net result is a three- to five-fold shift in the cytokine dose-response curve for promoting eosinophil survival. When coupled with the inhibition of production of these cytokines, this probably explains the profound decrease in eosinophils in tissues as well as in the circulation caused by glucocorticoid treatment. Studies by Kawabori et al. have shown in the rat that glucocorticoid treatment causes a rapid disappearance and phagocytosis of eosinophils in the intestine and other tissues (167). Although the process of apoptosis in eosinophils has been shown to be associated with fragmentation of eosinophil DNA and expression of adhesion molecules which render the eosinophil susceptible to phagocytosis, relatively little is known about the intracellular biochemical mechanisms which underlie this process (166,168). Apoptosis, and the role of glucocorticoids in its regulation, is discussed at length in Chapter 7. The combined suppression of eosinophil-priming cytokine production and the direct suppression of eosinophil survival by glucocorticoids probably synergize to produce the dramatic reduction of eosinophils in allergic diseases and allergic reactions.

B. Relevance of Chemokines to Allergic Inflammation and the Actions of Glucocorticoids

Over the last several years, a family of chemotactic cytokines termed chemokines has been recognized and studied intensively (169–172). These molecules are able to induce movement, and in some cases activation, of selected cell types. The family of chemokines is quite large and divided into two subfamilies: the α (C-X-C) family and the β (C-C) family. In general, these are 8- to 10- kDa cytokines which exhibit 25–75% homology at the amino acid level and contain four conserved cysteine residues. In the case of the C-X-C family, the first two cysteines have an intervening amino acid. Among the recognized chemokines, which now number over 30 in humans, are molecules which will induce selective migration of neutrophils or various combinations of lymphocytes, monocytes, eosinophils, and basophils. The growth of interest in the chemokines as being relevant to allergic diseases stems from the recognition that some of these molecules can induce basophil histamine release (e.g., MCP-1, MIP-1α, RANTES) (173,174) and eosinophil or lymphocyte migration (e.g., MCP-3, RANTES, MIP-1α) (175–177). Among the chemokines tested to date, RANTES and CKβ10 (also called MCP-4 from Human Genome Sciences) are the most effective in inducing eosinophil chemotaxis; MCP-3 and eotaxin (in guinea pigs) also have eosinophil chemotactic activity (177,178, and unpublished observations). RANTES is also a potent stimulus for eosinophil transendothelial migration and synergizes with eosinophil-priming cytokines such as IL-5 (179). Several laboratories have begun to analyze which cell types in the lung produce RANTES and under what conditions. These studies revealed that airway epithelial cells are a primary source of RANTES signals as measured by immunohistochemistry in nasal polyps and mucosa of the upper and lower airways (180). This result was somewhat unexpected, since in vitro studies reported in the literature had suggested that a major source would be lymphocytes and perhaps fibroblasts (181,182). Prompted by these findings, several laboratories have determined the expression of RANTES in cultured airway epithelial cells, its regulation by cytokines, and the effects of glucocorticoids on its expression (183–185). Various airway epithelial cell lines can express RANTES after stimulation with the cytokines TNF-α and γ-IFN; the combination of these two cytokines gives a profound induction of RANTES gene expression (183). Incubation of epithelial cells with glucocorticoid produces a marked suppression of RANTES expression. Thus, like the other classes of cytokines discussed in this chapter, glucocorticoids appear to act early by inhibiting expression of RANTES. Studies on various other chemokines, including IL-8, MCP-1, and MIP-1α, have demonstrated a similar inhibitory effect of glucocorticoids on expression (Fig. 4) (186).

With regard to the possible relevance of RANTES to eosinophil and mononuclear cell recruitment in vivo, studies in animals and more recently humans have demonstrated that injection of RANTES induces a marked infiltration of tissues with eosinophils and mononuclear cells including lymphocytes (187,188). In studies in humans, eosinophils are the predominant infiltrating cell type (188). Staining of biopsies from RANTES-challenged sites in humans with antibodies against either CD3 or CD45RO (which is found on the surface of both memory lymphocytes and eosinophils) revealed rich infiltrates of cells positive for these markers (188).

It has been postulated that the site of the inhibitory action of glucocorticoids is against the production of the cytokines and chemokines which induce activation of endothelium and leukocytes rather than the response of either endothelium or leukocytes to these cytokines (17). If this hypothesis is correct, then glucocorticoids should have relatively modest or no effect, when applied locally, on cell recruitment induced by injection of a chemoattractant. In fact, this is the case in studies done by Yancey et al. with C5a in which glucocorticoid treatment failed to inhibit infiltration of the skin by neutrophils (189) and in studies by Katori's group in which glucocorticoids did not prevent leukotriene B_4 (LTB$_4$)–induced rolling and adhesion (190). Interpretation is a bit complicated, since neutrophils are increased in number in the circulation following treatment with oral steroids (191,192). Planned experiments will determine

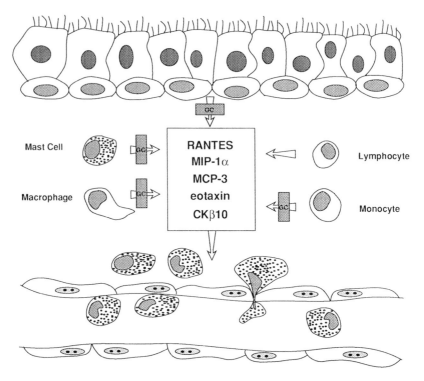

Figure 4 Chemokines and allergic disease. Chemokines derived from epithelial cells and elsewhere stimulate movement and localization of leukocytes. Glucocorticoids inhibit chemokine production. See legend for Figure 1 and text.

whether locally administered glucocorticoids inhibit RANTES-induced eosinophil infiltration. As far as the airways are concerned, we believe that an important role of RANTES may be localization of infiltrating cells to the epithelium and that inhaled glucocorticoids can prevent this event by blocking RANTES production (180).

IV. Summary

The objective of this chapter has been to discuss the effects of glucocorticoids on cell recruitment in allergic reactions and models of allergic diseases within the context of the role of cytokines and adhesion molecules. To be sure, inhibition of the infiltration of inflammatory cells by glucocorticoids is not the only important result of therapy with these drugs, and inhibition of the cytokine network is not the only mechanism by which glucocorticoids achieve this effect. However, cytokines play a central role in leukocyte recruitment, and many of the beneficial effects of glucocorticoid treatment, including changes in physiology, vascular tone, smooth muscle tone, and secretion, probably result in a diminution of the number of infiltrating inflammatory cells at the sites of exposure to antigen. We have concluded that cytokines mediate cellular recruitment in allergic reactions at a number of levels: they activate local vascular endothelial cells to play an active role in the recruitment of leukocytes, they activate leukocytes in the circulation, especially eosinophils, and they cause the movement of leukocytes once they have adhered to vascular endothelium. Glucocorticoids clearly inhibit the generation of all the classes of cytokines discussed, indirectly resulting in inhibition of endothelial activation, eosinophil priming, and adhesion and movement of leukocytes into the tissue. There is a relatively large accumulation of data supporting these statements in general, although many of the specific pieces of information are still missing. Unfortunately, this information does not assist us greatly in developing new drugs to replace glucocorticoids, since a clear conclusion is that glucocorticoids work at a multitude of sites, affecting a multitude of cytokines, and have no single mode of action. It is hoped that new studies on the intracellular mechanism of glucocorticoid action may result in the development of drugs which can achieve the same pleiotropic beneficial effects without the undesirable effects which, in some cases, work through subtly different molecular mechanisms.

Acknowledgements

The authors would like to thank Bonnie Hebden for her assistance in the preparation of this chapter.

Discussion

DR. BUSSE: With systemic corticosteroids, circulating levels of eosinophils decrease. Do you therefore feel that one mechanism by which systemic corticosteroids inhibit eosinophil migration during segmental antigen challenge is through an effect on the number of eosinophils available for migration.

DR. SCHLEIMER: Although the reduction in eosinophil recruitment by oral steroids must result, at least in part, from a decrease in circulating eosinophils, the fact that topical steroids inhibit eosinophil recruitment suggests that steroids also work locally.

DR. O'BYRNE: Inhaled corticosteroids (400 µg/day for 1 week) can prevent allergen-induced increases in blood eosinophils.

DR. BOCHNER: With the possible exception of modest effects of glucocorticoids on epithelial cell ICAM-1 expression, I'm not aware of any studies showing the effects of glucocorticoids on baseline leukocyte and/or tissue adhesion molecule expression. How single-dose steroids acutely affect circulating cell numbers is not clear, although it does not appear to be due to rapid changes in adhesion molecules. Intravital microscopy studies in the 1950s to 1960s suggest that the earliest steps in cell recruitment, namely, rolling or margination, are inhibited by systemic steroid treatment. We would predict that this effect is due to inhibition of the release of leukocyte-activating or endothelium-activating factors rather than an effect on adhesion molecules per se (e.g., inhibition of the release of stimuli that induce P-selectin expression).

DR. BUSSE: Do you have any information on the effect of corticosteroids on the function of eosinophils that have undergone transendothelial migration?

DR. SCHLEIMER: In vitro, glucocorticoids have minimal effects on cytokine-induced eosinophil transendothelial migration when either the eosinophils or the endothelial cells have been treated. We have not performed functional studies on transmigrated cells. Available evidence indicates that eosinophil functions such as adhesion and degranulation are not inhibited by steroids.

DR. GLEICH: The effects of glucocorticoids on eosinophil migration in the segmental antigen challenge of patients are very impressive. I would like to recount experiments which Dr. R. Egan and his colleagues at the Schering-Plough Corporation performed in mice. In essence, they showed that glucocorticoids block eosinophil accumulation in the antigen-challenged lung of the mouse and prevented eosinophil migration out of the bone marrow. Administration of an anti–IL-5 antibody caused precisely the same effects as the glucocorticoids. (T Kung, D Stelts, J Zurcher, et al. Mechanisms of allergic pulmonary eosinophilia in the mouse. J Allergy Clin Immunol 1994; 94:1217–1224.)

DR. DURHAM: What is the time course of the IL-4–induced and IL-13–induced increase in endothelial VCAM-1 expression? I ask because we recently showed that topical steroid inhibited nasal late responses and IL-4 mRNA and tissue eosinophilia at 24 hr. We speculated that this effect of IL-4 may be VCAM-1 dependent.

DR. SCHLEIMER: Both IL-4 and IL-13 induce VCAM-1 in vitro steadily over a 24-hr period.

DR. BARNES: You have demonstrated that glucocorticoids do not inhibit ICAM-1 expression in endothelial cells, but there is evidence that they may inhibit ICAM-1 expression in epithelial cells and monocytes in a NF-κB dependent mechanism. It is therefore important to consider differences in steroid control of cell adhesion in different cell types.

DR. SCHLEIMER: Cell type–selective effects of steroids are seen for other molecular targets as well (e.g., cytokine production).

DR. PERRETTI: Do you think that dexamethasone will affect RANTES-induced eosinophil accumulation? If so, do you expect the steroid to be effective locally and/or systemically?

DR. SCHLEIMER: I would expect that local steroids would not inhibit responses to injected RANTES. Dr. Beck is presently designing experiments to test this important question.

DR. GAULDIE: We have used a recombinant adenovirus expressing RANTES administered intratracheally into rats (Sprague-Dawley). This causes massive accumulation of mononuclear cells to the lung, but we do not see any significant presence of eosinophils. Can you comment?

DR. SCHLEIMER: The species differences of these chemokine responses are interesting. We learned the hard way that human RANTES has no effect in mice. Hugh Rosen showed that it induces a pronounced eosinophil accumulation in dogs previously exposed to parasites but not naive dogs. (Meurer et al. J Exp Med 1993; 178:1913–1921.) We anticipated that allergic disease status (perhaps eosinophil priming) might dramatically influence this response. Dr. Beck finds that normal individuals display eosinophil recruitment after RANTES skin challenge, which is much slower than in allergics.

DR. DENBURG: We have published results (Kanai et al. Am J Respir Crit Care Med 1994; 150:1094) on the effects of inhaled nasal budesonide on nasal polyp eosinophils. There was a decrease selectively in the activated (EG2 positive) eosinophil subpopulation compared with untreated polyps.

DR. SCHLEIMER: Within a polyp, it is difficult to isolate those effects on eosinophils from those which result indirectly from effects of steroids on the tissue milieu.

DR. DURHAM: Does intradermal RANTES induce macroscopic changes as well as local eosinophilia? What is the time course? Barry Kay has recently shown that allergen-induced late skin responses are accompanied by increased RANTES mRNA expression at 24 hr.

DR. BECK: Surprisingly enough, we have not seen any macroscopic changes, nor have the subjects experienced any symptoms referable to these sites at any of the doses used thus far (0.08–4.0 µg). We see significant tissue eosinophilia as early as 30 min after RANTES injection, but the plateau seems to occur between 6 and 24 hr in allergic subjects.

DR. LEUNG: Considering your stepwise model of adhesion preceding trans-endothelial migration of eosinophils into the skin, do you know whether

VCAM-1 or E-selectin is induced by RANTES directly on endothelial cells or whether saline injection (by disrupting keratinocytes and causing IL-1 or TNF release) leads to endothelial cell adhesion molecule expression which in concert with RANTES leads to eosinophil infiltration?

DR. SCHLEIMER: We are planning to determine the effect of RANTES injection on the state of endothelial activation. We have found that phenol-containing saline does activate endothelium, but injection of saline alone with a small-gauge needle causes minimal activation.

DR. LANE: PPD induces mononuclear and eosinophil infiltration into an inflammation site. In a double-blind, placebo-controlled study, we have shown that 10-day treatment with oral prednisolone, 40 mg, suppresses eosinophil/macrophage/T-cell infiltration into the site with no suppression of endothelial ICAM-1, VCAM-1 and ELAM-1. We have not looked at RANTES expression in this in vivo model.

DR. SCHLEIMER: I was not aware of those studies. Although, it is, of course, difficult to quantitate by immunohistochemistry, this is an intriguing result which parallels the lack of effect in vitro on endothelial activation. We would presume that production of endothelial activators is not inhibited in this case.

DR. GAULDIE: Since there are differences in tissue structure between lung and skin, there may be different mechanisms involved in eosinophil recruitment.

DR. THOMPSON: Your data show that eosinophils die when exposed to glucocorticoids while also exposed to a cytokine, but that higher concentrations of cytokine will protect them. In light of that, what do you mean in interpreting those results when you say that steroids have no "direct toxic effect"?

DR. SCHLEIMER: Simply that the steroid effect must result from a disruption of the pathway by which cytokines promote survival rather than by directly inducing the final common pathway of cell death.

Dr. Mauro Perretti presented some of his recent findings with lipocortin.

DR. LANE: (1) Are there data on the effect of lipocortin at the molecular level? (2) What is the interaction of lipocortin with phospholipases?

DR. PERRETTI: (1) The molecular mechanism responsible for lipocortin 1 action is not yet clear. As I said, we propose a selective interference with the degranulation process. We do not know whether this is the consequence of an inhibition of phospholipase A2 or not. Certainly, in our models of cytokine-induced leukocyte migration, lipocortin and dexamethasone are potent inhibitors of cell recruitment, whereas inhibitors of arachidonic acid metabolism are unable to modify cell trafficking. (2) In studies using porcine pancreatic phospholipase A2, lipocortin 1 was found not to inhibit the enzyme. However, in recent years, the importance of a cytosolic form of phospholipase A2 in regulating arachidonic acid release and metabolism has become evident. Kim et al. have published that lipocortin 1 inhibits the activity of cytosolic phospholipase A2 by direct interaction with the enzyme. (KM Kim, DK Kim, YM Park, C-K Kim, DS Na. Annexin-I inhibits phospholipase A2 by specific interaction, not by substrate depletion. FEBS Lett 1994; 343:251–255.) As I said, we do not have data on this subject, but certainly if you add lipocortin 1 to intact cells, you will observe inhibition of prostanoid release. Finally, I would like to stress that it is very unlikely that this mechanism is responsible for the lipocortin 1 effect on leukocyte recruitment.

DR. BRATTSAND: Katori and Oda described in their paper that after steroid treatment the neutrophils stuck in between the endothelial cells and the basement membrane. (T Oda, M Katori. Inhibition site of dexamethasone on extravasation of polymorphonuclear leukocytes in the hamster cheek pouch. J Leukoc. Biol 1992; 52:337–342.) The neutrophils need proteases for getting through the basement membrane and glucocorticoids blocks collagenase production. Thus, my question is whether the AP-1–mediated inhibition of metalloprotease synthesis is important for this block of locomotion.

DR. PERRETTI: It is very likely that enzymatic release occurs during leukocyte emigration and that this contributes to the chemotaxis in the subendothelial space. Our data with the lipocortin 1 peptide show an inhibitory action on the release of elastase from human neutrophils. I should also recall that old studies have shown that glucocorticoids selectively affect enzymatic release from macrophages with an inhibitory action on stimulated elastase release and no effect on the constitutive release of lysozyme. Therefore, glucocorticoids and the lipocortin 1 N-terminus peptide may selectively affect enzymatic release from leukocytes, and this may relate to the inhibition of leukocyte chemotaxis in the subendothelial space.

References

1. Brattsand R, Thalen A, Roempke K, Kallstrom L, Gruvstad E. Influence of 16α, 17α-acetal substitution and steroid nucleus fluorination on the topical to systemic activity ratio of glucocorticoids. J Steroid Biochem 1982; 16:779–786.
2. Brattsand R. Development of glucocorticosteroids with lung selectivity. Clin Exp Aspects 1989; 17–38.
3. Schleimer RP. Glucocorticosteroids: their mechanism of action and use in allergic diseases. In: Middleton E, Reed CE, Ellis EF, N.F. Adkinson J. Yunginger JW, Busse W, eds. Allergy Principles and Practice. 4th ed. St Louis: Mosby, 1993:893–925.

4. Munck A, Guyre PM, Holbrook NJ. Physiological functions of glucocorticoids in stress and their relation to pharmacological actions. Endocr Rev 1984; 5:25–44.

5. Besedovsky H, Rey AD, Sorkin E, Dinarello CA. Immunoregulatory feedback between interleukin-1 and glucocorticoid hormones. Science 1986; 233:652–654.

6. Persson CGA. Glucocorticoids for asthma—early contributions. Pulm Pharmacol 1989; 2:163–166.

7. Guyre PM, Munck A. Molecular biology of glucocorticoid hormone action. In: Schleimer RP, Claman HN, Oronsky AL, eds. Anti-inflammatory Steroid Action. Basic and Clinical Aspects. San Diego: Academic Press, 1989:199–225.

8. Flower RJ, Blackwell GJ. Anti-inflammatory steroids induce biosynthesis of a phospholipase A2 inhibitor which prevents prostaglandin generation. Nature 1979; 278:456–459.

9. Hirata F, Notsu Y, Iwata M, Parente L, DiRosa M, Flower RJ. Identification of several species of phospholipase inhibitory protein(s) by radioimmunoassay for lipomodulin. Biochem Biophys Res Commun 1982; 109:223–230.

10. Davidson FF, Dennis EA, Powel M, Glenney JR. Inhibition of phospholipase A_2 by "lipocortins" and calpactins. An effect of binding to substrate phospholipids. J Biol Chem 1987; 262:1698–1705.

11. Perretti M, Ahluwalia A, Harris JG, Goulding NJ, Flower RJ. Lipocortin-1 fragments inhibit neutrophil accumulation and neutrophil-dependent edema in the mouse. J Immunol 1993; 151:4306–4314.

12. Perretti M, Flower RJ. Modulation of IL-1-induced neutrophil migration by dexamethasone and lipocortin 1. J Immunol 1993; 150:992–999.

13. Wahl SM, Altman LC, Rosenstreich DL. Inhibition of in vitro lymphokine synthesis by glucocorticosteroids. J Immunol 1975; 115:476–481.

14. Werb Z. Biochemical actions of glucocorticoids on macrophages in culture. Specific inhibition of elastase, collagenase, and plasminogen activator secretion and effects on other metabolic functions. J Exp Med 1978; 147:1695–1712.

15. Gillis S, Crabtree GR, Smith KA. Glucocorticoid-induced inhibition of T-cell growth factor production. II. the effect on the in vitro generation of cytolytic T-cells. J Immunol 1979; 123:1632–1638.

16. Guyre PM, Girard MT, Morganelli PM, Manganiello PD. Glucocorticoid effects on the production and actions of immune cytokines. J Ster Biochem 1988; 30:89–93.

17. Schleimer RP. Effects of glucocorticoids on inflammatory cells relevant to their therapeutic applications in asthma. Am Rev Respir Dis 1990; 141:S59–S69.

18. Schüle R, Rangarajan P, Kliewer S, Ransome LJ, Bolado J, Yang N, Verma IM, Evans RM. Functional antagonism between oncoprotein c-Jun and the glucocorticoid receptor. Cell 1990; 62:1217–1226.

19. Yang-Yen H-F, Chambard J-C, Sun Y-L, Smeal T, Schmidt TJ, Drouin J, Karin M. Transcriptional interference between c-Jun and the glucocorticoid receptor: Mutual inhibition of DNA binding due to direct protein-protein interaction. Cell 1990; 62:1205–1215.

20. Drouin J, Charron J, Gagner JP, Jeanotte L, Nemer M, Plante RK, Wrange O. The pro-opio melanocortin gene: a model for negative regulation of transcription by glucocorticoids. J Cell Biochem 1987; 35:293.

21. Sakai DD, Helms S, Carlstedt-Duke J, Gustafsson JA, Rottman FM, Yamamoto KR. Hormone mediated repression: a negative glucocorticoid receptor element from the bovine prolactin gene. Genes Dev 1988; 2:1144.

22. Lee SW, Tsou A-P, Chan H, Thomas J, Petrie K, Eugui Em, Allison AC. Glucocorticoids selectively inhibit the transcription of the interleukin 1β gene and decrease the stability of interleukin 1β mRNA. Proc Natl Acad Sci USA 1988; 85:1204–1208.

23. Tobler A, Meier R, Seitz M, Dewald B, Baggiolini M, Fey MF. Glucocorticoids downregulate gene expression of GM-CSF, NAP-1/IL-8, and IL-6, but not of M-CSF in human fibroblasts. Blood 1992; 79:45–51.

24. Hogg JC. Pathology of asthma. J Allergy Clin Immunol 1993; 92:1–5.

25. Jeffrey PK, Wardlaw AJ, Nelson FC, Collins JV, Kay AB. Bronchial biopsies in asthma. An ultrastructural, quantitative study and correlation with hyperreactivity. Am Rev Respir Dis 1989; 140:1745–1753.

26. Bousquet J, Chanez P, Lacoste JY, Barneon G, Ghavanian N, Enander I, Venge P, Ahlstedt S, Simony-Lafontaine J, Godard P, Michel FB. Eosinophilic inflammation in asthma. N Engl J Med 1990; 323:1033–1039.

27. Bochner BS, Undem BJ, Lichtenstein LM. Immunological aspect of allergic asthma. Annu Rev Immunol 1994; 12:295–335.

28. Lundgren R, Söderberg M, Hörstedt P, Stenling R. Morphological studies of bronchial mucosal biopsies from asthmatics before and after ten years of treatment with inhaled steroids. Eur Respir J 1988; 1:883–889.

29. Laitinen LA, Laitinen A, Heino M, Haahtela T. Eosinophilic airway inflammation during exacerbation of asthma and its treatment with inhaled corticosteroids. Am Rev Respir Dis 1991; 143:423–427.

30. Adelroth E, Rosenhall L, Johansson S-A, Linden M, Venge P. Inflammatory cells and eosinophilic activity in asthmatics investigated by bronchoalveolar lavage. The effects of antiasthmatic treatment with budesonide or terbutaline. Am Rev Respir Dis 1990; 142:91–99.

31. Burke C, Power CK, Norris A, Condez A, Schmekel B, Poulter LW. Lung function and immunopathological changes after inhaled corticosteroid therapy in asthma. Eur Respir J 1992; 5:73–79.

32. Herxheimer H. Influence of cortisone on induced asthma and bronchial hyposensitization. Br Med J 1954; 1:184–187.

33. Pepys J, Hutchcroft BJ. Bronchial provocation tests in etiologic diagnosis and analysis of asthma. Am Rev Respir Dis 1975; 112:829–859.

34. Holgate ST, Hardy C, Robinson C, Agius RM, Howarth PH. the mast cell as a primary effector cell in the pathogenesis of asthma. J Allergy Clin Immunol 1986; 77:274–282.

35. Burge PS, Efthimiou J, Turner-Warwick M, Nelmes PTJ. Double-blind trials of inhaled beclomethasone dipropionate and fluocortin butyl ester in allergen-induced immediate and late asthmatic reactions. Clin Allergy 1982; 12:523–531.

36. Dahl R, Johansson SA. Importance of duration of treatment with inhaled budesonide on the immediate and late bronchial reaction. Eur J Respir Dis 1982; 122 (Suppl.):167–175.

37. Metzger WJ, Hunninghake GW, Richerson HB. Late asthmatic responses: inquiry into mechanisms and significance. Clin Rev Allergy 1985; 3:145-165.
38. De Monchy JGR, Kauffman HF, Venge P, Koeter GH, Jansen HM, Sluiter HJ, de Vries K. Bronchoalveolar eosinophilia during allergen-induced late asthmatic reactions. Am Rev Respir Dis 1985; 131:373-376.
39. Liu MC, Hubbard WC, Proud D, Stealey B, Galli S, Kagey-Sobotka A, Bleecker ER, Lichtenstein LM. Immediate and late inflammatory responses to ragweed antigen challenge of the peripheral airways in asthmatics: cellular, mediator, and permeability changes. Am Rev Respir Dis 1991; 144:51-58.
40. Dinarello CA. Interleukin-1 and its biologically related cytokines. Adv Immunol 1989; 44:153-205.
41. Beutler B, Cerami A. Cachectin: More than a tumor necrosis factor. N Engl J Med 1987; 316:379-385.
42. Ying S, Robinson DS, Varney V, Meng Q, Tsicopoulos A, Moqbel R, Durham SR, Kay AB, Hamid Q. TNFα mRNA expression in allergic inflammation. Clin Exp Allergy 1991; 21:745-750.
43. Bochner BS, Landy SD, Plaut M, Dinarello CA, Schleimer RP. Interleukin 1 production by human lung tissue. I. Identification and characterization. J Immunol 1987; 139:2297-2302.
44. Bochner BS, Lamas AM, Benenati SV, Schleimer RP. On the central role of vascular endothelium in allergic reactions. In: Dorsch R, eds. Late Phase Allergic Reactions. Boca Raton, FL: CRC Press, 1990:221-235.
45. Moser R, Schleiffenbaum B, Groscurth P, Fehr J. Interleukin 1 and tumor necrosis factor stimulate human vascular endothelial cells to promote transendothelial neutrophil passage. J Clin Invest 1989; 83:444-455.
46. Cybulsky MI, Colditz IG, Movat HZ. The role of interleukin-1 in neutrophil leukocyte emigration induced by endotoxin. Am J Pathol 1986; 124:367-372.
47. Briscoe D, Cotran R, Pober J. Effects of TNF, LPS, and IL-4 on the expression of VCAM-1 in vivo: correlation with CD3+ T cell infiltration. J Immunol 1992; 149:2954-2960.
48. Groves RW, Ross E, Barker JNWM, Ross JS, Camp RDR, MacDonald DM. Effect of in vivo interleukin-1 on adhesion molecule expression in norman human skin. J Invest Dermatol 1992; 98:384-387.
49. Groves RW, Allen MH, Ross EL, Barker JNWN, MacDonald DM. Tumour necrosis factor alpha is pro-inflammatory in normal human skin and modulates cutaneous adhesion molecule expression. Br J Dermatol 1995; 132:345-352.
50. Kyan-Aung U, Haskard DO, Poston RN, Thornhill MH, Lee TH. Endothelial leukocyte adhesion molecule-1 and intercellular adhesion molecule-1 mediate the adhesion of eosinophils to endothelial cells in vitro and are expressed by endothelium in allergic cutaneous inflammation in vivo. J Immunol 1991; 146:521-528.
51. Leung DYM, Pober JS, Cotran RS. Expression of endothelial-leukocyte adhesion molecule-1 in elicited late phase allergic reactions. J Clin Invest 1991; 87:1805-1809.
52. Benenati S, Bochner B, Horn T, Farmer E, Schleimer R. Endothelial-leukocyte adhesion molecule-1 (ELAM-1) expression following cutaneous allergen challenge (abstr.). J Allergy Clin Immunol 1991; 87:304.

53. Klein LM, Lavker RM, Matis WL, Murphy GF. Degranulation of human mast cells induces an endothelial antigen central to leukocyte adhesion. Proc Natl Acad Sci USA 1989; 86:8972–8976.

54. Walsh LJ, Trinchieri G, Waldorf HA, Whitaker D, Murphy GF. Human dermal mast cells contain and release tumor necrosis factor α, which induces endothelial leukocyte adhesion molecule 1. Proc Natl Acad Sci USA 1991; 88:4220–4224.

55. Georas SN, Liu MC, Newman W, Beall WD, Stealey BA, Bochner BS. Altered adhesion molecule expression and endothelial activation accompany the recruitment of human granulocytes to the lung following segmental antigen challenge. Am J Respir Cell Mol Biol 1992; 7:261–269.

56. Bentley AM, Durham SR, Robinson DS, Menz G, Storz C, Cornwell O, Kay AB, Wardlaw AJ. Expression of endothelial and leukocyte adhesion molecules intercellular adhesion molecule-1, E-selectin, and vascular cell adhesion molecule-1 in the bronchial mucosa in steady-state and allergen-induced asthma. J Allergy Clin Immunol 1993; 92:857–868.

57. Plaut M, Pierce JH, Watson CJ, Hanley-Hyde J, Nordan RP, Paul WE. Mast cell lines produce lymphokines in response to cross-linkage of FcεRI or to calcium ionophores. Nature 1989; 339:64–67.

58. Gordon JR, Galli SJ. Mast cells as a source of both preformed and immunologically inducible TNF-α/cachectin. Nature 1990; 346:274–276.

59. Mazingue C, Carriere V, Dessaint J-P, Detoeuf F, Turz T, Auriault C, Capron A. Regulation of IgE synthesis by macrophages expressing Fcε-receptors: role of interleukin 1. Clin Exp Immunol 1987; 67:587–593.

60. Borish L, Mascali JJ, Dishuck J, Beam WR, Martin RJ, Rosenwasser LH. Detection of alveolar macrophage-derived IL-1β in asthma. J Immunol 1992; 149:3078–3082.

61. Bieber T, Salle Hdl, Wollenberg A, Hakimi J, Chizzonite R, Ring J, Hanau D, de la Salle C. Human epidermal langerhans cells express the high affinity receptor for immunoglobulin E (FcεRI). J Exp Med 1992; 175:1285–1290.

61a. Barkans J, Grant JA, Taborda-Barata L, Ying S, Menz G, Pfister R, Durham SR, Kay AB, Humbert M. High affinity IgE receptor (FcεRI)-bearing cells in bronchial biopsies from atopic and nonatopic asthma. J Allergy Clin Immunol 1996; 97:308 (abstract).,

62. Smith KA. T cell growth factor. Immunol Rev 1980; 51:337–357.

63. Snyder DS, Unanue ER. Corticosteroids inhibit murine macrophage Ia expression and interleukin-1 production. J Immunol 1982; 129:1803–1805.

64. Beutler B, Krochin N, Milsark IW, Luedke C, Cerami A. Control of cachectin (tumor necrosis factor) synthesis: mechanisms of endotoxin resistance. Science 1986; 232:977–980.

65. Bochner BS, Rutledge BK, Schleimer RP. Interleukin 1 production by human lung tissue. II. Inhibition by antiinflammatory steroids. J Immunol 1987; 139:2303–2307.

66. Wershil BK, Furuta GT, Lavigne JA, Choudhury AR, Wang Z-S, Galli SJ. Dexamethasone of cyclosporin A suppress mast cell-leukocyte cytokine cascades. J Immunol 1995; 154:1391–1398.

67. Schleimer RP. The effects of anti-inflammatory steroids on mast cells. In: Kaliner

M, Metcalfe D, eds. The Mast Cell in Health and disease. New York: Dekker, 1992:483–511.

68. Staruch MJ, Wood DD. Reduction of serum interleukin-1-like activity after treatment with dexamethasone. J Leukoc Biol 1985; 37:193–207.

69. Liu MC, Proud D, Hubbard WC, Stealey BA, Bochner BS, Newman W, Lichtenstein LM, Ferraci L, Walinskas J, Schleimer RP. Effects of prednisone on inflammation at sites of segmental allergen challenge in allergic asthmatic subjects. J Clin Invest 1994;

70. Bachert C, Hauser U, Prem B, Rudack C, Ganzer U. Proinflammatory cytokines in allergic rhinitis. Eur Arch Otorhinolaryngol 1995; 252(suppl. 1):S44–S49.

71. Schleimer RP, Freeland HS, Peters SP, Brown KE, Derse CP. An assessment of the effects of glucocorticoids on degranulation, chemotaxis, binding to vascular endothelial cells and formation of leukotriene B4 by purified human neutrophils. J Pharmacol Exp Ther 1989; 250:598–605.

72. Kaiser J, Bickel C, Bochner BS, Schleimer RP. The effects of the potent glucocorticoid budesonide on adhesion of eosinophils to human vascular endothelium and on endothelial expression of adhesion molecules. J Pharmacol Exp Ther 1993; 267:245–249.

73. Lane SJ, Sousa AR, Poston RN. In vivo cutaneous tuberculin response to prednisolone in corticosteroid resistant bronchial asthma. J Allergy Clin Immunol 1991; 91:A221.

74. Montefort S, Roche WR, Howarth PH, Djukanovic R, Gratziou C, Carroll M, Smith L, Britten KM, Haskard D, Lee TH, Holgate ST. Intercellular adhesion molecule-1 (ICAM-1) and endothelial leukocyte adhesion molecule-1 (ELAM-1) expression in the bronchial mucosa of normal and asthmatic subjects. Eur Respir J 1992; 5:815–823.

75. Hus-Lin SC, Berman CL, Furie BC, August D, Furie B. A platelet membrane protein expressed during platelet activation and secretion. J Biol Chem 1984; 259:9121–9126.

76. McEver RP, Beckstead JH, Moore KL, Marshall-Carlson L, Bainton DF. GMP-140, a platelet α-granule membrane protein, is also synthesized by vascular endothelial cells and is localized in Weibel-Palade bodies. J Clin Invest 1989; 84:92–99.

77. McEver RP. GMP-140, a receptor that mediates interactions of leukocytes with activated platelets and endothelium. Trends Cardiovasc Med 1991; 1:152–156.

78. Hattori R, Hamilton KK, Fugate RD, McEver RP, Sims PJ. Stimulated secretion of endothelial von Willebrand factor is accompanied by rapid redistribution to the cell surface of the intracellular granule membrane protein GMP-140. J Biol Chem 1989; 264:7768–7771.

79. Lorant DE, Patel KD, Mcintyre TM, Mcever RP, Prescott SM, Zimmerman GA. Coexpression of GMP-140 and PAF by endothelium stimulated by histamine or thrombin—a juxtacrine system for adhesion and activation of neutrophils. J Cell Biol 1991; 115:223–234.

80. Palluy O, Morliere L, Gris JC, Bonne C, Modat G. Hypoxia/reoxygenation stimulates endothelium to promote neutrophil adhesion. Free Rad Biol Med 1992; 13:21–30.

81. Patel KD, Zimmerman GA, Prescott SM, McEver RP, McIntyre TM. Oxygen radicals induce human endothelial cells to express GMP-140 and bind neutrophils. J Cell Biol 1991; 112:749–759.

82. Gaboury JP, Anderson DC, Kubes P. Molecular mechanisms involved in superoxide-induced leukocyte-endothelial cell interaction in vivo. Am J Physiol 1994; 266:H637–H642.

83. Kunzendorf U, Notter M, Hock H, Distler A, Diamantstein T, Walz G. T cells bind to the endothelial adhesion molecule GMP-140 (P-selectin). Transplantation 1993; 56:1213–1217.

84. Vadas MA, Lucas CM, Gamble JR, Lopez AF, Skinner MP, Berndt MC. Regulation of eosinophil function by P-selectin. In: Gleich GJ, Kay AB, eds. Eosinophils in Allergy and Inflammation. New York: Dekker, 1993:69–80.

85. Wein M, Sterbinsky SA, Bickel CA, Schleimer RP, Bochner BS. Comparison of eosinophil and neutrophil ligands for P-selectin: ligands for P-selectin differ from those for E-selectin, Am J Respir Cell Mol Biol 1995; 12:315–319.

86. Geng JG, Bevilacqua MP, Moore KL, McIntyre TM, Prescott SM, Kim JM, Bliss GA, Zimmerman GA, McEver RP. Rapid neutrophil adhesion to activated endothelium mediated by GMP-140. Nature 1990; 343:757–759.

87. Thorlacius H, Raud J, Rosengren-Beezley S, Forrest MJ, Hedqvist P, Lindbom L. Mast cell activation induces P-selectin-dependent leukocyte rolling and adhesion in postcapillary venules in vivo. Biochem Biophys Res Commun 1994; 203:1043–1049.

88. Gaboury JP, Johnston B, Niu XF, Kubes P. Mechanisms underlying acute mast cell-induced leukocyte rolling and adhesion in vivo. J Immunol 1995; 154:804–813.

89. Asako H, Kurose I, Wolf R, DeFrees S, Zheng ZL, Phillips ML, Paulson JC, Granger DN. Role of H1 receptors and P-selectin in histamine-induced leukocyte rolling and adhesion in postcapillary venules. J Clin Invest 1994; 93:1508–1515.

90. Kubes P, Kanwar S. Histamine induces leukocyte rolling in post-capillary venules. J Immunol 1994; 152:3570–3577.

91. Lorant DE, Topham MK, Whatley RE, McEver RP, McIntyre TM, Prescott SM, Zimmerman GA. Inflammatory roles of P-selectin. J Clin Invest 1993; 92:559–570.

92. Weyrich AS, McIntyre TM, McEver RP, Prescott SM, Zimmerman GA. Monocyte tethering by P-selectin regulates monocyte chemotactic protein-1 and tumor necrosis factor-α secretion. J Clin Invest 1995; 95:2297–2303.

93. Gotsch U, Jager U, Dominis M, Vestweber D. Expression of P-selectin on endothelial cells is upregulated by LPS and TNF-α in vivo. Cell Adhes Commun 1994; 2:7–14.

94. Suzuki H, Zweifach BW, Forrest MJ, Schmid-Schonbein GW. Modification of leukocyte adhesion in spontaneously hypertensive rats by adrenal corticosteroids. J Leukoc Biol 1995; 57:20–26.

95. Osborn L, Hession C, Tizard R, Vassallo C, Luhowskyj S, Chi-Rosso G, Lobb R. Direct expression cloning of vascular cell adhesion molecule 1, a cytokine-induced endothelial protein that binds to lymphocytes. Cell 1989; 59:1203–1211.

96. Bochner BS, Luscinskas FW, Gimbrone MA Jr, Newman W, Sterbinsky SA,

Derse-Anthony C, Klunk D, Schleimer RP. Adhesion of human basophils, eosinophils, and neutrophils to IL-1-activated human vascular endothelial cells: contributions of endothelial cell adhesion molecules. J Exp Med 1991; 173:1553–1557.

97. Dobrina A, Menegazzi R, Carlos TM, Nardon E, Cramer R, Zacchi T, Harlan JM, Patriarca P. Mechanisms of eosinophil adherence to cultured vascular endothelial cells: eosinophils bind to the cytokine-induced endothelial ligand vascular cell adhesion molecule-1 via the very late activation antigen-4 integrin receptor. J Clin Invest 1991; 88:20–26.

98. Walsh GM, Mermod J, Hartnell A, Kay AB, Wardlaw AJ. Human eosinophil, but not neutrophil, adherence to IL-1-stimulated human umbilical vascular endothelial cells is α4β1 (very late antigen-4) dependent. J Immunol 1991; 146:3419–3423.

99. Weller PF, Rand TH, Goelz SE, Chi-Rosso G, Lobb RR. Human eosinophil adherence to vascular endothelium mediated by binding to vascular cell adhesion molecule 1 and endothelial leukocyte adhesion molecule 1. Proc Natl Acad Sci USA 1991; 88:7430–7433.

100. Sriramarao P, von Andrian UH, Butcher EC, Bourdon MA, Broide DH. L-selectin and very late antigen-4 integrin promote eosinophil rolling at physiological shear rates in vivo. J Immunol 1994; 153:4238–4246.

101. Luscinskas FW, Kansas GS, Ding H, Pizcueta P, Schleiffenbaum BE, Tedder TF, Gimbrone MA. Monocyte rolling, arrest and spreading on IL-4-activated vascular endothelium under flow is mediated via sequential action of L-selectin, β1-integrins, and β2-integrins. J Cell Biol 1994; 125:1417–1427.

102. Masinovsky B, Urdal D, Gallatin WM. IL-4 acts synergistically with IL-1β to promote lymphocyte adhesion to microvascular endothelium by induction of vascular cell adhesion molecule-1. J Immunol 1990; 145:2886–2895.

103. Thornhill MH, Kyan-Aung U, Haskard DO. IL-4 increases human endothelial cell adhesiveness for T cells but not for neutrophils. J Immunol 1990; 144:3060–3065.

104. Schleimer RP, Sterbinsky SA, Kaiser J, Bickel CA, Klunk DA, Tomioka K, Newman W, Luscinskas FW, Gimbrone MA Jr., McIntyre BW, Bochner BS. Interleukin-4 induces adherence of human eosinophils and basophils but not neutrophils to endothelium: association with expresion of VCAM-1. J Immunol 1992; 148:1086–1092.

105. Bochner BS, Klunk DA, Sterbinsky SA, Coffman RL, Schleimer RP. Interleukin-13 selectively induces vascular cell adhesion molecule-1 (VCAM-1) expression in human endothelial cells. J Immunol 1995; 154:799–803.

106. Tepper RI, Levinson DA, Stanger BZ, Campos-Torres J, Abbas AK, Leder P. IL-4 induces allergic-like inflammatory disease and alters T cell development in transgenic mice. Cell 1990; 62:457–467.

107. Tepper RI, Coffman RL, Leder P. An eosinophil-dependent mechanism for the antitumor effect of interleukin-4. Science 1992; 257:548–551.

108. Kyan-Aung U, Haskard DO, Lee TH. Vascular cell adhesion molecule-1 and eosinophil adhesion to cultured human umbilical vein endothelial cells In vitro. Am J Respir Cell Mol Biol 1991; 5:445–450.

109. Schleimer RP, Bochner BS. Letter to the editor. J Immunol 1991; 147:380–381.
110. Lee B-J, Naclerio RM, Bochner BS, Taylor TM, Lim MC, Baroody FM. Nasal challenge with allergen unregulates the local expression of vascular enothelial adhesion molecules. J Allergy Clin Immunol 1994; 94:1006–1016.
111. Zangrilli JG, Fish JE, Peters SP. Inflammation in allergic asthma: Findings from invasive studies. Allergy: Principles and Practice 1993; Update 16:1–15.
112. Ohkawara Y, Yamauchi K, Maruyama N, Hoshi H, Ohno I, Honma M, Tanno Y, Tamura G, Shirato K, Ohtani H. In situ expression of the cell adhesion molecules in bronchial tissues from asthmatics with air flow limitation: in vivo evidence of VCAM-1/VLA-4 interaction in selective eosinophil infiltration. Am J Respir Cell Molec Biol 1995; 12:4–12.
113. Beck LA, Stellato C, Beall LD, Schall TJ, Leopold D, Bickel CA, Baroody F, Bochner BS, Schleimer RP. Detection of the chemokine RANTES and endothelial adhesion molecules in nasal polyps. J Allergy Clin Immunol 1995;
114. Weg VB, Williams TJ, Lobb RR, Nourshargh S. A monoclonal antibody recognizing very late activation antigen-4 inhibits eosinophil accumulation in vivo. J Exp Med 1993; 177:561–566.
115. Abraham WM, Sielczak MW, Ahmed A, Cortes A, Lauredo IT, Kim J, Pepinsky B, Benjamin CD, Leone DR, Lobb RR, Weller PF. α_4-integrins mediate antigen-induced late bronchial responses and prolonged airway hyperresponsiveness in sheep. J Clin Invest 1994; 93:776–787.
116. Metzger WJ, Ridger V, Tollefson V, Arrhenius T, Gaeta FCA, Elices M, Anti-VLA-4 antibody and CS-1 peptide inhibitor modifies airway inflammation and bronchial airway hyperresponsiveness (BHR) in the allergic rabbit (abstr.). J Allergy Clin Immunol 1994; 93:183.
117. Nakajima H, Sano H, Nishimura T, Yoshida S, Iwamoto I. Role of vascular cell adhesion molecule-1/very late activation antigen-4 and intercellular adhesion molecule-1/lymphocyte function-associated antigen-1 interactions in antigen-induced eosinophil and T-cell recruitment into the tissue. J Exp Med 1994; 179:1145–1154.
118. Kay AB, Ying S, Varney SR, Gaga M, Durham SR, Moqbel R, Wardlaw AJ, Hamid Q. Messenger RNA expression of the cytokine gene cluster, interleukin-3 (IL-3), IL-4, IL-5, and granulocyte/macrophage colony-stimulating factor, in allergen-induced late-phase cutaneous reactions in atopic subjects. J Exp Med 1991; 173:775–778.
119. Durham SR, Ying S, Varney VA, Jacobson MR, Sudderick RM, Mackay IS, Kay AB, Hamid A. Cytokine messenger RNA expression for IL-3, IL-4, IL-5, and granulocyte-macrophage colony-stimulating factor in the nasal mucosa after local allergen provacation—relationship to tissue eosinophilia. J Immunol 1992; 148:2390–2394.
120. Ying S, Durham SR, Barkans J, Masuyama K, Jacobson M, Rak S, Löwhagen O, Moqbel R, Kay Ab, Hamid QA. T cells are the principal source of interleukin-5 mRNA in allergen-induced rhintis. Am J Respir Cell Mol Biol 1993; 9:356–360.

121. Ying S, Durham SR, Jacobson MR, Rak S, Masuyama K, Lowhagen O, Kay AB, Hamid QA. T lymphocytes and mast cells express messenger RNA for interleukin-4 in the nasal mucosa in allergen-induced rhinitis. Immunology 1994; 82:200-206.

122. Bradding P, Feather IH, Howarth PH, Meuller R, Roberts JA, Britten K, Bews JPA, Hunt TC, Okayama Y, Heusser CH, Bullock GR, Church MK, Holgate ST. Interleukin-4 is localized to and released by human mast cells. J Exp Med 1992; 176:1381-1386.

123. Bradding P, Feather IH, Wilson S, Bardin PG, Heusser CH, Holgate ST, Howarth PH. Immunolocalization of cytokines in the nasal mucosa of normal and perennial rhinitic subjects. J Immunol 1993; 151:3853-3865.

124. Brunner T, Heusser C, Dahinden C. Human peripheral blood basophils primed by interleukin 3 produce IL-4 in response to immunoglobulin E receptor stimulation. J Exp Med 1993; 177:605-612.

125. Schroeder JT, MacGlashan DW, Kagey-Sobotka A, White JM, Lichtenstein LM. IgE-dependent IL-4 secretion by human basophils - the relationship between cytokine production and histamine release in mixed leukocyte cultures. J Immunol 1994; 153:1808-1817.

126. Iwamoto I, tomoe S, Tomioka H, Takatsu K, Yoshida S. Role of CD4+ T lymphocytes and interleukin-5 in antigen-induced eosinophil recruitment into the site of cutaneous late-phase reaction in mice. J Leukoc Biol 1992; 52:572-578.

127. Nakajima H, Iwamoto I, Tomoe S, Matsumura R, Tomioka H, Takatsu K, Yoshido S. CD4+ T-lymphocytes and interleukin-5 mediate antigen-induced eosinophil infiltration into the mouse trachea. Am Rev Respir Dis 1992; 146:374-377.

128. Robinson D, Hamid Q, Ying S, Bentley A, Assoufi B, Durham S, Kay AB. Prednisolone treatment in asthma is associated with modulation of bronchoalveolar lavage cell interleukin-4, interleukin-5, and interferon-γ cytokine gene expression. Am Rev Respir Dis 1993; 148:401-406.

129. Masuyama K, Jacobson MR, Rak S, meng Q, Sudderick RM, Kay AB, Lowhagen O, Hamid Q, Durham SR. Topical glucocorticosteroid (fluticasone propionate) inhibits cells expressing cytokine mRNA for interleukin-4 in the nasal mucosa in allergen-induced rhinitis. Immunology 1994; 82:192-199.

130. Liu MC, Xiao HQ, Lichtenstein LM, Huang SK. Prednisone inhibits TH$_2$-type cytokine gene expression at sites of allergen challenge in subjects with asthma. Am Rev Respir Dis 1994; 149:A944.

131. Wu CY, Fargeas C, Nakajima T, Delespesse G. Glucocorticoids suppress the production of interleukin 4 by human lymphocytes. Eur J Immunol 1991; 21:2645-2647.

132. Campbell HD, Tucker WQJ, Hort Y, Martinson ME, Mayo G, Clutterbuck EJ, Sanderson CJ, Young IG. Molecular cloning, nucleotide sequence, and expression of the gene encoding human eosinophil differentiation factor (interleukin 5). Proc Natl Acad Sci USA 1987; 84:6629-6633.

133. Clutterbuck EJ, Hirst EMA, Sanderson CJ. Human interleukin-5 (IL-5) regulates the production of eosinophils in human bone marrow cultures: Comparison and interaction with IL-1, IL-3, IL-6, and GMCSF. Blood 1989; 73:1504-1512.

134. Yamaguchi Y, Suda T, Suda J, Eguchi M, Miura Y, Harada N, Tominaga A,

Takatsu K. Purified interleukin 5 supports the terminal differentiation and proliferation of murine eosinophilic precursors. J Exp Med 1988; 167:43–56.

135. Sanderson CJ. Interleukin-5, eosinophils, and disease. Blood 1992; 79:3101–3109.

136. Lopez AF, Williamson DJ, Gamble JR, Begley CG, Harlan JM, Klebanoff SJ, Waltersdorph A, Wong G, Clark SC, Vadas MA. Recombinant human granulocyte-macrophage colony-stimulating factor stimulates in vitro mature human neutrophil and eosinophil function, surface receptor expression, and survival. J Clin Invest 1986; 78:1220–1228.

137. Lopez AF, Sanderson CJ, Gamble JR, Campbell HD, Young IG, Vadas MA. Recombinant human interleukin 5 is a selective activator of human eosinophil function. J Exp Med 1988; 167:219–224.

138. Lopez AF, Eglinton JM, Gillis D, Park LS, Clark S, Vadas MA. Reciprocal inhibition of binding between interleukin 3 and granulocyte-macrophage colony-stimulating factor to human eosinophils. Proc Natl Acad Sci USA 1989; 86:7022–7026.

139. Rothenberg ME, Owen WF Jr., Silberstein DS, Woods J, Soberman RJ, Austen KF, Stevens RL. Human eosinophils have prolonged survival, enhanced functional properties, and become hypodense when exposed to human interleukin 3. J Clin Invest 1988; 81:1986–1992.

140. Warringa RAJ, Koenderman L, Kok PTM, Kreukniet J, Bruijnzeel PLB. Modulation and induction of eosinophil chemotaxis by granulocyte-macrophage colony-stimulating factor and interleukin-3. Blood 1991; 77:2694–2700.

141. Tomioka K, MacGlashan DW Jr., Lichtenstein LM, Bochner BS, Schleimer RP. GM-CSF regulates human eosinophil responses to F-Met peptide and platelet activating factor. J Immunol 1993; 151:4989–4997.

142. Ebisawa M, Liu MC, Yamada T, Kato M, Lichtenstein LM, Bochner BS, Schleimer RP. Eosinophil transendothelial migration induced by cytokines II. The potentiation of eosinophil transendothelial migration by eosinophil-active cytokines. J Immunol 1994; 152:4590–4597.

143. Broide DH, Firestein GS. Endobronchial allergen challenge in asthma. Demonstration of cellular source of granulocyte macrophage colony-stimulating factor by in situ hybridization. J Clin Invest 1991; 88:1048–1053.

144. Kato M, Liu MC, Stealey BA, Friedman B, Lichtenstein LM, Permutt S, Schleimer RP. Production of granulocyte/macrophage colony-stimulating factor in human airways during allergen-induced late-phase reactions in atopic subjects. Lymphokine Cytokine Res 1992; 11:287–292.

145. Sedgwick JB, Calhoun WJ, Gleich GJ, Kita H, Abrams JS, Schwartz LB, Volovitz B, Ben-Yaakov M, Busse WW. Immediate and late airway response of allergic rhinitis patients to segmental antigen challenge. Am Rev Respir Dis 1991; 144:1274–1281.

146. Massey W, Friedman B, Kato M, Cooper P, Kagey-Sobotka A, Lichtentein LM, Schleimer RP. Appearance of IL-3 and GM-CSF activity at allergen-challenged cutaneous late-phase reaction sites. J Immunol 1993; 150:1084–1092.

147. Wong GG, Witek JS, Temple PA, Wilkens KM, Leary AC, Luxenberg DP, Jones SS, Brown EL, Kay RM, Orr EC, Shoemaker C, Gold DW, Kaufman RJ, Hewick RM, Wang EA, Clark SC. Human GM-CSF: Molecular cloning of the

complementary DNA and purification of the natural and recombinant proteins. Science 1985; 228:810–815.

148. Lieschke GH, Burgess AW. Granulocyte colony-stimulating factor and granulo-cyte-macrophage colony-stimulating factor. New Engl J Med 1992; 327:28–35.

149. Robinson DS, Hamid Q, Ying S, Tsicopoulos A, Barkans J, Bentley AM, Corrigan C, Durham SR, Kay AB. Predominant T$_{H2}$-like bronchoalveolar T-lym-phocyte population in atopic asthma. N Engl J Med 1992; 326:298–304.

150. Wodner-Filipowicz A, Heusser CH, Moroni C. Production of the haemopoietic growht factors GM-CSF and interleukin-3 by mast cells in response to IgE recep-tor-mediated activation. Nature 1989; 339:150–152.

151. Desreumaux P, Janin A, Dubucquoi S, Copin MC, Torpier G, Capron A, Capron M, Prin L. Synthesis of interleukin-5 by activated eosinophils in patients with eosinophilic heart diseases. Blood 1993; 82:1553–1560.

152. Rolfe FG, Hughes JM, Armour CL, Sewell WA. Inhibition of interleukin-5 gene expression by dexamethasone. Immunology 1992; 77:494–499.

153. Culpepper JA, Lee F. Regulation of IL-3 expression by glucocorticoids in cloned murine T-lymphocytes. J Immunol 1985; 135:3191–3197.

154. Churchill L, Friedman B, Schleimer RP, Proud D. Production of granulocyte-macrophage colony-stimulating factor by cultured human tracheal epithelial cells. Immunology 1992; 75:189–195.

155. Kato M, Schleimer RP. Antiinflammatory steroids inhibit GM-CSF production by human lung tissue. Lung 1994; 172:113–124.

156. Hartnell A, Kay AB, Wardlaw AJ. Interleukin-3-induced up-regulation of CR3 expression on human eosinophils is inhibited by dexamethasone. Immunology 1992; 77:488–493.

157. Kita H, Abu-Ghazaleh R, Sanderson CJ, Gleich GJ. Effect of steroids on immu-noglobulin-induced eosinophil degranulation. J Allergy Clin Immunol 1991; 87:70–77.

158. Fijisawa T, Atsuta J, Terada A, Iguchi K, kamiya H, Ueno K. IL-5 alone is suf-ficient to induce eosinophil degranulation. J Allergy Clin Immunol 1995; 95:A338.

159. Sedgwick JB, Geiger KM, Busse WW. Superoxide generation by hypodense eosi-nophils from patients with asthma. Am Rev Respir Dis 1990; 142:120–125.

160. Sedgwick JB, Calhoun WJ, Vrtis RF, Bates ME, McAllister PK, Busse WW. Comparison of airway and blood eosinophil function after in vivo antigen chal-lenge. J Immunol 1992; 149:3710–3718.

161. Lamas AM, Marcotte GV, Schleimer RP. Human endothelial cells prolong eosi-nophil survival. Regulation by cytokines and glucocorticoids. J Immunol 1989; 142:3978–3984.

162. Lamas AM, Leon OG, Schleimer RP. Glucocorticoids inhibit eosinophil responses to granulocyte-macrophage colony-stimulating factor. J Immunol 1991; 147:254–259.

163. Cox G, Ohtoshi T, Vanceri C, Denbura JA, Dolovich J, Gauldie J, Jordana M. Promotion of eosinophil survival by human bronchial epithelial cells and its modu-lation by steroids. Am J Respir Cell Mol Biol 1991; 4:525–531.

164. Wallen N, Kita H, Weiler D, Gleich GJ. Glucocorticoids inhibit cytokine-mediated eosinophil survival. J Immunol 1991; 147:3490–3495.

165. Hallsworth MP, Litchfield TM, Lee TH. Glucocorticoids inhibit granulocyte-macrophage colony-stimulating factor and interleukin-5 enhanced in vitro survival of human eosinophils. Immunology 1992; 75:382–385.

166. Her E, Frazer J, Austen KF, Owen WF. Eosinophil hematopoietins antagonize the programmed cell death of eosinophils—cytokine and glucocorticoid effects on eosinophils maintained by endothelial cell conditioned medium. J Clin Invest 1991; 88:1982–1987.

167. Kawabori S, Soda K, Perdue MH, Bienenstock J. The dynamics of intestinal eosinophil depletion in rats treated with dexamethasone. Lab Invest 1991; 64:224–233.

168. Schleimer RP, Bochner BS. The effects of blucocorticoids on human eosinophils. J Allergy Clin Immunol 1994; 94:1202–1213.

169. Oppenheim JJ, Zachariae COC, Mukaida N, Matsushima K. Properties of the novel proinflammatory supergene "intercrine" cytokine family. Annu Rev Immunol 1991; 9:617–648.

170. Schall TJ. Biology of the RANTES/SIS cytokine family. Cytokine 1991; 3:165–183.

171. Baggiolini M, Deward B, Walz A. Interleukin-8 and related chemotactic cytokines. In: Gallin JI, Goldstein IM, Snyderman R, eds. Inflammation: Basic Principles and Clinical Correlates. New York: Raven Press, 1992:247–263.

172. Miller MD, Krangel MS. Biology and biochemistry of the chemokines: A family of chemotactic and inflammatory cytokines. Crit Rev Immunol 1992; 12:17–46.

173. Kuna P, Reddigari SR, Schall TJ, Rucinski D, Sadick M, Kaplan AP. Characterization of the human basophil response to cytokines, growth factors, and histamine releasing factors of the intercrine/chemokine family. J Immunol 1993; 150:1932–1943.

174. Alam R, Forsythe P, Stafford S, Heinrich J, Bravo R, Proost P, Van Damme L. Monocyte chemotactic protein-2, monocyte chemotactic protein-3, and fibroblast-induced cytokine - three new chemokines induce chemotaxis and activation of basophils. J Immunol 1994; 153:3155–3159.

175. Kameyoshi Y, Dorschner A, Mallet AI, Christophers E, Schroder JM. Cytokine RANTES released by thrombin-stimulated platelets is a potent attractant for human eosinophils. J Exp Med 1992; 176:587–592.

176. Rot A, Krieger M, Brunner T, Bischoff SC, Schall TJ, Dahinden CA. RANTES and macrophage inflammatory protein 1α induce the migration and activation of normal human eosinophil granulocytes. J Exp Med 1992; 176:1489–1495.

177. Dahinden CA, Geiser T, Brunner T, von Tscharner V, Caput D, Ferrara P, Minty A, Baggiolini M. Monocyte chemotactic protein 3 is a most effective basophil- and eosinophil-activating chemokine. J Exp Med 1994; 179:751–756.

178. Jose PJ, Griffiths-Johnson DA, Collins PD, Walsh DT, Moqbel R, Totty NF, Truong O, Hsuan JJ, Williams TF. Eotaxin: a potent eosinophil chemoattractant cytokine detected in a guinea pig model of allergic airways inflammation. J Exp Med 1994; 179:881–887.

179. Ebisawa M, Yamada T, Bickel C, Klunk D, Schleimer RP. Eosinophil trans-endothelial migration induced by cytokins III. Effect of the chemokine RANTES. J Immunol 1994; 153:2153-2160.

180. Beck LA, Schall TJ, Beall LD, Leopold D, Bickel C, Baroody F, Naclerio RM, Schleimer RP. Detection of the chemokine RANTES and activation of vascular endothelium in nasal polyps. J Allergy Clin Immunol 1994; 93:A234.

181. Schall TJ, Jongstra J, Dyer BJ, Jorgensen J, Clayberger C, Davis MM, Krensky AM. A human T cell–specific molecule is a member of a new gene family. J Immunol 1988; 141:1018-1025.

182. Rathanaswami P, Hachicha M, Sadick M, Schall TJ, McColl SR. Expression of the cytokine RANTES in human rheumatoid synovial fibroblasts. J Biol Chem 1993; 268:5834-5839.

183. Stellato C, Beck LA, Gorgon GA, Proud D, Schall TJ, Ono SJ, Lichtenstein LM, Schleimer RP. Expression of the chemokine RANTES by a human bronchial epithelial cell line: Modulation by cytokines and glucocorticoids. J Immunol 1995;

184. Davis RJ, Wang JH, Trigg CJ, Devalia JF. Expression of GM-CFS, IL-8 and RANTES bronchial epithelium of mild asthmatics is down regulated by inhaled beclomethasone dipropionate. Intl Arch Allergy 1994;

185. Kwon OJ, Jose PJ, Robbins RA, Schall TJ, Williams TJ, Barnes PJ. Glucocorticoid inhibition of RANTES expression in human lung epithelial cells. Am J Respir Cell Mol Biol 1995; in press:

186. VanOtteren GM, Standiford TJ, Kunkel SL, Danford JM, Burdick MD, Abruzzo LV, Strieter RM. Expression and regulation of macrophage of inflammatory proetin-1α by murine alveolar and peritoneal macrophages. Am J Respir Cell Mol Biol 1994; 10:8-15.

187. Meurer R, Van Riper G, Feeney W, Cunningham P, Hora D Jr., Springer MS, MacIntyre DE, Rosen H. Formation of eosinphilic and monocytic intradermal inflammatory sites in the dog by injection of human RANTES but not human monocyte chemoattractant protein 1, human macrophage inflammatory protein 1α, or human interleukin 8. J Exp Med 1993; 178:1913-1921.

188. Beck L. Bickel C, Sterbinsky S, Stellato C, Hamilton R, Rosen H, Bochner B, Schleimer R. Injection of human subjects with RANTES causes dermal infiltration of eosinophils (EOS) and mononuclear cells (MNC). FASEB J 1995; 9:A804.

189. Yancey KB, Hammer CH, Harvath L, Renfer L, Frank MM, Lawley TJ. Studies of human C5a as a mediator of inflammation in normal human skin. J Clin Invest 1985; 75:486-495.

190. Oda T, Katori M. Inhibition site of dexamethasone on extravasation of poly-mophonuclear leukocytes in the hamster cheek pouch microcirculation. J Leukoc Biol 1992; 52:337-342.

191. Boggs DR, Athens JW, Cartwright GE, Wintrobe MM. The effect of adrenal glucocorticosteroids upon the cellular composition of inflammatory exudates. Am J Pathol 1964: 44:763-773.

192. Mishler JM, Emerson PM. Development of neutrophilia by serially increasing doses of dexamethasone. Br J Haematol 1977; 36:249-257.

193. Laitinen LA, Laitinen A, Haahtela T. A comparative study of the effects of an

inhaled corticosteroid, budesonide, and a β_2-agonist, terbutaline, on airway inflammation in newly diagnosed asthma: a randomized, double-blind, parallel-group controlled trial. J Allergy Clin Immunol 1992; 90:32–42.

194. Laitinen LA, Laitinen A, Haahtela T. Airway mucosal inflammation even in patients with newly diagnosed asthma. Am Rev Respir Dis 1993; 147:697–704.

195. Haahtela T, Jarvinen M, Kava T, Kiviranta K, Koskinen S, Lehtonen K, Nikander K, Persson T, Reinikainen K, Selroos O, Sovijarvi A, Steniusaarniala B, Svahn T, Tammivaara R, Laitinen LA. Comparison of β2-agonist, terbutaline, with an inhaled corticosteroid, budesonide, in newly detected asthma. N Engl J Med 1991; 325:388–392.

196. Djukanovic R, Wilson JW, Britten KM, Wilson SJ, Walls AF, Roche WR, Howarth PH, Holgate ST. Effect of an inhaled corticosteroid on airway inflammation and symptons in asthma. Am Rev Respir Dis 1992; 145:669–674.

197. Jeffrey PK, Godfrey RW, Ådelroth E, Nelson F, Rogers A, Johansson S-Å. Effects of treatment on airway inflammation and thickening of reticular collagen in asthma: a quantitative light and electron microscopic study and correlation with BAL. In: Ådelroth E, ed. Cells, Mediators and Mucosal Inflammation in Asthma. Umeå, Sweden: Nyheternas Tryckeri, 1990:

198. Jeffrey PK, Godfrey RW, Adelroth E, Nelson F, Roger A, Johannson SA. Effects of treatment on airway inflammation and thickening of basement membrane reticular collagen in asthma. A quantitative light and electron microscopic study. Am Rev Respir Dis 1992; 145:890–899.

199. Wilson JW, Djukanovic R, Howarth PH, Holgate ST. Inhaled beclomethasone dipropionate downregulates airway lymphocyte activation in atopic asthma. Am J Respir Crit Care Med 1994; 149:86–90.

200. Claman DM, Boushey HA, Liu J, Wong H, Fahy JV. Analysis of induced sputum to examine the effects of prednisone on airway inflammation in asthmatic subjects. J Allergy Clin Immunol 1994; 94:861–869.

201. Duddridge M, Ward C, Hendrick DJ, Walters EH. Changes in bronchoalveolar lavage inflammatory cells in asthmatic patients treated with high dose inhaled beclomethasone dipropionate. Eur Respir J 1993; 6:489–497.

202. Bentley AM, Robinson DS, Assoufi B, Kay AB, Durham SR. The effect of prednisolone treatment on the local bronchial cellular infiltrate in asthma—reduction in eosinophils, T-lymphocytes and mast cells. J Allergy Clin Immunol 1993; 91:222–.

203. Holgate ST, Wilson JR, Howarth PH. New insights into airway inflammation by endobronchial biopsy. Am Rev Respir Dis 1992; 145:S2–S6.

204. Pipkorn U, Proud D, Lichtenstein LM, Kagey-Sobotka A, Norman PS, Naclerio RM. Inhibition of mediator release in allergic rhinitis by pretreatment with topical glucocorticosteroids. N Engl J Med 1987; 316:1506–1510.

205. Pipkorn U, Proud D, Lichtenstein LM, Schleimer RP, Peters SP, Adkinson NF Jr., Kagey-Sobotka A, Norman PS, Naclerio RM. Effect of short-term systemic glucocorticoid treatment on human nasal mediator release after antigen challenge. J Clin Invest 1987; 80:957–961.

206. Bascom R, Wachs M, Naclerio RM, Pipkorn U, Galli SJ, Lichtenstein LM. Basophil influx occurs after nasal antigen challenge: effects of topical corticosteroid pretreatment. J Allergy Clin Immunol 1988; 81:580–589.
207. Bascom R, Pipkorn U, Lichtenstein LM, Naclerio RM. The influx of inflammatory cells into nasal washings during the late response to antigen challenge. Am Rev Respir Dis 1988; 138:406–412.
208. Jacobson MR, Rak S, Sudderick RM, Masuyama K, Kay AB, Lowhagen P, Hamid Q, Hamid SR. Influence of prolonged treatment with topical corticosteroid on allergen-induced cellular infiltration in the nasal mucosa. Clin Exp Allergy 1994; 24:
209. Slott RI, Zweiman B. Histologic studies of human skin test responses to ragweed and compound 48/80. II. Effects of corticosteroid therapy. J Allergy Clin Immunol 1975; 55:232–240.
210. Massey W, Ebisawa M, Bochner B, Cooper P, Kagey-Sobotka A, Lichtenstein L, Schleimer R. Systemic prednisone inhibits allergen (AG)-induced cutaneous GM-CSF production. J Allergy Clin Immunol 1994; 93:A287.
211. Rebuck JW, Smith RW, Margulis RR. The modification of leukocytic function in human windows by ACTH. Gastroenterol 1951; 19:644–657.
212. Rebuck JW, Mellinger RC. Interruption by topical cortisone of leukocytic cycles in acute inflammation in man. Ann NY Acad Sci 1953; 56:715–732.
213. Mancini RE, Colombi PA, Galli H, Orcivoli L. Effect of glucocorticoid hormones on experimentally induced allergic reactions on human skin. J Allergy 1961; 32:471–482.
214. Charlesworth EN, Kagey-Sobotka A, Schleimer RP, Norman PS, Lichtenstein LM. Prednisone inhibits the appearance of inflammatory mediators and the influx of eosinophils and basophils associated with the cutaneous late-phase response to allergen. J Immunol 1991; 146:671–676.
215. Djukanovic R, Wilson JW, Britten KM, Wilson SJ, Walls AF, Roche WR, Howarth PH, Holgate ST. Effect of an inhaled corticosteroid on airway inflammation and symptoms in asthma. Am Rev Respir Dis 1992; 145:669–674.

11

Airway Lymphocytes

STEPHEN R. DURHAM, CHRIS J. CORRIGAN, DOUGLAS S. ROBINSON, and A. B. KAY

National Heart and Lung Institute
Imperial College
London, England

QUTAYBA HAMID

McGill University
Montreal, Quebec, Canada

I. Introduction

Bronchial asthma may be defined in terms of (1) reversible airflow limitation either spontaneously or with treatment, (2) the presence of bronchial hyper-responsiveness (heightened sensitivity to nonspecific irritants), and (3) airway inflammation. Clearly asthma is not a disease of smooth muscle constriction alone. The role of inflammatory changes, including altered vascular permeability, epithelial changes, cellular recruitment activation, and secretion of mediators and cytokines, is increasingly being recognized. Whereas the traditional view in allergy and asthma has highlighted the role of IgE-dependent events, mast cells, basophils, and eosinophils, more recent studies have focused on the important effector function of T lymphocytes, T-lymphocyte activation, and secretion of specific cytokines in these disorders. Moreover, abnormal T-cell function has been shown to be a feature of both extrinsic (IgE-mediated) asthma and so-called "intrinsic asthma" where no extrinsic allergic cause may be identified, although the profile of cytokines secreted may differ between these two forms of asthma. This chapter summarizes recent evidence for the role of T lymphocytes in asthma. There follows some observations from our group regarding the effects of corticosteroids on T lymphocytes, both in vitro and from in vivo studies of the upper and lower respiratory tract. Finally, the implications with regard to future (possibly more targeted) therapy are discussed.

II. T Lymphocytes and Asthma

Murine studies have indicated the role of so-called "TH2-type" $CD4^+$ T-helper lymphocytes in response to environmental allergens and parasitic infestation (1). More recent in vitro observations in humans have supported the functional dichotomy between $CD4^+$ T lymphocytes based on their profile of cytokine secretion into TH1-type and TH2-type cells (2,3). TH1 cells produce predominantly interleukin-2 (IL-2) and γ-interferon, whereas TH2-type cells produce IL-4 and IL-5. IL-3 and granulocyte-macrophage colony-stimulating factor (GM-CSF) are produced by both types. Several studies have now confirmed that human allergen-specific T-lymphocyte clones, when cultured in vitro, produce predominantly IL-4 and IL-5 (2). Earlier human studies in vivo focused on the skin model, specifically the allergen-induced late-phase response. By use of immunohistology cutaneous biopsies obtained at 24 hr after allergen provocation demonstrated increased numbers of $CD4^+$ T lymphocytes, an increase in $CD25^+$ (IL-2 receptor–bearing) cells presumably T lymphocytes, and increased numbers of eosinophils (4). In situ hybridization studies confirmed that the principal cytokines expressed during human late skin responses at least at mRNA levels were IL-4, IL-5, IL-3, and GM-CSF, consistent with activation of a distinct TH2-type T-lymphocyte subset (5). Additional studies examined the influence of successful grass pollen immunotherapy on these changes (6). Following immunotherapy, inhibition of the late cutaneous response was accompanied not by inhibition of TH-2 type cytokines mRNA expression but rather an increase in IL-2 and γ-interferon mRNA (7). These studies suggested that immunotherapy may act by stimulating an additional TH1 response, possibly with reciprocal inhibition of TH2 lymphocytes and their effects.

T lymphocytes are prominent in the epithelial layer and submucosa of the human respiratory tract. We have tested the hypothesis that T-lymphocyte recruitment, activation, and cytokine secretion may contribute to eosinophil recruitment and activation and IgE-dependent events resulting in airway narrowing and bronchial hyperresponsiveness during naturally occurring day to day asthma. Specifically, we asked the questions: What is the evidence for T lymphocytes and T-lymphocyte activation in patients with extrinsic asthma compared with healthy normal nonatopic control subjects? Does the presence and activation of T lymphocytes relate to asthma severity? Are these changes consistent in different forms of asthma, including occupational asthma and so-called "intrinsic" asthma? How specific are these changes for asthma compared with other airway diseases? Is it possible to provoke these changes in vivo using bronchial provocation? Is the disease (and associated T-lymphocytes changes) ameliorated by successful treatment with corticosteroids?

A. Asthma Versus Controls

Peripheral blood total T-lymphocyte numbers in asthmatics did not differ from control subjects. When T-lymphocyte "activation" was assessed by flow cytometry, increased percentages of CD25$^+$ (IL-2 receptor–bearing) and HLA-DRH CD4$^+$ T lymphocytes were observed in the asthmatic group (8,9). In contrast, no differences were observed in CD8 T-lymphocyte numbers or their activation status. The degree of T-lymphocyte activation correlated with disease severity. Clinical improvement following corticosteroid treatment was accompanied by a decrease in T-cell activation markers with a time course that paralleled improvements in peak flow. Peripheral blood and T-lymphocytes from asthmatics who were clinically resistant to corticosteroid therapy were also shown to express these markers in vivo and to be refractory to the inhibitory effects of corticosteroids in vitro (10,11).

Immunohistochemical studies of fiberoptic bronchoscopic bronchial mucosal biopsies from patients with mild atopic extrinsic asthma demonstrated increased numbers of "activated" EG2$^+$ (ECP-secreting) eosinophils and increased numbers of CD25$^+$ cells, presumed to be T lymphocytes (12). Subsequent double-immunostaining techniques have confirmed that the majority (approximately 65–80%) of CD25$^+$ cells in mucosal biopsies from asthmatics are T lymphocytes with fewer numbers of CD25$^+$ macrophages and eosinophils (13). In situ hybridization studies demonstrated an increase in IL-5 mRNA$^+$ cells (14). Subsequent studies involving bronchoalveolar lavage of asthmatic patients compared with normal controls demonstrated a characteristic "TH2-type" phenotype with increased expression in BAL cells of mRNA for IL-4, IL-5, IL-3, GM-CSF but not for IL-2 or γ-interferon (15). GM-CSF has also been identified in asthmatic bronchial epithelium (16). Immunomagnetic separation demonstrated that the majority of cells expressing IL-4 and IL-5 were CD2$^+$; i.e., were indeed T lymphocytes. Very recent studies from our group have employed the technique of sequential immunocytochemistry followed by in situ hybridization of bronchial biopsies from allergic asthmatics. The majority of cells expressing IL-4 and IL-5 (70–80%) were T lymphocytes with lesser contributions from mast cells and eosinophils (17). IL-5 and GM-CSF mRNA have also been colocalized to eosinophils (18,19). Others have identified mast cells as an alternative source of these cytokines (20), and also monocytes and epithelial cells as well as CD4$^+$ T lymphocytes (21). Taken together these studies involving peripheral blood, bronchial mucosal biopsies, and bronchoalveolar lavage confirm that T lymphocytes are activated in bronchial asthma and express TH2-type cytokines, and this is accompanied by eosinophil recruitment and activation.

B. Relationship to Asthma Severity

In patients with extrinsic asthma with a wide spectrum of disease from mild to moderately severe (Aas score 1–4), the number of CD25/CD4$^+$ T lymphocytes in bronchoalveolar lavage correlated significantly with an asthma symptom severity score, baseline 1-sec forced expiratory volume (FEV$_1$), and the level of airway responsiveness (methacholine PC20, provocation concentration that caused a 20% reduction in FEV$_1$) (22). Immunocytochemistry of bronchial biopsies from atopic subjects with or without asthma and normal controls demonstrated that T-lymphocyte activation and eosinophil activation were features of asthma rather than atopy per se (23). A significant correlation was also observed between CD25$^+$ T lymphocytes and EG2$^+$ eosinophils and between eosinophils and airway methacholine responsiveness. Similar studies have documented a relationship between the percentages of BAL CD4$^+$ T lymphocytes expressing messenger RNA for IL-4 and IL-5, asthma symptom severity, and the level of airway responsiveness (24).

C. Asthma of Diverse Etiology

Immunopathological studies have been performed on fiberoptic bronchoscopic biopsies obtained from patients with occupational asthma and patients with intrinsic asthma. Mucosal biopsies from patients with isocyanate-induced asthma revealed increased CD25$^+$ cells and increases in eosinophils comparable to those observed in patients with extrinsic asthma (25). Similar studies were performed in patients who were skin prick test negative common aeroallergens and in whom no extrinsic cause could be identified. Biopsies from these patients were characterized by greater numbers of CD4$^+$ T lymphocytes and macrophages in the submucosa and similar evidence of recruitment and activation of T lymphocytes and eosinophils (26). Bronchoalveolar lavage studies in patients with intrinsic asthma have also shown evidence for T-lymphocyte activation with increased CD25 expression. However, the profile of cytokines expressed by BAL lymphocytes differed in that in addition to increases in cells expressing mRNA for IL-5, increases in IL-2 but not IL-4$^+$ cells were observed (27,28).

D. Specificity for Asthma

These studies are ongoing. Fiberoptic bronchoscopy and bronchoalveolar lavage from patients with tuberculosis have shown an increase in T-lymphocyte activation and preferential expression of TH1-type cytokines, particularly IL-2 and γ-interferon with no increases in IL-4 or IL-5 (29).

E. Allergen Provocation

Allergen bronchial challenge is artificial when compared with natural environmental allergen exposure. Bronchial provocation involves the administration of large quantities of allergen in soluble form over short periods of time. This is in contrast to natural exposure to low allergen concentrations in particulate form over prolonged periods. Nevertheless, allergen inhalation may result in the development of late asthmatic responses (6–24 hr) and associated increases in bronchial hyperresponsiveness (30). These increases in responsiveness have been shown to precede the late response and correlate with airway inflammatory changes. Drugs which inhibit late responses, for example, corticosteroids and disodium cromoglycate, in general have been shown to be effective in the prophylaxis of day to day asthma (31). Previous studies involving measurements in peripheral blood demonstrated that the late response was associated with increases in mediators of hypersensitivity (32), activation of neutrophils (33) and eosinophils (34,35), and increases in peripheral T-lymphocyte IL-2 receptor expression (36,37). Studies of bronchoalveolar lavage following allergen provocation have also shown increases in eosinophils which correlated with the size of the late response (38,39). Late responses have also been associated with increases in BAL CD4$^+$ cells up to 48 hr after challenge (40). In contrast, patients who developed "single early responses" showed increased numbers of CD8$^+$ T lymphocytes in BAL at 6–8 hr, which suggested that recruitment of CD8$^+$ cells may have some "protective" value against the development of late responses (41). More recent studies from our own (42,43) and other groups (19,44–47) have shown that T-lymphocyte recruitment activation and expression of eosinophil-modifying cytokines at both the mRNA and protein levels occur during human late asthmatic responses. We identified a close correlation between the numbers of activated (CD25$^+$) CD4$^+$ lymphocytes, IL-5 mRNA expression, and the number of activated eosinophils in bronchoalveolar lavage (43). Bronchoalveolar eosinophilia in turn correlated with the magnitude of the late response. Similar findings were confirmed in bronchial biopsies from the same subjects (42).

III. Corticosteroids and T Lymphocytes in Asthma

A. In Vitro Effects

Corticosteroids have extremely potent effects on human T lymphocytes in vitro (48). For example, dexamethasone and budesonide were effective in picomolar concentrations in inhibiting T-lymphocyte proliferation in response to mitogen (Fig. 1). The IC$_{50}$ (inhibitory concentration that caused 50% inhibition compared with control) for dexamethasone was 5×10^{-9} molar and approximately

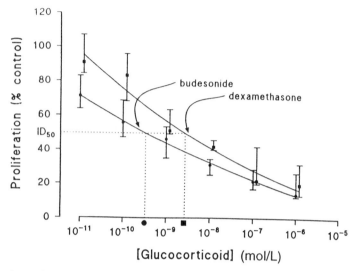

Figure 1 Inhibition of PHA-induced proliferation of peripheral blood T lymphocytes from asthmatic patients (n=8) by budesonide (circles) and dexamethasone (squares). Data are presented as median ± SIQR. Square and circle on the x-axis show the ID_{50} concentrations (inhibitory dose that caused a 50% inhibition of proliferation) of dexamethasone and budesonide, respectively.

10-fold lower for budesonide. Corticosteroids have also been shown to be effective in inhibiting transcription of cytokine genes relevant to asthma (49). This is in contrast to the relative lack of effect of corticosteroids on the degranulation and release of preformed mediators from mast cells (50,51) and their weak effect on degranulation of eosinophils (52). Thus, it seems likely that the potent eosinophil-modifying properties of corticosteroids in human studies in vivo are likely to be indirect either via modification of cytokine production from cells such as T lymphocytes and other cells or by inhibiting the permissive effect of cytokines on eosinophil survival (53–55).

B. T Lymphocytes in the Upper Airway

There are similarities but also differences between the ultrastructure of the nasal and bronchial mucosae. For example, the nasal mucosa lacks smooth muscle, whereas submucosal glands are more prominent. Whereas epithelial disruption is a characteristic feature of asthma, the epithelium in rhinitis appears relatively well preserved. The effects of drugs are also different. Antihistamines are effective in rhinitis but not bronchial asthma. In contrast, beta-sympathomimetic drugs reverse smooth muscle constriction and bronchospasm, whereas they have little effect on the nasal mucosa. However, there are also marked similarities. For example, we and others have demonstrated large numbers of T lymphocytes in the epithelium and nasal submucosa (56), although numbers do not differ between subjects with and without rhinitis. Allergen-induced late responses occurring in the nose are accompanied by increases in CD4[+] cells and CD25[+] cells (57). Double immunostaining has confirmed that the majority of these cells are T lymphocytes (13). Late responses are accompanied by increases in cells expressing mRNA for IL-4 and IL-5 (58). The principal cells expressing TH2-type cytokines in our studies are T lymphocytes (59,60), although we and others have demonstrated that mast cells are also capable of expressing IL-4 and IL-5 (59–62). We have extended these studies to examine the effect of topical corticosteroids on the nasal mucosa during both allergen provocation (63) and natural seasonal exposure (64). Six weeks of treatment with topical corticosteroid (fluticasone propionate) was effective in inhibiting both early and late nasal responses. Inhibition of the late response was accompanied by fewer T lymphocytes, CD25[+] cells, and activated eosinophils in the nasal mucosa (figure 2). Submucosal mast cell counts were also decreased, whereas, surprisingly, increased numbers of submucosal neutrophils were observed. In situ hybridization studies indicated that prolonged treatment with topical corticosteroids resulted in a selective decrease in allergen-induced increases in cells expressing mRNA for IL-4 but not for IL-5 (63). These results indicated that corticosteroids may be effective in inhibiting late responses following a decrease in T lymphocytes and/or mast cells and their products (particularly IL-4) with a consequent reduction in tissue eosinophilia and possibly other local IgE-mediated events. Natural seasonal allergen exposure to grass pollen in the same sub-

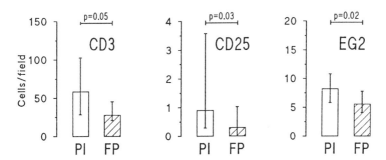

Figure 2   Cell infiltration (median cell counts ± IQ range) at allergen challenged sites (24 hr) in nasal biopsies from patients who had received 6 weeks treatment with fluticasone propionate aqueous nasal spray (hatched boxes) or matched placebo nasal spray (open boxes). Numbers of T cells (CD3[+]), activated cells (CD25[+]), and eosinophils (EF2[+]) are shown. *P* values are shown (Mann-Whitney U-test).

jects the following year resulted in increases in T lymphocytes, eosinophils, and epithelial migration of mast cells, all of which were inhibitable by pretreatment with topical corticosteroids (64).

C. T Lymphocytes in the Lower Airway

Several studies have now examined the effects of topical corticosteroids on bronchial mucosal lymphocytes (65–67). In an uncontrolled study, 6 weeks of treatment with beclomethasone dipropionate did not reduce airway T-lymphocyte numbers (65,66). We have undertaken a double-blind placebo-controlled trial of oral prednisolone, 0.6 mg/kg, for 14 days in a group of patients with moderately severe asthma in whom an elective trial of oral corticosteroid therapy was indicated (68). None of the patients had taken inhaled corticosteroids in the preceding month or steroid tablets in the preceding 6 months. Compared with placebo, prednisolone resulted in clinical improvement and a marked reduction in airway methacholine responsiveness (two- to fourfold increase in methacholine PC20). Fiberoptic bronchoscopy, bronchoalveolar lavage, and bronchial biopsy were performed before and after treatment with each subject acting as his or her own control. Cells were counted in BAL cytocentrifuge preparations and the number of cells expressing cytokine mRNA were assessed by in situ hybridization using radioactive ^{35}S-labeled RNA probes. There was a trend for reduction in CD25$^+$ cells and a significant reduction in eosinophils and eosinophil-modifying cytokines, including IL-4 and IL-5 (Fig. 3). Immunohistology was performed on cryostat sections from bronchial mucosal biopsies using selected monoclonal antibodies. Cells expressing cytokine mRNA were assessed by in situ hybridization (69). Reductions in CD3$^+$ T lymphocytes, activated EG2$^+$ eosinophils, and tryptase-only positive (mucosal type) mast cells ($P < .02$) cells were observed only in prednisolone-treated patients. There was also a reduction in cells expressing mRNA for IL-4 and IL-5 (see Fig. 3) and increases in γ-interferon, changes which were virtually identical to those observed in bronchoalveolar cells. These data provide strong support in vivo for the view that corticosteroid treatment in asthma may act by modulation of cytokine expression with consequent inhibition of the local bronchial cellular infiltrate particular tissue eosinophilia.

IV. Summary

Studies from our own and other groups have confirmed that bronchial asthma is accompanied by T-lymphocyte activation in peripheral blood, bronchoalveolar lavage, and bronchial biopsies from patients with a wide range of disease severity. Bronchial asthma is also characterised by the production of TH2-type cytokines with eosinophil-modifying properties, which may in large measure

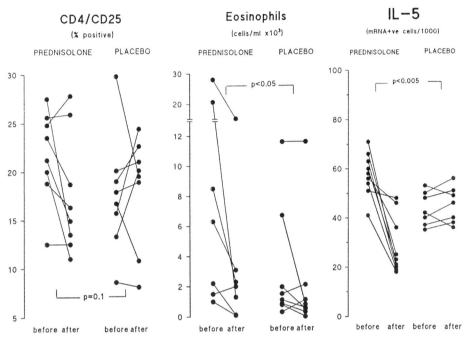

Figure 3 Bronchoalveolar lavage studies in patients with moderately severe asthma before/after an elective trial of 2 weeks' prednisolone, 0.6 mg/kg per day. Numbers of activated T lymphocytes (flow cytometry, CD4/CD25$^+$ cells), eosinophils (cells/ml $\times$ 10^3), and number of cells mRNA$^+$/1000 for interleukin-5 are shown. Results are compared with placebo-treated patients (Mann-Whitney U-test, *P* values shown).

account for the tissue eosinophilia characteristic of the disease. The principal cell source of these cytokines may be the T lymphocyte with contributions from other cells, including mast cells, epithelial cells, and eosinophils. In vitro studies have confirmed that corticosteroids are extremely potent in inhibiting T-lymphocyte proliferation and cytokine production. These changes are mirrored by the in vivo effects of corticosteroids on human T lymphocytes and eosinophils in the upper and lower airways. Thus, corticosteroids are extremely potent in suppressing T lymphocytes and, particularly in the upper airway, cytokine mRNA expression for IL-4 with a consequent reduction in local IgE-dependent events, including tissue eosinophilia during late responses. In the lower airway, corticosteroids may act by inhibiting both IL-4 and IL-5 expression. These observations highlight specific targets for future pharmacological modulation, including a potentially wider role for immunosuppressive agents (70) and strategies directed against specific cytokines, particularly IL-4 and IL-5.

Discussion

DR. BUSSE: In your introduction, you indicated that it is critical to address the specificity of your findings to asthma. In that regard, have you studied eosinophilic pneumonia?

DR. DURHAM: No. The only data we have at present on the specificity of the changes for asthma relate to tuberculosis where many BAL lymphocytes are CD25$^+$ but are TH1 and express mRNA for IFN-γ. (DS Robinson, S Ying, IK Taylor, et al. Evidence for a Th1-like bronchoalveolar T cell subset and predominance of interferon-gamma gene activation in pulmonary tuberculosis. Am J Respir Crit Care Med 1994; 149:989–993.) It would be of interest to look at other diseases which cause airway obstruction such as sarcoid or bronchiectasis.

DR. LAITINEN: (1) It is difficult to get many lymphocytes from BAL in our experience. (2) What was the dose response of prednisolone employed in your study. Were any side effects reported by the patients?

DR. DURHAM: (1) I agree. We consistently get about 60% fluid recovery, including 1 × 10^7 cells, of which approximately 10% are lymphocytes. For some purposes, the use of segmental allergen challenge may increase lymphocyte yield up to 10-fold. (2) We employed 0.6 mg/kg (approximately 40 mg prednisolone daily) for 2 weeks. No side effects, either local or systemic, were reported by the patients.

DR. SZEFLER: In the study on the prednisolone effect on cytokine profiles, are the outlier patients among the various cytokine profiles the same patients for each cytokine?

DR. DURHAM: Yes, these were the same patients.

DR. JORDANA: Have you had a chance to investigate immunoreactive IL-4 and IL-5 as opposed to mRNA in the tissue or IL-4 and IL-5 protein in the BAL?

DR. DURHAM: These studies are ongoing. Bradding et al. have demonstrated IL-4 and IL-5 protein, principally from mast cells, in bronchial biopsies from asthmatics (P Bradding, IH Feather, PH Howarth, et al. Interleukin-4 is localized to and released by human mast cells. J Exp Med 1992; 176:1381–1386). They did not identify IL-4 or IL-5 protein from T lymphocytes, although this may have been due to (1) the method of fixation used, and (2) T lymphocytes do not store cytokines, which presumably are rapidly released and are not therefore stainable, in contrast to mast cells (and eosinophils), which store cytokines in the cytoplasmic granules.

DR. SCHLEIMER: (1) Do you have evidence of epithelial cells producing IL-5? (2) What is the correlation between IL-4 and eosinophils? (3) How can you explain the improvement of reactivity seen with systemic glucocorticoids?

DR. DURHAM: (1) I know of no published data supporting epithelial cells as a source of IL-5. (2) In the late nasal response model, 6 weeks of treatment with topical corticosteroid inhibited allergen-induced increases in IL-4, and these changes correlated with the associated decrease in eosinophils. We speculate the IL-4 effect may be VLA-4/VCAM-1 dependent. (3) The improvements in reactivity were very consistent, as were the changes in cytokine gene expression for IL-4 and IL-5. This does not prove a casual association. However, I believe that modulation by corticosteroids of gene expression which influences tissue eosinophils and IgE synthesis may well account for the observed improvements in airway reactivity in our study.

DR. MCFADDEN: The first few studies that examined the influence of glucocorticoids on airway reactivity used oral agents and found negative results as have others subsequently. I don't know how important these observations are. It is very unlikely that the route of administration confers any particular selectivity for this effect. More likely, issues such as dose and duration of treatment are driving the findings.

DR. HARGREAVE: Have you looked at the number of B cells in BAL, or do you know of any such measurements?

DR. DURHAM: No. We have identified B cells (CD20$^+$) in the nasal mucosa of patients with atopic rhinitis but not in the skin. We have not looked in the bronchial mucosa or BAL fluid.

DR. HOWARTH: Can you clarify the discrepancy between T-cell activation marker and T-cell cytokine production? You describe approximately 30% of T cells from the airways expressing IL-2 receptor (CD25$^+$) but only 30/1000 cells (3%) are IL-4 or IL-5 mRNA positive. What do the other activated T cells generate? The reason I ask is that we have tried to address the difficult question you raised in your talk about identifying products in T cells. Using monensin blockade of Golgi secretion and stimulation of lavage T cells from asthmatics, we find that approximately 70% of lavage T cells have the potential to generate IFN-γ, suggestive of T-cell anergy, whereas like you, we find $\leq 1\%$ are IL-4 or IL-5 generating. I believe we need to know more about the meaning of IL-2 receptor expression in airway T cells.

DR. DURHAM: I have no data, but speculate that the small proportion of activated T cells which do express message for TH2 cytokines are allergen specific.

DR. GLEICH: First, I must compliment you on a lucid, well-integrated presentation. Second, I am curious about your thoughts concerning the overall mechanisms of LPR. For example, in cutaneous LPRs, eosinophils infiltrate the skin within a very few hours and even at 30 min. Dr. K.M Leiferman (KM Leiferman, T Fujisawa, BH Gray, GJ Gleich. Extracellular deposition of eosinophil and neutrophil granule proteins in the IgE-mediated cutaneous late phase reaction. Lab Inves 1990; 62:579–589) noted eosinophil migration and infiltration which was marked by 2 hr. These events appear to be very rapid and seem difficult to explain on a T-cell basis. Third, in the skin LPRs, neutrophils infiltrate and degranulate at the same rate as eosinophils. Do you have data on neutrophils from the work of your group?

DR. DURHAM: In our study, biopsies were obtained at 24 hr after allergen and control challenges, with each subject acting as his or her own control. I assume that early recruitment of eosinophils at 1–2 hr after allergen is likely to be mast cell dependent rather than dependent on T cells. We see allergen-induced recruitment of neutrophils at 24 hr in the nose (S Rak, MR Jacobson, RM Sudderick, et al. Influence of prolonged treatment with topical corticosteroid (fluticasone propionate) on early and late phase nasal responses and cellular infiltration in the nasal mucosa after allergen challenge. Clin Exp Allergy 1994; 24:930–939) and lung (AM Bentley, D Meng, DS Robinson, et al. Increases in activated T-lymphocytes, eosinophils, and cytokine messenger RNA expression for interleukin-5 and granulocyte/macrophage colony-stimulating factor in bronchial biopsies after allergen inhalation challenge in atopic asthmatics. Am J Respir Cell Molec Biol 1993; 8:35–42, 1993). Paradoxically, in the nose, inhibition of the late nasal response by topical corticosteroid is accompanied by an increase in allergen-induced neutrophilia in the nasal mucosa, which questions the role of neutrophils in human late responses.

DR. LEMANSKE: In allergic asthmatic patients, one would anticipate finding a TH2-like cytokine profile in the airways. Have you any data comparing and contrasting BAL or biopsy results from allergic asthmatic patients with similar results obtained from nonatopic or so-called "intrinsic" asthma?

DR. DURHAM: Walker et al. (C Walker, JJ-C Virchow, PLB Bruijnzeel, K Blaser. T cell subsets and their soluble products regulate eosinophilia in allergic and nonallergic asthma. J Immunol 1991; 146:1829–1835) has shown increases in activated T lymphocytes in BAL fluid from patients with so-called intrinsic asthma, although their profile of cytokines appear to be different with IL-5 and IL-2 production and no IL-4. We are currently evaluating cytokine expression in atopic and nonatopic asthmatics by the use of bronchial biopsies. Interestingly, by both in situ studies and by PCR, the findings for both groups are comparable; that is, we see increased mRNA expression for both IL-4 and

IL-5 in the bronchial mucosa in atopic and nonatopic asthmatics (unpublished observations).

DR. LEUNG: *Comment*: With regard to the recovery of T cells from segmental allergen challenges, in studies published from our group on homing receptors of T cells infiltrating into the lung, the more vigorous the allergen response the less specific were the infiltrating T cells. (L. Picker, R Martin, A Trumble et al. Control of lymphocyte recirculation in man: differential expression of homing-associated adhesion molecules by memory/effector T cells in pulmonary vs cutaneous effector sites. Eur J Immunol 1994; 24:1269–1277.) Thus, increasing cell yield may be a double-edged sword. The observation that most T cells in the LPR are TH2-like in cytokine expression may reflect the differentiation capacity of local tissue milieu; that is, dominance of IL-4 and IL-13 inducing TH2 cells. (1) Can you define for us what a TH2-like cell is in 1994? Specifically, do TH2-like cells in humans express IL-2 as well? (2) Can you review briefly whether the activated T cells in the peripheral blood of asthmatics have similar cytokine profiles to those seen in their airways?

DR. DURHAM: (1) There are no consistent phenotypic markers for TH2-type cells, so one is left with identifying the profile of cytokines produced. The TH1 versus TH2 dichotomy is helpful but not absolute and not strictly comparable between mice and humans. For example, human TH2 cells may produce IL-2. (2) Dr. Chris Corrigan in our group has shown that asthmatics have activated $CD25^+/CD4^+$ T lymphocytes (by flow cytometry) which correlate with disease severity and are inhibitable by oral corticosteroid treatment (CJ Corrigan, A Hartnell, AB Kay. T lymphocyte activation in acute severe asthma. Lancet 1988; 1:1129–1132; CJ Corrigan, AB Kay. CD4 T-lymphocyte activation in acute severe asthma. Relationship to disease severity and atopic status. Am Rev Respir Dis 1990; 141:970–977, 1990).

DR. A. LAITINEN: Have you looked at what happens when you stop treatment? Could there be a difference between oral and inhaled steroid treatment concerning the duration of downregulatory effect? With inhaled steroid treatment we can get restoration of damaged epithelium in asthmatics. We do not know if this happens with oral steroids.

DR. DURHAM: We have not done a steroid withdrawal study to answer your question. I know of no direct comparison between oral and inhaled steroids and their effects on airway mucosa.

DR. LIU: Are the same T cells producing IL-4 and IL-5? *Comment*: In the model of segmental challenge, we have observed that the marked increase in BAL T cells recruited to the inflammatory site is associated with a marked and specific induction of IL-4 and IL-5 mRNA expression with no induction of IL-

2 and IFN-γ. Analysis was performed using a semiquantitative reverse transcription polymerase chain reaction (RT-PCR) assay. This specific profile of TH2 cytokine gene expression may indicate selective recruitment or activation of T cell subsets at the site of allergic inflammation.

DR. DURHAM: The answer to your question lies in performing double in situ hybridization of BAL/biopsies using alternatively labeled antisense riboprobes directed against IL-4 an IL-5. We have no data at present.

DR. ROCKLIN: Have you stained biopsies/BALF for the present of CD45 RO$^+$ cells?

DR. DURHAM: A very high proportion of tissue (as opposed to circulating) T lymphocytes are of memory (CD45 RO) phenotype in the skin LPR. (AJ Frew, AB Kay. UCHL1+ (CD45RO+) memory T-cells predominate in the CD4 + cellular infiltrate associated with allergen-induced late-phase skin reactions in atopic subjects. Clin Exp Immunol 1991; 84:270–274.)

References

1. Mossman TR, Coffman RI. Th1 and Th2 cells: different patterns of lymphokine secretion lead to different functional properties. Annu Rev Immunol 1989; 7:145–173.
2. Wierenga EA, Snock M, de Groot C, Chretien L, Bos JD, Jansen HM, Kapsenberg MI. Evidence for compartmentalisation of functional subsets of CD4+ T lymphocytes in atopic patients. J Immunol 1990; 144:4651–4656.
3. Cher DJ, Mossmann TR. Two type of murine helper T-cell clone. II. Delayed-type hypersensitivity is mediated by Th1 clones. J Immunol 1987; 138:3688–3694.
4. Frew AJ, Kay AB. The relationship between infiltrating CD4+ T lymphocytes activated eosinophils and the magnitude of the allergen-induced late phase cutaneous reaction. J Immunol 1988; 141:4158.
5. Kay AB, Sun Ying, Varney V, Gaga M, Durham SR, Moqbel R, Wardlaw AJ, Hamid Q. Messenger RNA expression of the cytokine gene cluster, IL-3, IL-4, IL-5 and GM-CSF in allergen-induced late-phase cutaneous reactions in atopic subjects. J Exp Med 1991; 173:775–778.
6. Varney V, Gaga M, Frew AJ, Aber VA, Kay AB, Durham SR. Usefulness of immunotherapy in patients with severe summer hayfever uncontrolled by antiallergic drugs. Br Med J 1991; 302:265–269.
7. Varney VA, Hamid QA, Gaga M, Sun Ying, Jacobson M, Frew AJ, Kay AB, Durham SR. Influence of grass pollen immunotherapy on cellular infiltration and cytokine mRNA expression during allergen-induced late-phase cutaneous responses. J Clin Invest 1993; 92:644–651.
8. Corrigan CJ, Hartnell A, Kay AB. T lymphocyte activation in acute severe asthma. Lancet 1988; 1:1129–1131.

9. Corrigan CJ, Kay AB. CD4 T lymphocyte activation in acute severe asthma. Relationship to disease severity and atopic status. Am Rev Respir Dis 1990; 141:970–977.

10. Corrigan CJ, Brown PH, Barnes NC, Tsai JJ, Kay AB. Glucocorticosteroid resistance in chronic asthma: glucocorticoid pharmacokinetics, glucocorticoid receptor characteristics and inhibition of peripheral blood T-cell proliferation by glucocorticoids in vitro. Am Rev Respir Dis 1991; 144:1016–1025.

11. Corrigan CJ, Brown PH, Barnes NC, Tsai JJ, Kay AB. Glucocorticosteroid resistance in chronic asthma: peripheral blood T lymphocyte activation and a comparison of the T lymphocyte inhibitory effects of glucocorticoids and cyclosporin A. Am Rev Respir Dis 1991; 144:1026–1032.

12. Azzawi M, Bradley B, Jeffery PK, Frew A, Wardlaw AJ, Knowles G, Assoufi B, Collins JV, Durham S, Kay AB. Identification of activated T lymphocytes and eosinophils in bronchial biopsies in stable atopic asthma. Am Rev Respir Dis 1990; 142:1407–1413.

13. Hamid Q, Barkans J, Robinson DS, Durham SR, Kay AB. Co-expression of CD25 and CD3 in atopic allergy and asthma. Immunology 1992; 75:659–663.

14. Hamid Q, Azzawi M, Sun Ying, Moqbel R, Wardlaw AJ, Corrigan CJ, Bradley B, Durham SR, Collins JV, Jeffery PK, Quint DJ, Kay AB. Expression of mRNA for interleukin-5 in mucosal bronchial biopsies from asthma. J Clin Invest 1991; 87:1541–1546.

15. Robinson DS, Hamid Q, Sun Ying, Tsicopoulos A, Barkans J, Bentley AM, Corrigan CJ, Durham SR, Kay AB. Predominant Th2-type bronchoalveolar lavage T-lymphocyte population in atopic asthma. N Engl J Med 1992; 326:298–304.

16. Sousa AR, Poston RN, Lane SJ, Nakhosteen JA, Lee TA. Detection of GM-CSF in asthmatic bronchial epithelium and decrease by inhaled corticosteroids. Am Rev Respir Dis 1993; 147:1557–1561.

17. Kay AB, Hamid Q, Durham SR. Phenotype of cells expressing cytokine messenger RNA in atopic allergy and asthma. Int Arch Allergy Appl Immunol 1995; 107:208–210.

18. Broide DH, Lotz M, Cuomo AJ, Cobum DA, Federman EC, Wasserman SI. Cytokines in symptomatic asthma airways. J Allergy Clin Immunol 1992; 89:958–967.

19. Broide DH, Firestein GS. Endobronchial allergen challenge in asthma: Demonstration of cellular source of granulocyte macrophage colony-stimulating factor by in situ hybridization. J Clin Invest 1991; 88:1048–1053.

20. Bradding P, Roberts JA, Britten KM, et al. Interleukin-4, -5, and -6 and tumor necrosis factor-α in normal and asthmatic airways: evidence for the human mast cell as a source of these cytokines. Am J Respir Cell Mol Biol 1994; 10:471–480.

21. Ackerman V, Marini M, Vittori E, et al. Detection of cytokines and their cell sources in bronchial biopsy specimens from asthmatic patients. Chest 1994; 105:687–696.

22. Robinson, D.S., Bentley, A.M., Hartnell, A., Kay, A.B., Durham, S.R. Activated memory T helper cells in bronchoalveolar lavage from atopic asthmatics. Relation-

ship to asthma symptoms, lung function and bronchial responsiveness. Thorax
1993; 48:26–32.

23. Bradley BL, Azzawi M, Jacobson M, Assoufi B, Collins JV, Irani A-MA,
Schwartz LB, Durham SR, Jeffery PK, Kay AB Eosinophils, T-lymphocytes, mast
cells, neutrophils and macrophages in bronchial biopsy specimens from atopic subjects with asthma: Comparison with biopsy specimens from atopic subjects without
asthma and normal control subjects and relationship to bronchial
hyperresponsiveness. J Allergy Clin Immunol. 1991; 88:661–674.

24. Robinson DS, Sun Ying, Bentley AM, Qiu Meng, North J, Durham SR, Kay AB,
Hamid Q. Relationships among numbers of bronchoalveolar lavage cells expressing messenger ribonucleic acid for cytokines, asthma symptoms, and airway
methacholine responsiveness in atopic asthma. J Allergy Clin Immunol 1993;
92:397.

25. Bentley AM, Maestrelli P, Saetta M, Fabbri LM, Robinson DS, Bradley BL,
Jeffery PK, Durham SR, Kay AB. Activated T-lymphocytes and eosinophils in the
bronchial mucosa in isocyanate-induced asthma. J Allergy Clin Immunol 1992;
89:877–883.

26. Bentley AM, Menz G, Storz Chr, Robinson DS, Bradley B, Jeffery PK, Durham
SR, Kay AB. Identification of T-lymphocytes, macrophages and activated eosinophils in the bronchial mucosa in intrinsic asthma: relationship to symptoms and
bronchial responsiveness. Am Rev Respir Dis 1992; 146:500–506.

27. Walker C, Virchow J-C, Bruijnzeel PLB, Blaster K. T cell subsets and their
soluble products regulate eosinophilia in allergic and non-allergic asthma. J
Immunol 1991; 146:1829–1835

28. Walker C, Bode E, Boer L, Hansel TT, Blaser K, Virchow J-C. Allergic and non-
allergic asthmatics have distinct patterns of T cell activation and cytokine production in peripheral blood and bronchoalveolar lavage. Am Rev Respir Dis 1992;
146:109–115.

29. Robinson DS, Sun Ying, Taylor IK, Wangoo A, Mitchell DM, Kay AB, Hamid Q,
Shaw RJ. Evidence of a TH1-like bronchoalveolar T-cell subset and predominance
of interferon-gamma gene activation in pulmonary tuberculosis. Am J Respir Crit
Care Med 1994; 149:989–993.

30. Durham SR. The significance of late responses in asthma. Clin and Exp All 1991;
21:3–7.

31. Cockcroft DW, Murdock KY. Comparative effects of inhaled salbutamol, sodium
cromoglycate, and beclomethasone dipropionate on allergen-induced early asthmatic
responses, late asthmatic responses, and increased bronchial responsiveness to histamine. J Allergy Clin Immunol 1987; 79:734–740.

32. Durham SR, Lee TH, Cromwell O, Shaw RJ, Merrett TG, Merrett J, Cooper P,
Kay AB. Immunologic studies in allergen-induced late-phase asthmatic reactions.
J Allergy Clin Immunol 1984; 74:49–60.

33. Durham SR, Carroll M, Walsh GM, Kay AB. Leukocyte activation during allergen-induced late-phase asthmatic reactions. N Engl J Med 1984; 311:1398–1402.

34. Durham SR, Kay AB. Eosinophils, bronchial hyperreactivity and late-phase asthmatic reactions. Clin Allergy 1985; 15:411–418.

35. Durham SR, Loegering DA, Dunnette S, Gleich GJ, Kay AB. Blood eosinophils

and eosinophil-derived proteins in allergic asthma. J Allergy Clin Immunol 1989; 84:931–936.

36. Gerblich A, Salik H, Schuyler MR. Dynamic changes in peripheral blood and bronchoalveolar lavage after antigen bronchoprovocation in asthmatics. Am Rev Respir Dis 1991; 143:533–537.

37. Gerblich A, Campbell A, Schuyler MR. Changes in T lymphocyte subpopulations after antigenic bronchial provocation in asthmatics. N Engl J Med 1984; 310:1349–1352.

38. De Monchy JGR, Kauffman HF, Venge P, Koeter GH, Jansen HM, Sluiter HJ, De Vries K. Bronchoalveolar eosinophilia during allergen-induced late asthmatic reactions. Am Rev Respir Dis 1985; 131:373–376.

39. Aalbers R, Kaufmann HF, Vrugt B, et al. Bronchial lavage and bronchoalveolar lavage in allergen-induced single early and dual asthmatic responders. Am Rev Respir Dis 1993; 147:76–81.

40. Metzger WJ, Zavala D, Richerson HB, Moseley P, Iwamota P, Monick M, Sjoerdsma K, Humminghake GW. Local allergen challenge and bronchoalveolar lavage of allergic asthmatic lungs: description of the model and local airway inflammation. Am Rev Respir Dis 1987; 135:433–440.

41. Gonzalez MC, Diaz P, Galleguillos FR, Ancic P, Cromwell O, Kay AB. Allergen-induced recruitment of bronchoalveolar helper (OKT4) and suppressor (OKT8) T-cells in asthma. Am Rev Respir Dis 1987; 136:600–604.

42. Bentley AM, Qiu Meng, Robinson DS, Hamid Q, Kay AB, Durham SR. Increases in activated T lymphocytes, eosinophils and cytokine messenger RNA for IL-5 and GM-CSF in bronchial biopsies after allergen inhalation challenge in atopic asthmatics. Am J Resp Cell Mol Biol 1993; 8:35–42.

43. Robinson DS, Hamid Q, Bentley A, Sun Ying, Kay AB, Durham SR. Activation of CD4+ T cells, increased Th2-type cytokine mRNA expression, and eosinophil recruitment in bronchoalveolar lavage after allergen inhalation challenge in atopic asthmatics. J Allergy Clin Immunol 1993; 92:313–324.

44. Liu MC, Walter C, Hubbard DP, et al. Immediate and late inflammatory responses to ragweed antigen challenge of the peripheral airways in allergic asthmatics. Am Rev Respir Dis 1991; 144:51–58.

45. Gratziou C, Carroll M, Walls A, Howarth PH, Holgate ST. Early changes in T lymphocytes recovered by bronchoalveolar lavage after local allergen challenge of asthmatic airways. Am Rev Respir Dis 1992; 145:1259–1264.

46. Ohnishi T, Kita H, Weiler D, Sur S, Sedgwick JB, Calhoun WJ, Busse WW, Abrams JS, Gleich GJ. IL-5 is the predominant eosinophil-active cytokine in the antigen-induced pulmonary late-phase reaction. Am Rev Respir Dis 1993; 147:901–907

47. Broide DH, Paine MM, Firestein GS. Eosinophils express interleukin-5 and granulocyte macrophage-colony-stimulating factor mRNA at sites of allergic inflammation in asthmatics. J Clin Invest 1992; 90:1414–1424.

48. Haczku A, Bentley A, Brown P, Assoufi B, Baiqing L, Kay AB, Corrigan C. The effect of dexamethasone, cyclosporine and rapamycin on T lymphocyte proliferation in vitro: comparison of cells from patients with glucocorticoid sensitive and

glucocorticoid-resistant chronic asthma. J Allergy Clin Immunol 1994; 93:510–519.

49. Guyre PM, Girard MT, Morganelli PM, Manginiello PD. Glucocorticoid effects on the production and action of immune cytokines. J Steroid Biochem 1988; 30:89–93.

50. Schleimer RP, Schulman ES, Macglashan DW, Peter SP, Adams GK, Lichtenstein LM, Adkinson NF. Effects of dexamethasone on mediator release from human lung fragments and purified human lung mast cells. J Clin Invest 1983; 81:1830–1835.

51. Cohan VL, Undem BJ, Fox CC, Adkinson NF, Lichtenstein LM, Schleimer RP. Dexamethasone does not inhibit the release of mediators from human lung mast cells residing in airway, intestine, or skin. Am Rev Respir Dis 1989; 140:951–954.

52. Kita H, Abu-Ghazaleh R, Sanderson CJ, Gleich GJ. Effects of steroids on immunoglobulin-induced eosinophil degranulation. J Allergy Clin Immunol 1991; 87:70–77.

53. Lamas AM, Leon OG, Schleimer RP. Glucocorticoids inhibit eosinophil responses to granulocyte-macrophage colony-stimulating factor. J Immunol 1991; 147:254–259.

54. Waller N, Kita H, Weiller D, Gleich GJ. Glucocorticoids inhibit cytokine-mediated eosinophil survival. J Immunol 1991; 147:3490–3495.

55. Hallsworth MP, Litchfeld TM, Lee /TH. Glucocorticoids inhibit granulocyte-macrophage colony-stimulating factor and interleukin-5 enhanced in vitro survival of human eosinophils. Immunology 1992; 75:382–385.

56. Rak S, Jacobson MR, Sudderick RM, et al. Influence of prolonged treatment with topical corticosteroid (fluticasone propionate) on early and late phase nasal responses and cellular infiltration in the nasal mucosa after allergen challenge. Clin Exp Allergy 1994; 24:930–939.

57. Varney VA, Jacobson MR, Sudderick RM, Robinson DS, Irani A-MA, Schwartz LB, Mackay IS, Kay AB, Durham SR. Immunohistology of the nasal mucosa following allergen-induced rhinitis. Identification of activated T lymphocytes, eosinophils and neutrophils. Am Rev Respir Dis 1992; 145:170–176.

58. Durham SR, Sun Ying, Varney VA, Jacobson MR, Sudderick RM, Mackay IS, Kay AB, Hamid QA. Cytokine messenger RNA expression for IL-3, IL-4, IL-5 and GM-CSF in the nasal mucosa after local allergen provocation: relationship to tissue eosinophilia. J Immunol 1992; 148:2390–2394.

59. Sun Ying, Durham SR, Barkans J, Masuyama K, Jacobson M, Rak S, Löwhagen O, Moqbel R, Kay AB, Hamid QA. T cells are the principal source of interleukin-5 mRNA in allergen-induced rhinitis. Am J Respir Cell Mol Biol 1993; 9:356.

60. Sun Ying, Durham SR, Jacobson MR, Rak S, Lowhagen O, Kay AB, Hamid QA. T lymphocytes and mast cells express messenger for the interleukin-4 in the nasal mucosa in allergen-induced rhinitis. Immunology 1994; 82:200–206.

61. Britten KM, Howarth PH, Roche WE. Immunohistochemistry on resin sections, a comparison of resin embedding techniques for small mucosal biopsies. Biotech Histochem 1993; 68:271–280.

62. Bradding P, Feather IH, Howarth PH, et al. Interleukin 4 is localised to an released by human mast cells. J Exp Med 1992; 176:1381–1386.

63. Masuyama K, Jacobson MR, Rak S, Qiu Meng, Sudderick RM, Kay AB, Lowhagen O, Hamid Q, Durham SR. Topical glucocorticosteroid (fluticasone pro-

pionate) inhibits cytokine mRNA expression for interleukin-4 (IL-4) in the nasal mucosa in allergic rhinitis. Immunology 1994; 82:192–199.

64. Jacobson MR, Rak S, Sudderick RM, Masuyama K, Kay AB, Lowhagen O, Hamid Q, Durham SR. Influence of prolonged treatment with topical corticosteroid on allergen-induced cellular infiltration in the nasal mucosa. Clin Exp Allergy 1994; 24:930–939.

65. Djukanovic R, Wilson JW, Britten KM, et al. Effect of an inhaled corticosteroid on airway inflammation and symptoms in asthma. Am Rev Respir Dis 1992; 145:669–674.

66. Wilson JW, Djukanovic R, Howarth PH, Holgate ST. Inhaled beclomethasone dipropionate downregulated airway lymphocyte activation in atopic asthma. J Respir Crit Care Med 1994; 149:86–90.

67. Laitinen LA, Laitinen A, Haahtela T. A comparative study of the effects of an inhaled corticosteroid, budesonide, and of a β_2-agonist, terbutaline, on airway inflammation in newly diagnosed asthma. J Allergy Clin Immunol 1992; 90:32–42.

68. Robinson DS, Hamid Q, Sun Ying, Bentley AM, Assoufi B, North J, Qui Meng, Durham SR, Kay AB. Prednisolone treatment in asthma is associated with modulation of bronchoalveolar lavage cell IL-4, IL-5 and IFN-gamma cytokine gene expression. Am Rev Respir Dis 1993; 148:401–406.

69. Bentley AM, Robinson DS, Assoufi B, Kay AB, Durham SR. A controlled trial of prednisolone treatment in asthma: reduction in eosinophils, T lymphocytes and mast cells within the bronchial mucosa. Clin Exp Allergy 1993;23 (Suppl. 1):75 (FC30).

70. Alexander AG, Barnes NC, Kay AB. Trial of cyclosporin A in corticosteroid-dependent chronic severe asthma. Lancet 1992; 339:324–328.

12

Effects of Corticosteroids on Basophils and Mast Cells

JUDAH A. DENBURG

McMaster University
Hamilton, Ontario, Canada

I. Introduction

This chapter will review the effects of corticosteroids on the metachromatic cell subsets, basophils and mast cells. Although this subject has been reviewed extensively by Schleimer as recently as 1993 (1), aspects of basophil and mast cell biology have come to light since that time which are quite relevant to understanding how corticosteroids may affect these cells both in vitro and in vivo. Accordingly, this chapter deals with the effects of corticosteroids on the survival and proliferation of basophils and mast cells in vitro; effects on cell function, including mediator release and cytokine gene expression and production; effects in vivo on various types of allergic reactions (anaphylaxis, urticaria/angioedema, and tissue-specific responses to allergen); and effects on diseases in which basophils or mast cells proliferate (various forms of leukemia and mast cell proliferative disorders). Special emphasis is placed on work that has emanated from our laboratory exploring basophil and mast cell development using assays to detect progenitor cells for these and related myeloid lineages. The complex circuitry of corticosteroid effects on hemopoietic cytokine production during the course of allergic inflammatory reactions, with consequent effects on basophil and mast cell lineages both in vitro and in vivo, is given special attention.

II. Basic Biology: In Vitro Studies

This section focuses on corticosteroid effects on the proliferation, survival, and function of basophils and mast cells. Further, corticosteroid modulation of basophil and mast cell function is addressed. The reader is also referred to extensive reviews on these topics by Schleimer and Denburg (1–4). An overall summary of the effects of corticosteroids on basophils and mast cells is provided in Table 1.

A. Effects on Cell Survival and Proliferation

Mast cells can be propagated in vitro in large numbers through the use of specific cytokines: Interleukin-3 (IL-3), primarily in rodent systems, supports the continued proliferation of mast cell lines of various stages of commitment and maturation and the ligand for c-*kit* (KL), also known as stem cell factor, induces the differentiation of human mast cells from bone marrow, cord blood,

Table 1 Effects of Corticosteroids on Basophils and Mast Cells

	Basophils		Mast cells	
Model/function	human	animal	human	animal
In Vitro				
Mediator release				
Histamine	↓	U	NE	↓
Prostanoids/leukotrienes	↓	U	NE	↓
Proteases	↓	U	U	↓
Cytokines	↓	U	U	↓
Survival/activation	NE	U	U	U
Proliferation/differentiation	↓	U	U	↓
In Vivo				
Mediator release	U	U	↓ or NE	↓
Tissue numbers	↓	U	↓	↓

Abbreviations: NE, no consistent effect; U, unknown/unclear.

or fetal liver progenitors (5-7). KL (8) can also induce rodent mast cells of the serosal type to differentiate both in vitro and in vivo (9-10). More recently, it has been shown that KL can also prevent apoptosis in rodent mast cells (11), thus representing a survival-inducing factor for serosal mast cells, with IL-3 its counterpart for the mucosal mast cell subtype. Rodent basophils have been more difficult to propagate in vitro in pure cultures, although there are some cell lines originally thought to be basophilic but now known to represent subtypes of mucosal mast cells (e.g., rat basophilic leukemia, or RBL, cells). In human culture systems, IL-3, IL-5, and granulocyte-macrophage colony-stimulating factor (GM-CSF) support the growth and differentiation of basophil-eosinophil colonies, which are derived from a common basophil-eosinophil progenitor (12-15). In contrast to findings in rodents, IL-3 is not a human mast cell differentiation factor, since it binds only to basophils (16,17).

In all of these systems, corticosteroids can be shown to have suppressive effects on the survival and proliferation of basophils or mast cells. For example, T-cell production of IL-3 can be downregulated by corticosteroids in vitro (1,2), thus effectively interfering with the continued survival of IL-3–dependent mast cell lines. Dexamethasone causes a reversible inhibition of immortalized murine mast cell line growth (18) as well as decreases in vitro of protease (RMCPII) production by RBL-2H3 cells (19).

Recently, we have shown that budesonide at concentrations as low as 10^{-10} M in vitro can inhibit both GM-CSF production and the formation of basophil-containing colonies derived from progenitors in human peripheral blood (20-22). The dose-response curve of budesonide is steep, and at 10^{-8} M there is virtual complete inhibition of colony formation in vitro (22). Although this effect may be mediated by inhibition of GM-CSF production by accessory cells present in these cultures, which conceivably interact with progenitors via this and other hemopoietic cytokine release, it is also possible that the effects are directly on the progenitors themselves. This is supported in part by cultures of HL-60 cells, representing a myeloid leukemic cell which can be induced to differentiate along several lineages, including basophilic (23-25). Budesonide has direct effects in blocking the differentiation of HL-60 myeloid cells to the basophil lineage in vitro at similar concentrations to its effect on colony-forming cells in methylcellulose cultures or on cytokine production by structural cells (26, 27). There are some reports of enhanced histamine production and maturation induced by micromolar doses of dexamethasone added to murine bone marrow–derived mast cells in vitro (28), but these are the minority.

Suppressive effects of corticosteroids can also be demonstrated in vitro on human mast cell lines, such as HMC-1, which represents a poorly differentiated mast cell derived from a patient with mast cell leukemia (29). It is not yet clear whether in any of these systems there is downregulation by corticosteroids of specific cytokines—produced by the cells themselves in autocrine fashion—on which the survival and proliferation of the progenitors and their ensuing progeny depend. More work needs to be done on purified hemopoietic progenitors which are now available in large quantity in a number of species, including human, based on cell surface immunophenotype with markers such as CD34 (30) and c-*kit* (31–33).

B. Effects on Cell Function

Mediator Release

Mast cell lines in vitro can be induced to release mediators through IgE-dependent and IgE-independent pathways. It appears that there are distinct differences among species, triggering mechanisms, and types of mediator release as well as differences between basophils and mast cells in terms of whether or not corticosteroids can suppress cell function (1,2,34). For example, human mast cells derived from the lung are particularly resistant to corticosteroid-mediated inhibition of mediator release (35), whereas those in rodents by and large are sensitive to the effects of corticosteroids (1–3, 36,37). However, even among various rodent species, IgE-dependent mediator release can be differentially affected by corticosteroids in vitro compared with calcium ionophore or other nonspecific secretagogues; this is probably related to specific effects of corticosteroids on signal transduction in mast cell subtypes (38,39). The results depend on the subtype of mast cell. Differences between mast cells and basophils have also been pointed out; for example, basophils are sensitive to downregulation of mediator release by corticosteroids both in vitro and in vivo (1–3), whereas epithelial mast cells, which represent the mucosal subtype, are in general more inhibitable than serosal mast cells by corticosteroids (40,41). Recently, evidence has been provided that rat mast cell protease II (RMCPII) production by RBL cells, a mucosal mast cell phenotype, shows a dose-dependent downregulation by corticosteroids in vitro (19), mirroring in vivo effects on RMCPII and histamine production in the rat treated with corticosteroids after infection with the nematode *Nippostrongylus brasiliensis* (40,41).

Cytokine Gene Expression and Production

Basophils and Mast Cells

The effects of corticosteroids on cytokine gene expression and production by mast cells in rodents and humans are now beginning to be explored, offering potentially a much more exciting possibility for assessing the effects of corticosteroids on mast cell-dependent leukocyte cascades (42–44). Thus, IL-1 and tumor necrosis factorα (TNF-α) are both produced by mast cells during IgE-dependent reactions in the skin in mice; the reaction can be partially inhibited by antibody to TNF-α (44); subsequent abrogation of leukocyte infiltration by corticosteroids may represent the mechanism responsible for their effects on the late-phase response in vivo (1–3,36,45,46). The effects of corticosteroids on other cytokines, such as IL-4, IL-5, and IL-6, involved in allergic inflammatory reactions and derived, at least in part, from mast cells or basophils (47–50), as well as the effects of corticosteroids on KL-induced mast cell and basophil mediator release, remain to be fully explored.

Airway Structural Cells

In our laboratory, we have concentrated on the production of hemopoietic and proinflammatory cytokines by the structural cells involved in allergic inflammatory or other chronic inflammatory reactions. Corticosteroids can be shown in vitro to inhibit IL-1, IL-6, GM-CSF, and IL-8 gene expression and production by upper and lower airway epithelial cells and fibroblasts (26,27,51–53). These effects of corticosteroids on such structural cells may underlie the down-regulatory effects of corticosteroids in vivo on mast cell and basophil numbers, which are discussed below.

C. Effects of Corticosteroids on Signal Transduction Pathways

The effects of corticosteroids on various signaling pathways leading to mediator release and/or cytokine expression in mast cells and basophils have been briefly mentioned above (36–39) and are beyond the scope of this chapter. For further references on this area, see the reviews by Schleimer (2) as well as MacGlashan (54,55).

III. Applied Biology: Ex Vivo and In Vivo Studies

We now turn to the effects of corticosteroids in vivo and ex vivo in situations where IgE-dependent reactions involving mast cells and basophils occur. The effects of corticosteroids in vivo on proliferative responses of these cells during bone marrow disorders such as leukemia and mast cell proliferation will also be explored.

A. Effects of IgE-dependent Reactions in Allergic Inflammation

The IgE-dependent response exhibits a typical early phase which lasts several minutes to an hour followed by a late-phase response several hours later. This has been demonstrated in human IgE-dependent reactions in several different tissues, including the upper and lower airways and skin (1,35,46,56). The clinical conditions associated with these reactions include allergic rhinitis, asthma, some forms of urticaria and angioedema, and some cases of anaphylaxis.

In animal models, these IgE-dependent reactions, involving both early- and late-phase responses, can also be defined, and the roles of mast cells and basophils have been proposed to be similar, if not identical, to those in the human. Principally, much evidence points to the involvement of mast cell mediators such as histamine, tryptase, and prostaglandin E2 during the early-phase response, whereas basophil mediators such leukotrienes and histamine characterize the late-phase response (56). Steroids given *orally* have very little effect on a variety of mast cell–mediated, IgE-dependent or IgE-independent reactions in humans (1,2,36), including cold urticaria, ongoing anaphylaxis, and early-phase responses in the skin and the airways (1,2). However, *topical* corticosteroids appear to have an effect in reducing IgE-dependent responses (such as whealing in the skin) in these tissues and in causing a change either in the distribution or in the numbers of mast cells in several species during the chronic phase of inflammatory responses in the airways (57–63).

Only rarely are corticosteroids ineffective in reducing mast cell numbers when given topically (64). Thus, in work done by our group, it was shown that the numbers of mast cells in the nasal mucosa in allergic rhinitis and polyposis are reduced after 1 or 2 weeks of treatment with inhaled budesonide (61,65). Similar results have been noted in nasal biopsies of patients with seasonal allergic rhinitis (S Durham et al., personal communication, May 1995); prolonged exposure to topical corticosteroids inhibits the appearance of c-*kit*–positive mast cells in the submucosa (66).

The mechanism for these changes in mast cell numbers is not clear, but it may involve downregulation of cytokines such as KL, which is involved in preventing apoptosis of these cells (11). Indeed, recently we have shown that the structural cells derived from human nasal polyps express the gene for and produce KL (67,68). Another mechanism targeted by both steroids and cyclosporin A is an IgE-dependent and mast cell/TNF-α–dependent leukocyte cascade in a mouse model (69). Whether or not these are the mechanisms in vivo for the corticosteroid effect on mast cell numbers during the chronic inflammatory phase of allergy-type reactions is still not known. Soda et al., in elegant studies in rats infected with *Nippostrongylus brasiliensis*, had shown that mast cell and eosinophil numbers were markedly reduced in the gastrointestinal mucosa 7 hr after systemic dexamethasone treatment (60,70); the mechanism for this appeared to be macrophage engulfment, a process which was not dependent on T cells (70). Apoptosis of mast cells as a result of the corticosteroid treatment is likely to have occurred. Whether or not cytokine-induced survival of mast cells in vivo is interfered with by corticosteroids in this model has not yet been fully clarified.

There are clearly species differences in the ability of corticosteroids to interfere with either mast cell or basophil numbers or mediator release in vivo. Moreover, there are differences dependent on the immunization protocol such that if antigen is given with aluminum hydroxide as an adjuvant in the guinea pig, inducing IgE antibody responses, there is greater likelihood that corticosteroid treatment will block bronchial responses to the relevant antigen (2).

B. Effects of Corticosteroids on Mast Cells and Basophils in Asthma

Models

Work by several investigators in our group has focused over the past few years on the effects of inhaled corticosteroids on inflammatory indices and bronchial responses in human asthma. Two distinct models have been examined: the controlled withdrawal of corticosteroids by inhalation to induce a mild asthma exacerbation (71,72) and allergen challenge studies in mild to moderate asthmatics (73,74).

Steroid Withdrawal

Several interesting observations which have direct relevance to the assessment of effects on mast cells and basophils emerge from these studies of inhaled corticosteroids. First, inhaled corticosteroids markedly diminish the numbers of peripheral blood basophils and eosinophils as well as their progenitors (72,74), together with decreases in sputum eosinophils and several cytokines associated with these reactions (72–77). The effect of withdrawal of inhaled corticosteroid revealed the converse: An increase in sputum eosinophils and eosinophil mediators, an increase in blood progenitors, and changes in peak flow rates as well as bronchial responsiveness (71,72,77). These changes could be restored by inhaled corticosteroids (71), suggesting that these corticosteroids were exerting direct effects on the airway and inflammatory responses associated with it; in addition, direct or indirect effects were exerted on the circulating blood compartments, especially those of progenitors, which presumably have emanated from the bone marrow. These results are consistent with and expand on previous observations on the effects of topical steroids on basophils and eosinophils during late-phase responses in a number of tissues (1–3,35,46,56,57).

Allergen Provocation

In more recent studies, using a canine model of induced bronchial hyperresponsiveness and pulmonary airflow obstruction consequent on inhalation of *Ascaris suum* in sensitized dogs (78), inhaled budesonide given for 7 days prior to antigen challenge abrogated bone marrow increases in the output of granulocyte progenitors as well as the inflammatory infiltrate in the airway (79). Preliminary observations indicate that a serum factor with hemopoietic activity is released following airway antigen challenge in these dogs; this serum factor can induce increased proliferation of granulocyte progenitors from naive bone marrow taken prior to antigen challenge ex vivo (22,80). If, indeed, the myeloid progenitor population examined includes both basophil and mast cell progenitors, then one of the effects of corticosteroids given by inhalation during IgE-dependent reactions could be to block the release from the bone marrow of progenitor cells destined to be recruited to and populate the airways or other relevant tissues targeted by the allergic reaction with terminally differentiated inflammatory effector cells.

Recently, in a similar allergen challenge model, Gauvreau (81) in our group has explored the effects of inhaled budesonide in humans on the expression of cells and cytokines in the blood and airways, as measured by colony-forming assays and staining of cells in induced sputum, respectively. Allergen challenge induces increases in both sputum and blood eosinophils, as well as mast cells, within 24 hr after challenge; in addition, increases in blood basophil-eosinophil progenitors are observed. All of these effects are prevented by pretreatment with budesonide but not with salbutamol (a β_2-agonist).

Progenitors

Studies of the effects of inhaled budesonide on bone marrow progenitor responses in humans following allergen challenge are currently underway. The latter can be measured both in the blood and marrow using immunophenotypic markers such as CD34 and flow cytometry (82). Preliminary evidence indicates that circulating $CD34^+$ cells are increased in atopics compared with nonatopics; they are also increased following allergen challenge within the atopic asthmatic population compared with prior to allergen (82). Since the $CD34^+$ population contains a subpopulation of basophil/eosinophil progenitors, the effects of inhaled corticosteroids may be to reduce basophil/eosinophil progenitor release from the marrow and access to the airway after allergen challenge.

There is still conflicting evidence as to whether or not corticosteroids can directly suppress basophil/eosinophil or mast cell progenitor growth and differentiation. Using either HL-60 cells or methylcellulose colony assays, we have demonstrated dose-dependent inhibitory effects of budesonide on basophil/eosinophil differentiation in vitro beginning at concentrations as low as 10^{-10} M (21). This is in accord with previous data on the suppressive effects of hydrocortisone on eosinophil but not neutrophil differentiation in vitro (83). In contrast, Shalit found no suppressive effect of dexamethasone on eosinophil differentiation from CD34-enriched human progenitor cell populations stimulated with Il-5 in vitro (84); these findings need to be confirmed using less primitive progenitor cell populations. Recently, Butterfield has examined the effects of several differentiation-inducing agents on HMC-1 cells, a human mast cell leukemia line, in vitro; only minimal effects were noted (85). No information is available on the effect of corticosteroids on HMC-1 cells or nontransformed human mast cells derived from bone marrow after stimulation with KL.

It is important to note that certain allergic types of reactions do respond clinically to systemic (oral) corticosteroids, including reactions to contrast media and dyes where pretreatment with corticosteroids systemically can markedly reduce the incidence of anaphylactoid reactions and some cases of delayed pressure angioedema/urticaria, in which corticosteroid treatment can have a major therapeutic benefit (86).

C. Effects on Proliferative Diseases

Mast cell and basophil mediator release as a consequence of systemic mastocytosis or its cutaneous counterpart and urticaria pigmentosa (both part of a spectrum of mast cell proliferative disorders, MCPD) as well as chronic myeloid leukemia with basophilic crisis involving hyperhistaminemia (87) and reactions mimicking anaphylactic episodes can be partially treated by systemic or topical corticosteroids (88). Topical treatment of urticaria pigmentosa in the skin with corticosteroids or systemic steroid treatment in other forms of cutaneous mastocytosis has been shown to have beneficial clinical effects (88,89). A combination of antihistamines, nonsteroidal anti-inflammatory agents, and possibly systemic corticosteroids can partially to fully block idiopathic syncopy and anaphylaxis related to increased mast cell numbers or MCPD. In some cases, the addition of systemic corticosteroids to a chemotherapeutic regimen for MCPD has been shown to have a beneficial effect by being cytotoxic to mast cells (88).

IV. Summary

Mast cells and basophils are prominent in allergic types of reactions and their survival, proliferation, and function are a result of a complex circuitry of cytokines and triggering events by cytophilic antibodies in response to antigen. Corticosteroids can be shown to have inhibitory effects at many stages of mast cell and basophil development and function (Fig. 1), but great differences exist among species, triggering events, sensitization protocols, and even among subsets of mast cells and basophils. The advent of inhaled or topical corticosteroids for allergic diseases of the airways and skin has heralded a much more effective and consistent approach to the management of these disorders, including asthma and allergic rhinitis. Inhaled corticosteroids appear to have profound effects on mast cell, basophil, and other granulocyte progenitors in the peripheral blood and bone marrow as well as on mature cell accumulation and survival both in vivo and in vitro. These mechanisms, rather than mediator release per se, may be crucial for the overall beneficial therapeutic effects of corticosteroids in allergy.

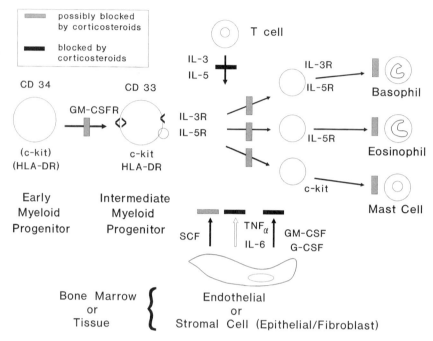

Figure 1   Effects of corticosteroids on inflammatory cell differentiation. Depicted here are the known and possible points in the differentiative process of basophils, eosinophils, and mast cells where corticosteroids can act. Blockade of tissue-derived proinflammatory cytokines, which also possess hemopoietic activity, such as TNF-α, IL-6, GM-CSF, and G-CSF or T-cell–derived IL-3 and IL-5, is known. Less clear is whether corticosteroids block stages of progenitor differentiation, shown here schematically as an orderly sequence of development from CD34+ cells to mature, end-stage cells. Recent acquisition of techniques to isolate and quantitate pure progenitor populations may facilitate approaches to answering this question.

Discussion

DR. LIU: Regarding the question of how topical steroids in the lung suppress circulating cell precursors, is it known how much circulating budesonide is needed to directly affect the bone marrow?

DR. DENBURG: The hemopoietic signal(s) which are present in serum 24 hr after allergen challenge to dog lung has not yet been characterized. Whether or not a systemic (spillover) effect of budesonide is required to suppress the marrow response is currently being addressed.

Dr. Lane: What are the characteristics of the allergen-induced steroid sensitive, colony-forming activity in the dog model in either physicochemical terms or in terms of antibody neutralization?

Dr. Denburg: We have not yet fully characterized the serum factor(s). It does withstand freezing and thawing. Work is in progress defining the activity; for example, we have tried neutralization experiments with anti-human GM-CSF with no effect.

Dr. Schleimer: I have a comment and then a question. An important point is that although mast cell degranulation is not inhibited by steroids in humans, both Galli's lab and Krangel's lab have recently shown inhibition of cytokine production (TNF and MCP-1, respectively) in mast cells. (BK Wershil, GT Furuta, JA Lavigne, et al. Dexamethasone or cyclosporin A suppress mast cell–leukocyte cytokine cascades. J Immunol 1995; 154:1391–1398; RS Selvan, JH Butterfield, MS Krangel. Expression of multiple chemokine genes by a human mast cell leukemia. J Biol Chem 1994; 269:13893–13898.) Regarding eosinophil colony formation, Meir Shalit has shown that the development of eosinophil colonies using purified CD34 cells and IL-5 is not affected by steroids (M Shalit, S Sekhsari, HL Malech. Modulation of growth and differentiation of eosinophils from human peripheral blood CD34+ cells by IL5 and other growth factors. J Allergy Clin Immunol 1994; 93:268). In your system, where steroids do work, have you used purified progenitors or are there accessory cells which generate cytokines that are necessary for colony formation and whose actions are inhibited by steroids?

Dr. Denburg: Not in the CFU assays. However, in the HL-60 assay system, these are all myeloid progenitors. Even in a so-called purified progenitor system, it may be difficult to distinguish between direct and indirect effects.

Dr. Gauldie: Are there any data implicating a specific chemotaxis factor(s) that brings in precursor cells to the lung or does the final differentiation have to occur before the mature cell migrated to the tissue?

Dr. Denburg: CD34 is a potential adhesion molecule that may mediate tissue migration of progenitors; it is also found on endothelial cells. Other adhesion molecules potentially involved in progenitor migration may include L-selectin. In the dog model presented, we have attempted to use retroviral markers or thymidine-analogue (BRDU) labeling to follow the traffic and fate of bone marrow–derived progenitors. Our preliminary findings suggest that the progenitor cells move from marrow to blood and possibly into the lung (in the BAL fluid). These data require confirmation.

Dr. Brattsand: with 10 nM concentration, it remains to be studied for how long that concentration is needed in plasma for modulating progenitors and stem cells.

Dr. Pedersen: When was the last dose of budesonide given prior to the level measurement?

Dr. Denburg: One hour prior to allergen challenge.

Dr. Barnes: Could you be more explicit about the involvement of basophils in asthma? Are there any specific markers that can be used?

Dr. Denburg: Basophils have been shown to be important contributors to the late-phase allergic response in the skin, nose, and lung. Basophils are seen in these reactions, and their mediators are increased. Both basophils and eosinophils can be shown to increase in vivo in the blood and tissues in tandem; there are even congenital anomalies of basophil and eosinophil granules or common absence. Last, the basophils and eosinophils derive from a common hemopoietic progenitor.

Dr. Rocklin: Have you studied whether steroids affect the expression of cytokine receptors on myeloid progenitor cells or the response of progenitor cells to cytokines?

Dr. Denburg: Not yet. Using purified CD34/45–positive cells, we may be able to answer that question.

Dr. Gleich: I should comment on the problem of basophil granule proteins. To investigate basophil granule proteins, one needs very large numbers of basophils and thus basophil granules. We have been able to obtain about 5×10^{11} basophils from a patient with basophil leukemia, have purified the granules, lysed the granules, and begun analyses of granule proteins. In conjunction with C. Wilde of Incyte Corp., we have found that the basophil granule contains a very large number of proteins, including several potent proteases. Many of the sequences found are novel. These granule proteins need to be purified in large quantity to generate reagents useful for basophil localization. Once such reagents are available, perhaps basophil localization will be simple.

Dr. Liu: With regard to the role of basophils in asthma, MacGlashan and Lichtenstein have shown that basophils make and release IL-4 and probably IL-13. On a per cell basis, the production of IL-4 by basophils may be equal to or greater than that of the lymphocyte. (D MacGlashan, JM White, S-K Huang, et al. Secretion of IL-4 from human basophils. J Immunol 1994; 152:3006.)

Dr. Schleimer: In fact, I believe that basophils make considerably more IL-4 per cell than do lymphocytes. In addition, a Japanese group recently did a careful study of basophils in BAL in asthma and found significant numbers of cells that had the characteristics of basophils (T Koshino, TS Teshima, N Fukushima, et al. Identification of basophils by immunohistochemistry in the airways of post-mortem cases of fatal asthma. Clin Exp Allergy 1993; 23:919–925).

References

1. Schleimer RP. The effects of anti-inflammatory steroids on mast cells. In: Kaliner MA, Metcalfe DD, eds. The Mast Cell in Health and Disease. New York: Dekker 1993:483-511.
2. Schleimer RP. The effects of glucocorticoids on mast cells and basophils. In: Schleimer RP, Claman HN, Oronsky A, eds. Anti-inflammatory Steroid Action: Basic and Clinical Aspects. San Diego: Academic Press, 1989:226-258.
3. Denburg JA. Basophil and mast cell lineages in vitro and in vivo. Blood 1992; 79:846-860.
4. Denburg JA. Differentiation of human basophils and mast cells. In: Marone G, ed. Human Basophils and Mast Cells: Biological Aspects. Basel: Karger, 1995:49-71.
5. Mitsui H, Furitsu T, Dvorak AM, et al. Development of human mast cells from umbilical cord blood cells by recombinant human and murine c-kit ligand. Proc Natl Acad Sci USA 1993; 90:735-739.
6. Irani AM, Nilsson G, Miettinen U, et al. Recombinant human stem cell factor stimulates differentiation of mast cells from dispersed human fetal liver cells. Blood 1992; 80:3009-3021.
7. Valent P, Spanblochl E, Sperr WR, et al. Induction of differentiation of human mast cells from bone marrow and peripheral blood mononuclear cells by recombinant human stem cell factor/kit-ligand in long-term culture. Blood 1992; 80:2237-2245.
8. Zsebo KM, Williams DA, Geissler EN, et al. Stem cell factor is encoded at the S1 locus of the mouse and is the ligand for the c-kit tyrosine kinase receptor. Cell 1990; 63:213-224.
9. Tsai M, Shih L-S, Newlands GFJ, et al. The rat c-kit ligand, stem cell factor, induces the development of connective tissue-type and mucosal mast cells in vivo. Analysis by anatomical distribution, histochemistry, and protease phenotype. J Exp Med 1991; 174:125-131.
10. Galli SJ, Iemura A, Garlick DS, Gamba-Vitalo C, Zsebo KM, Andrews RG. Reversible expansion of primate mast cell populations in vivo by stem cell factor. J Clin Invest 1993; 91:148-152.
11. Iemura A, Tsai M, Ando A, Wershil BK, Galli SJ. The c-kit ligand, stem cell factor, promotes mast cell survival by suppressing apoptosis. Am J Pathol 1994; 144:321-328.
12. Denburg JA, Silver JE, Abrams JS. Interleukin-5 is a human basophilopoietin: Induction of histamine content and basophilic differentiation of HL-60 cells and of peripheral blood basophil-eosinophil progenitors. Blood 1991; 77:1462-1468.

13. Leary AG, Ogawa M. Identification of pure and mixed basophil colonies in culture of human peripheral blood and marrow cells. Blood 1984; 64:78-83.
14. Mayer P, Valent P, Schmidt G, Liehl E, Bettelheim P. The in vivo effects of recombinant human interleukin-3: demonstration of basophil differentiation factor, histamine producing activity, and priming of GM-CSF responsive progenitors in nonhuman primates. Blood 1989; 74:613–621.
15. Valent P, Schmidt G, Besemer J, et al. Interleukin-3 is a differentiation factor for human basophils. Blood 1989; 73:1763–1769.
16. Valent P, Besemer J, Sillaber C, et al. Failure to detect IL-3 binding sites on human mast cells. J Immunol 1990; 145:3432–3437.
17. Valent P, Besemer J, Muhm M, Lechner K, Bettelheim P. Interleukin-3 activates human blood basophils via high affinity binding sites. Proc Natl Acad Sci USA 1989; 86:5542–5546.
18. Tchekneva E, Serafin WE. Kirsten sarcoma virus-immortalized mast cell lines. Reversible inhibition of growth by dexamethasone and evidence for the presence of an autocrine growth factor. J Immunol 1994; 152:5912–5921.
19. Saunders PR, Marshall JS. Dexamethasone induces a down regulation of rat mast cell protease II content in rat basophilic leukaemia cells. Agents Actions 1992; 36:4–10.
20. Linden M, Brattsand R. Effects of a corticosteroid, budesonide, on alveolar macrophage and blood monocyte secretions of cytokines: differential sensitivity of GM-CSF, IL-1 beta, and IL-6. Pulm Pharmacol 1994; 7:43–47.
21. Linden M, Svensson C, Andersson M, et al. Increased numbers of circulating leucocyte progenitors in patients with allergic rhinitis during natural allergen exposure (abstr). Annual Meeting of the American Thoracic Society, Boston, May 22–25, 1994.
22. Denburg JA, Woolley M, Leber B, Linden M, O'Byrne P. Basophil and eosinophil differentiation in allergic reactions. J Allergy Clin Immunol 1994; 94:1135–1141.
23. Hutt-Taylor SR, Harnish D, Richardson M, Ishizaka T, Denburg JA. Sodium butyrate and a T lymphocyte cell line-derived differentiation factor induce basophilic differentiation of the human promyelocytic leukemia cell line HL-60. Blood 1988; 71:209–215.
24. Tsuda T, Wong D, Dolovich J, Bienenstock J, Marshall J, Denburg JA. Synergistic effects of nerve growth factor and granulocyte-macrophage colony-stimulating factor on human basophilic cell differentiation. Blood 1991; 77:971–979.
25. Tsuda T, Switzer J, Bienenstock J, Denburg JA. Interactions of hemopoietic cytokines on differentiation of HL-60 cells. Nerve growth factor is a basophilic lineage-specific co-factor. Int Arch Allergy Appl Immunol 1990; 91:15–21.
26. Denburg J, Dolovich J, Kanai N, et al. Microenvironmental control of inflammatory cell differentiation. Int Arch Allergy Appl Immunol 1992; 99:330–332.
27. Denburg JA, Gauldie J, Dolovich J, Ohtoshi T, Cox G, Jordana M. Structural cell-derived cytokines in allergic inflammation. Int Arch Allergy Appl Immunol 1991; 94:127–132.
28. Pitton C, Michel L, Salem P, et al. Biochemical and morphological modifications

in dexamethasone-treated mouse bone marrow-derived mast cells. J Immunol 1988; 141:2437–2444.

29. Butterfield JH, Weiler D, Dewald G, Gleich GJ. Establishment of an immature mast cell line from a patient with mast cell leukemia. Leukoc Res 1988; 12:345–355.

30. Lansdorp PM, Sutherland HJ, Eaves CJ. Selective expression of CD45 isoforms on functional subpopulations of CD34+ hemopoietic cells from human bone marrow. J Exp Med 1990; 172:363–366.

31. Broudy VC, Lin N, Zsebo KM, et al. Isolation and characterization of a monoclonal antibody that recognizes the human c-kit receptor. Blood 1992; 79:338–346.

32. Briddell RA, Broudy VC, Bruno E, Brandt JE, Srour EF, Hoffman R. Further phenotypic characterization and isolation of human hematopoietic progenitor cells using a monoclonal antibody to the *c-kit* receptor. Blood 1992; 79:3159–3167.

33. Lerner NB, Nocka KH, Cole SR, et al. Monoclonal antibody YB5.B8 identifies the human c-kit protein product. Blood 1991; 77:1876–1883.

34. Schleimer RP, Derse CP, Friedman B, et al. Regulation of human basophil mediator release by cytokines. I. Interaction with antiinflammatory steroids. J Immunol 1989; 143:1310–1317.

35. Cohen VL, Undem BJ, Fox CC, Adkinson NF, Jr., Lichtenstein LM, Schleimer RP. Dexamethasone does not inhibit the release of mediators from human mast cells residing in airway, intestine or skin. Am Rev Respir Dis 1989; 140:951–954.

36. Collado-Escobar D, Cunha-Melo JR, Beavan MA. Treatment with dexamethasone down-regulates IgE-receptor-mediated signals and up-regulates adenosine-receptor--mediated signals in a rat mast cell (RBL-2H3) line. J Immunol 1990; 144:244–250.

37. White MV, Igarashi Y, Lungren JD, Shelhamer J, Kaliner M. Hydrocortisone inhibits rat basophilic leukemia cell mediator release induced by neutrophil-derived histamine releasing activity as well as by anti-IgE. J Immunol 1991; 147:667–673.

38. Collado-Escobar D, Ali H, Beaven MA. On the mechanism of action of dexamethasone in a rat mast cell line (RBL-2H3 cells). Evidence for altered coupling of receptors and G-proteins. J Immunol 1990; 144:3449–3457.

39. Hide M, Ali H, Price SR, Moss J, Beaven MA. GTP -binding protein G alpha Z: its down-regulation by dexamethasone and its credentials as a mediator of antigen-induced responses in RBL-2H3 cells. Mol Pharmacol 1991; 40:473–479.

40. King SJ, Miller HR, Newlands GF, Woodbury RG. Depletion of mucosal mast cell protease by corticosteroids: effect on intestinal anaphylaxis in the rat. Proc Natl Acad Sci USA 1985; 82:1214–1218.

41. Huntley JF, Mackellar A, Miller HR. Altered expression of mast cell proteases in the rat. Quantitative and immunohistochemical analysis of the distribution of rat mast cell proteases I and II during helminth infection. APMIS 1991; 101:953–962.

42. Gordon JR, Galli SJ. Mast cells as a source of both preformed and immunologically inducible TNF-alpha/cachectin. Nature 1990; 346:274–276.

43. Gordon JR, Galli SJ. Release of both preformed and newly synthesized tumor necrosis factor alpha (TNF-alpha)/cachectin by mouse mast cells stimulated via the Fc epsilon RI. A mechanism for the sustained action of mast cell-derived TNF-alpha during IgE-dependent biological responses. J Exp Med 1991; 174:103–107.

44. Wershil BK, Wang ZS, Gordon JR, Gali SJ. Recruitment of neutrophils during IgE-dependent cutaneous late phase reactions in the mouse is mast cell-dependent. Partial inhibition of the reaction with antiserum against tumor necrosis factor-alpha. J Clin Invest 1991; 87:446–453.

45. Galli SJ, Gordon JR, Wershil BK. Mast cell cytokines in allergy and inflammation. Agents Actions 1993; 43(Suppl.):209–220.

46. Baroody FM, Cruz AA, Lichtenstein LM, Kagey-Sobotka A, Proud D, Naclerio RM. Intranasal beclomethasone inhibits antigen-induced nasal hyperresponsiveness to histamine. J Allergy Clin Immunol 1992; 90;373–376.

47. Bradding P, Feather IH, Howarth PH, et al. Interleukin 4 is localized to and released by human mast cells. J Exp Med 1992; 176:1381–1386.

48. Bradding P, Feather IH, Wilson S, et al. Immunolocalization of cytokines in the nasal mucosa of normal and perennial rhinitis subjects. The mast cell as a source of IL-4, IL-5, and IL-6 in human allergic mucosal inflammation. J Immunol 1993; 151:3853–3865.

49. Seder RA, Plaut M, Barbieri S, Urban J, Jr., Finkelman FD, Paul WE. Purified Fc epsilon R+ bone marrow and splenic non-B, non-T cells are highly enriched in the capacity to produce IL-4 in response to immobilized IgE, IgG2a, or ionomycin. J Immunol 1991; 147:903–909.

50. MacGlashan D, Jr., White JM, Huang SK, Ono SJ, Schroeder JT, Lichtenstein LM. Secretion of IL-4 from human basophils. The relationship between IL-4 mRNA and protein in resting and stimulated basophils. J Immunol 1994; 152:3006–3016.

51. Ohtoshi T, Xaubet A, Andersson B, et al. Nasal inflammation mediated by human structural cell-derived GM-CSF: effect of budesonide (abstr.). J Allergy Clin Immunol 1990; 85:297.

52. Jordana M, Dolovich J, Ohno I, Finotto S, Denburg J. Nasal polyposis: a model for chronic inflammation. In: Busse WW, Holgate ST, eds. Asthma and Rhinitis. Boston: Blackwell, 1995:156–164.

53. Cox G, Ohtoshi T, Vancheri C, et al. Promotion of eosinophil survival by human bronchial epithelial cells and its modulation by steroids. Am J Respir Cell Mol Biol 1991; 4:525–531.

54. MacGlashan D, Jr. Signal mechanisms in the activation of basophils and mast cells. Immunology Series 1992; 57:273–299.

55. Warner JA, MacGlashan DW, Jr. Signal transduction events in human basophils. A comparative study of the role of protein kinase C in basophils activated by anti-IgE antibody and formyl-methionyl-leucyl-phenylalanine. J Immunol 1990; 145:1897–1905.

56. Sheth KK, Lemanske RF, Jr. The early and late asthmatic response to allergen. In: Busse WW, Holgate ST, eds. Asthma and Rhinitis. Boston: Blackwell, 1995: 946–960.

57. Pipkorn U, Hammarlund A, Enerback L. Prolonged treatment with topical gluco-corticoids results in an inhibition of the allergen-induced weal-and-flare response and a reduction in skin mast cell numbers and histamine content. Clin Exp Allergy 1989; 19:19–25.

58. Lawlor F, Black AK, Murdoch RD, Greaves MW. Symptomatic dermographism: wealing, mast cells and histamine are decreased in the skin following long-term application of a potent topical corticosteroid. Br J Dermatol 1989; 121:629–634.

59. Sheth KK, Sorkness RL, Clough JJ, McAllister PK, Castleman WL, Lemanske RFJ. Reversal of persistent post bronchiolitis airway abnormalities with dexamethasone in rats. J Appl Physiol 1994; 76:333–338.

60. Soda K, Kawabori S, Perdue MH, Bienenstock J. Macrophage engulfment of mucosal mast cells in rats treated with dexamethasone. Gastroenterology 1991; 100:929–937.

61. Otsuka H, Denburg JA, Befus AD, et al. Effect of beclomethasone dipropionate on nasal metachromatic cell subpopulations. Clin Allergy 1986; 16:589–595.

62. Kawabori S, Denburg JA, Schwartz LB, et al. Histochemical and immunohistochemical characteristics of mast cells in nasal polyps. Am J Respir Cell Mol Biol 1992; 6:37–43.

63. Duddridge M, Ward C, Hendrick DJ, Walters EH. Changes in bronchoalveolar lavage inflammatory cells in asthmatic patients treated with high dose inhaled beclomethasone dipropionate. Eur Respir J 1993; 6:489–497.

64. Juliusson S, Holmberg K, Karlsson G, Enerback L, Pipkorn U. Mast cells and mediators in the nasal mucosa after allergen challenge. Effects of four weeks' treatment with topical glucocorticoid. Clin Exp Allergy 1993; 23:591–599.

65. Kanai N, Denburg JA, Evans S, Conway M, Jordana M, Dolovich J. Nasal polyp inflammation: effect of topical nasal steroid. Am Rev Respir Dis 1994; 150:1094–1100.

66. Rak S, Jacobson MR, Sudderick RM, et al. Influence of prolonged treatment with topical corticosteroid (fluticasone propionate) on early and late phase nasal responses and cellular infiltration in the nasal mucosa after allergen challenge. Clin Exp Allergy 1994; 24:930–939.

67. Nakagawa N, Howie K, Switzer J, Marshall JS, Denburg JA. Human nasal polyp fibroblasts produce stem cell factor (SCF) (abstr.). J Allergy Clin Immunol 1995; 95:292.

68. Denburg JA. Microenvironmental influences on inflammatory cell differentiation. Allergy 1995; 50(Suppl 25):25–28.

69. Wershil BK, Furuta GT, Lavigne JA, Roy Choudhury A, Wang Z-S, Galli SJ. Dexamethasone or cyclosporin A suppress mast cell-leukocyte cytokine cascades. Multiple mechanisms of inhibition of IgE- and mast cell-dependent cutaneous inflammation in the mouse. J Immunol 1995; 154:1391–1398.

70. Soda K, Kawabori S, Kanai N, Bienenstock J, Perdue MH. Steroid-induced depletion of mucosal mast cells and eosinophils in intestine of athymic nude rats. Int Arch Allergy Appl Immunol 1993; 101:39–46.

71. Gibson PG, Wong BJ, Hepperle MF, et al. A research method to induce and examine a mild exacerbation of asthma by withdrawal of inhaled corticosteroid. Clin Exp Allergy 1992; 22:525–532.

72. Gibson PG, Dolovich J, Girgis-Gabardo A, et al. The inflammatory response in asthma exacerbation: changes in circulating eosinophils, basophils and their progenitors. Clin Exp Allergy 1990; 20:661–668.

73. Pin I, Freitag AP, O'Byrne PM, et al. Changes in the cellular profile of induced sputum after allergen-induced asthmatic responses. Am Rev Respir Dis 1992; 145:1265–1269.
74. Gibson PG, Manning PJ, O'Byrne PM, et al. Allergen-induced asthmatic responses: relationship between increases in airway responsiveness and increases in circulating eosinophils, basophils, and their progenitors. Am Rev Respir Dis 1991; 143:331–335.
75. Choudry NB, Watson R, Denburg J, O'Byrne PM. Time course of circulating inflammatory cells and their progenitors after allergen inhalation in asthmatics subjects (abstr.). Am Rev Respir Dis 1992; 145:A35.
76. Hargreave FE, Gibson PG, Ramsdale EH, Dolovich J, Denburg J. Evaluation of asthma and airway hyperresponsiveness by cytology of bronchoalveolar lavage or sputum. In: Pichler WJ, Stadler BM, Dahinden C, et al., Progress in Allergy and Clinical Immunology. Toronto: Hogrefe & Huber, 1989:179–182.
77. Pin I, Gibson PG, Kolendowicz R, et al. Use of induced sputum cell counts to investigate airway inflammation in asthma. Thorax 1992; 47:25–29.
78. Woolley MJ, Wattie J, Ellis R, et al. Effect of an inhaled corticosteroid on airway eosinophils and allergen-induced airway hyperresponsiveness in dogs. J Appl Physiol 1994; 77:1303–1308.
79. Woolley MH, Denburg JA, Ellis R, Dahlback M, O'Byrne PM. Allergen-induced changes in bone marrow progenitors and airway responsiveness in dogs and the effect of inhaled budesonide on these parameters. Am J Respir Cell Mol Biol 1994; 11:600–606.
80. Inman MD, Ellis R, Wattie J, et al. Stimulation of canine bone marrow granulocyte progenitor growth by a serum factor present at 24 hours after allergen inhalation (abstr.). J Allergy Clin Immunol 1995; 95:376.
81. Gauvreau GM, Watson RM, Doctor J, Denburg JA, O'Byrne PM. Inhaled budesonide, but not salbutamol, reduces allergen-induced increases in circulating eosinophils and their progenitors (abstr.). J Allergy Clin Immunol 1995; 95:299.
82. Sehmi R, Howie K, Denburg JA. Elevated levels of CD34+ hemopoietic progenitor cells in atopic subjects (abstr.). J Allergy Clin Immunol 1995; 95:382.
83. Bjornson BH, Harvey JM, Rose L. Differential effect of hydrocortisone on eosinophil and neutrophil proliferation. J Clin Invest 1985; 76:924–929.
84. Shalit M, Sekhsaria S, Malech HL. Modulation of growth and differentiation of eosinophils from human peripheral blood CD34+ cells by IL5 and other growth factors (abstr). J Allergy Clin Immunol 1994, 93:268.
85. Nilsson G, Blom T, Kusche-Gullberg M, Kjellen L, Butterfield JH, Sundstrom C, Nilsson K, Hellman L. Phenotypic characterization of the human mast-cell line HMC-1. Scand J Immunol 1994; 39:489–498.
86. Wasserman SI, Marquardt DL. Anaphylaxis. In: Middleton E, Jr, Reed CE, Ellis EF, Adkinson NF, Jr., Yunginger JW, eds. Principles and Practice. 3rd ed. St Louis: Mosby, 1988:1365–1376.
87. Rosenthal S, Schwartz JH, Canellos GP. Basophilic chronic granulocytic leukemia with hyperhistaminaemia. Br J Haematol 1977; 36:367–372.

88. Denburg JA, Rosenthal DM. Mast cell disease. In: Brain M, Carbone P, eds. Current Therapy in Hematology-Oncology. 5th ed. St. Louis: Mosby-Year Book, 1994:120–124.
89. Guzzo C, Lavker R, Roberts LJ, Fox K, Schechter N, Lazarus G. Urticaria pigmentosa. Systemic evaluation and successful treatment with topical steroids. Arch Dermatol 1991; 127:191–196.

13

Glucocorticoid Effects on Human Eosinophils

GERALD J. GLEICH and
LOREN W. HUNT

Mayo Clinic and Mayo Foundation
Rochester, Minnesota

BRUCE S. BOCHNER and
ROBERT P. SCHLEIMER

The Johns Hopkins Asthma and Allergy Center
The Johns Hopkins University School of
    Medicine
Baltimore, Maryland

I. Introduction

This chapter provides an overview of the present literature on the influence of glucocorticoids on human eosinophils. Eosinophilic leukocytes are thought to be critically involved in both chronic allergic diseases and in experimental allergic reactions (1,2). Eosinophils are now suspected of being responsible for many of the pathological features of asthma; toxic eosinophilic granule proteins, such as major basic protein (MBP) and eosinophil-derived leukotrienes, have been implicated in airways reactivity, vascular leak syndromes, destruction and sloughing of epithelium, and other inflammatory changes which are pathognomonic of asthma (3,4). Clearly, eosinophils contain the glucocorticoid receptor and are important targets of glucocorticoid action (5,6). In the following discussion, we emphasize the effects of glucocorticoids on the production, function, and survival of human eosinophils. In vitro studies are considered first, then in vivo findings; where appropriate, studies in animals are also discussed. We also discuss a potential glucocorticomimetic agent.

II. In Vitro Studies

A. Effects of Glucocorticoids on Generation of Eosinophils in Vitro

Numerous studies have established that the formation of eosinophil-rich colonies in bone marrow colony assays is inhibited by the presence of glucocorticoids in the culture system (7–9). Interpretation of the reported findings is difficult owing to the intrinsic nature of colony-forming assays which often involve several cell types in addition to the relevant progenitor cells. Bjornson et al. (7) showed that glucocorticoids reduced the numbers of eosinophilic colonies generated from bone marrow or peripheral blood when a conditioned medium derived from activated peripheral blood mononuclear cells was used as the source of the growth factor. If glucocorticoids were added during preparation of the conditioned medium, a large decrease in colony-stimulating activity was also observed (7). Slovick et al. (8) likewise demonstrated that glucocorticoids inhibit eosinophil colony formation induced by exogenously added growth factors. Interestingly, when the growth factors were derived from either activated peripheral blood mononuclear cells or the MO cell line, the inhibitory effect was much less than when supernatants from a macrophage-like cell line (GCT) were used, possibly because the former contain more "eosinophil colony-stimulating factor" (EO-CSF) [perhaps now known as interleukin-5 (IL-5) or granulocyte-macrophage colony-stimulating factor (GM-CSF)] than the latter. These investigators also showed that glucocorticoids inhibit EO-CSF production by monocytes and that glucocorticoids had no effect on colony formation when purified progenitors were used (at that time, mononuclear-depleted and T-cell–depleted bone marrow). Slovick et al. concluded that glucocorticoids inhibit eosinophil colony formation indirectly by diminishing the release of cytokines (IL-1, IL-2) by cells in the colony assay (8). Recent studies by Shalit et al. have shown that the formation of eosinophil colonies by stimulation of purified $CD34^+$ primitive hematopoietic progenitor cells with purified cytokines (IL-5, IL-3, GM-CSF) is not inhibited by glucocorticoids, supporting the concept that glucocorticoid effects on eosinophil colony formation result from an inhibition of the release of factors that induce eosinophil colony growth (10). The most direct hypothesis to explain the above-described results is that glucocorticoid inhibition of the production of IL-5 and other eosinophilopoietic factors by bone marrow cells is responsible for the suppression of colony growth (11–14).

B. Adhesion

Leukocyte adhesion can be induced by stimulation of leukocytes, stimulation of endothelium, or both (15–18). Both processes appear to be involved in vivo in allergic reactions. In vitro, endothelial expression of adhesion molecules can be activated by the cytokines IL-1 and tumor necrosis factor (TNF). These cytokines induce expression of intercellular adhesion molecule 1 (ICAM-1), E-selectin, and vascular cell adhesion molecule 1 (VCAM-1), all of which can bind to their respective counterligands on the surfaces of leukocytes, including eosinophils (18,19). IL-4 and IL-13 can induce endothelial cells to express VCAM-1 and not the other adhesion molecules (20–22). VCAM-1 binds to very late antigen (VLA)-4 on the surface of eosinophils and causes adhesion (21–26). Because VLA-4 is not found on the surface of neutrophils, it has been proposed that IL-4 (or IL-13) activation of VCAM-1 expression may be one mechanism by which selective recruitment of eosinophils occurs. Several investigators (22,27–30; and Dr. C. Dunn, Upjohn; Dr. J. White, SmithKline Beecham; and Dr. J. Pober, Yale University, personal communications, 1995) have now shown that glucocorticoid treatment of endothelial cells prior to stimulation with these cytokines does not inhibit the expression or function of these adhesion molecules. Glucocorticoids also failed to inhibit neutrophil or basophil adhesion to endothelial cells stimulated by either endothelial activators or leukocyte activators (27,28). In contrast, Cronstein et al. reported that glucocorticoids inhibit endothelial E-selectin expression (31). The reason for the disparity of results between Cronstein and many others is unknown. A recent study showed that glucocorticoids did not inhibit eosinophil adhesion to endothelial cells induced by IL-4 or other endothelial activators or by leukocyte activators, including platelet-activating factor (PAF) and formyl-methionyl-leucyl-phenylalanine (FMLP) (29).

Eosinophils cultured with GM-CSF or other cytokines show strikingly increased adhesion, transendothelial migration, and expression of the adhesion molecule CD11b in response to chemoattractants like PAF or FMLP (32–36). Glucocorticoids did not inhibit the increase in adhesion molecule expression or changes in intracytoplasmic calcium which followed activation with chemoattractants (35). Glucocorticoids are known to be potent inhibitors of the release of factors that activate both endothelium, including IL-1, TNF-α, IL-4 (and likely IL-13), and leukocytes, including chemokines (Table 1). On the other hand, glucocorticoids inhibit cytokine-induced expression of ICAM-1 on eosinophils (53); in these experiments, GM-CSF, IL-3, and IL-5 stimulated eosinophil ICAM-1 expression, and dexamethasone, 10^{-9} to 10^{-7} M, inhibited this response in a dose-related manner. Thus, although glucocorticoids do not appear directly to inhibit activation of eosinophils or endothelial cells by these cytokines, with exception of ICAM-1 expression, it is likely that they indirectly inhibit the activation of eosinophils and endothelial cells by depressing the generation of these cytokines.

Recently, at the 5th International Conference on Human Leukocyte Differentiation Antigens, where CD designations are assigned, approximately 475

Table 1   The Effect of Glucocorticoids on the Production of Cytokines Relevant to
Eosinophil Recruitment and Activation

Cytokine	Relevant action	Effect of glucocorticoids on synthesis	Reference
Endothelial activators			
IL-1, TNF-α	Induce E-selectin, VCAM-1 and ICAM-1, induce chemokine release	Inhibition	37–41
IL-4	Induces VCAM-1 expression	Inhibition	42–45
IL-13	Induces VCAM-1 expression	Unknown	
Eosinophil activators			
IL-3, IL-5, GM-CSF	Prime eosinophil responses, prolong eosinophil survival	Inhibition	14, 42, 44 46–50
RANTES, MIP-1α	Eosinophil chemoattractant	Inhibition	51, 52
MCP-2, MCP-3 Eotaxin	Eosinophil chemoattractant	Unknown	
LCF	Eosinophil chemoattractant	Unknown	

monoclonal antibodies were tested for reactivity towards purified human eosinophils (54). Of these, 350 were negative. Thirty-five pools, each containing 10 negative antibodies, were analyzed for increased staining in eosinophils cultured overnight in the presence of either medium alone or the potent glucocorticoid budesonide. Budesonide failed to induce expression of negative markers detectable with the pooled antibodies (C. Bickel, B. Bochner, and R. Schleimer, unpublished observations).

C. Chemotaxis

Glucocorticoid treatment in vivo (24 hr) has been shown by Clark et al. to inhibit subsequent in vitro migration of these eosinophils (55). In contrast, Altman et al. found no effect on eosinophil chemotaxis 4 hr after glucocorticoid treatment (56). Because glucocorticoids may lead to alterations in subsets of eosinophils in vivo, as seen with lymphocytes and basophils, it is difficult to interpret the results of these studies. As in the case of human neutrophils, in vitro studies indicate that eosinophils are resistant to the effects of glucocorticoids on chemotaxis. Kurihara et al. reported that incubation of purified human eosinophils with glucocorticoid for up to 6 hr had no effect on migration of eosinophils in response to PAF in vitro (57). Prin et al. claimed that glucocorticoids induce a modest inhibition of chemotaxis, but the concentration of dexamethasone used was high (4×10^{-6} M) (5). Although glucocorticoids may not inhibit the chemotactic cellular response itself (i.e., either actual cell motility or the expression of adhesion molecules on either eosinophils or endothelium), they are powerful and specific inhibitors of the release of most members of the families of inflammatory mediators that induce both chemotaxis and adhesion (e.g. PAF [58]; leukotriene B_4 [LTB$_4$] [59]; peptides, including members of the chemokine family [60], especially RANTES [51]; MCP-3 and eotaxin; chemotactic hematopoietic cytokines, such as IL-5 [14]; and others). No information is yet available on the effects of glucocorticoids on the release of MCP-3 or eotaxin; in all of the other cases mentioned above, glucocorticoids are potent and effective inhibitors of their release. Thus, one can speculate that in vivo treatment with glucocorticoids inhibits eosinophil migration indirectly by decreasing or completely preventing the production of chemoattractants for eosinophils. Howe et al. have shown that glucocorticoids inhibit the release of a uterus-derived eosinophil chemotactic factor suspected to be involved in eosinophil infiltration during estrus (61). Another example, more relevant to allergic diseases of the airways, is the effect of glucocorticoids on the release and production of the chemokine RANTES from epithelial cells. Recent immunohistochemical studies have identified epithelium as a primary source of this eosinophilic chemotactic chemokine (62). Studies in nasal polyps, nasal biopsies, and human central airways have all shown epithelial cell production of RANTES. In vitro studies have established that glucocorticoids inhibit the epithelial production of RANTES dramatically (51). Thus, on the one hand, epithelium may be the source of chemoattractants which ultimately lead to the migration of eosinophils and destruction of airway epithelium. On the other hand, epithelium, which is an immediate target of topically applied glucocorticoids in either the nose or lung, appears to be extremely susceptible to the profound suppressive effects of steroids on the release of the RANTES chemoattractant.

D. MHC Class II Expression

Although blood eosinophils from normal persons do not express major histocompatibility complex (MHC) class II antigens, the expression of this marker can be induced in vitro by stimulation with cytokines (63,64). These class II–positive eosinophils can present antigen to and activate T lymphocytes (63–65). Surprisingly, glucocorticoids and IL-5 were synergistic in stimulating eosinophils to express the MHC class II antigens HLA-DR and HLA-DP (53). Furthermore, steroids enhanced GM-CSF–induced and IL-3–induced but not γ-interferon (IFN-γ)–induced expression of these class II antigens. Analyses of the effects of glucocorticoids on antigen presentation showed that dexamethasone, 10^{-8} M, caused an enhancement of antigen presentation. Thus, glucocorticoids enhance both cytokine-induced class II antigen expression on eosinophils and antigen presentation to T cells by eosinophils.

E. Degranulation

The effects of glucocorticoids on degranulation vary among different cell types (e.g., glucocorticoids inhibit degranulation of human basophils, rat mast cells, and rat basophilic leukemia [RBL] cells but not human mast cells) (66,67). Although a study by Hallam et al. showed an inhibitory effect of high concentrations of glucocorticoid on eosinophil antibody-dependent cellular cytotoxicity (68), a careful and detailed study by Kita et al. failed to find an effect of glucocorticoids on eosinophil degranulation (69). In the latter case, glucocorticoids did not inhibit immunoglobulin-induced degranulation of eosinophils which had been primed by cytokines. These findings are similar to studies in human neutrophils in which dexamethasone failed to inhibit degranulation or LTB_4 release (27).

F. Survival/Apoptosis

An intensively studied area in biology, in general, and in inflammatory cells, in particular, is programmed cell death; that is, apoptosis (70–72). In contrast to necrotic cell death, apoptosis is characterized by defined changes, such as condensation of chromatin and the nucleus, shrinkage of the cell, expression of as yet incompletely understood adhesion molecules on the cell surface that facilitate engulfment, and the orderly destruction of the apoptotic cell by phagocytic cells in vivo. Also associated with apoptosis is a destruction of cellular DNA by endonucleases which cleave in the internucleosomal regions forming a "laddering" of DNA. All types of circulating granulocytes appear to undergo programmed cell death, and, when cultured in the absence of enriched medium, they die rather quickly. In vitro, granulocytes are phagocytosed by macrophage-like cells through a process that appears to involve the vitronectin receptor on the phagocytic cells and unknown ligands on the apoptotic leukocyte (73–75). Engulfment of apoptotic neutrophils may also involve phosphatidylserine on the outer leaflet of the neutrophil plasma membrane as an important recognition ligand (76). When eosinophils are cultured with appropriate cytokines (IL-3, IL-5, or GM-CSF), their survival in vitro can be prolonged for days or weeks (77–79). If glucocorticoids are added to such cultures, the eosinophils will die despite the presence of survival-prolonging cytokines (80–84). This is a dynamic process, and when greater concentrations of cytokine are added to the culture, the inhibitory effects of glucocorticoids are overcome. Interestingly, one cytokine, which can prolong eosinophil survival, IFN-γ, is unable to overcome completely the inhibitory effect of glucocorticoids on eosinophil survival (82). The ability of glucocorticoids to prevent the survival-prolonging effects of cytokines is probably important in their usefulness in diseases accompanied by eosinophilia. Unfortunately, programmed cell death in eosinophils has made study of the effects of glucocorticoids on other functions difficult, because glucocorticoid effects usually require many hours. Because glucocorticoids begin to diminish the survival of these cells only after about 24 hr, it is important that the effects of glucocorticoids on survival be distinguished from any possible effects on function. Eosinophils express on their surface *fas* (APO-1, CD95), which is a molecule that can trigger programmed cell death in many cell types. Cross linking of *fas* with an antibody induces eosinophilic apoptosis (85). It is not known whether *fas* ligand–expressing cells can induce this process and what effect glucocorticoids may have. Recently, CD69 has also been shown to induce eosinophil apoptosis following cross linking (86).

The molecular mechanisms by which glucocorticoids accelerate eosinophil apoptosis and antagonize the survival-prolonging effect of cytokines are unknown. Recent studies on the effects of glucocorticoids on induction of the synthesis of inflammatory proteins, such as collagenase, have revealed that the glucocorticoid receptor complex can bind directly to the transcription factor AP-1, which is a heterodimer of members of the c-*jun* and c-*fos* oncogene families (87,88). By directly binding to AP-1, the glucocorticoid receptor complex prevents AP-1 from inducing the synthesis of collagenase and other inflammatory genes. Perhaps, therefore, the antagonism of the survival-prolonging effect of cytokines in eosinophils results from a similar interaction between the glucocorticoid receptor complex and a transcription factor. In addition to AP-1, several other transcription factors have been described for which there is evidence for either a direct or indirect interaction with the glucocorticoid receptor complex. A list of some of these transcription factors is found in Table 2. For eosinophils, the following may be of interest: CREB, the cyclic AMP response transducer; GATA-1, a member of a family of transcription factors, some of which induce genes in eosinophils; NF-AT, which is involved in T-cell activation; NF-κB, involved in many inflammatory responses; and NF IL-6, which has been shown to be involved in the induction of the transcription of acute phase proteins. Details of the molecular actions of the cytokines that prolong eosinophil survival must be obtained before the precise mechanism of the glucocorticoid effect can be determined. Of note, several groups have recently shown activation of tyrosine kinases in eosinophils stimulated by IL-5 and other survival-prolonging cytokines (103–106). Furthermore, it was recently reported that glucocorticoids block this response (107). The recent recognition that both cytokine generation and activation of tyrosine kinases accompany eosinophil stimulation implies that transcription factor pathways are likely to be induced in these cells and thus must be considered as potential targets of glucocorticoid action.

Table 2 DNA Binding Proteins Suspected to Interact with the Glucocorticoid-Receptor Complex

DNA binding protein	Possible functional relevance	Reference
AP-1	Cell growth, inflammatory gene activation	87–91
NF-κB	Immune and inflammatory responses	92
NF IL-6	Induces acute phase proteins	93, 94
OTF-1	Important in cell cycle	95
CREB	Mediates some cAMP responses	96
GATA-1	Involved in erythroid differentiation	97
NF-AT	Involved in T cell activation	98, 99
X Box protein	Control of MHC expression	100
OCT-2A	Lymphocyte-specific factor	101
OAP	Octomer-associated protein involved in IL-2 transcription important in lymphocyte activation	102

There are numerous sites at which glucocorticoids may modify eosinophil survival (Fig. 1). Besides their ability to reduce the synthesis by other cell types of survival-promoting cytokines, glucocorticoids must also work within the eosinophil to antagonize the action of these cytokines. This may occur either by antagonism of the cytokine-induced transcription factors or perhaps also by inhibition of autocrine production of the same cytokines. Alternatively, glucocorticoids may reduce levels of expression of the cytokine receptors themselves. The pathway by which survival-promoting cytokines prevent triggering of the programmed cell death pathway may also be disrupted by glucocorticoids. It is not yet known whether these are active or passive pathways. Cohen and Duke have distinguished between *induction* mechanisms, in which protein synthesis is required, and *release* mechanisms in which protein synthesis is necessary to maintain survival (70). Because HL-60 cells fall into the latter category, and can differentiate into eosinophils, it seems likely that eosinophils have a "release" mechanism (70). This is in contrast to certain lymphocytes and other cell types in which protein synthesis inhibitors often do not induce apoptosis. Interestingly, studies by Cox have shown that glucocorticoids actually prolong neutrophil survival in contradiction to their effects on eosinophils (108). Numerous intracellular molecules have been identified which may participate in programmed cell death. Although it has been suggested that eosinophil survival-promoting cytokines maintain hematopoietic cell growth by suppressing apoptosis (109), little is presently known regarding the molecular details in eosinophils. In T cells, a glucocorticoid receptor–like molecule, Nur77, is essential in triggering the final common pathway of programmed cell death (110,111). In addition, a family of intracellular molecules, including

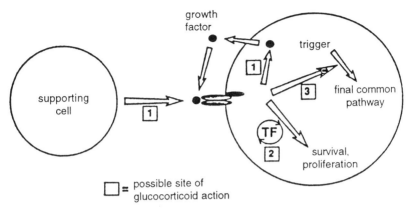

Figure 1 A model describing possible sites of glucocorticoid action on eosinophil survival. The model shows a supporting cell (left) and eosinophil (right); both are capable of producing growth factors that can maintain eosinophil survival. Possible sites of glucocorticoid action are indicated by boxes with numbers and are (1) inhibition of the production of eosinophil survival-promoting cytokines including GM-CSF, IL-3, and IL-5 by the supporting cell and direct inhibition of autocrine production of survival-promoting factors by the eosinophil itself; (2) prevention of the action of transcription factors whose activity is induced by the engagement of the hematopoietic cytokine receptor, thus preventing transcription factor (TF)-dependent processes which induce survival and proliferation in less mature cells; and (3) eosinophils may have an active process by which the trigger for the final common pathway of programmed cell death is suppressed. Glucocorticoids may prevent this active suppression of triggering of the final common pathway and thus facilitate entry into apoptosis. (From Schleimer RP, Bochner BS. The effects of glucocorticoids on human eosinophils. J Allergy Clin Immunol 1994; 94:1202–1213 with permission.)

Bcl-2, Bcl-xL, Bcl-xS, and Bax, are profound regulators in triggering this final pathway (112–115). Other intracellular molecules, such as IL-1–converting enzyme (72,116,117), p53 (118,119), S1, c-*myc* (120), and cyclins (121–123), probably participate in apoptosis in many cell types; at present, no information is available in the eosinophil.

III. In Vivo Studies

A. Effects of Glucocorticoids on Circulating Eosinophils

A single dose of a potent glucocorticoid causes a profound fall in circulating levels of eosinophils (124). This change in cell numbers occurs within a few hours, reaching a nadir at 4–8 hr, at which point usually less than 20% of the initial value remains. Prolonged administration of glucocorticoids is not always associated with eosinopenia, however; it is unclear how important the allergic disease process is in maintaining their presence in spite of ongoing glucocorticoid treatment. The mechanism for the fall in eosinophil numbers is not entirely known, but it is probably multifactorial. As discussed above, glucocorticoids inhibit the formation of the primary eosinophil colony-forming factors IL-5, IL-3, and GM-CSF both in vitro (14,46–49) and in vivo (42,50,125). Although IL-5 is probably the key factor, all of these cytokines can stimulate eosinophil growth in some instances. In rats, glucocorticoids have been shown to cause a sequestration of eosinophils in primary and secondary lymphoid tissues, including spleen and lymph nodes (126). The mechanism of this effect is unknown, but it may contribute to the rapid fall in circulating eosinophil numbers after glucocorticoid treatment. The ability of glucocorticoids to hasten programmed cell death in eosinophils may also explain the phenomenon. Studies in rats found glucocorticoid-induced engulfment of eosinophils in the gut (127); unfortunately, analogous human studies are lacking. The administration of glucocorticoids to patients with eosinophilia usually causes a marked reduction in circulating eosinophil numbers (128–131). This reduction is likely an important mechanism of the beneficial effect of glucocorticoids in hypereosinophilic diseases and is likely to occur by the same mechanisms described above.

B. Effects of Glucocorticoids on Recruitment of Eosinophils to Allergic Reaction Sites

Several studies have shown that glucocorticoid treatment decreases the number of eosinophils in the airways of patients with asthma undergoing bronchoscopy and biopsy (132–135). Glucocorticoids also reduce the presence of eosinophil proteins in bronchoalveolar lavage fluids (132). Most studies have examined glucocorticoid effects on antigen challenge reactions in which prior treatment with either oral or topical glucocorticoids also decreased the influx of eosinophils into the nose, the skin, and the lungs (136–139). For glucocorticoids administered orally, this probably results, in part, from reduced circulating levels of eosinophils. However, local recruitment mechanisms are certainly also quite sensitive because topical glucocorticoids are extremely effective (136). Although topical corticosteroid treatment at commonly used doses does not greatly diminish blood eosinophils, it does reduce the percentage of low-density eosinophils (140). Furthermore, local endobronchial challenge results in an increase in the levels of circulating eosinophils and eosinophil progenitors in humans (141), and glucocorticoids can block a similar response in dogs (142). One explanation for these findings is that lung cells release cytokines which activate the bone marrow and that glucocorticoids inhibit the local release of bone marrow–activating cytokines. It seems quite likely, therefore, that the ability of glucocorticoids to inhibit recruitment of eosinophils in vivo can result from both local effects on tissue cells at the challenge site as well as from systemic effects. Of interest are the findings of Kung et al., who showed that glucocorticoids inhibited eosinophil infiltration into BAL fluids of sensitized and challenged mice and concurrently inhibited eosinophil egress from the bone marrow (143); anti–IL-5 showed identical results. These findings suggest another glucocorticoid effect; that is, inhibition of eosinophil release from the bone marrow.

Although the roles of adhesion molecule expression in the inflammation of lung and other tissues have not been clearly established in humans, it is known that VCAM-1, E-selectin, and ICAM-1 can be increased following experimental antigen challenge (144–147) and, in perennial rhinitis, that VCAM-1 and ICAM-1 are chronically elevated (148). Studies in monkeys, sheep, guinea pigs, and mice have implicated the VLA-4/VCAM-1 pathway and ICAM-1 in eosinophil recruitment to the lungs (149–153). Although in vivo studies clearly demonstrate an inhibition by glucocorticoids of eosinophil and basophil recruitment, the precise mechanism and especially the role of adhesion molecules have not been completely delineated. Numerous adhesion molecules and their counterligands have been characterized, but others are as yet unknown. Furthermore, the in vitro models are often inadequate to assess the effects of inflammatory stimuli or anti-inflammatory drugs. Clearly, when viewed by intravital microscopy, the treatment of animals with glucocorticoids causes disruption of the leukocyte adhesion to local vasculature (154–158). In these reports, the leukocytes that are adherent subsequently have essentially normal transendothelial migration and chemotaxis within the tissue, suggesting that the primary target of the glucocorticoids was the inhibition of the initial adhesion response itself. Although glucocorticoids do not appear to inhibit endothelial adhesion molecule expression directly, they may do so indirectly in vivo, because they are potent and effective inhibitors of the secretion of cytokines which induce endothelial activation including IL-1, TNF, and IL-4 (37,159,160). Although this hypothesis has yet to be tested directly in experimental allergen challenge reactions, considerable data presently exists to support the concept. For example, the treatment of human lung tissue in vitro with glucocorticoids inhibits IL-1 release (37). Furthermore, in vivo studies found that the release of endothelium-activating cytokines, IL-1, TNF, and IL-4, is inhibited in the lungs by glucocorticoids (38,42–44,161,162). Individuals pretreated with prednisone for 3 days had dramatically diminished levels of soluble E-selectin in BAL fluids 20 hr after antigen challenge, providing circumstantial evidence for inhibition of endothelial activation (139,163). Glucocorticoids may also directly or indirectly inhibit the expression or function of adhesion molecules acting early to induce rolling such as P-selectin and its counterligands. Glucocorticoid treatment of patients with eosinophilic disorders reduces the level of the eosinophil-activating cytokines, IL-5 and GM-CSF, in parallel with a decline in circulating eosinophil numbers and disease activity (124,126). The cytokines thought to be of potential importance in recruitment of eosinophils during allergic inflammation and the effect of glucocorticoids on their production are listed in Table 1.

IV. Lidocaine as a Glucocorticomimetic Agent

The observation that eosinophils die in vitro by undergoing apoptosis and that eosinophil active growth factors permit eosinophil survival has led to the use of the eosinophil-survival assay as a means to detect eosinophil active cytokines (164). The eosinophil-survival assay, as a test for cytokines, is exquisitely sensitive and detects GM-CSF at concentrations as low as 1 pg/ml (165). Using this assay, it has been possible to measure eosinophil active cytokines in a variety of clinical situations (165–168), including allergen-induced pulmonary late-phase reactions (168) where evidence for both IL-5 and GM-CSF was found. In order to detect such activities in asthma, BAL fluids from hospitalized patients ill with severe asthma were tested (169). Among 40 BAL fluids analyzed, only 15 produced an enhancement of eosinophil survival above background; the remaining 25 caused a reduction is eosinophil survival. Although initially it was speculated that this decrease in eosinophil survival was due to glucocorticoids which were administered to all patients as part of their care, it was not possible to detect glucocorticoids in the BAL fluids using high-performance liquid chromatography. Because lidocaine is used for topical anesthesia of the airways and might be present in these BAL fluids, it was tested in the eosinophil-survival assay to determine if it could alter the effects of eosinophil active growth factors. Surprisingly, lidocaine was able to antagonize potently the effects of IL-5, IL-3, and GM-CSF at concentrations present in the BAL fluids. Lidocaine was not directly toxic for eosinophils, and its effect(s) on eosinophil survival mediated by IL-5, IL-3, and GM-CSF, like those of glucocorticoids, was overcome by increasing concentrations of the growth factors. Similarly, lidocaine antagonized the ability of IFN-γ to enhance eosinophil survival in vitro, but there the effect of lidocaine, again like those of glucocorticoids, could not be overcome by increasing concentrations of IFN-γ. Therefore, lidocaine appeared to be glucocorticomimetic, because it produced essentially the same results in the eosinophil survival assay as did glucocorticoids.

Because the eosinophil is believed to be a critical mediator cell in bronchial asthma (170–172), and because eosinophil active cytokines stimulate eosinophil-associated inflammation, the possibility that lidocaine might be a useful treatment of asthma was tested. Twenty patients who had severe, glucocorticoid-dependent asthma requiring both topical and systemic glucocorticoids to control symptoms of airflow obstruction were treated with nebulized lidocaine initially using a dose of 2 ml of a 2% solution (40 mg) four times daily (total daily dose, 160 mg) (173). After 2–4 weeks of treatment, some patients were increased to 3 ml of a 2% solution (60 mg), four times daily (total daily dose, 240 mg), but most patients were changed to a 4% solution at a dose of 2.5 ml (100 mg) four times daily (total daily dose, 400 mg). Patients were treated for up to 26 months. Initially, all topical and systemic glucocorticoids were maintained at the doses used prior to lidocaine therapy; only when peak flow rates were stable and symptoms well controlled were oral steroids cautiously reduced. Before lidocaine treatment, all but three of the patients had evidence of side effects of glucocorticoid treatment with prominent weight gain and cushingoid habitus, and several had glucose intolerance, myopathy, osteoporosis, cataracts, glaucoma, mood alteration or peptic ulcer disease. During lidocaine treatment (mean of 13.5 months), 17 of the 20 patients reduced prednisone by 90–100% of the initial maintenance dose. The other three patients did not noticeably improve. Overall, 13 of the 17 patients who responded to lidocaine were able to stop oral glucocorticoids entirely and the side effects of steroid therapy disappeared. Interestingly, the factor limiting prednisone reduction was the occurrence of glucocorticoid withdrawal symptoms. Patients experienced profound deep aching of the extremities and long bones with generalized myalgias, fatigue, listlessness, and occasional mood alteration, most commonly depression. Following lidocaine nebulization, one patient experienced subjective chest tightness. Lidocaine was stopped in this patient because of this reaction and because the patient did not appear to benefit from the lidocaine. Several patients had upper respiratory infections with exacerbations of asthma requiring 7- to 10-day periods of increased dosages of prednisone; these exacerbations of asthma did not affect the overall rate of withdrawal of prednisone in these patients.

Although this was an open clinical trial, the results in these patients with glucocorticoid-requiring asthma encourage the belief that the patients truly were benefited. This conclusion is underscored by the fact that some patients had been treated with glucocorticoids for up to 32 years; the mean duration of steroid use was 6.5 years and the median was 3.0 years. Moreover, patients such as these are the most difficult to treat effectively and are exceedingly difficult to wean from glucocorticoids. To gain more accurate information on the effectiveness of lidocaine in asthma, double-blind placebo-controlled studies with lidocaine have commenced. However, blinding is difficult, because all patients inhaling lidocaine experience topical anesthesia of the larynx and the pharynx. If the results of the double-blind placebo-controlled studies corroborate the results of this open trial, then lidocaine would appear to be a glucocorticomimetic drug, and its use would permit patients to experience the benefit of glucocorticoids without their side effects.

V. Summary

It is readily apparent that eosinophils are important targets of glucocorticoid effects. Disruption of the cytokine network by glucocorticoids can indirectly diminish eosinophil generation, survival, and function. In addition, glucocorticoids appear to have direct effects on the survival and perhaps function of these cells. Rapid advances in our knowledge of the biochemistry of signal transduction, as well as the interaction between cell surface receptors and RNA transcription machinery, will allow detailed analyses of the mechanisms by which the functions and life cycle of eosinophils are influenced by glucocorticoids.

Acknowledgments

This chapter has been taken in part and used with permission from R.P. Schleimer and B.S. Bochner: The effects of glucocorticoids on human eosinophils. J Allergy Clin Immunol 1994; 94:1202–1213.

We would like to thank Bonnie Hebden, Cheryl Adolphson, and Linda Arneson for their assistance in the preparation of this manuscript and Carol Bickel for assistance in the analysis of eosinophil phenotype.

Discussion

DR. BUSSE: Several doses of oral prednisone, that is 20–30 mg, will cause profound eosinopenia and presumably an improvement in asthma. In in vitro studies, suppression of various eosinophil responses occurs at 10^{-5} M concentration of corticosteroid. This suggests that the eosinophil is rather insensitive to the steroid effects. How do you explain the sensitivity to in vivo administration of steroids and relative insensitivity to in vitro steroid?

DR. GLEICH: Note that concentrations of dexamethasone slightly $\geq 10^{-8}$ M were effective in inhibiting the response of the eosinophil to IL-5. Presumably glucocorticoids produce eosinopenia by their ability to either reduce cytokine production and/or their effect on target cells.

DR. SCHLEIMER: According to the results that were shown, dexamethasone was active. This is certainly achievable in vivo at 10^{-8} M. Although in most in vitro systems the IC_{50} for dexamethasone is $1–2 \times 10^{-9}$ M, this assay utilizes cytokines (e.g., IL-5), which at high concentrations antagonize the action of the steroid, perhaps shifting the steroid dose response curve to the right.

DR. THOMPSON: Have you studied the metabolism of hydrocortisone in your assay.

DR. GLEICH: No.

DR. BARNES: Is the effect of lidocaine on eosinophil survival shared by other local anesthetics which work via a Na^+ channel? Some asthmatic patients show an unexpected increase in bronchoconstriction after nebulized lidocaine, so it may be dangerous to use in some patients. Have you seen any adverse effects with nebulized lidocaine in your patients with severe asthma?

DR. GLEICH: Concerning the lidocaine inhibition of eosinophil-cytokine interactions, we have found that other topical anesthetics have the same effect. The mechanism of this effect is presumably through the Na^+ channel. Concerning lidocaine-induced asthma exacerbations, Dr. Hunt has not noted this problem, possibly because the patients with asthma are under intensive therapy with glucocorticoid when lidocaine therapy is begun.

DR. LAITINEN: (1) Do other anesthetics have similar effects as lidocaine? If so, should we be very suspicious toward all results received with BAL technique? (2) Why did you study estradiol?

DR. GLEICH: (1) Concerning your first question, other topical anesthetics have similar effects as lidocaine. Because high concentrations of lidocaine or other topical anesthetics may be present in the lung after the performance of a BAL, investigators should exert caution in the use of such fluids in experiments employing bioassays. Concerning question 2, estradiol was tested in the experiments on degranulation and on glucocorticoid inhibition of cytokine-mediated eosinophil survival as a control steroid without glucocorticoid effect.

DR. BOCHNER: Do you know yet whether the clinical improvement you are seeing with inhaled lidocaine is associated with a reduction in airways and/or peripheral blood eosinophils? Do you achieve concentrations of lidocaine in the lung that approach what appears to be needed in vitro to affect eosinophil survival?

DR. GLEICH: We have not made any systematic observations on the lidocaine-treated patients. Remember that blood eosinophils are not a terribly useful index of asthma severity. Analyses of eosinophil numbers are included in an ongoing prospective blinded study.

DR. LEUNG: (1) Aside from its effects on eosinophils, do you know from the BAL studies whether lidocaine has effects on other cell types; for example, T cells and cytokine expression. (2) Do you know the mechanisms of lidocaine-induced inhibition of eosinophil survival?

DR. GLEICH: Presently, we do not have data on the effect of lidocaine on other immune functions. The mechanism of the lidocaine effect on eosinophils is under investigation.

DR. THOMPSON: (1) What are the tissue concentrations of IL-5, GM-CSF, and IFN-γ? (2) Do eosinophils contain estrogen receptors? This would be critical to know so as to interpret the lack of effect of estrogen on eosinophil survival.

DR. GLEICH: We do not have any data on the effect of lidocaine on cytokine levels, such as IL-2 or IFN-γ. Data in the literature suggest that the eosinophil possesses an estrogen receptor, although these data were obtained many years ago.

DR. SZEFLER: (1) Have you measured lidocaine concentrations in BALF? (2) How is the lidocaine administered in the clinical studies of patients with asthma?

DR. GLEICH: Indeed, and in the study with Dr. David Broide (169), concentrations of lidocaine up to 2.5 mg/ml were measured. Lidocaine was administered by nebulization.

DR. LIU: During bronchoscopy, lidocaine is routinely instilled into airways as boluses of liquid. The amount of lidocaine recovered in BAL fluids probably does not reflect the amount delivered to the whole lung by nebulization.

DR. MCFADDEN: (1) Are you advocating using inhaled lidocaine for the treatment of asthma? (2) Have any of your patients aspirated because of the anesthetic effects of lidocaine in the swallowing mechanism?

DR. GLEICH: Yes, I am suggesting, based on our preliminary results, that nebulized lidocaine may be an effective treatment for steroid-resistant asthma. After lidocaine nebulization, patients notice a numb mouth, and these patients have been advised to refrain from eating or drinking for 1–2 hours after this therapy. With this precaution, none has aspirated.

DR. LANE: (1) Does lidocaine bronchodilate or does it protect in challenge procedures? (2) Have you demonstrated direct glucocorticoid receptor binding by lidocaine on eosinophils?

DR. GLEICH: We have not measured any bronchodilatory effect of lidocaine nor have we tested the effect of lidocaine on eosinophil glucocorticoid receptors.

DR. HERSCHMAN: Does nebulized lidocaine have any effect on steroid-resistant asthma?

DR. GLEICH: Essentially all of the patients treated by Dr. Loren Hunt (173) required moderate (10–30 mg) or high (30-100 mg/day) prednisone administration and thus could be regarded as steroid resistant.

DR. JORDANA: It is clear that glucocorticosteroids powerfully inhibit the survival of peripheral blood eosinophils. We have isolated eosinophils directly from nasal polyp tissues and found that glucocorticoids do not actually inhibit very well their survival ex vivo. Also, we measured the amount of GM-CSF in nasal polyp fragments and found levels of GM-CSF that one would predict override the inhibitory effect of GC. Thus, the response to steroids of eosinophils within an inflamed microenvironment might be quite different than that of peripheral blood eosinophils.

DR. LEUNG: Although your data on lidocaine effects in asthma are very intriguing, given the concerns over β-agonist overuse masking airway inflammatory effects, it will be important to monitor other parameters of airway inflammation, including T-cell activation, to be certain the anesthetic treatment is not masking other parameters of inflammation. Thus, aside from steroid reduction and improvement in clinical effects, BAL and biopsy studies are needed.

DR. GLEICH: These issues are presently under investigation.

DR. PEDERSEN: Have you performed a controlled study to compare the effect of lidocaine delivered from a nebulizer which generates particles of a size that will not enter the lungs with the effects of a nebulizer which delivers a high dose of lidocaine to the intrapulmonary airways?

DR. GLEICH: This study is presently underway.

DR. LAITINEN: If I remember correctly, anesthetics like lidocaine have anti-inflammatory effects in the intestine. Dr. Edsbacker should know about that.

DR. EDSBACKER: A few reports have appeared on the beneficial effect of lidocaine and lidocaine analogues in inflammatory bowel disease, more specifically enema formulations for the treatment of proctitis. Symptoms and inflammatory markers are reduced following treatment.

DR. SMALDONE: Compared with the amount of lidocaine given to a patient by instillation during bronchoscopy (approximately 100 mg), the amount delivered by nebulizer is greatly reduced—for a 40-mg dose in the nebulizer, the lung or airway dose would be $\leq$ 4 mg.

DR. GLEICH: I agree that this is likely the case.

References

1. Gleich GJ, Kita H, Adolphson CR. Eosinophils. In: Frank MM, Austen KF, Claman HN, Unanue ER, eds. Samter's Immunologic Diseases. Boston: Little, Brown, 1994:205–245.
2. Kay AB. Eosinophils and asthma (letter to the editor). N Engl J Med 1991; 324:1514–1515.

3. Flavahan NA, Slifman NR, Gleich GJ, Vanhoutte PM. Human eosinophil major basic protein causes hyperreactivity of respiratory smooth muscle. Am Rev Respir Dis 1988; 138:685–688.

4. Gundel RH, Letts LG, Gleich GJ. Human eosinophil major basic protein induces airway constriction and airway hyperresponsiveness in primates. J Clin Invest 1991; 87:1470–1473.

5. Prin L, Lefebvre PP, Gruart V, Capron M, Storme L, Formstecher P, Loiseau S, Capron A. Heterogeneity of human eosinophil glucocorticoid receptor expression in hypereosinophilic patients: absence of detectable receptor correlates with resistance to corticotherapy. Clin Exp Immunol 1989; 78:383–389.

6. Schleimer RP. Glucocorticosteroids: their mechanism of action and use in allergic diseases. In: Middleton E, Reed CE, Ellis EF, Adkinson NF Jr, Yunginger JW, Busse W, eds. Allergy: Principles and Practice. 4th ed. St. Louis: Mosby, 1993:893–925.

7. Bjornson BH, Harvey JM, Rose L. Differential effect of hydrocortisone on eosinophil and neutrophil proliferation. J Clin Invest 1985; 76:924–929.

8. Slovick FT, Abboud CN, Brennan JK, Lichtman MA. Modulation of in vitro eosinophil progenitors by hydrocortisone: role of accessory cells and interleukins. Blood 1985; 66:1072–1079.

9. Butterfield JH, Ackerman SJ, Weiler D, Eisenbrey AB, Gleich GJ. Effects of glucocorticoids on eosinophil colony growth. J Allergy Clin Immunol 1986; 78:450–457.

10. Shalit M, Sekhsaria S, Malech HL. Modulation of growth and differentiation of eosinophils from human peripheral blood CD34+ cells by IL5 and other growth factors. Cell Immunol 1995; 160:50–57.

11. Sanderson CJ, Warren DJ, Strath M. Identification of a lymphokine that stimulates eosinophil differentiation in vitro. J Exp Med 1985; 162:60–74.

12. Yamaguchi Y, Suda T, Suda J, Eguchi M, Miura Y, Harada N, Tominaga A, Takatsu K. Purified interleukin 5 supports the terminal differentiation and proliferation of murine eosinophilic precursors. J Exp Med 1988; 167:43–56.

13. Sher A, Coffman RL, Hieny S, Cheever AW. Ablation of eosinophil and IgE responses with anti–IL-5 or anti–IL-4 antibodies fails to affect immunity against *Schistosoma mansoni* in the mouse. J Immunol 1990; 145:3911–3916.

14. Rolfe FG, Hughes JM, Armour CL, Sewell WA. Inhibition of interleukin-5 gene expression by dexamethasone. Immunology 1992; 77:494–499.

15. Butcher EC. Leukocyte-endothelial cell recognition: three (or more) steps to specificity and diversity. Cell 1991; 67:1033–1036.

16. Harlan J, Liu D. Adhesion: Its Role in Inflammatory Disease. New York: Freeman, 1992.

17. Springer TA. Adhesion receptors of the immune system. Nature 1990; 346:425–434.

18. Bochner BS, Schleimer RP. The role of adhesion molecules in human eosinophil and basophil recruitment. J Allergy Clin Immunol 1994; 93:427–438.

19. Albelda SM, Buck CA. Integrins and other cell adhesion molecules. FASEB J 1990; 4:2868–2880.

20. Thornhill MH, Kyan-Aung U, Haskard DO. IL-4 increases human endothelial cell adhesiveness for T cells but not for neutrophils. J Immunol 1990; 144:3060–3065.
21. Schleimer RP, Sterbinsky SA, Kaiser J, Bickel CA, Klunk DA, Tomioka K, Newman W, Luscinskas FW, Gimbrone MA Jr, McIntyre BW, Bochner BS. Interleukin-4 induces adherence of human eosinophils and basophils but not neutrophils to endothelium: association with expression of VCAM-1. J Immunol 1992; 148:1086–1092.
22. Bochner BS, Klunk DA, Sterbinsky SA, Coffman RL, Schleimer RP. Interleukin-13 selectively induces vascular cell adhesion molecule-1 (VCAM-1) expression in human endothelial cells. J Immunol 1995; 154:799–803.
23. Bochner BS, Luscinskas FW, Gimbrone MA Jr, Newman W, Sterbinsky SA, Derse-Anthony C, Klunk D, Schleimer RP. Adhesion of human basophils, eosinophils, and neutrophils to IL-1–activated human vascular endothelial cells: contributions of endothelial cell adhesion molecules. J Exp Med 1991; 173:1553–1557.
24. Dobrina A, Menegazzi R, Carlos TM, Nardon E, Cramer R, Zacchi T, Harlan JM, Patriarca P. Mechanisms of eosinophil adherence to cultured vascular endothelial cells: eosinophils bind to the cytokine-induced endothelial ligand vascular cell adhesion molecule-1 via the very late activation antigen-4 integrin receptor. J Clin Invest 1991; 88:20–26.
25. Walsh GM, Mermod J, Hartnell A, Kay AB, Wardlaw AJ. Human eosinophil, but not neutrophil, adherence to IL-1-stimulated human umbilical vascular endothelial cells is α4β1 (very late antigen-4) dependent. J Immunol 1991; 146:3419–3423.
26. Weller PF, Rand TH, Goelz SE, Chi-Rosso G, Lobb RR. Human eosinophil adherence to vascular endothelium mediated by binding to vascular cell adhesion molecule 1 and endothelial leukocyte adhesion molecule 1. Proc Natl Acad Sci USA 1991; 88:7430–7433.
27. Schleimer RP, Freeland HS, Peters SP, Brown KE, Derse CP. An assessment of the effects of glucocorticoids on degranulation, chemotaxis, binding to vascular endothelial cells and formation of leukotriene B4 by purified human neutrophils. J Pharmacol Exp Therap 1989; 250:598–605.
28. Bochner BS, Peachell PT, Brown KE, Schleimer RP. Adherence of human basophils to cultured umbilical vein vascular endothelial cells. J Clin Invest 1988; 81:1355–1360.
29. Kaiser J, Bickel C, Bochner BS, Schleimer RP. The effects of the potent glucocorticoid budesonide on adhesion of eosinophils to human vascular endothelium and on endothelial expression of adhesion molecules. J Pharmacol Exp Therap 1993; 267:245–249.
30. Moser R, Schleiffenbaum B, Groscurth P, Fehr J. Interleukin 1 and tumor necrosis factor stimulate human vascular endothelial cells to promote transendothelial neutrophil passage. J Clin Invest 1989; 83:444–455.
31. Cronstein BN, Kimmel SC, Levin RI, Martiniuk F, Weissman G. A mechanism for the antiinflammatory effects of glucocorticosteroids: the glucocorticoid receptor regulates leukocyte adhesion to endothelial cells and expression of endothelial-

leukocyte adhesion molecule 1 and intercellular adhesion molecule 1. Proc Natl Acad Sci USA 1992; 89:9991–9995.

32. Lopez AF, Sanderson CJ, Gamble JR, Campbell HD, Young IG, Vadas MA. Recombinant human interleukin 5 is a selective activator of human eosinophil function. J Exp Med 1988; 167:219–224.

33. Yamaguchi Y, Hayashi Y, Sugama Y, Miura Y, Kasahara T, Kitamura S, Torisu M, Mita S, Tominaga A, Takatsu K, Suda T. Highly purified murine interleukin 5 (IL-5) stimulates eosinophil function and prolongs in vitro survival. J Exp Med 1988; 167:1737–1742.

34. Walsh GM, Hartnell A, Wardlaw AJ, Kurihara K, Sanderson CJ, Kay AB. IL-5 enhances the in vitro adhesion of human eosinophils, but not neutrophils, in a leukocyte integrin (CD11/18)-dependent manner. Immunology 1990; 71:258–265.

35. Tomioka K, MacGlashan DW Jr, Lichtenstein LM, Bochner BS, Schleimer RP. GM-CSF regulates human eosinophil responses to F-Met peptide and platelet activating factor. J Immunol 1993; 151:4989–4997.

36. Ebisawa M, Liu MC, Yamada T, Kato M, Lichenstein LM, Bochner BS, Schleimer RP. Eosinophil transendothelial migration induced by cytokines. II. The potentiation of eosinophil transendothelial migration by eosinophil-active cytokines. J Immunol 1994; 152:4590–4597.

37. Bochner BS, Rutledge BK, Schleimer RP. Interleukin 1 production by human lung tissue. II. Inhibition by antiinflammatory steroids. J Immunol 1987; 139:2303–2307.

38. Borish L, Mascali JJ, Dishuck J, Beam WR, Martin RJ, Rosenwasser LH. Detection of alveolar macrophage-derived IL-1β in asthma. J Immunol 1992; 149:3078–3082.

39. Snyder DS, Unanue ER. Corticosteroids inhibit murine macrophage Ia expression and interleukin-1 production. J Immunol 1982; 129:1803–1805.

40. Smith KA. T cell growth factor. Immunol Rev 1980; 51:337–357.

41. Beutler B, Krochin N, Milsark IW, Luedke C, Cerami A. Control of cachectin (tumor necrosis factor) synthesis: mechanisms of endotoxin resistance. Science 1986; 232:977–980.

42. Robinson D, Hamid Q, Ying S, Bentley A, Assoufi B, Durham S, Kay AB. Prednisolone treatment in asthma is associated with modulation of bronchoalveolar lavage cell interleukin-4, interleukin-5, and interferon-γ cytokine gene expression. Am Rev Respir Dis 1993; 148:401–406.

43. Masuyama K, Jacobson MR, Rak S, Meng Q, Sudderick RM, Kay AB, Lowhagen O, Hamid Q, Durham SR. Topical glucocorticosteroid (fluticasone propionate) inhibits cells expressing cytokine mRNA for interleukin-4 in the nasal mucosa in allergen-induced rhinitis. Immunology 1994; 82:192–199.

44. Liu MC, Xiao HQ, Lichtenstein LM, Huang SK. Prednisone inhibits TH_2-type cytokine gene expression at sites of allergen challenge in subjects with asthma (abstr). Am Rev Respir Dis 1994; 149:A944.

45. Wu CY, Fargeas C, Nakajima T, Delespesse G. Glucocorticoids suppress the production of interleukin 4 by human lymphocytes. Eur J Immunol 1991; 21:2645–2647.

46. Culpepper JA, Lee F. Regulation of IL-3 expression by glucocorticoids in cloned murine T-lymphocytes. J Immunol 1985; 135:3191–3197.

47. Churchill L, Friedman B, Schleimer RP, Proud D. Production of granulocyte-macrophage colony-stimulating factor by cultured human tracheal epithelial cells. Immunology 1992; 75:189–195.

48. Kato M, Schleimer RP. Antiinflammatory steroids inhibit granulocyte/macrophage colony-stimulating factor production by human lung tissue. Lung 1994; 172:113–124.

49. Tobler A, Meier R, Seitz M, Dewald B, Baggiolini M, Fey MF. Glucocorticoids downregulate gene expression of GM-CSF, NAP-1/IL-8, and IL-6, but not of M-CSF in human fibroblasts. Blood 1992; 79:45–51.

50. Massey W, Kato M, Kagey-Sobotka A, Cooper P, Lichenstein L, Schleimer R. Topical corticosteroids inhibit allergen (AG)-induced cutaneous GM-CSF production (abstr). J Allergy Clin Immunol 1993; 91:317.

51. Stellato C, Beck LA, Gorgone GA, Proud D, Schall TJ, Ono SJ, Lichtenstein LM, Schleimer RP. Expression of the chemokine RANTES by a human bronchial epithelial cell line: Modulation by cytokines and glucocorticoids. J Immunol 1995; 155:410–418.

52. Van Otteren GM, Standiford TJ, Kunkel SL, Danforth JM, Burdick MD, Abruzzo LV, Strieter RM. Expression and regulation of macrophage inflammatory protein-1α by murine alveolar and peritoneal macrophages. Am J Respir Cell Mol Biol 1994; 10:8–15.

53. Guida L, O'Hehir RE, Hawrylowicz CM. Synergy between dexamethasone and interleukin-5 for the induction of major histocompatibility complex class II expression by human peripheral blood eosinophils. Blood 1994; 84:2733–2740.

54. Ebisawa M, Schleimer RP, Bickel C, Bochner BS. Phenotyping of purified human peripheral blood eosinophils using the blind panel of monoclonal antibodies. In: Schlossman S, Boumsell L, Gilks W, Harlan J, Kishimoto T, Morimoto C, Ritz J, Shaw S, Silverstein R, Springer T, Tedder T, Todd R, eds. Leukocyte Typing V: White Cell Differentiation Antigens. Oxford, UK: Oxford University Press, 1995:1036–1038.

55. Clark RAF, Gallin JI, Fauci AS. Effects of in vivo prednisone on in vitro eosinophil and neutrophil adherence and chemotaxis. Blood 1979; 53:633–641.

56. Altman LC, Hill JS, Hairfield WM, Mullarkey MF. Effects of corticosteroids on eosinophil chemotaxis and adherence. J Clin Invest 1981; 67:28–36.

57. Kurihara K, Wardlaw AJ, Moqbel R, Kay AB. Inhibition of platelet-activating factor (PAF)–induced chemotaxis and PAF binding to human eosinophils and neutrophils by the specific ginkgolide-derived PAF antagonist BN 52021. J Allergy Clin Immunol 1989; 83:83–90.

58. Andersson P, Chignard M, Brange C, Nilsson T, Juhlin M, Le-Couedic JP. Effect of glucocorticosteroid treatment on antigen-induced mediator release from sensitized guinea pig lungs. In: Hogg JC, Ellul-Micallef R, Brattsand R, eds. Glucocorticoids, Inflammation and Bronchial Hyperreactivity. Amsterdam: Excerpta Medica, 1985:132–135.

59. Flower RJ. Glucocorticoids and the inhibition of phospholipase A$_2$. In: Schleimer

RP, Claman HN, Oronsky A, eds. Anti-inflammatory Steroid Action. Basic and Clinical Aspects. San Diego: Academic Press, 1989:48–66.

60. Wertheim WA, Kunkel SL, Standiford TJ, Burdick MD, Becker FS, Wilke CA, Gilbert AR, Strieter RM. Regulation of neutrophil-derived IL-8: the role of prostaglandin E_2, dexamethasone, and IL-4. J Immunol 1993; 151:2166–2175.

61. Howe RS, Lee YH, Fischkoff SA, Teuscher C, Lyttle CR. Glucocorticoid and progestin regulation of eosinophil chemotactic factor and complement C3 in the estrogen-treated rat uterus. Endocrinology 1990; 126:3193–3199.

62. Beck LA, Schall TJ, Beall LD, Leopold D, Bickel C, Baroody F, Naclerio RM, Schleimer RP. Detection of the chemokine RANTES and activation of vascular endothelium in nasal polyps (abstr). J Allergy Clin Immunol 1994; 93:A234.

63. Lucey DR, Nicholson-Weller A, Weller PF. Mature human eosinophils have the capacity to express HLA-DR. Proc Natl Acad Sci USA 1989; 86:1348–1351.

64. Hansel TT, De Vries IJM, Carballido JM, Braun RK, Carballido-Perrig N, Rihs S, Blaser K, Walker C. Induction and function of eosinophil intercellular adhesion molecule-1 and HLA-DR. J Immunol 1992; 149:2130–2136.

65. Weller PF, Rand TH, Barrett T, Elovic A, Wong DTW, Finberg RW. Accessory cell function of human eosinophils. HLA-DR–dependent, MHC-restricted antigen-presentation and IL-1 alpha expression. J Immunol 193; 150:2554–2562.

66. Schleimer RP. The effects of glucocorticoids on mast cells and basophils. In: Schleimer RP, Claman HN, Oronsky A, eds. Anti-inflammatory Steroid Action. Basic and Clinical Aspects. San Diego: Academic Press, 1989:226–258.

67. Schleimer RP. The effects of anti-inflammatory glucocorticoids on mast cells. In: Kaliner M, Metcalfe D, eds. The Mast Cell in Health and Disease. New York: Marcel Dekker, 1992:483–511.

68. Hallam C, Pritchard DI, Trigg S, Eady RP. Rat eosinophil-mediated antibody-dependent cellular cytotoxicity: investigations of the mechanisms of target cell lysis and inhibition by glucocorticoids. Clin Exp Immunol 1982; 48:641–648.

69. Kita H, Abu-Ghazaleh R, Sanderson CJ, Gleich GJ. Effect of steroids on immunoglobulin-induced eosinophil degranulation. J Allergy Clin Immunol 1991; 87:70–77.

70. Cohen JJ, Duke RC. Apoptosis and programmed cell death in immunity. Ann Rev Immunol 1992; 10:267–293.

71. Williams GT, Smith CA. Molecular regulation of apoptosis: Genetic controls on cell death (review). Cell 1993; 74:777–779.

72. Vaux DL, Haecker G, Strasser A. An evolutionary perspective on apoptosis (review). Cell 1994; 76:777–779.

73. Stern M, Meagher L, Savill J, Haslett C. Apoptosis in human eosinophils. Programmed cell death in the eosinophil leads to phagocytosis by macrophages and is modulated by IL-5. J Immunol 1992; 148:3543–3549.

74. Savill J, Hogg N, Ren Y, Haslett C. Thrombospondin cooperates with CD36 and the virtonectin receptor in macrophage recognition of neutrophils undergoing apoptosis. J Clin Invest 1992; 90:1513–1522.

75. Savill J, Fadok V, Henson P, Haslett C. Phagocyte recognition of cells undergoing apoptosis. Immunol Today 1993; 13:131–136.

76. Fadok VA, Savill JS, Haslett C, Bratton DL, Doherty DE, Campbell PA, Henson PM. Different populations of macrophages use either the vitronectin receptor or the phosphatidylserine receptor to recognize and remove apoptotic cells. J Immunol 1992; 149:4029–4035.

77. Lopez AF, Williamson DJ, Gamble JR, Begley CG, Harlan JM, Klebanoff SJ, Waltersdorph A, Wong G, Clark SC, Vadas MA. Recombinant human granulocyte-macrophage colony-stimulating factor stimulates in vitro mature human neutrophil and eosinophil function, surface receptor expression, and survival. J Clin Invest 1986; 78:1220–1228.

78. Silberstein DS, Owen WF Jr, Gasson JC, DiPersio JF, Golde DW, Bina JC, Soberman R, Austen KF, David JR. Enhancement of human eosinophil cytotoxicity and leukotriene synthesis by biosynthetic (recombinant) granulocyte-macrophage colony-stimulating factor. J Immunol 1986; 137:3290–3294.

79. Rothenberg ME, Owen WF Jr, Silberstein DS, Woods J, Soberman RJ, Austen KF, Stevens RL. Human eosinophils have prolonged survival, enhanced functional properties, and become hypodense when exposed to human interleukin 3. J Clin Invest 1988; 81:1986–1992.

80. Lamas AM, Marcotte GV, Schleimer RP. Human endothelial cells prolong eosinophil survival. Regulation by cytokines and glucocorticoids. J Immunol 1989; 142:3978–3984.

81. Lamas AM, Leon OG, Schleimer RP. Glucocorticoids inhibit eosinophil responses to granulocyte-macrophage colony-stimulating factor. J Immunol 1991; 147:254–259.

82. Wallen N, Kita H, Weiler D, Gleich GJ. Glucocorticoids inhibit cytokine-mediated eosinophil survival. J Immunol 1991; 147:3490–3495.

83. Cox G, Ohtoshi T, Vanceri C, Denburg JA, Dolovich J, Gauldie J, Jordana M. Promotion of eosinophil survival by human bronchial epithelial cells and its modulation by glucocorticoids. Am J Respir Cell Mol Biol 1991; 4:525–531.

84. Hallsworth MP, Litchfield TM, Lee TH. Glucocorticoids inhibit granulocyte-macrophage colony-stimulating factor and interleukin-5 enhanced in vitro survival of human eosinophils. Immunology 1992; 75:382–385.

85. Matsumoto K, Schleimer RP, Saito H, Iikura Y, Bochner BS. Induction of apoptosis in human eosinophils by anti-fas antibody treatment in vitro. Blood 1995; 86:1437–1443.

86. Walsh CM, Williamson ML, Symon FA, Wardlaw AJ. Inhibition of cytokine-induced eosinophil survival and induction of apoptosis by ligation of CD69 (abstr). Am J Respir Crit Care Med 1995; 151:A241.

87. Schüle R, Rangarajan P, Kliewer S, Ransome LJ, Bolado J, Yang N, Verma IM, Evans RM. Functional antagonism between oncoprotein c-Jun and the glucocorticoid receptor. Cell 1990; 62:1217–1226.

88. Yang-Yen H-F, Chambard J-C, Sun Y-L, Smeal T, Schmidt TJ, Drouin J, Karin M. Transcriptional interference between c-Jun and the glucocorticoid receptor: mutual inhibition of DNA binding due to direct protein-protein interaction. Cell 1990; 62:1205–1215.

89. Radler-Pohl A Geberl S, Sachsenmaier C, Konig H, Kramer M, Oehler T, Streile M, Ponta H, Rapp U, Rahmsdorf HJ, Cato ACB, Angel P, Herrlich P. The activation and activity control of AP-1 (Fos/Jun). Ann NY Acad Sci 1993; 684:127–148.

90. Jonat C, Rahmsdorf HJ, Park K-K, Cato ACB, Gebel S, Ponta H, Herrlich P. Antitumor promotion and antiinflammation: Down-modulation of AP-1 (Fos/Jun) activity by glucocorticoid hormone. Cell 1990; 62:1189–1204.

91. Schüle R, Rangarajan P, Yang N, Kliewer S, Ransome LJ, Bolado J, Verma IM, Evans RM. Retinoic acid is a negative regulator of AP-1-responsive genes. Proc Natl Acad Sci USA 1991; 88:6092–6096.

92. Mukaida N, Morita M, Ishikawa Y, Rice N, Okamoto S, Kasahara T, Matsushima K. Novel mechanism of glucocorticoid-mediated gene repression. Nuclear factor-κB is target for glucocorticoid-mediated interleukin 8 gene repression. J Biol Chem 1994; 269:13289–13295.

93. Nishio Y, Isshiki H, Kishimoto T, Akira S. A nuclear factor for interleukin-6 expression (NF-IL6) and the glucocorticoid receptor synergistically activate transcription of the rat α1-acid glycoprotein gene via direct protein-protein interaction. Mol Cell Biol 1993; 13:1854–1862.

94. Hoke GM, Barry D, Fey GH. Synergistic action of interleukin-6 and glucocorticoids is mediated by the interleukin-6 response element of the rat α2 macroglobulin gene. Mol Cell Biol 1992; 12:2282–2294.

95. Kutoh E, Strömstedt P-E, Poellinger L. Functional interference between the ubiquitous and constitutive octamer transcription factor 1 (OTF-1) and the glucocorticoid receptor by direct protein-protein interaction involving the homeo subdomain of OTF-1. Mol Cell Biol 1992; 12:4960–4969.

96. Chatterjee VKK, Madison LD, Mayo S, Jameson JL. Repression of the human glycoprotein hormone α-subunit gene by glucocorticoids: evidence for receptor interactions with limiting transcriptional activators. Mol Endocrinol 1991; 5:100–110.

97. Chang T-J, Scher BM, Waxman S, Scher W. Inhibition of mouse GATA-1 function by the glucocorticoid receptor: possible mechanism of glucocorticoid inhibition of erythroleukemia cell differentiation. Mol Endocrinol 1993; 7:528–542.

98. Paliogianni F, Raptis A, Ahuja SS, Najjar SM, Boumpas DT. Negative transcriptional regulation of human interleukin 2 (IL-2) gene by glucocorticoids through interference with nuclear transcription factors AP-1 and NF-AT. J Clin Invest 1993; 91:1481–1489.

99. Vacca A, Felli MP, Farina AR, Martinotti S, Maroder M, Screpanti I, Meco D, Petrangeli E, Frati L, Gulino A. Glucocorticoid receptor-mediated suppression of the interleukin 2 gene expression through impairment of the cooperativity between nuclear factor of activated T cells and AP-1 enhancer elements. J Exp Med 1992; 175:637–646.

100. Celada A, McKercher S, Maki RA. Repression of major histocompatibility complex IA expression by glucocorticosteroids: the glucocorticoid receptor inhibits the DNA binding of the X box DNA binding protein. J Exp Med 1993; 177:691–698.

101. Wieland S, Döbbeling U, Rusconi S. Interference and synergism of glucocorticoid receptor and octamer factors. EMBO J 1991; 10:2513–2521.

102. Northrop JP, Crabtree GR, Mattila PS. Negative regulation of interleukin-2 transcription by the glucocorticoid receptor. J Exp Med 1992; 175:1235–1245.
103. Bates ME, Bertics PJ, Busse WW. IL-5 induces tyrosine (Y) phosphorylation of peripheral blood eosinophil (EOS) proteins including a 45-kDa protein immunoreactive with MAP-kinase antibodies (abstr). J Allergy Clin Immunol 1994; 93:268.
104. Pazdrak K, Forsythe P, Alam R. Involvement of RAF-1 kinase in intracellular signaling of interleukin-5 in eosinophils and partially differentiated HL-60 cells (abstr). J Allergy Clin Immunol 1994; 93:267.
105. Schreiber D, Forsythe P, Alam R. Activation of eosinophils and partially differentiated HL-60 cells by IL-5 utilizes MAP kinase as an intermediate step in signal transduction. J Allergy Clin Immunol 1994; 93:267.
106. Pazdrak K, Schreiber D, Forsythe P, Justement L, Alam R. The intracellular signal transduction mechanism of interleukin-5 in eosinophils: the involvement of lyn tyrosine kinase and the Ras-Raf-1-MEK-microtubule-associated protein kinase pathway. J Exp Med 1995; 181:1827–1834.
107. Schweizer RC, Welmers-van Kessel BAC, Raaijmakers HAM, Lammers J-WJ, Koenderman L. Effect of dexamethasone on eosinophil migration and tyrosine phosphorylation in vitro (abstr). Am J Respir Crit Care Med 1995; 151:A239.
108. Cox G. Glucocorticoid treatment inhibits apoptosis in human neutrophils. J Immunol 1995; 154:4719–4725.
109. Williams GT, Smith CA, Spooncer E, Dexter TM, Taylor DR. Haemopoietic colony stimulating factors promote cell survival by suppressing apoptosis. Nature 1990; 343:76–79.
110. Liu Z-G, Smith SW, McLaughlin KA, Schwartz LM, Osborne BA. Apoptotic signals delivered through the T-cell receptor of a T-cell hybrid require the immediate-early gene nur77. Nature 1994; 367:281–284.
111. Woronicz JD, Calnan B, Ngo V, Winoto A. Requirement for the orphan steroid receptor Nur77 in apoptosis of T-cell hybridomas. Nature 1994; 367:277–281.
112. Nunez G, London L, Hockenbery D, Alexander M, McKearn JP, Korsmeyer SJ. Deregulated Bcl-2 gene expression selectively prolongs survival of growth factor-deprived hemopoietic cell lines. J Immunol 1990; 144:3602–3610.
113. Sentman CL, Shutter JR, Hockenbery D, Kanagawa O, Korsmeyer SJ. bcl-2 Inhibits multiple forms of apoptosis but not negative selection in thymocytes. Cell 1991; 67:879–888.
114. Boise LH, González-Garcia M, Postema CE, Ding L, Lindsten T, Turka LA, Mao X, Nunez G, Thompson CB. bcl-x, a bcl-2–related gene that functions as a dominant regulator of apoptotic cell death. Cell 1993; 74:597–608.
115. Oltvai ZN, Milliman CL, Korsmeyer SJ. Bcl-2 heterodimerizes in vivo with a conserved homolog, Bax, that accelerates programmed cell death. Cell 1993; 74:609–619.
116. Barinaga M. Cell suicide: by ICE, not fire. Science 1994; 263:754–756.
117. Wilson KP, Black JF, Thomson JA, Kim EE, Griffith JP, Navia MA, Murcko MA, Chambers SP, Aldape RA, Raybuck SA, Livingston DJ. Structure and mechanism of interleukin-1β converting enzyme. Nature 1994; 370:270–275.
118. Yonish-Rouach E, Resnitzky D, Lotem J, Sachs L, Kimchi A, Oren M. Wild-

type p53 induces apoptosis of myeloid leukaemic cells that is inhibited by interleukin-6. Nature 1991; 352:345–347.

119. Lowe SW, Schmitt EM, Smith SW, Osborne BA, Jacks T. p53 is required for radiation-induced apoptosis in mouse thymocytes. Nature 1993; 362:847–849.

120. Shi Y, Glynn JM, Guilbert LJ, Cotter TG, Bissonnette RP, Green DR. Role for c-myc in activation-induced apoptotic cell death in T cell hybridomas. Science 1992; 257:212–214.

121. Sherr CJ. Mammalian G1 cyclins. Cell 1993; 73:1059–1065.

122. Nasmyth K, Hunt T. Dams and sluices. Nature 1993; 366:634–635.

123. Shi L, Nishioka WK, Th'ng T, Bradbury EM, Litchfield DW, Greenberg AH. Premature p34^{cdc2} activation required for apoptosis. Science 1994; 263:1143–1145.

124. Saunders RH, Adams E. Changes in circulating leukocytes following the administration of adrenal cortex extract (ACE) and adrenocorticotropic hormone (ACTH) in infectious mononucleosis and chronic lymphatic leukemia. Blood 1950; 5:732–741.

125. Sousa AR, Poston RN, Lane SJ, Nakhosteen JA, Lee TH. Detection of GM-CSF in asthmatic bronchial epithelium and decrease by inhaled corticosteroids. Am Rev Respir Dis 1993; 147:1557–1561.

126. Sabag N, Castrillon MA, Tchernitchin A. Cortisol-induced migration of eosinophil leukocytes to lymphoid organs. Experientia 1978; 34:666–667.

127. Kawabori S, Soda K, Perdue MH, Bienenstock J. The dynamics of intestinal eosinophil depletion in rats treated with dexamethasone. Lab Invest 1991; 64:224–233.

128. Gleich GJ, Schroeter AL, Marcoux JP, Sachs MI, O'Connell EJ, Kohler PF. Episodic angioedema associated with eosinophilia. N Engl J Med 1984; 310:1621–1626.

129. Butterfield JH, Leiferman KM, Abrams J, Silver JE, Bower J, Gonchoroff N, Gleich GJ. Elevated serum levels on interleukin-5 in patients with the syndrome of episodic angioedema and eosinophilia. Blood 1992; 79:688–692.

130. Zora J, O'Connell EJ, Sachs MI, Hoffman AD. Eosinophilic gastritis: a case report and review of the literature. Ann Allergy 1984; 53:45–47.

131. Bochner BS, Friedman B, Krishnaswami G, Schleimer RP, Lichtenstein LM, Kroegel C. Episodic eosinophilia-myalgia–like syndrome in a patient without L-tryptophan use: association with eosinophil activation and increased serum levels of granulocyte-macrophage colony-stimulating factor. J Allergy Clin Immunol 1991; 88:629–636.

132. Adelroth E, Rosenhall L, Johansson S-A, Linden M, Venge P. Inflammatory cells and eosinophilic activity in asthmatics investigated by bronchoalveolar lavage. The effects of antiasthmatic treatment with budesonide or terbutaline. Am Rev Respir Dis 1990; 142:91–99.

133. Laitinen LA, Laitinen A, Haahtela T. A comparative study of the effects of an inhaled corticosteroid, budesonide, and a β_2 agonist, terbutaline, on airway inflammation in newly diagnosed asthma: a randomized, double-blind, parallel-group controlled trial. J Allergy Clin Immunol 1992; 90:32–42.

134. Djukanovic R, Wilson JW, Britten KM, Wilson SJ, Walls AF, Roche WR, Howarth PH, Holgate ST. Effect of an inhaled corticosteroid on airway inflammation and symptoms in asthma. Am Rev Respir Dis 1992; 145:669–674.

135. Jeffrey PK, Godfrey RW, Adelroth E, Nelson F, Roger A, Johannson SA. Effects of treatment on airway inflammation and thickening of basement membrane reticular collagen in asthma. A quantitative light and electron microscopic study. Am Rev Respir Dis 1992; 145:890–899.

136. Pipkorn U, Proud D, Lichtenstein LM, Kagey-Sobotka A, Norman PS, Naclerio RM. Inhibition of mediator release in allergic rhinitis by pretreatment with topical glucocorticosteroids. N Engl J Med 1987; 316:1506–1510.

137. Pipkorn U, Proud D, Lichtenstein LM, Schleimer RP, Peters SP, Adkinson NJ Jr, Kagey-Sobotka A, Norman PS, Naclerio RM. Effect of short-term systemic glucocorticoid treatment on human nasal mediator release after antigen challenge. J Clin Invest 1987; 80:957–961.

138. Charlesworth EN, Kagey-Sobotka A, Schleimer RP, Norman PS, Lichtenstein LM. Prednisone inhibits the appearance of inflammatory mediators and the influx of eosinophils and basophils associated with the cutaneous late-phase response to allergen. J Immunol 1991; 146:671–676.

139. Liu MC, Proud D, Lichtenstein LM, Stealey BA, Hubbard WC, Ferracci L, Walinskas J, Kato M, Schleimer RP. Effects of prednisone on the airway inflammation following allergen challenge in subjects with allergic asthma (abstr). Am Rev Respir Dis 1993; 147:A521.

140. Evans PM, O'Connor BJ, Fuller RW, Barnes PJ, Chung KF. Effect of inhaled corticosteroids on peripheral blood eosinophil counts and density profiles in asthma. J Allergy Clin Immunol 1993; 91:643–650.

141. Gibson PG, Manning PJ, O'Byrne PM, Girgis-Gabardo A, Dolovich J, Denburg JA, Hargreave FE. Allergen-induced asthmatic responses—relationship between increases in airway responsiveness and increases in circulating eosinophils, basophils, and their progenitors. Am Rev Respir Dis 1991; 143:331–335.

142. Woolley MJ, Denburg JA, Ellis R, Dahlback M, O'Byrne PM. Allergen-induced changes in bone marrow progenitors and airway responsiveness in dogs and the effect of inhaled budesonide on these parameters. Am J Respir Cell Mol Biol 1994; 11:600–606.

143. Kung TT, Stelts D, Zurcher JA, Watnick AS, Jones H, Mauser PJ, Fernandez X, Umland S, Kreutner W, Chapman RW, Egan RW. Mechanisms of allergic pulmonary eosinophilia in the mouse. J Allergy Clin Immunol 1994; 94:1217–1224.

144. Kyan-Aung U, Haskard DO, Poston RN, Thornhill MH, Lee TH. Endothelial leukocyte adhesion molecule-1 and intercellular adhesion molecule-1 mediate the adhesion of eosinophils to endothelial cells in vitro and are expressed by endothelium in allergic cutaneous inflammation in vivo. J Immunol 1991; 146:521–528.

145. Leung DYM, Pober JS, Cotran RS. Expression of endothelial-leukocyte adhesion molecule-1 in elicited late phase allergic reactions. J Clin Invest 1991; 87:1805–1809.

146. Montefort S, Gratziou C, Goulding D, Polosa R, Haskard DO, Howart PH, Holgate ST, Carroll MP. Bronchial biopsy evidence for leukocyte infiltration and upregulation of leukocyte-endothelial cell adhesion molecules 6 hours after local allergen challenge of sensitized asthmatic airways. J Clin Invest 1994; 93:1411–1421.
147. Lee B-J, Naclerio RM, Bochner BS, Taylor RM, Lim MC, Baroody FM. Nasal challenge with allergen upregulates the local expression of vascular endothelial adhesion molecules. J Allergy Clin Immunol 1994; 94:1006–1016.
148. Montefort S, Feather IH, Wilson SJ, Haskard DO, Lee TH, Holgate ST, Howarth PH. The expression of leukocyte-endothelial adhesion molecules is increased in perennial allergic rhinitis. Am J Respir Cell Mol Biol 1992; 7:393–398.
149. Gundel RH, Wegner CD, Torcellini CA, Clarke CC, Haynes N, Rothlein R, Smith CW, Letts LG. Endothelial leukocyte adhesion molecule-1 mediates antigen-induced acute airway inflammation and late-phase airway obstruction in monkeys. J Clin Invest 1991; 88:1407–1411.
150. Wegner CD, Gundel RH, Reilly P, Haynes N, Letts LG, Rothlein R. Intercellular adhesion molecule-1 (ICAM-1) in the pathogenesis of asthma. Science 1990; 247:456–459.
151. Abraham WM, Sielczak MW, Ahmed A, Cortes A, Lauredo IT, Kim J, Pepinsky B, Benjamin CD, Leone DR, Lobb RR, Weller PF. α_4-integrins mediate antigen-induced late bronchial responses and prolonged airway hyperresponsiveness in sheep. J Clin Invest 1994; 93:776–787.
152. Metzger WJ, Ridger V, Tollefson V, Arrhenius T, Gaeta FCA, Elices M. Anti-VLA-4 antibody and CS-1 peptide inhibitor modifies airway inflammation and bronchial airway hyperresponsiveness (BHR) in the allergic rabbit (abstr) J Allergy Clin Immunol 1994; 93:183.
153. Nakajima H, Sano H, Nishimura T, Yoshida S, Iwamoto I. Role of vascular cell adhesion molecule-1/very late activation antigen-4 and intercellular adhesion molecule-1/lymphocyte function-associated antigen-1 interactions in antigen-induced eosinophil and T-cell recruitment into the tissue. J Exp Med 1994; 179:1145–1154.
154. Michael M, Whorton CM. Delay of the early inflammatory response by cortisone. Proc Soc Exp Biol Med 1951; 76:754–757.
155. Moon VH, Tershakovec GA. Influence of cortisone upon acute inflammation. Proc Soc Exp Biol Med 1952; 79:63–65.
156. Ebert RH, Barclay WR. Changes in connective tissue reaction induced by cortisone. Ann Intern Med 1952; 37:506–518.
157. Barclay WR, Ebert RH. The effect of cortisone on the vascular reactions to serum sickness and tuberculosis. Ann NY Acad Sci 1953; 56:634–636.
158. Allison F, Smith MR, Wood WB. Studies on the pathogenesis of acute inflammation. I. The inflammatory reaction to thermal injury as observed in the rabbit ear chamber. J Exp Med 1955; 102:655.
159. Schleimer RP. Effects of glucocorticoids on inflammatory cells relevant to their therapeutic applications in asthma. Am Rev Respir Dis 1990; 141:S59–S69.

160. Schleimer RP, Kato M, Kaiser J, Lichtenstein LM, Bochner BS, Liu MC. Antiinflammatory steroid actions in human lung. In: Holgate ST, Austen KF, Lichtenstein LM, Kay AB, eds. Asthma: Physiology, Immunopharmacology, and Treatment, Fourth International Symposium. London: Academic Press, 1993:375–389.

161. Mier JW, Vachino G, Klempner MS, Aronson FR, Noring R, Smith S, Brandon EP, Laird W, Atkins MB. Inhibition of interleukin-2-induced tumor necrosis factor release by dexamethasone: prevention of an acquired neutrophil chemotaxis defect and differential suppression of interleukin-2–associated side effects. Blood 1990; 76:1933–1940.

162. Waage A, Bakke O. Glucocorticoids suppress the production of tumour necrosis factor by lipopolysaccharide-stimulated human monocytes. Immunology 1988; 63:299–302.

163. Georas SN, Liu MC, Newman W, Beall WD, Stealey BA, Bochner BS. Altered adhesion molecule expression and endothelial activation accompany the recruitment of human granulocytes to the lung following segmental antigen challenge. Am J Respir Cell Mol Biol 1992; 7:261–269.

164. Begley CG, Lopez AF, Nicola NA, Warren DJ, Vadas MA, Sanderson CJ, Metcalf D. Purified colony-stimulating factors enhance the survival of human neutrophils and eosinophils in vitro: a rapid and sensitive microassay for colony-stimulating factors. Blood 1986; 68:162–166.

165. Ohnishi T, Kita H, Weiler D, Sur S, Sedgwick JB, Calhoun WJ, Busse WW, Abrams JS, Gleich GJ. IL-5 is the predominant eosinophil-active cytokine in the antigen-induced pulmonary late-phase reaction. Am Rev Respir Dis 1993; 147:901–907.

166. Owen WF Jr, Rothenberg ME, Petersen J, Weller PF, Silberstein D, Sheffer AL, Stevens RL, Soberman RJ, Austen KF. Interleukin 5 and phenotypically altered eosinophils in the blood of patients with the idiopathic hypereosinophilic syndrome. J Exp Med 1989; 170:343–348.

167. Owen WJ Jr, Petersen J, Shef DM, Fokerth RD, Anderson RJ, Corson JM, Sheffer AL, Austen KF. Hypodense eosinophils and interleukin 5 activity in the blood of patients with the eosinophilia-myalgia syndrome. Proc Natl Acad Sci USA 1990; 87:8647–8651.

168. Ohnishi T, Sur S, Collins DS, Fish JE, Gleich GJ, Peters SP: Eosinophil survival activity identified as interleukin-5 is associated with eosinophil recruitment and degranulation and lung injury twenty-four hours after segmental antigen lung challenge. J Allergy Clin Immunol 92:607–615, 1993.

169. Ohnishi T, Kita H, Mayeno AN, Sur S, Broide DH, Gleich GJ. Lidocaine in bronchoalveolar lavage fluid is an inhibitor of eosinophil-active cytokines. Clin Exp Immunol, in press.

170. Gleich GJ, Adolphson CR. The eosinophilic leukocyte: structure and function. Adv Immunol 1986; 39:177–253.

171. Djukanovic R, Roche WR, Wilson JW, Beasley CRW, Twentyman OP, Howarth PH, et al. State of the Art: mucosal inflammation in asthma (review). Am Rev Respir Dis 1990; 142:434–57.

172. Ohashi Y, Motojima S, Fukuda T, Makino S. Airway hyperresponsiveness, increased intercellular spaces of bronchial epithelium, and increased infiltration of eosinophils and lymphocytes in bronchial mucosa in asthma. Am Rev Respir Dis 1992; 145:1469–76.
173. Hunt LW, Swedlund HA, Gleich GJ. The effect of nebulized lidocaine on severe glucocorticoid-dependent asthma. Mayo Clin Proc, in press.

14

Cytokines and Growth Factors in Asthma

STEPHEN J. LANE, DAVID J. COUSINS, ANA R. SOUSA, DONTCHO Z. STAYNOV, and TAK H. LEE

UMDS
Guy's and St. Thomas' Hospitals
London, England

I. Introduction

The pathology of bronchial asthma demonstrates a multicellular process. Even in the mildest of cases, there is in vivo evidence for infiltration of the bronchial mucosa with mononuclear cells and granulocytes of which the eosinophil is prominent. In order to understand more fully the nature of the cellular infiltrate, it is critical to understand the regulation of the factors which cause these cells to be preferentially activated and recruited to the site of airway inflammation. Recent data suggests that the central role of bronchial inflammation in asthma is mediated in part by an increasing array of cytokines and growth factors of which interleukin-4 (IL-4), IL-5, and granulocyte-macrophage colony-stimulating factor (GM-CSF) are central. This chapter examines the evidence implicating cytokines in the pathogenesis of bronchial asthma, their pharmacological regulation by corticosteroids, and recent advances in their molecular regulation. In addition, the mechanisms contributing to failure to respond to corticosteroids are addressed.

II. What Are Cytokines and Growth Factors?

Cytokines are glycoprotein molecules which mediate and regulate the cell-cell communication of immune response (lymphokines and monokines), viral infections (interferons), inflammation, and hematopoeisis (colony-stimulating factors) (1). Molecular cloning of cytokine cDNAs in the 1980s has allowed the definitive identification of the structures and biological activities of individual cytokine molecules. Cytokines can act on many different cell types, are produced by diverse cell types, and have overlapping activities. They act in hormonal, autocrine, and paracrine fashions on sequentially expressed surface receptor molecules, and via linked second-messenger systems to effect specific gene transcription and thereby cellular responses; for example, differentiation and activation. Cytokines are synthesized transiently and are secreted rapidly, as needed. Cytokines function through a cytokine network rather than colinearly and can act as either positive or negative signals, depending on the target cell type. This network can be controlled either at the activation phase (when the production of cytokines is induced) or at the effector phase (when cytokines exert their functions through their receptors).

III. Criteria for Cytokine Involvement in Asthma

In order for a cytokine to be implicated in the pathogenesis of asthma its synthesis, storage, and/or secretion should be detectable in a relevant biological sample. Changes in these parameters should reflect the clinical expression of the disease either in response to challenge procedures in the laboratory, baseline airflow obstruction, and spontaneous clinical asthma, including responses to therapeutic interventions. In addition, the administration of the cytokine should mimic some component of the asthmatic response in vitro and subsequently in vivo in animal and human models of asthma. Finally, administration of a specific antagonist should reverse a component of the asthmatic response in the in vivo situation of spontaneous clinical asthma. Increasing numbers of cytokines and growth factors are being implicated to varying degrees in the pathogenesis of asthma and, although the evidence for some of these molecules is compelling, their central pathogenic role has yet to be confirmed. Based on our current knowledge of the pathogenesis of asthma, prime candidates are the cytokines IL-5, GM-CSF, and IL-4.

IV. Specific Cytokine Involvement in Asthma

A. GM-CSF

GM-CSF is produced from monocytes-macrophages, T cells, mast cells, eosinophils, and epithelial cells (2). It stimulates the proliferation and differentiation of normal granulocytic and monocytic stem cells and modulates the function of mature granulocytes leading to enhancement of the expression of CD11a, CD11b, and CD11c (3–5). GM-CSF induces histamine release from basophils and is chemotactic for and enhances eosinophil survival in culture (6–8). We have demonstrated that peripheral blood monocytes (PBMs) from atopic subjects generate an eosinophil viability–enhancing factor which is mainly accounted for by GM-CSF (9). In addition, we have observed that alveolar macrophage-derived GM-CSF primes eosinophils for enhanced leukotriene C_4 (LTC$_4$) generation in atopic asthmatic individuals (10). Thus, the presence of GM-CSF in the lung may precondition eosinophils for enhanced proinflammatory functions on subsequent stimulation and either alone or in concert with other cytokines may lead to eosinophil colony formation from bone marrow progenitors.

B. IL-5

IL-5 is produced from T cells, mast cells, and eosinophils, and, in addition to its action on eosinophils, IL-5 also promotes the differentiation of and is proinflammatory for basophils and is an important cofactor for IgE synthesis (11,12). Eosinophilic infiltration of the bronchial mucosa is characteristic of asthma. Early differentiation of eosinophil precursors depends on IL-3 and GM-CSF, and IL-5 produces terminal differentiation of the committed eosinophil precursors (13,14). All three cytokines activate mature eosinophils in terms of enhanced phagocytosis, increased secretion of proinflammatory molecules, and prolonged viability in culture (15–17). Unlike GM-CSF and IL-3, IL-5 is relatively specific in its action for eosinophils indicating that it may be a critical mediator in the asthmatic process. It is interesting that exogenous IL-5 applied topically to the upper airway mucosa was associated with eosinophilic infiltrate and increased histamine responsiveness. In addition, anti–IL-5 monoclonal antibodies blocked the eosinophilic response to parasitic infestation in mice and also inhibited lung eosinophilic infiltration in experimental animal antigen challenge models of asthma (18–20).

C. IL-4

IL-4 is produced by T cells, mast cells, and basophils, and it is an essential factor for IgE generation (21,22). The evidence is strongly suggestive that IgE plays a central role in the pathogenesis of atopic asthma. This evidence comes from epidemiological association, animal models, and in vitro studies. A complex array of cytokines is implicated in the control of IgE synthesis by B cells. Isotype switching to mature IgE transcripts in antigen-specific plasma cells is dependent on IL-4 and is enhanced by cognate and noncognate T-cell interaction, the local cytokine milieu (IL-5, IL-6, IL-13, tumor necrosis factor α [TNF-α]), hydrocortisone, Epstein-Barr virus, and activation of the CD40 B-cell receptor, whereas it is inhibited by γ–interferon (INF-γ) and IL-8

(12,23–25). Circulating IgE then binds to high- and low-affinity receptors on mast cells, basophils, platelets, and mononuclear cells priming them for subsequent activation on allergen exposure with the development of target organ inflammation. Human T cells are unable to differentiate into T-helper (TH) type 2 cells in the absence of IL-4 in the microenvironment. These data are strongly reinforced by the observation that mice with germline disruption of the IL-4 gene fail to generate TH2 cells and IgE in vivo (26). Whereas both IL-4 and IL-13 are able to exert switching signals on B cells for IgE production, the positive activity of IL-4 on the TH2 development is not shared by any other cytokine. The cellular source of IL-4 in the endogenous microenvironment of the lymphoid tissues, where the interaction between the antigen-presenting cells (APCs) allergen peptides, and the T cell occurs is unclear. It may be that IL-4 is produced by TH precursors or by a particular subset of T cells as can occur in the mouse; that is, the α-β T-cell receptor (TCR) positive CD4 CD8 double-negative, CD44$^+$ T cells (27). In addition, IL-4 may be produced by cells other than T cells. Human bone marrow non-B, non-T cells, belonging to mast cells and/or basophil lineages, when activated by anti-IgE antibodies could express mRNA for and produce IL-4 (28,29). In addition, human IgE synthesis in B cells has been induced in vitro by mast cells and basophils (29). Therefore, whether TH2 expansion occurs as a result of mast cell or basophil activation with subsequent IL-4 and IgE generation occurs or vice versa is a relevant question, as mast cells can be activated by IgE-independent mechanisms through complement receptors or via proteolytic enzymes as can occur in parasitic infestation. This situation, however, pertains to the atopic as well to the nonatopic state and does not explain the basal difference at the molecular level between these two groups; however, it may be important in the pathogenesis of parasitic infestation.

D. IL-1β and IL-1 Receptor Antagonists (IL-1ra)

Recent evidence for the existence of naturally occurring cytokine antagonists has added to the complexity of the cytokine network involved in the immunopathology of bronchial asthma. The IL-1 family consists of three structurally related polypeptides, that is, IL-1α, IL-1β, and IL-1ra, which inhibits the activities of both IL-1α and IL-1β by blocking the binding of IL-1 to its cell surface receptors but with no subsequent biological activity (30,31). The genes encoding these peptides have been localized to the long arm of chromosome 2 (32,33). The two forms of IL-1, IL-1α and IL-1β, are the product of separate genes. They have different amino acid sequences, but they are structurally related at the three-dimensional level, act through the same cell surface receptors, and share biological activities (34). Recombinant IL-1ra shows 26% amino acid sequence homology to human IL-1β and 19% homology to IL-1α. Also,

IL-1ra exhibits similar hydrophilicity plots. Thus, IL-1ra shows some structural similarity to the two described forms of IL-1. The degree of homology between IL-1α and IL-1β is similar to that between IL-1ra and the two other forms of IL-1 (35). IL-1α and IL-1β are produced by many different cell types, such as monocytes, tissue macrophages, alveolar macrophages, lymphocytes, smooth muscle, and endothelium (36–41). IL-1α and β act on most cells; among their most important functions in asthma are stimulation of granulocyte activity, B cell proliferation, and differentiation. They also activate T cells and stimulate their proliferation, activate endothelium and epithelium, and stimulate in vivo hematopoiesis (42–44). IL-1ra is produced mainly by monocytes, macrophages, neutrophils, fibroblasts, and keratinocytes (45–48). Although IL-1 and IL-1ra can be produced by the same cell, their expression is differentially regulated (32,49). This differential regulation will contribute to the balance of IL-1 and IL-1ra production during disease. Over 100 times excess of IL-1ra is needed to inhibit the action of IL-1 (50). Furthermore, only about 5% of IL-1 receptors need to be bound to IL-1 in order to give rise to a biological response.

It has been demonstrated that IL-1β directly contributes to the pathology of asthma (51). Intratracheal administration of IL-1β to Brown-Norway rats induces inflammatory changes which are characterized by an increase in neutrophil counts in the bronchoalveolar lavage (BAL) fluid and increased airway responsiveness to bradykinin. IL-1β expression on alveolar macrophages is upregulated with increased levels being detectable in the BAL from asthmatic individuals as compared with nonasthmatic control subjects, which correlates with clinical severity of the disease (52–54). There is also evidence involving IL-1ra in the pathology of bronchial asthma. Exposure of ovalbumin-sensitized guinea pigs to an aerosol of IL-1ra immediately before antigen challenge resulted in a marked protection against bronchial hyperreactivity and pulmonary eosinophil accumulation compared with IL-1ra vehicle pretreated animals (55).

E. Other Cytokines

Many other cytokines are being increasingly implicated in the pathogenesis of the asthmatic process, although their roles are less well defined. The monocyte chemoattractant peptide-1 (MCP-1) is produced by lymphocytes, monocytes, macrophages, endothelium, smooth muscle cells, and fibroblasts (56). It is a member of the low molecular weight chemokine family and is chemotactic for monocytes and eosinophils and is proinflammatory for basophils (57). MCP-1 is an 8- to 15-kDa basic peptide which is encoded by the human homologue of the mouse JE gene, the first platelet-derived growth factor (PDGF) early-response gene to be identified (56,57). It belongs to the IL-8 gene superfamily of small molecular weight cytokines known as chemokines. However, it belongs to the same subfamily as RANTES and MIP-1α and β, the C-C subfamily, which is distinct from the IL-1/NAP-1/C-X-C subfamily. MCP-1 is known to activate different inflammatory cells, such as monocytes, and can be produced by different cell types, including monocytes, macrophages, and pulmonary alveolar macrophages (58–64). In addition, interest has recently been focused on other members of this family; that is, IL-8 and RANTES, both of which are chemotactic for eosinophils.

The pathological changes of asthma include epithelial shedding, thickening of the reticular layer beneath the basal lamina of the epithelium, dilatation of the bronchial blood vessels, mucosal edema, submucosal gland edema, and smooth muscle hypertrophy and hyperplasia (65). In addition, there is thickening of the basement membrane and a cellular infiltrate of eosinophils and mononuclear cells in the bronchial mucosa (66). Increased levels of potent profibrogenic cytokines such as transforming growth factor β (TGF-β) and basic fibroblast growth factor (bFGF) have recently been described in bronchial biopsies from mildly symptomatic asthmatic subjects supporting the hypothesis that chronic release of these molecules may contribute to the structural changes seen in the airway wall in asthma (67).

V. T-Helper Cytokine Profile in Asthma

There is compelling evidence for the central role of activated CD4$^+$ T-helper cells in the pathogenesis of asthma. Examination of the cytokine profile generated by murine TH clones in vitro has shown that different clones produce different patterns of cytokines (68). These different patterns should have different functional effects, and so may determine the nature of the ensuing inflammatory response (69). At one extreme, the TH1 pattern was characterized by IL-2 and IFNγ production but with little or no IL-4 or IL-5 generation. Transfer of TH1 clones to donor mice produced delayed-type hypersensitivity reactions which were not seen with TH2 clones, and this could be blocked with antibodies to IFNγ (70,71). The TH2 clones, however, generated IL-4 and IL-5 with no IL-2 or IFN-γ. Both subsets produced GM-CSF and IL-3. TH1 products were poor at helping antibody synthesis in vitro, whereas TH2 products enhanced immunoglobulin synthesis leading to IgE generation (72).

TH1-like cell lines were subsequently isolated from animals infected with *Brucella abortus*, which produces a delayed-type hypersensitivity response, whereas TH2 cell lines dominated in animals parasitized with *Nippostrongylus brasiliensis*, which produces a pronounced eosinophilia and IgE response (73). The development of either a TH1 or TH2 pattern of cytokine synthesis by both murine and human T cells expanded in vitro is enhanced by IFN-γ or IL-4 in the culture medium, respectively, and TGF-β and PDGFβ inhibit TH2 cytokine production in the murine system (74–80). Therefore, different T cell cytokine responses determine the inflammatory response in animals. What is the relevance of this to bronchial asthma?

Initial analysis of human T-cell clones failed to show a TH1 or TH2 pattern, but it is now clear that certain antigens can direct a TH1 or TH2 response. Allergen-specific T-cell clones produce a preponderance of IL-4 and IL-5, but little IL-2 or IFN-γ, and might be expected to participate in IgE and eosinophilic responses in allergic disease. Such TH2-like clones have been derived from the conjunctiva of subjects with vernal conjunctivitis and the skin of subjects with atopic dermatitis (81–82). By in situ hybridization, the cells expressing mRNA for IL-3, IL-4, IL-5, and GM-CSF, but not IL-2 or IFN-γ, were detected after cutaneous and nasal allergen provocation, whereas IL-2 and IFN-γ mRNA-positive cells were predominant in the cutaneous tuberculin response (83–85). More recently, IL-2 and IFN-γ mRNA were detected in tuberculoid leprosy skin lesions by polymerase chain reaction (PCR) amplification, whereas IL-4 and IL-5 were present in lepromatous lesions, supporting the concept that the production of different patterns of cytokines may lead to different immunopathological responses in vivo (86).

It appears in the murine model that TH1 and TH2 lymphocytes have a common precursor, called TH0 cells, which produce both patterns of cytokines. Kamogawa and co-workers generated a transgenic mouse model which expressed the herpes simplex virus 1 (HSV-1) thymidine kinase gene under the transcriptional control of a murine IL-4 promoter (87). This rendered the IL-4–producing cells sensitive to the cytotoxic effects of the antiviral drug gancyclovir. Activation of transgenic T cells in the presence of gancyclovir eliminated IL-4 and IFN-γ production, demonstrating that IL-4 and IFN-γ–producing cells express IL-4 or have expressed IL-4 at one time. These results strongly suggest that effector cells producing either IL-4 or IFN-γ have a common precursor which expresses the IL-4 gene and that TH1 and TH2 cells in the murine model differentiate from a common precursor which can be termed TH0. In the human, however, indirect evidence suggests that this is not the case. When a human TH2 cell clone was treated with IL-12, it was shown to produce IFN-γ, which implies that IL-12 converts a TH2 cell to that of a TH0 or TH1 phenotype (88). This evidence indicates that, in the human, the pattern of TH1 and TH2 cytokine production may be determined by the local cytokine milieu rather than through an irreversible differentiation step per se.

VI. In Vivo Evidence for Cytokine Involvement in Asthma

Strong evidence implicating the role of cytokines and growth factors in the pathogenesis of bronchial asthma has been generated in the last few years from studies on the fluid and cellular components of bronchoalveolar lavage (BAL) and on airway histology obtained from asthmatic subjects in vivo. Using techniques of immunohistochemistry and in situ hybridization, these studies have demonstrated increased synthesis and storage of these molecules whose levels can be significantly altered in response to challenge procedures and therapeutic intervention. In addition, these changes in the expression of some of these molecules correlate with clinical symptoms.

A. Evidence from BAL

Using the techniques of in situ hybridization, Robinson et al. demonstrated increased proportions of cells positive for IL-4 and IL-5 mRNA in atopic asthmatic subjects (89,90). They subsequently showed that symptomatic asthmatic subjects had greater proportions of cells positive for IL-3, IL-4, IL-5, and GM-CSF mRNA in BAL fluid as compared with asymptomatic asthmatics (91). No differences between the groups in numbers of cells expressing IL-2 and IFN-γ mRNA were detected. In addition, they demonstrated significant associations between the number of cells expressing mRNA for IL-4, IL-5, and GM-CSF with baseline airflow obstruction, nonspecific bronchial hyperresponsiveness (BHR), and asthmatic symptoms. Further evidence comes from Broide et al., who demonstrated increased levels of TNF-α, GM-CSF, and IL-6 in the BAL fluid of symptomatic as compared with asymptomatic asthmatic subjects (92).

Evidence from challenge models of asthma further supports cytokine involvement in asthma. Increases have been shown in the number of cells expressing mRNA for the TH2 cytokines IL-4, IL-5, and GM-CSF but not IL-3, IL-2, or IFN-γ after allergen challenge as compared with diluent and the IL-4 and IL-5 mRNAs were associated with activated CD4$^+$ T cells (93,94). Furthermore, in a double-blind placebo-controlled study, it has been shown that a decrease in BHR in asthma after treatment with prednisolone orally for 2 weeks significantly correlated with a decrease in BAL eosinophilia, a reduction in the number of BAL cells expressing mRNA for IL-4 and IL-5, and an increase in cells expressing mRNA for IFN-γ (95).

B. Evidence from In Vivo Bronchial Histology

Using immunohistochemical analysis of bronchial biopsies obtained from 12 asthmatic and 12 normal subjects, we have shown upregulation of MCP-1 staining in the bronchial epithelium (96). Using hue saturation intensity (HSI) color image analysis in order to quantify the reactions of the monoclonal antibody in asthmatic biopsies, we have shown significant increases in the expression in the epithelium, whereas normal subjects were much less immunoreactive. Likewise, staining was increased in the subepithelium in asthmatic airway biopsies. The staining of the epithelium showed a significant negative correlation with the percentage of FEV_1 predicted, which supports its potential functional significance in asthma. MCP-1 is a potent chemoattractant and activating agent for monocytes. Expression in the bronchial epithelium can therefore be implicated in the accumulation of interepithelial macrophages and probably in the formation of macrophage-rich exudate that can be sampled in BAL. Furthermore, its production in the bronchial wall might assist in the activation of macrophages and in the degranulation and release of LTC_4 by basophils, thereby leading to increased inflammation and bronchospasm.

Immunohistochemical analysis of bronchial biopsies from symptomatic and asymptomatic atopic and nonatopic asthmatics revealed increased immunoreactivity with IL-1, IL-2, IL-3, IL-4, and IL-5, GM-CSF, and TNF-α as opposed to asymptomatic control subjects (97–99). It was interesting that tissue eosinophilia and BHR correlated with IL-5 immunoreactivity in the atopic subjects but with IL-2 and GM-CSF in the nonatopic asthmatics. In addition, supernatants from bronchial epithelial cells derived from asthmatic subjects cultured 48 hr in serum-free medium generated a chemotactic activity for T lymphocytes which was enhanced by the addition of histamine to the culture medium which was partly mediated by IL-8 (100). Residual chemotactic activity was mediated by a single protease-sensitive substance with an apparent molecular weight of 56 kDa and an estimated isoelectric point of 8.9–9.1. The partially purified chemoattractant specifically enhanced the migration of $CD4^+$ T lymphocytes, and its activity was inhibited by the univalent Fab fragment of a monoclonal antibody to CD4.

Bronchial biopsies from atopic asthmatic subjects obtained after allergen challenge demonstrated an increased influx of activated eosinophils and activated $CD4^+$ T cells and an increase in the number of cells expressing mRNA for IL-5 and GM-CSF (101). There was a significant inverse correlation between the numbers of cells expressing mRNA for IL-4 and IFN-γ. This supports the hypothesis that allergen-induced late asthmatic responses are accompanied by T-cell activation, cytokine mRNA expression for IL-5 and GM-CSF, and local recruitment and activation of eosinophils in the bronchial mucosa. In addition, Montefort et al. demonstrated that local endobronchial allergen installation leads to an increased inflammatory cell infiltrate of the airway mucosa that involved upregulation of intercellular adhesion molecule 1 (ICAM-1) and E-selectin expression in the microvasculature (102). Upregulation of these endothelial adhesion molecules was associated with a marked increase in the numbers of leukocytes expressing the β_2-integrin and leukocyte function antigen (LFA-1), which correlated with ICAM-1 expression, suggesting a mechanism for leukocyte recruitment.

C. In Vivo Pharmacological Modulation of Cytokine Expression in Asthma

Cytokine expression in bronchial biopsies correlates with response to therapeutic intervention. We have shown that asthmatic airway epithelial cells stain strongly for GM-CSF as compared with those from nonasthmatic control subjects. In addition, when these subjects are treated with inhaled beclomethasone, 1-mg daily for 8 weeks, or with matching placebo, there was a significant reduction in the expression of GM-CSF in the epithelium in the patients who were given corticosteroids, whereas the group of subjects who were given placebo showed no significant change in GM-CSF staining (103). There was a correlation between the percentage suppression of GM-CSF staining by inhaled corticosteroids and the percentage increase in FEV_1 and the percentage decrease in carbachol responsiveness. These findings suggest that GM-CSF plays a role in the inflammatory process of bronchial asthma and that the epithelial cells may be a target for drug action. These findings were also observed by Wang et al., who observed that after 4 months of treatment with inhaled beclomethasone dipropionate there was decreased expression of GM-CSF, IL-8, and activated eosinophils in the bronchial epithelium (104). The changes in GM-CSF and IL-8 expression correlated with the changes in eosinophil infiltration seen after treatment. These results further support the importance of GM-CSF in eosinophil activation in the epithelium in vivo and in the pathogenesis of BHR in mild asthma. In addition, they have shown increased expression of RANTES in bronchial biopsies from asthmatic subjects which was downregulated by treatment with beclomethasone in vivo (105). RANTES is produced by T cells, platelets, and epithelial cells (106) and is chemotactic for memory T cells and eosinophils. It is a member of the small cytokine superfamily which, in addition to IL-8 and MCP-1, is increased in bronchial epithelium in bronchial asthma.

In a study involving 12 normal and 18 asthmatic individuals, we have demonstrated increased expression of both IL-1β and IL-1ra in the asthmatic bronchial epithelium (107). The finding of elevated levels of IL-1ra in asthmatic bronchial epithelium suggests that antagonism to IL-1 is part of the host's natural response to disease. Disease might result in part from the failure to produce sufficient amounts of these physiological inhibitors. Furthermore, when asthmatic subjects are treated with inhaled beclomethasone, 1 mg daily for 8 weeks, or with matching placebo, there was a significant decrease in the percentage change in epithelial expression of IL-1β by beclomethasone but not of IL-1ra. These data suggest that beclomethasone may have an anti-inflammatory effect by preferentially inhibiting IL-1β epithelial expression without appreciable effect on Il-1ra.

Glucocorticoid therapy improves symptoms, reduces BHR, and improves lung function in asthma. Glucocorticoids are now widely used as first-line anti-inflammatory agents in asthma. The above in vitro and in vivo studies suggest that corticosteroids may act to inhibit cytokine production and thereby help to improve asthma (108–110). Cytokines have been detected in BAL fluid and cells and in bronchial biopsies from asthmatic subjects, and their levels correlate with baseline airflow obstruction, BHR, and symptom scores. In addition, the levels are increased after allergen challenge and correlate with an improvement in symptoms and lung function after therapeutic intervention with corticosteroids. As yet, this does not prove a cause and effect relationship; however, the evidence supporting their central role in asthma pathogenesis is compelling.

VII. Failure to Respond to Corticosteroid Therapy in Asthma: Relevance to Cytokine Networks

The airflow obstruction of the majority of patients with chronic and severe bronchial asthma will improve following treatment with corticosteroids. The mechanism of steroid action is unknown. One way in which the mechanism can be explored is to study a subgroup of patients in whom systemic or inhaled treatment with steroids, even when given in large doses, does not lead to any improvement in airflow obstruction. The asthma in such patients is usually severe, and they are seriously disabled for long periods of time. We have defined corticosteroid-resistant (CR) asthma as an improvement in FEV_1 of less than 15% after a 14-day course of 40-mg of prednisolone orally, whereas corticosteroid-sensitive (CS) asthma has been defined as an improvement of greater than 30% in FEV_1 after a similar course of prednisolone (111). CR asthma is associated with disease chronicity, a more frequent family history of asthma, and impaired in vitro responsiveness of peripheral blood mononuclear cells (PBMCs) to the suppressive effects of glucocorticoids (112–115). We have demonstrated in vitro defects in monocyte steroid responsiveness in CR asthmatics. In contrast to nonasthmatic controls, monocyte supernatants from asthmatic subjects generated a neutrophil-priming activity (NPA) which was selectively suppressed in vitro in a dose-dependent and rank-order fashion by corticosteroid treatment in the CS but not in the CR group (111,116,117). The degree of in vitro suppression by corticosteroids of NPA correlated significantly with in vivo airways responsiveness to oral prednisolone. In addition, we have demonstrated that the enhanced monocyte expression of the activation antigens, complement receptors 1 and 3, and class 2 molecules seen in bronchial asthma is suppressed by hydrocortisone in CS but not in CR asthmatic patients (114). Furthermore, we have provided evidence for an in vivo defect in the responsiveness of the macrophage–T cell interaction to the suppressive effects of corticosteroids in CR asthma and that resistance to glucocorticoids is not organ specific. The classic tuberculin-driven cell-mediated immune response was used to investigate the in vivo responsiveness of mononuclear cells to oral prednisolone in CS and CR asthma in a double-blind, crossover, placebo-controlled study (118). Prednisolone suppressed the cutaneous tuberculin response and infiltration of macrophages, eosinophils, and T-memory cells in the CS but not in the CR group. There was no significant suppression by prednisolone of the number of neutrophils, monocytes/immature macrophages, or adhesion molecules in either group.

Glucocorticoids mediate their effects through a soluble receptor protein that acts by transcriptionally regulating a small number of target genes (119,120). Glucocorticoids bind the cytoplasmic glucocorticoid receptor (GR) causing it to dephosphorylate, to dissociate two 90-kDa-associated heat shock proteins (hsps), to form dimers, and to translocate to the nucleus. When in the nucleus, the GR may interact with other transcription peptides at protein level, most notably AP-1, NF-κB, NF-κ, cyclic AMP response element binding protein and calreticulin, in order to suppress the increased gene transcription associated with these proinflammatory transcription factors (121–123). Alternatively, free GR may bind to sequences of DNA known as glucocorticoid-response elements (GREs) in the promoter regions of the glucocorticoid-responsive genes resulting in enhancement of gene transcription. The resultant effects on gene transcription depend critically on tissue-specific and activator-dependent interaction with *cis* elements present in the promoter regions of these genes. For example, IL-8 gene transcription is enhanced by phorbol myristate acetate (PMA; also known as 12-O-tetradecanoylphorbol-13-acetate [TPA]), IL-1β, and TNF-α by interaction with its minimal enhancer region at –94 to –71 base pair (bp) of the IL-8 promoter (124–126). Dexamethasone directly suppresses this activation through its GRE (–330 to –325 bp) in a fibrosarcoma cell line but by transcriptional interference with the NF-κB recognition site (–80 to –69 bp) in a glioblastoma cell line independently of the GRE. Several mechanisms have been shown to result in direct gene repression by glucocorticoids (120,121). First, the GR can neutralize the binding of a basal tissue-specific enhancer. Second, the GR can transcriptionally interfere with other transcription factors, and vice versa, at a protein-protein level. Third, the GR can displace other transcription factors at overlapping DNA binding sites. Resistance to glucocorticoids may occur at several levels (Fig. 1). These include (1) altered bioavailability of the administered drug; (2) a consistent polymorphism in one or more of the functional domains of the GR; (3) defective interaction between the GR and other transcriptional factors at the protein or DNA level; (4) impaired regulation of specific genes; and (5) abnormalities of as yet ill-defined local chromatin structure. We have shown that CR asthma is not due to altered bioavailability in CR patients or to impaired ligand binding and subsequent nuclear translocation of the GR (116,127). Using a gel retardation assay, we have demonstrated impaired binding of the GR to its GRE in CR patients. This defect is associated with decreased numbers of nuclear translocated GRs available for GRE binding, although their binding affinity is normal (128). We have provided evidence that the GR is structurally normal in these patients and have shown that this defect in CR asthma does not result from a consistent polymorphism in one or more of the functional domains of the GR cDNA (129). The fact that dexamethasone-GR binding experiments indicate normal quantities of nuclear translocated receptors and that GR-DNA binding assays indicate reduced numbers of structurally normal GRs available for GREs suggests transcriptional interference with the nuclear translocated GR and may indicate that transcriptional interference of GR-mediated repression of steroid-responsive genes is occurring at the protein-protein level or more distally at the protein-DNA level.

Glucocorticoids have different actions in different cell types which depend on the tissue-specific expression of steroid-responsive genes and on the presence or absence of inflammation in the tissue and on the state of cellular differentiation. Kam et al. have shown that a reversible decreased ligand binding affinity of the nuclear translocated GR, but not of the cytoplasmic GR, can be induced in vitro by CD4-positive lymphocytes derived from normal subjects by incubation with a combination of both IL-2 and IL-4 and can be reversed by serum deprivation for 48 hr (130). These data suggest that factors present in the nucleus inducible by IL-2 and IL-4 can interfere with the binding affinity of the nuclear translocated GR for its ligand which may affect the efficiency of subsequent gene transcription. In addition, we have demonstrated that the addition of lipopolysaccharide (LPS) to peripheral blood monocytes derived from CS asthmatic patients in culture decreased the subsequent responsiveness of NPA to dexamethasone suppression by 30-fold (116,117). This "inflammation-dependent" in vitro glucocorticoid resistance may give insights into why CR asthmatics are not clinically "Addisonian" in that the anti-inflammatory responsiveness of an individual to glucocorticoids may be determined locally at the site of inflammation and may depend on the relative concentrations of transcriptionally active molecules generated locally at the site of the inflammatory insult.

A putative transcription factor responsible for transcriptional interference with the GR in CR asthma is the proinflammatory AP-1 (119,121,131,132). AP-1 is the heterodimeric product of Fos and Jun proteins and is formed in activated cells by expression of the c-*fos* proto-oncogene. AP-1 binds to its DNA binding site (the TRE- or TPA-responsive element, TGACTCA) in order to effect gene transcription of certain proinflammatory peptides; for example, collagenase and α-fetoprotein. The induction of AP-1 is enhanced by the cytokines IL-2, TNF-α, TGF-β, and FGF, and PDGF, PMA, anti-CD3, LTB$_4$, and A23187. Its induction in human monocytes is suppressed by IL-4 and IFN-

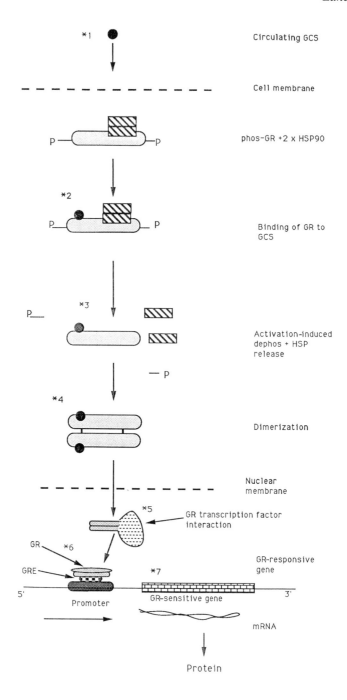

γ at the transcriptional and posttranscriptional levels, respectively (133–134). AP-1 and GR mutually repress each other's DNA binding and transactivating functions by (1) direct protein-protein interaction between amino acid residues $GR_{440-553}$ and Fos_{40-110} independently of DNA binding and (2) by AP-1–GR competition at mutually exclusive or overlapping DNA binding sites ("composite GRE") (121,131). It is interesting that AP-1, a central proinflammatory peptide, and GR, a central ligand-activated anti-inflammatory peptide, interact directly at these levels in order to reciprocally affect gene transcription. AP-1 is one of an increasing number of transcription factors which interfere with the GR at the protein-protein and protein-DNA levels. It is therefore likely that eventual gene transcription by the GR is affected by the ratio of interacting proinflammatory and anti-inflammatory transcription factors present in the nuclei of inflamed cells. We have shown that PMA fails to enhance AP-1/TRE binding in PBMCs as effectively in CR as opposed to CS patients (15 vs 115%, respectively) (128). In addition, dexamethasone fails to suppress PMA-induced AP-1/TRE binding as effectively in CR as opposed to CS patients (–25 vs. –52%, respectively), which may indicate that there are qualitative or quantitative defects of the Fos and/or Jun components of AP-1 or defects in their regulation in patients with CR asthma.

VIII.   Molecular Regulation of Cytokines in Bronchial Asthma

A.   GM-CSF and IL-5

The above in vivo studies have suggested that IL-5 and GM-CSF may be central to the mechanisms of airways eosinophilia in asthma and prompt an evaluation of the regulatory control of the production of these two molecules. The human GM-CSF and IL-5 genes are located on the long arm of chromosome 5 in a small segment (5q23) in close proximity with the genes of IL-3, IL-4, IL-13 (135–145), interferon regulatory factor 1 (IRF-1), and several as yet unidentified genes (146). There is a similar location of these genes on the mouse chromosome 11 (147–149). This suggests a common origin and/or some com-

---

Figure 1   Schematic representation of the mechanism of corticosteroid action. GCS, glucocorticosteroid, GR, glucocorticoid receptor protein; hsp, heat shock protein; p, phosphate group; GRE, glucocorticoid response element. Resistance to the anti-inflammatory actions of glucocorticoids may occur at the levels marked by the asterixes. *1, bioavailability; *2, ligand binding; *3, dephosphorylation and hsp release; *4, dimerization; *5, transcription factor interaction; *6, GR-DNA binding; *7, specific gene defect.

mon regulatory mechanisms of expression for these genes. Indeed, all these cytokines are expressed by the TH2-type lymphocytes, although some are also expressed by other cells. Some of them (IL-3, IL-5, and GM-CSF) share β chains of their corresponding receptors, which implies overlapping functions (150–152).

None of these genes is expressed in quiescent T cells, but they can be expressed after specific as well as nonspecific activation. Although GM-CSF can be expressed in blood mononuclear cells, purified T cells, monocytes, macrophages, fibroblasts, endothelial cells, and a number of cell lines, IL-5 is expressed only by some subsets of T cells, eosinophils, and mast cells (153–159).

Activation of T cells via the antigen receptor triggers sequential expression of a large number of genes for transcription factors (c-*fos*, c-*myc*, NF-AT, and NF-κB), cytokines (including IL-2, IL-3, IL-4, IL-5, and GM-CSF), and surface molecules (IL-2r, insulin receptor), and leads to the activation of the various biological functions of these cells (160). This activation proceeds via inositol trisphosphate, diacylglycerol, Ca^{2+} influx, and the protein kinase C (PKC) activation pathway and can be substituted by Ca^{2+} ionophore (A23187) and activators of PKC such as PMA (161–163). The chain of events that follow and the genes which are expressed in order to activate IL-5 and GM-CSF transcription remains to be identified.

IL-5 can also be activated by anti-CD3 antibody, IL-2, IL-4, phytohemagglutinin (PHA), and concanavalin A (ConA) (164–169). GM-CSF cannot be activated by IL-2 or IL-4 (165). Activation of both IL-5 and GM-CSF expression requires protein synthesis in T cells (165), whereas in mouse peritoneal macrophages, cycloheximide fails to inhibit GM-CSF production (170). Cyclosporin A (CsA) does not inhibit IL-5 expression in T cells (165). However, it does inhibit GM-CSF in T cells, mouse spleen cells, thymoma cells, and mast cell lines (159,171,172). Dexamethasone inhibits GM-CSF and IL-5 mRNA accumulation (170,173). Whether activated by αCD3 or PMA, GM-CSF and IL-5 display different time courses of expression (165,168). The regulation of GM-CSF is both transcriptional and posttranscriptional (169,174–176). There are no data on postranscriptional regulation of IL-5, and there is less likely to be any, because there are not conserved AU sequences in the 3′ untranslated region (UTR) of the mRNA (177).

Transient expression and in vitro transcription of reporter gene plasmids controlled by the GM-CSF promoter have identified several cis-acting sequences. Gasson and co-workers (178–180) identified two elements; one positive (from –47 to –29) element which is active in fibroblasts and T cells and one negative (from –188 to –174) element which is active in HTLV-1–infected T cells which constitutively produce several cytokines (including GM-CSF and IL-5). The function of the –47- to –29-bp element is tissue specific. It has no effect in nonproducers of GM-CSF (COS cells and adenovirus-transformed human kidney cell line 293) but is active in Jurkat cells and endothelial cells after activation with PHA and PMA. In human fibroblasts, PMA activation leads to increased GM-CSF transcription under the control of this element, whereas TNF-α and IL-1 activation of the GM-CSF expression is regulated postranscriptionally via the 3' untranslated region (UTR) of the mRNA. The −47 to −29 region contains a 15-bp sequence ATTAATCATTTCCTC 100% conserved between mouse and human GM-CSF which differs by only one nucleotide (underlined, T in IL-5) from a corresponding region in the IL-5 promoter. Shannon and co-workers (181,182) have identified two protein binding motifs. The first, cytokine-1 (CK-1, binds NF-GMa), is a 10-bp sequence GAGATTCCAC, −95 to −86 bp from the transcription initiation site. This element belongs to a very degenerate motif known as the lymphokine consensus sequence GRGRTTYCAY (where R is A or G and Y is T or C) which is found in the promoters of mouse and human IL-2, IL-3, IL-4, IL-5, and IFN-γ (183). In embryonic fibroblasts, they have shown that, in response to TNFα, NF-GMa binding is induced and that the CK-1 in the granulocyte colony–stimulating factor (G-CSF) gene is a TNF-α, but not PMA, responsive enhancer. The second element, cytokine-2 (CK-2, binds NF-GMb), is a 7-bp sequence TCAGGTA −82 to −76 bp from the transcription initiation site. Both of these elements were shown to bind specific nuclear proteins from cells able to produce GM-CSF (HUT78 and U5637 cells) whether or not they were stimulated to express GM-CSF. They were not present in cells which cannot express GM-CSF. This implies that these factors define tissue specificity and not an activation pathway. Using a transient transfection assay, Kaushansky (184) identified an additional positive regulatory element between −58 and −44 bp. This element was required for the upregulation of reporter gene expression in response to IL-1 in endothelial cells or ConA/PMA in T cells. No significant effect on transcriptional regulation was detected when the CK-1 element was deleted in either T cells or endothelial cells. Low-level reporter gene expression was seen in unstimulated cells of all types tested; however, this activity was abolished when the 3' UTR from GM-CSF was included in the construct. This supports the observations (170,174–176) that GM-CSF regulation is both transcriptional and postranscriptional.

The most extensive work on the GM-CSF promoter has been carried out by Arai and collaborators (185–190). They have used the mouse promoter (highly conserved between mouse and human GM-CSF) with the human T-cell line Jurkat in numerous transfection, in vitro transcription, footprinting, and gel retardation experiments. They have identified four *cis* elements responsible for efficient transcription. CLE1 (mouse −108 to −99, identical to human CK-1 −95 to −86), CLE2 (mouse −94 to −88, identical to human CK-2 −82 to −76), a GC box (mouse –84 to –73, corresponding to human –72 to –61) and CLE0 (mouse –54 to –40, corresponding to human –42 to –28). The CLE1 motif is required for induction of GM-CSF transcription by the p40^x transactivating protein (from HTLV-1) but has no effect on PMA/A23187 induction. Both the CLE2 and GC box motifs are required together for efficient activation by PMA/A23187 or p40^x. They have also shown that the region spanning CLE2/GC box contains two protein binding motifs, the GM2 sequence GGTAGTTCCC, which binds the PMA/A23187–inducible factor NF-GM2, and CCGCCC which binds constitutive factors A$_1$, A$_2$, and B. NF-GM2 appears to be NF-κB, or a very closely related factor, and A$_1$ appears to be Sp1. In the human sequence, the GM2 motif is identical to the mouse, but the GC box is CCGCCT; this C to T mutation may be important, since a mutation from C to A abolishes binding of all three constitutive factors and also causes loss of transcriptional inducibility. In addition to the CLE2/GC box domain, they have also identified the CLE0 element. This region is the same as that previously identified by Nimer et al. (179,180) and Heike et al. (191), who reported that it was required for PMA/A23187 induction of GM-CSF. Miyatake et al. (189) showed that this region binds two factors NF-CLE0a and NF-CLE0b, and that this complex is induced severalfold on activation with PMA/A23187. The recognition sequences of these factors overlap; NF-CLE0a binds TCATTTCC (human –37 to –30) and NF-CLE0b binds TTAATCAT (human –41 to –34). It would appear that NF-CLE0a plays a positive role in the induction of GM-CSF, whereas NF-CLE0b acts as a suppressor. Interestingly this CLE0 element is found very highly conserved in several genes, notably IL-4, IL-5, and G-CSF. The proteins NF-CLE0a and NF-CLE0b can bind to the CLE0 element from IL-5 and IL-4 but not G-CSF, which is not produced by T-cells. This suggests that the CLE0 element plays a role in the coordinate induction of these cytokines in T cells. However, the IL-5 CLE0 element, despite its very high homology to GM-CSF, binds NF-CLE0 weaker than the IL-4 CLE0, which is less homologous. Since this experiment was performed using nuclear proteins from Jurkat cells, which do not make IL-5, it implies that other factor(s) are also involved in this complex.

Using DNAse 1 footprinting and gel retardation assays, we have studied the transcription factors involved in the activation of IL-5 gene expression (192). We have found several cis-acting elements in the promoter region of the IL-5 gene: (1) a 15-nucleotide sequence ATTA_TTCATTTAATC. This sequence is fully conserved between mouse and human IL-5 and differs in only one nucleotide (underlined T) from GM-CSF. Although this sequence is not found in other genes it binds transcription factors found in many different cells; (2) AAGATCTTC, which is present with low homology in the promoter regions of many lymphokine genes; (3) GAGGAA, which binds transcription factors of the ets family and is different from the ets-1/ets-2 factors found in activated T cells.

The accumulated results are not sufficient to fully explain the complex mechanisms of expression of GM-CSF and IL-5. However, some conclusions can be drawn; (1) GM-CSF is expressed in a wide variety of differentiated and nondifferentiated cell types unlike IL-5, which is only expressed by a limited group of fully differentiated cells. In T cells, however, more stringent activation conditions are required for the expression of GM-CSF than for IL-5; (2) the regulation of GM-CSF in T cells and non–T cells occurs by different combinations of transcriptional and posttranscriptional controls; (3) in T cells there is at least one mechanism of IL-5 activation that is different to those of GM-CSF; (4) there are highly conserved motifs found in the promoters of IL-5 and GM-CSF, which suggests that there is a shared pathway of regulation. However, the IL-5 promoter does not contain a motif homologous to the CLE2/GC box, which implies that the PMA activation pathways may be different.

We have studied the levels of IL-5 and GM-CSF mRNA in PBMCs of a number of atopic and nonatopic individuals. In order to obtain quantitative results, we have developed a quantitative PCR analysis of the corresponding cDNAs (168). Activation of the cells with PMA (5 ng/ml) for 20 hr led to expression of high levels of IL-5 and GM-CSF mRNA. There was a marked difference between the levels of mRNA for both genes in some atopic patients as compared with nonatopic control subjects, suggesting that in some atopic patients IL-5 and GM-CSF may contribute to eosinophilia. There was a significant correlation between the levels of IL-5 and GM-CSF mRNA in activated cells.

Thus, high IL-5 producers are also high GM-CSF producers. Transcription of IL-5 and GM-CSF started about 3 hr after activation and increased well over 15 hr after which time it remained stable for another 24 hr. There was a small but significant lag period of 3 hr between the kinetics of GM-CSF and IL-5 mRNA levels, suggesting that the transcription of the two genes may be regulated by different mechanisms and that expression of GM-CSF may be required for the increase in the IL-5 mRNA level. In order to test the latter possibility, we incubated mononuclear cells in the presence of (1) GM-CSF for 3 and 20 hr, (2) GM-CSF and PMA for 2 and 20 hr; (3) anti–GM-CSF monoclonal antibody and PMA for 20 hr, and (4) PMA alone. IL-5 mRNA was not detected for up to 20 hr with rhGM-CSF alone. After 2 hr of activation with PMA, the presence of rhGM-CSF did not result in the appearance of IL-5 mRNA and the GM-CSF mRNA level was as weak as it was after activation with PMA alone. Finally, the presence of anti–GM-CSF antiserum did not inhibit PMA activation of either.

B. IL-4

In addition to IL-5 and GM-CSF, the gene coding for IL-4 is located on the long arm of chromosome 5 at band q23-31 and shares the common four-exon and three-intron structure. IL-4 is produced by TH2 cells, mast cells, and basophils and several potential mechanisms governing control of its expression have recently been described in murine and in human T cells. The transcription of the IL-4 gene is regulated by multiple promoter elements acting together after being bound by the correspondingly activated or newly synthesized transcription factors (193). Some cis-acting elements have now been located in the proximal promoter, the most important of which to date appears to be the 11-bp positive regulatory P sequence located at –79 to –69 bp from the transcription initiation site (TIS) (194). Other P sites have been described in the murine promoter and show high conversion with the known human sequence. The human and murine P sites are bound by family of transcription factors which are T-cell specific but not T-cell subset–specific, termed NF(P). A novel positive regulatory element, positive regulatory element 1 (PRE-1), which possesses a strong basal enhancing effect on gene transcription has been identified in the distal promoter of the human IL-4 gene at –239 to –224 bp from the TIS (195). PRE-1 is ubiquitous and is not restricted to T cells. It is bound by the two transcription factors, POS-1 and POS-2, and it is suppressed in a cis fashion by a T-cell–specific negative regulatory element (NRE) located 45 bp upstream of PRE-1. Two transcription factors, NEG-1 and NEG-2, bind to the NRE in order to effect repression of IL-4 gene transcription (195–197). Impairment of the function of this repressor element could lead to uncontrolled hyperactivity of the PRE and may be of importance in the overexpression of the IL-4 gene which can be seen in atopic subjects. As yet, there is no definite explanation for the restriction of IL-4 expression to human T cells, mast cells, and basophils. It is important to note that overexpression of IL-5 and GM-CSF also occurs in atopic disease states, indicating that impairment of a common regulating mechanism may be present in these subjects.

C. Mechanisms of Steroid Suppression

Cellular activation stimuli generate transcriptionally active molecules which increase proinflammatory cytokine gene expression and so contribute to the inflammation characteristic of bronchial asthma. It is becoming more apparent that glucocorticoids suppress cytokine gene expression by interference with the regulation of effector functions of these transcription factors which may differ from cytokine to cytokine. In order to understand how glucocorticoids act to suppress the transcription of a specific proinflammatory gene, it is important to determine what factors upregulate the expression of that gene. To date, there is no information available about the mechanisms by which corticosteroids act to suppress the transcription of the cytokines IL-4, IL-5, and GM-CSF. Potentially, the glucocorticoid receptor may alter transcription of these genes by interfering at a protein-protein level with any of the transcription factors described above. However, it is likely that the GR will interfere with the factors that bind to CLE0, since these proteins are very closely related to NF-AT, which contains AP-1, to which the GR is known to bind (198). Since this element is present in the promoters of all three cytokines and is involved in their coordinate activation, interference by the GR at this point would indeed downregulate their transcription. Another potential site of GR interference is the P sequence of the IL-4 promoter which also appears to interact with NF-AT or a closely related protein (195,199). The CLE2 region of the GM-CSF promoter binds to NF-κB, which has also been shown to interact with the GR, thus providing another route for glucocortcoid action on GM-CSF transcription (200). It is also possible that the GR may affect the novel double-palindromic element we have described and thus downregulate all three genes in a coordinated manner (201). The GR may also act to downregulate expression of the transcription factors required for cytokine production; for example, NF-AT. Unfortunately, since the genes for NF-AT$_c$ and NF-AT$_p$ were only recently cloned, it will be some time before these potential mechanisms of action are elucidated (202).

IX. Summary

It is becoming increasingly apparent that cytokines and growth factors are central to the inflammatory response seen in asthma. They are present in increased amounts in both BAL and in the airway epithelium and submucosa in spontaneous asthma. Their levels change after challenge procedures and therapeutic intervention and correlate significantly with symptom scores, baseline airflow obstruction, and BHR. GM-CSF, IL-5, and IL-4 are at present prime candidates and evidence supporting their central role in the pathogenesis of asthma is now compelling. However, recent evidence has implicated an increasing number of molecules such as MCP-1, RANTES, IL-8, TGF-β, and bFGF in the inflammatory process. It is now critical to understand the molecular regulation of these cytokines in order to determine whether common regulatory mechanisms exist which may be amenable to subsequent pharmacological manipulation.

Acknowledgment

This chapter was taken with permission from Proceedings of Topical Glucocorticoids in Asthma—Mechanisms and Clinical Actions. In: Lung Biology in Health and Diseases, Longboat Key, Florida, December 1994.

Discussion

DR. BUSSE: (1) Is there a parallel between the tissue expression of IL-1β and IL-1ra in asthma? If so, do you speculate that the increase in IL-1ra is a compensatory reaction to protect against the IL-1β effects? (2) In subjects treated with corticosteroids, is there a parallel fall in IL-1β and IL-1ra?

DR. LANE: (1) Asthmatic subjects show an increase in IL-1β and IL-ra in the bronchial epithelium. This may reflect an anti-inflammatory physiological attempt by the induction of IL-1ra in response to increased levels of IL-1 in asthma. (2) Expression of IL-1β in bronchial epithelium decreases in all of the asthmatic subjects studied. It is interesting that only three of these asthmatic subjects showed reduction by steroids in IL-1ra expression. This heterogeneity of response of IL-1RA to glucocorticoids in some asthmatics may be clinically relevant in terms of disease severity or response to therapeutic intervention and may reflect an inflammatory/anti-inflammatory imbalance in these subjects. There is a correlation between IL-1β and IL-1ra expression in the bronchial epithelium in asthmatic subjects.

DR. THOMPSON: (1) There have been a few reports of accessory proteins which cooperate in GR : DNA binding. One accessory protein is approximately 130,000 M_r and another quite small—a few thousand daltons. Have you tested for such factors in your patients showing decreased GR and GRE binding? (2) Historically, your resistant patients have the same GR concentration as sensitive patients. From that, one would conclude the decreased GR and GRE binding you describe is not due to decreased GR content of your cell extracts. But have you carried out GR and ligand binding and GR and DNA binding in parallel on preparations from resistant patients?

DR. LANE: Binding analysis of the reduced glucocorticoid-resistant and GRE interaction in GR asthma indicate that reduced numbers of GR are effectively available for GRE interaction. In the presence of a structurally normal GR, this would indicate transcriptional interference of the GR and GRE interaction. To date, we do not know how this transcriptional interference is occurring and what contribution known or novel transcriptionally active molecules are making. This experiment is of critical importance. The GR-ligand binding experiments were not carried out in parallel preparations.

DR. O'BYRNE: (1) Glucocorticoid-induced inhibition of GM-CSF is modest compared with GM-CSF staining. Please comment. (2) Did you correlate GM-CSF inhibition with eosinophil infiltration?

DR. LANE: (1) GM-CSF is important in asthma in vivo, as it is detectable in a relevant biological sample, that is, the airway epithelium and submucosa, in increased amounts as compared with nonasthmatic controls. In addition, changes in its expression reflect a clinical expression of the disease in that they correlate with improvement in bronchial hyperresponsiveness and changes in FEV_1 to 8 weeks of treatment with inhaled BDP, 1 mg/BD. The magnitude of its involvement is not yet possible to quantitate as GM-CSF has not been administered in vivo in an animal model of asthma or in the laboratory in human subjects. In addition, a specific antagonist is not available at the present time. (2) In this study, we did not correlate the extent of GM-CSF inhibition by glucocorticoids with eosinophil infiltration.

DR. GAULDIE: (1) You have shown staining in epithelium for IL-1β and IL-1ra. Does the epithelium make both of these? (2) Do you have in vitro evidence for IL-1 production by epithelium? Is it secreted or released?

DR. LANE: (1 and 2) Cultured epithelial cells from patients with asthma generate IL-1α, IL-1β, IL-6, IL-8, and GM-CSF, mRNA, and protein. To my knowledge, it is not known whether cultured epithelial cells secrete IL-1ra. We can extrapolate from these in vitro data that the increase in IL-1 staining of the bronchial epithelium in vivo is indeed coming from the epithelial cells, although this would really need to be confirmed by demonstrating mRNA with in situ hybridization.

DR. SMALDONE: (1) Clinically, were the asthmatics symptomatic at the time of biopsy? (2) Did you differentiate between atopic and nonatopic asthmatic patients?

DR. LANE: (1) These patients were mild asthmatic subjects clinically and on the basis of the baseline FEV_1 and carbachol responsiveness. (2) All the subjects studied were atopic.

DR. HARGREAVE: How disease-specific is the cytokine staining pattern you observed?

DR. LANE: These cytokines are important in asthma, because changes in their expression reflect clinical expression of disease in response to challenge procedures in the laboratory, baseline airflow obstruction, and response in FEV_1 to glucocorticoid therapy. This would indicate specificity for the asthmatic process.

DR. GLEICH: *Comment* 1: During analyses of eosinophil-active cytokines, we have been impressed by the occurrence of IL-5 and GM-CSF in BAL fluids (from allergic patients undergoing antigen challenge and from eosinophilic pneumonitis) and in skin blisters in several eosinophil-associated diseases. In contrast, IL-5 is usually present in the blood in the absence of GM-CSF. *Comment* 2: A caveat regarding occurrence of GM-CSF from PBMCs in culture:

One must be very careful to exclude LPS, which will strikingly increase macrophage GM-CSF production.

DR. LANE: (1) We have not measured GM-CSF in the peripheral blood. Our studies on atopic asthmatic subjects with eosinophilia have shown that cultured peripheral blood monocyte supernatants from asthmatic subjects enhance eosinophil viability secondary to GM-CSF. In addition, we have shown that alveolar macrophages from asthmatic subjects are proinflammatory for eosinophils, which is mediated in large part by GM-CSF

DR. DENBURG: (1) How much staining for GM-CSF is due to cells other than macrophages and epithelial cells? Other cells, for example eosinophils, produce GM-CSF (I Ohno, R Lea, S Finotto, et al. Granulocyte/macrophage colony-stimulating factor [GM-CSF] gene expression by eosinophils in nasal polyposis. Am J Respir Cell Molec Biol 1991; 5:505–510.) (2) After inhaled corticosteroids, which cells are most responsible for the decrease in GM-CSF immunostaining?

DR. LANE: We have not looked at double staining for macrophages and GM-CSF in the submucosa before and after steroids. (2) The majority of GM-CSF–secreting cells were macrophages on the basis of double immunostaining. We did not double stain after steroid therapy.

DR. HERSCHMAN: (1) Regarding the GR-resistance model, in the time course studies of GR-GRE binding, what is the time frame involved? Was this concluded from gel shifts? (2) Did you look in cell extracts for a GR inhibitor?

DR. LANE: (1) In these studies, peripheral blood monocytes were extracted from steroid-sensitive and steroid-resistant subjects and cultured for 60 min in the presence or absence of dexamethasone. Cells were taken at different intervals, the reaction stopped, and nuclear protein extracted and quantitated by Bradford assay and used for the gel shift assay with double-stranded radiolabeled GRE. (2) This is a critical experiment which we are currently addressing.

DR. LEUNG: (1) Can you clarify in your 60-min incubation experiments of steroid-resistant cells whether the GRE binding abnormalities were induced only in the presence of dexamethasone? (2) Although your data using chemical mutation analysis of glucocorticoid receptor cDNA indicate normal DNA sequences, can you rule out the possibility that an alternatively spliced glucocorticoid receptor is generated which may alter DNA receptor binding?

DR. LANE: (1) In our studies of GR and GRE binding, we have found that there is basal GR and GRE binding. Our values are in response to coincubation with dexamethasone and are presented as percentage increase from baseline. No differences were detected between the two groups in terms of baseline values. (2) If there was a defect of alternate splicing of glucocorticoid receptor, this would be reflected by changes at the RNA level. We have performed chemical mutational analysis of glucocorticoid receptor from six corticosteroid-resistant subjects and have found no base pair differences from wild-type control cDNA. In addition, we have found no differences in steroid-sensitive subjects.

DR. DURHAM: By use of in situ hybridization, Dr. Chris Corrigan has shown an increase in GM-CSF mRNA-positive peripheral blood mononuclear cells from asthmatic children versus controls which is inhibitable by inhaled treatment with corticosteroids. (V Gemou-Engesaeth, Q. Hamid, A Bush, et al. Elevated expression of Th2-type cytokine mRNA in peripheral blood mononuclear cells [PBMC] from child asthmatics: effect of inhaled glucocorticoid therapy (abstr.). J Allergy Clin Immunol 1995; 95:366.). Immunomagnetic separation (positive selection) has shown CD4$^+$ T lymphocytes (not CD8$^+$ cells) as the source of GM-CSF mRNA. GM-CSF expression at the protein level has also been confirmed by increased eosinophil survival-promoting activity of CD4$^+$ cell supernatants which is inhibitable selectively by monoclonal antibody against GM-CSF.

DR. SCHLEIMER: Drs. Leung and Szefler and their colleagues have shown that glucocorticoid resistance can be acquired or induced by exposure of cells to certain cytokines. Can you please comment on how such an induced resistance (presumably resulting from competition at the GR/transcription factor level) may have influenced your findings?

DR. LANE: The concept of inducibility or reversibility by cytokines and serum deprivation is very interesting and indeed Dr. Leung's work indicates that there may be heterogeneity in steroid-resistant subjects. In our neutrophil priming assay, we have shown that addition of LPS to cultured monocytes in steroid-sensitive individuals decreases the steroid responsiveness of neutrophil priming activity (NPA) and so can induce a degree of steroid resistance. This phenomenon may be important in the clinical area of steroid-dependent asthma, which is more likely to be a secondary phenomenon as a consequence of a more severe disease phenotype, rather than in steroid resistance, which is more likely to represent a primary phenomenon.

DR. SEVERINSEN: How was it determined that the amount of glucocorticoid receptor was the same in steroid-resistant and steroid-sensitive patients? A difference in the amount of receptor could potentially explain the lack of GRE binding in cells from steroid-resistant patients?

DR. LANE: We have not detected defects in dexamethasone binding or in nuclear translocation of the activated glucocorticoid receptor complex in unstimulated peripheral blood monocytes derived from steroid-resistant asthmatics. In addition, receptor density was similar to corticosteroid-sensitive controls. This would be unexpected as one would expect defects in ligand binding to be reflected in biochemical evidence of end-organ steroid resistance as in the familial cortisol-resistant syndrome. In addition, using chemical mutational analysis, we have failed to detect differences of glucocorticoid receptor at the RNA level in these subjects.

DR. PERSSON: Do you have any information on effects of steroids on GM-CSF in patients with steroid-resistant asthma as compared with normal asthmatics?

DR. LANE: We have shown no differences between CS and corticosteroid-resistant subjects in GM-CSF expression at the mRNA level by Northern analysis or at the protein level by ELISA in response to glucocorticoids in peripheral blood monocytes unstimulated or stimulated with LPS.

References

1. Masuda ES, Naito Y, Arai K et al. Expression of lymphokine genes in T cells. Immunologist 1993; 198–203.
2. Nicola NA, Metcalf M, Johnson GR, Burgess AW. Separation of functionally distinct human granulocyte-macrophage colony-stimulating factor. Blood 1979; 54:614–627.
3. Kapp A, Zeck-Kapp G, Donner M, et al. Human granulocyte-macrophage colony stimulating factor: an effective direct activator of human polymorphonuclear neutrophilic granulocytes. J Invest Dermatol 1988; 91:49–55.
4. Morrisey PJ, Bressler L, Park LS, et al. Granulocyte macrophage colony stimulating factor augments the primary antibody response by enhancing the function of antigen presenting cells. J Immunol 139:1113–1119.
5. Sullivan R, Griffin JD, Simons ER, et al. Effects of recombinant human granulocyte and macrophage colony-stimulating factor on signal transduction pathways in human granulocytes. J Immunol 1987; 139:3422–3430.
6. Haak-Frendscho M, Arai K-I et al. Human recombinant granulocyte-macrophage colony stimulating factor and interleukin 3 cause basophil histamine release. J Clin Invest 1988; 82:17–19.
7. Lopez AF, Williamson DJ, Gamble JR, et al. Recombinant human granulocyte-macrophage colony-stimulating factor stimulates in vitro mature human neutrophil and eosinophil function, surface receptor expression and survival. J Clin Invest 1986; 78:1220–1228.
8. Owen WF, Rothenberg ME, Silberstein DR, et al. Regulation of human eosinophil viability, density and function by granulocyte/macrophage colony-stimulating factor in the presence of 3T3 fibroblasts. J Exp Med 1987; 166:129–141.
9. Burke LA, Hallsworth MP, Litchfield TM, et al. Identification of the major activity derived from cultured human peripheral blood mononuclear cells, which

enhances eosinophil viability, as granulocyte-macrophage colony-stimulating factor (GM-CSF). J Allergy Clin Immunol 1991; 2:226–235.

10. Howell CJ, Pujol JL, Crea AEG, et al. Indentification of an alveolar macrophage-derived activity in bronchial asthma which enhanced leukotriene C4 generation by human eosinophils stimulated by ionophore (A23187) as granulocyte-macrophage colony-stimulating factor (GM-CSF). Am Rev Respir Dis 1987; 140:1340–1347.

11. Campbell HD, Tucker WQJ, Hort Y, et al. Molecular cloning, nucleotide sequence, and expression of the gene encoding human eosinophil differentiation factor (interleukin 5). Proc Natl. Acad Sci USA 1987; 84:6629–6623.

12. Pene J, Rousset F, Briere F, et al. Interleukin 5 enhances interleukin 4-induced IgE production by normal human B cells. The role of soluble CD23 antigen. Eur J Immunol 1988; 18:929–935.

13. Saito H, Hatake K, Dvorak AM, et al. Selective differentiation and proliferation of haematopoietic cells induced by recombinant human interleukins. Proc Natl Acad Sci USA 1988; 85:2288–2292.

14. Walsh GM, Hartnell A, Wardlaw AJ, et al. IL-5 enhances the *in vitro* adhesion of human eosinophils, but not neutrophils, in a leucocyte integrin (CD11/18)-dependent manner. Immunology 1990; 71:258–265.

15. Lopez AF, Sanderson CJ, Gamble JR, et al. Recombinant human interleukin 5 is a selective activator of human eosinophil function. J Exp Med 1988; 167:219–224.

16. Sehmi R, Wardlaw AJ, Cromwell O, et al. Interleukin-5 selectively enhances thechemotactic response of eosinophils obtained from normal but not eosinophilic subjects. Blood 1992; 79:2952–2959.

17. Warrings RAJ, Koenderman L, Kok PTM, et al. Modulation and induction of eosinophi chemotaxis by granulocyte-macrophage colony-stimulating factor and interleukin-3. Blood 1991; 77:2694–2700.

18. Coffman RL, Seymour BWP, Hudak S, et al. Antibody to interleukin-5 inhibits helminth-induced eosinophilia in mice. Science 1989; 245:308–310.

19. Gulbenkian AR, Egan RW, Fernandez X, et al. Interleukin-5 modulates eosinophil accumulation in allergic guinea-pig lung. Am Rev Respir Dis 1992; 146:263–265.

20. Robinson DS, Durham R, Kay AB. Cytokines in asthma. Thorax 1993: (48):845–853.

21. Geha RS. Regulation of IgE synthesis in humans. J Allergy Clin Immunol 1992; 90:143–150.

22. Schroeder JT, MacGlashan DW, Kagey-Sobotka A, et al. IgE-dependent IL-4 secretion by human basophils. The relationship between cytokine production and histamine release in mixed leukocyte cultures. J Immunol 1994; 153:1808–1817.

23. Del Prete G, Maggi E, Parronchi P, et al. IL-4 is an essential factor for the IgE synthesis induced *in vitro* by human T cell clones and their supernatants. J Immunol 1988; 140:4193–4198.

24. Vercelli D, Jabara HH, Arai K, et al. Endogenous IL-6 plays an obligatory role in the IL-4-induced human IgE synthesis. Eur J Immunol 1989; 19:1419–1424.

25. Kimata H, Yoshida A, Ishioka C, et al. Interleukin 8 (IL-8) selectively inhibits

immunoglobulin E production induced by IL-4 in human B cells. J Exp Med 1992; 176:1227–1231.

26. Kopf M, Le Gros G, Bachmann M, et al. Disruption of the murine IL-4 gene blocks Th2 cytokine responses. Nature 1993; 362:245–248.

27. Zlotnik A, Godfrey DI, Fischer M, et al. Cytokine production by mature and immature CD4-CD8 T cells. J Immunol 1992; 149:1211–1215.

28. Piccinni MP, Macchia D, Parronchi P, et al. Human bone marrow non-B, non-T cells produce IL-4 in response to cross-linkage of FC_ϵ and FC_γ treceptor. Proc Natl Acad Sci USA 1991; 88:8656–8660.

29. Brunner T, Heusser CH, Dahinden CA. Human peripheral blood basophils primed by interleukin 3 (IL-3) produce IL-4 in response to IgE receptor stimulation. J Exp Med 1993; 177:605–611.

30. Arend WP. Interleukin 1 receptor antagonist: anew member of the interleukin 1 family. J Clin Invest 1991; 88:1445–1451.

31. Dinarello CA, Thompson RC. Blocking IL-1: Interleukin 1 receptor antagonist in vivo and in vitro. Immunol Today 1991; 12:404–410.

32. Arend WP. interleukin-1 receptor antagonist. Adv Immunol 1993; 54:167–227.

33. Patterson D, Jones C, Hart I, et al. The human interleukin-1 receptor antagonist (IL-1RN) gene is located in chromosome 2q14 region. Genomics 1993; 15:173–176.

34. Dinarello CA. Interleukin-1 and interleukin-1 antagonism. Blood 1991; 77:1627–1652.

35. Steinkasserer A, Solari R, Mott HR, et al. Human interleukin-1 receptor antagonist. High yield expression in E. coli and examination of cysteine residues. FEBS Lett 1992; 310:63–65.

36. Bailly S, Fay M, Ferrua B, et al. Comparative production of IL-1β and Il-1α by LPS-stimulated human monocytes: Elisas measurements revisited. Cytokine 1994; 6:111–115.

37. Ackerman V, Marini M, Vittori E, et al. Detection of cytokines and their cell sources in bronchial biopsy specimens from asthmatic patients. Relationship to atopic status, symptoms, and level of airway hyperresponsiveness. Chest 1994; 105:687–696.

38. Simon PL, and Willoughby WF. The role of subcellular factors in pulmonary immune function: physicochemical characterisation of two distinct species of lymphocyte-activating factor produced by rabbit alveolar macrophages. J Immunol 1981; 126:1534–1541.

39. Tartakovsky B, Kovacs B, Takacs L, et al. T cell clone producing an IL-1 like activity after stimulation by antigen-presenting B cells. J Immunol 1986; 137:160–166.

40. Matsushima K, Procopio A, Abe H, et al. Production of interleukin 1 activity by normal human peripheral blood B lymphocytes. J Immunol 1985; 135:1132–1136.

41. Libby P, Ordovas JM, Birinyi LK, et al. Inducible interleukin-1 gene expression in human vascular smooth muscle cells. J Clin Invest 1986; 78:1432–1438.

42. Oppenheim JJ, Kovacs EJ, Matsushima K, et al. There is more than one interleukin 1. Immunol Today 1986; 7:45–56.

43. Weaver CT, Unanue ER. The costimulatory function of antigen-presenting cells. Immunol Today 1990; 11:49–54.
44. Tosi MF, Staark JM, Smith CW, et al. Induction of ICAM-1 expression on human airway epithelial cells by inflammatory cytokines: effects on neutrophil-epithelial cell adhesion. Am J Respir Cell Mol Biol 1992; 7:214–221.
45. Janson RW, Hance KR, and Arend WP. Production of IL-1 receptor antagonist by human in vitro-derived macrophages. Effects of lipopolysaccharides and granulocyte-macrophage colony-stimulating factor. J Immunol 1991; 147:4218.
46. Galve-De Rochemonteix B, Nicod LP, Junod AF, et al. Characterization of a specific 20- to 25-KD interleukin-1 inhibitor from cultured human lung macrophages. Am J Respir Cell Mol Biol 1990; 3:355–361.
47. McColl SR, Paquin R, Menard C, et al. Human neutrophils produce high levels of the interleukin 1 receptor antagonist in response to granulocyte/macrophage colony-stimulating factor and tumor necrosis factorα. J Exp Med 1992; 176:593–598.
48. Chan LS, Hammerberg C, Kan K, et al. Human dermal fibroblast interleukin-1 receptor antagonist (IL-1ra) and interleukin IL-1β mRNA and protein are co-stimulated by phorbol eater: implication for homeostatic mechanism. J Invest Dermatol 1992; 99:315–322.
49. Dinarello C, Wolff SM. The role of interleukin-1 in disease. N Engl J Med 1993; 328:106–113.
50. Carter DB, Deibel Jr MR, Dunn CJ, et al. Purification, cloning, expression, and biological characterization of an interleukin-1 receptor antagonist. Nature 1990; 344:633–637.
51. Tsukagoshi H, Sakamoto T, Xu W, et al. Effect of interleukin-1β on airway hyperresponsiveness and inflammation in sensitized and nonsensitized Brown Norway rats. J Allergy Clin Immunol 1994; 93:464–469.
52. Pujol JL, Cosso B, Daures JP, et al. Interleukin-1 release by alveolar macrophages in asthmatic patients and healthy subjects. Int Arch Allergy Appl Immunol 1990; 91:207–210.
53. Mattoli S, Mattoso VL, Soloperto M, et al. Cellular and biochemical characteristics of bronchoalveolar lavage fluid in symptomatic nonallergic asthma. J Allergy Clin Immunol 1991; 87794–802.
54. Broide DH, Lotz M, Cuomo AJ, et al. Cytokines in symptomatic asthma airways. J Allergy Clin Immunol 1992; 89:958–967.
55. Watson ML, Smith D, Bourne AD, et al. Cytokines contribute to airway dysfunction in antigen-challenged Guinea pigs: inhibition of airway hyperreactivity, pulmonary eosinophil accumulation, and tumour necrosis factor generation by pretreatment with an interleukin-1 receptor antagonist. Am J Respir Cell Mol Biol 1993; 8:365–369.
56. Leonard EJ, Yoshimura T. Human monocyte chemoattractant protein-1 (MCP-1). Immunol Today 1990; 11:97–101.
57. Rollins BJ, Walz A, Baggioline M. Recombinant human MCP-1/JE induces chemotaxis, calcium flux, and the respiratory burst in human monocytes. Blood 1991; 78:1112–1116.

58. Jiang B, Beller DI, Frendl G, et al. Monocyte chemoattractant protein-1 regulates adhesion molecule expression and cytokine production in human monocytes. J Immunol 1992; 148:2423–2428.
59. Yoshimura T, Yunk N, Moore SK, et al. Human monocyte chemoattractant factor-1 (MCP-1). Full length cDNA cloning, expression in mitogen-stimulated blood mononuclear leukocytes, and sequence similarities to mouse competence gene JE. FEBS Lett 1989; 244:487–493.
60. Colotta F, Borre A, Wang JM, et al. Expression of monocyte chemotactic cytokine by human mononuclear phagocytes. J Immunol 1992; 148:760–765.
61. Martin CA, Dorf ME. Differential regulation of interleukin-6, macrophage inflammatory protein-1 and JE/MCP-1 cytokine expression in macrophage cell lines. Cell Immunol 1991; 135:245–258.
62. Antoniades HN, Neville-Golden J, Galanopoulos T, et al. Expression of monocyte chemoattractant protein-1 mRNA in human idiopathic pulmonary fibrosis. Proc Natl Acad Sci USA 1992; 89:5371–5375.
63. Brieland JK, Jones ML, Clarke SJ, et al. Effect of acute inflammatory lung injury on the expression of monocyte chemoattractant protein-1 (MCP-1) in rat pulmonary alveolar macrophages. Am J Respir Cell Mol Biol 1992; 7:134–139.
64. Denholm EM, Wolber FM, Phan SH. Secretion of monocyte chemotactic activity by alveolar macrophages. Am J Pathol 1989; 135:571–580.
65. Jeffrey PK, Wardlaw AJ, Nelson FC, et al. Bronchial biopsies in asthma: An ultrastructural, quantitative study and correlation with hypereactivity. Am Rev Respir Dis 1989; 140:1745–1753.
66. Jeffrey PK, Godfrey RW, Adelroth E, et al. Effects of treatment on airway inflammation and thickening of basement membrane reticular collagen in asthma. A quantiative light and electron microscopic study. Am Rev Respir Dis 1992; 145:890–899.
67. Redington AE, Madden J, Frew AJ, et al. Basic fibroblast growth factor in asthma: immunolocalization in bronchial biopsies and measurement in bronchoalveolar lavage fluid at baseline and following allergen challenge. Am J Respir Crit Care Med 1995; 151:A702.
68. Mosmann TR, Coffan RL. Two types of mouse helper T-cell clone. Implications for immune regulation. Immunol Today 1987; 8:223–227.
69. Mosmann TR, Coffan RL. T_{h1} and T_{h2} cells: different patterns of lymphokine secretion lead to different functional properties. Annu Rev Immunol 1989; 7:145–173.
70. Cher DJ, Mosman TR. Two types of murine helper T cell clone II. Delayed type hypersensitivity is mediated by T_{h1} clones. J Immunol 1987; 138:3688–3694.
71. Fong TAT, Mosman TR. The role of IFN_γ in delayed type hypersensitivity is mediated by T_{h1} clones. J Immunol 1989; 143:2887–2893.
72. Stevens TK, Bossie A, Sanders VM, et al. Regulation of antibody isotype secretion by subsets of antigen-specific helper T cells. Nature 1988; 334:255–258.
73. Street NE, Schumacher JH, Fong TAT, et al. Heterogeneity of mouse helper T cells: evidence from bulk culture and limiting dilution cloning for precursors of Th1 and Th2 cells. J Immunol 1990; 144:1629–1639.

74. Coffman RL, Varkila K, Scott P, et al. Role of cytokines in the differentiation of CD4+ subsets in vivo. Immunol Rev 1991; 123:189–207.

75. Swain SL, Weinberg AD, English M, et al. IL-4 directs the development of T_{h2}-like effectors. J Immunol 1990; 145:3796–3806.

76. Gajewski TF, Fitch FW. Anti-proliferative effect of IFN_γ in immune regulation. III. Differential selection of T_{h1} and T_{h2} murine T helper T lymphocyte clones using recombinant IL-2 and IFN_γ. J Immunol 1988; 143:15–22.

77. Maggi E, Parronchi P, Manetti R, et al. Reciprocal regulatory effects of IFN and IL-4 on the *in vitro* development of human T_{h1} and T_{h2} clones. J Immunol 1992; 148:2142–2147.

78. Paliard X, de Waal Malefijt R, Yssel H, et al. Simultaneous production of IL-2, IL-4 and IFN_γ by activated human CD4$^+$ and CD8$^+$ T cell clones. J Immunol 1988; 141:849–855.

79. Wierenga EA, Snock M, de Groot C, et al. Evidence for compartmentalization of functional subsets of CD4$^+$ T lymphocytes in atopic patients. J Immunol 1990; 144:4651–4656.

80. Swain SL, Huston G, Tonkonogy S, et al. Transforming growth factor beta and IL-4 cause helper T cell precursors to develop into distinct effector helper cell that differ in lymphokine secretion pattern and cell surface phenotype. J Immunol 1991; 147:2991–3000.

81. Maggi E, Biswas P, Del Prete G, et al. Accumulation of T_{h2}-like helper T cells in the conjunctiva of patients with vernal conjunctivitis. J Immunol 1991; 146:1169–1174.

82. van Reijsen FC, Bruijnzeel-Koomen CAFM, Kalthoff FS, et al. Skin-derived aeroallergen-specific T cell clones of T_{h2} phentype in patients with atopic dermatitis. J Allergy Clin Immunol 1992; 90:184–192.

83. Kay AB, Sun Ying, Varney VA, et al. Messenger RNA expression of the cytokine gene cluster interleukin 3 (IL-3), IL-4, IL-5 and granulocyte/macrophage colony-stimulating factor, in allergen-induced late-phase cutaneous reactions in atopic subjects. J Exp Med 1991; 173:775–778.

84. Durham SR, Sun Ying, Varney VA, et al. Cytokine messenger RNA expression for IL-3, IL-4, IL-5, and granulocyte/macrophage colony-stimulating factor in the nasal mucosa after local allergen provocation: relationship to tissue eosinophilia. J Immunol 1992; 148:2390–2394.

85. Tsicopoulos A, Hamid Q, Varney V, et al. Preferential messenger RNA expression of T_{h1} type cells (IFN-$_{\gamma+}$, IL-2$^+$) in classical delayed-type (tuberculin) hypersensitivity reactions in human skin. J Immunol 1992; 148:2058–2061.

86. Yamamura M, Uyemura K, Deans RJ, et al. Defining protective responses to pathogens: cytokine profiles in leprosy patients. Science 1991; 254:277–279.

87. Kamogawa Y, Minasi LE Carding SR, et al. The relationship of IL-4 and IFN_γ-producing T cells studied by lineage ablation of IL-4-producing cells. Cell 1993; 75:985–995.

88. Manetti R, Gerosa F, Giudisi MG, et al. Interleukin 12 induces stable priming for interferon$_\gamma$ (IFN_γ) production during differentiation of human T helper (Th) cells

and transient IFN_γ production in established T_{h2} clones. J Exp Med 1994; 179:1273-1283.

89. Robinson DS, Hamid Q, Sun Y, et al. Evidence for a predominant T_{h2}-type bronchoalveolar T-lymphocyte population in atopic asthma. N Engl J Med 1992; 326:298-304.

90. Walker C, Virchow J-C, Bruijnzeel PLB, et al. T cell subsets and their soluble products regelate eosinophilia in allergic and nonallergic asthma. J Immunol 1991; 146:1829-1835.

91. Robinson DS, Sun Ying, Bentley AM, et al. Relationships among numbers of bronchoalveolar lavage cells expressing mRNA for cytokines, asthma symptoms, and airway methacholine responsiveness to atopic asthma. J Allergy Clin Immunol 1993; 92:397-403.

92. Broide DH, Lotz D, Cuomo AJ, et al. Cytokines in symptomatic asthma airways. J Allergy Clin Immunol 1992; 89:958-967.

93. DeMonchy JGR, Kauffman HF, Venge P, et al. Bronchoalveolar eosinophilia during allergen-induced late asthmatic responses. Am Rev Respir Dis 1985; 131:373-376.

94. Robinson DS, Hamid Q, Bentley AM, et al. Activation of CD4[+] T cells and increased IL-4, IL-5 and GM-CSF mRNA positive cells in bronchoalveolar lavage fluid (BAL) 24 hours after allergen inhalation challenge of atopic asthmatic patients. J Allergy Clin Immunol 1993; 92:313-326.

95. Robinson D, Hamid Q, Ying S, et al. Prednisolone treatment in asthma is associated modulation of bronchoalveolar lavage interleukin 4, interleukin 5, and interferon-$_\gamma$ cytokine gene expression. Am Rev Respir Dis 1993; 148:401-406.

96. Sousa AR, Lane SJ, Nakhosteen JA, Yoshimura T, Lee TH, Poston RN. Increased expression of the monocyte chemoattractant protein-1 in bronchial tissue from asthmatic subjects. Am J Respir Cell Mol Biol 1994; 10:142-147.

97. Sun Ying, Robinson DS, Varney V, et al. TNF-α mRNA expression in allergic inflammation. Clin Exp Allergy 1991; 21:745-750.

98. Hamid Q, Azzawi M, Sun Ying et al. Expression of mRNA for interleukin-5 in mucosal bronchial biopsies from asthma. J Clin Invest 1991; 87:1541-1546.

99. Ackerman V, Marini M, Vittori E, et al. Detection of cytokines and their cell sources in bronchial biopsy specimens from asthmatic patients: relationship to atopic status, symptoms, and level of airway hyperresponsiveness. Chest 1994; 105:687-696.

100. Bellini A, Yoshimura H, Vittori E, et al. Bronchial epithelial cells of patients with asthma release chemoattractant factors for T-lymphocytes. J Allergy Clin Immunol 1993; 412-424.

101. Bentley AM, Meng Q, Robinson DS, et al. Increases in activated T-lymphocytes, and cytokine mRNA expression for interleukin-5 and granulocyte/macrophage colony-stimulating factor in bronchial biopsies after allergen challenge in atopic asthmatics. Am J Respir Cell Mol Biol 1993; 35-42.

102. Montefort S, Gratziou C, Goulding D, et al. Bronchial biopsy evidence for leukocyte infiltration and upregulation of leukocyte-endothelial cell adhesion molecules 6 hours after local allergen challenge of sensitized asthmatic airways. J Clin Invest 1994; 93:1411-1421.

103. Sousa AR, Poston RN, Lane SJ, et al. GM-CSF expression in bronchial epithelium in asthmatic airways: decrease by inhaled corticosteroids. Am Rev Respir Dis 1993; 147:1557–1561.

104. Wang JH, Trigg CJ, Devalia JL, et al. Effect of inhaled beclomethasone dipropionate on expression of proinflammatory cytokines and activated eosinophils in the bronchial epithelium of patients with mild asthma. J Allergy Clin Immunol 1994; 94:1025–1034.

105. Devalia JL, Wang JH, Sapsford RJ, et al. Expression of RANTES in human bronchial epithelial cells is down-regulated by beclomethasone dipropinate. Clin Exp Allergy 1994; 24:992A.

106. Berkman N, Robichaud A, Krishnan VL, et al. RANTES is expressed by human airway epithelium in-vitro and in-vivo. Am J Respir Crit Care Med 1995; 151:A191.

107. Sousa AR, Lane SJ, Nakhosteen JA, et al. Upregulation of IL-1β and IL-1 receptor antagonist (IL-1ra) in asthmatic bronchial epithelium: Effect of steroids. Am J Respir Crit Care Med 1995; 151:A368.

108. Haahtela T, Jarvinen M, Kava T, et al. Comparison of a β_2 agonist, terbutaline, with an inhaled corticosteroid, budesonide, in newly-detected asthma. N Engl J Med 1991; 325:388–392.

109. British Thoracic Society Guidelines for management of asthma in adults. Br Med J 1990; 142:434–437.

110. Adelroth E, Rosenhall L, Johansson S-A, et al. Inflammatory cells and eosinophilic activity in asthmatics investigated in asthmatics by bronchoalveolar lavage. The effects of antiasthmatic treatment with budesonide or terbutaline. Am Rev Respir Dis 1990; 142:91–99.

111. Wilkinson JRW, Crea AEG, Clark TJH, et al. Identification and characterization of a monocyte-derived neutrophil-activating factor in corticosteroid-resistant bronchial asthma. J Clin Invest 1989; 84:1930–1941.

112. Carmichael J, Paterson IC, Diaz P, et al. Corticosteroid resistance in chronic asthma. Br Med J 1981; 282:1419–1422.

113. Kay AB, Diaz P, Carmichael J, et al. Corticosteroid-resistant chronic asthma and monocyte complement receptors. Clin Exp Immunol 1981; 44:576–580.

114. Wilkinson JR, Lane SJ, Lee TH. The effects of corticosteroids on cytokine generation and expression of activation antigens by monocytes in bronchial asthma. Int Arch Allergy Appl Immunol 1991; 94:220–221.

115. Corrigan CJ, Brown PH, Barnes NC, et al. Peripheral Blood T lymphocyte activation and comparison of the T lymphocyte inhibitory effects of glucocorticoids and cyclosporin A. Am Rev Respir Dis 1991; 144:1026–1032.

116. Lane SJ, Lee TH. 1991. Glucocorticoid receptor characteristics in monocytes of patients with corticosteroid resistant bronchial asthma. Am Rev Respir Dis 143; 1020–1024.

117. Lane SJ, Wilkinson JRW, Cochrane GM, et al. Differential *in vitro* regulation by glucocorticoids of monocyte-derived cytokine generation in glucocorticoid resistant bronchial asthma. Am Rev Respir Dis 1993; 147:690–696.

118. Lane SJ, Sousa AR, Poston RN, et al. *In vivo* cutaneous tuberculin response to

prednisolone in corticosteroid resistant bronchial asthma (abstr.). J Allergy Clin Immunol 1991; 91(1):221.

119. Gronemeyer H. Control of transcription activation by steroid hormone receptors. FASEB J 1992; 6:2524–2529.

120. Beato M. Gene regulation by steroid hormones. Cell 1989; 56:335–344.

121. Diamond MI, Miner JN, Yoshinaga SK, et al. Transcription factor interactions: selectors of positive or negative regulation from a single DNA element. Science 1990; 249:1266–1272.

122. Yang-Yen JF, Chambard JC, Sun YL, et al. Transcriptional interference between c-Jun and the glucocorticoid receptor: mutual inhibition of DNA binding due to direct protein-protein interaction. Cell 1990; 62:1205–1214.

123. Burns K, Duggan B, Atkinson BA, et al. Modulation of gene expression by calreticulin binding to the glucocorticoid receptor. Nature 1994; 367:476–480.

124. Mukaido N, Morita M, Ishikawa Y, et al. Novel mechanism of glucocorticoid-mediated gene repression; NFκB is target for glucocorticoid-mediated gene IL-8 gene repression. J Biol Chem 1994; 269:13289–13295.

125. Mukaido N, Mahe Y and Matsushima K. Cooperative interaction of NFκB and cis-regulatory enhancer binding protein-like factor binding elements in activating the IL-8 gene by pro-inflammatory cytokines. J Biol Chem 1990; 265:21128–21133.

126. Mukaido N, Gussella GL, Kasahara T, et al. Molecular analysis of the inhibition of IL-8 production by dexamethasone in a human fibrosarcoma cell line. Immunology 1992; 75:674–679.

127. Lane SJ, Palmer JBD, Skidmore IF, et al. Corticosteroid pharmakokinetics in asthma. Lancet 1991; 336:1265.

128. Adcock IM, Lane SJ, Brown CR, et al. Differences in binding of glucocorticoid receptor to DNA in steroid-resistant asthma. J Immunol 1995; 154:3500–3505.

129. Lane SJ, Arm JP, Staynoz DZ, et al. Chemical mutational analysis of the human glucocorticoid receptor cDNA in glucocorticoid-resistant bronchial asthma. Am J Res Molec Cell Biol 1994; 11:42–48.

130. Kam JC, Szefler SJ, Surs et al. Combination of IL-2 and IL-4 reduces glucocorticoid binding affinity and T cell response to glucocorticoids. J Immunol 1993; 151:3460–3466.

131. Kerrpola TK, Luk D, Curran T. Fos is a preferential target of glucocorticoid receptor inhibition of AP-1 activity *in vitro*. Mol Cell Biol 1993; 13:3782-790.

132. Jonat J, Rahmsdorf HJ, Park KK, et al. Antitumor promotion and anti-inflammation: down modulation of AP-1 (fos/jun) activity by glucocorticoid hormone. Cell 1990; 62:1189–1204.

133. Dokter WHA, Esselink MT, Halie MR, et al. Interleukin-4 inhibits the liposaccaride-induced expression of c-jun and c-fos mRNA and AP-1 binding activitity in human monocytes. Blood 1993; 81:337–343.

134. Radzioch D, Varesio L. c-fos mRNA expression in macrophages is down-regulated by interferon-γ at the post-transcriptional level. Mol Cell Biol 1991; 11:2718–2722.

135. Huebner K, Isobe M, Croce CM, et al. The human gene encoding GM-CSF is at

5q21-q32, the chromosome region deleted in the 5q- anomaly. Science 1985; 230:1282-1285.

136. Yang Y-C, Kovacic S, Kriz R, et al. The human genes for GM-CSF and IL-3 are closely linked in tandem on chromosome 5. Blood 1988; 71:958-961.

137. Sutherland GR, Baker E, Callen DF, et al. Interleukin-5 is at 5q31 and is deleted in the 5q-syndrome. Blood 1988; 71:1150-1152.

138. Van Leeuwen BH, Martinson ME, Webb GC, et al. Molecular organization of the cytokine gene cluster, involving the human IL-3, IL-4, IL-5 and GM-CSF genes, on human chromosome 5. Blood 1989; 73:1142-1148.

139. Huebner K, Nagarajan L, Besa E, et al. Order of genes on human chromsome 5q with respect to 5q interstitial deletions. Am J Hum Genet 1990; 46:26-36.

140. Wasmuth JJ, Park C, Ferrell RE. Report of the committee on the genetic constitution of chromosome 5. Cytogenet Cell Genet 1989; 51:137-148.

141. LeBeau MM, Lemons RS, Espinosa III R, et al. Interleukin-4 and Interleukin-5 map to human chromosome 5 in a region encoding growth factors and receptors and are deleted in myeloid leukemias with a del(5q). Blood 1989; 73:647-650.

142. Chandrasekharappa SC, Rebelsky MS, Firak TA, et al. A long-range restriction map of the Interleukin-4 and Interleukin-5 linkage group on chromosome 5. Genomics 1990; 6:94-99.

143. Warrington JA, Hall JV, Hinton LM, et al. Radiation hybrid map of 13 loci on the long arm of chromosome 5. Genomics 1991; 11:701-708.

144. Warrington JA, Bailey SK, Armstrong E, et al. A radiation hybrid map of 18 growth factor, growth factor receptor, hormone receptor, or neurotransmitter receptor genes on the distal region of the long arm of chromosome 5. Genomics 1992; 13:803-808.

145. Minty A, Chalon P, Derocq J-M, et al. IL-13 is a new human lymphokine regulating inflammatory and immune responses. Nature 1993; 362:248-250.

146. Morgan JG, Dolganov GM, Robins SE, et al. The selective isolation of novel cDNAs encoded by the regions surrounding the human interleukin 4 and 5 gene. Nucleic Acids Res 1992; 20:5173-5179.

147. D'Eustachio P, Brown M, Watson C, et al. The IL-4 gene maps to chromosome 11, near the gene encoding IL-3. J Immunol 1988; 141:3067-3071.

148. Takahashi M, Yoshida MC, Satoh H, et al. Chromosomal mapping of the mouse IL-4 and human IL-5 genes. Genomics 1989; 4:47-52.

149. Lee JS, Campbell HD, Kozak CH, et al. The IL-4 and Il-5 genes are closely linked and are part of a cytokine gene cluster on mouse chromosome 11. Somatic Cell Mol Genet 1989; 15:143-152.

150. Tominaga A, Takaki S, Hitoshi Y, et al. Role of the Interleukin 5 receptor system in hematopoiesis: molecular basis for overlapping function of cytokines. Biol Essays 1992; 14:527-533.

151. Lopez AF, Elliott MJ, Woodcock J, et al. Cross-competition on human haemopoietic cells. Immunol Today 1992; 13:495-500.

152. Cosman D. The hematopoietin receptor superfamily. Cytokine 1993; 5:95-106.

153. Clark SC, Kamen R. The human hematopoetic colony-stimulating factors. Science 1987; 236:1229-1237.

154. Yokota T, ARai N, deVries J, et al. Molecular biology of interleukin 4 and interleukin 5 genes and biology of their products that stimulate B cells, T cells and hemopoietic cells. Immunol Rev 1988; 102:137–187.

155. Devereux S, Linch D. Haemopoietic growth factors. Q J Med New Series 1990; 75:537–550.

156. Mosman TR, Moore KW. The role of IL-10 in cross-regulation of Th1 and Th2 responses. Immunol Today 1991; 12:A49–53.

157. Desreumaux P, Janin A, Colombel JF, et al. IL-5 mRNA expression by eosinophils in the intestinal mucosa of patients with coeliac disease. J Exp Med 1992; 175:293–296.

158. Broide DH, Paine MM, Firestein GS. Eosinophils express Interleukin-5 and granulocyte macrophage-colony-stimulating factor mRNA at sites of allergic inflammation in asthmatics. J Clin Invest 1992; 90:1414–1424.

159. Plaut M, Pierce JH, Watson CJ, et al. Mast Cell Lines Produce Lymphokines in Response to Cross-Linkage of FcεRI or to Calcium Ionophores. Nature 1989; 339:64–67.

160. Ullman K, Northrop J, Verweij C, et al. Transmission of signals from the T lymphocyte antigen receptor to the genes responsible for cell proliferation and immune function: the missing link. Ann Rev Immunol 1990; 8:421–452.

161. Klausner RD, Samelson LE. T cell antigen receptor activation pathways: the tyrosine kinse connection. Cell 1991; 64:875–878.

162. Weiss A, Imboden JB. Cell surface molecules and early events involved in human T lymphocyte activation. Adv Immunol 1987; 41:1–38.

163. Berridge MJ. Inositol triphosphate and diacylglycerol: two interacting second messengers. Ann Rev Biochem 1987; 56:159–193.

164. Tominaga A, Matsumoto M, Harada N, et al. Molecular properties and regulation of mRNA expression for murine T cell–replacing factor/IL-5. J Immunol 1988; 140:1175–1181.

165. Bohjanen PR, Okajima M, Hodes RJ. Differential regulation of interleukin 4 and interleukin 5 gene expression: a comparison of T-cell gene induction by anti-CD3 antibody or by exogenous lymphokines. Proc Natl Acad Sci USA 1990; 87:5283–5287.

166. Cardell S, Sander B. Interleukin 2, 4 and 5 are sequentially produced in mitogen-stimulated murine spleen cell cultures. Eur J Immunol 1990; 20:389–395.

167. Sander B, Cardell S, Moller G, et al. Differential regulation of lymphokine production in mitogen-stimulated murine spleen cells. Eur J Immunol 1991; 21:2495–2500.

168. Staynov DZ, Lee TH. Expression of IL-5 and GM-CSF in human peripheral blood mononuclear cells after activation with phorbol myristate acetate. Immunology 1992; 75:196–201.

169. Lindsten T, June CH, Ledbetter JA, et al. Regulation of lymphokine mRNA stability by a surface mediated T-cell activation pathway. Science 1989; 244:339–343.

170. Thorens B, Mermod J-J, Vassali P. Phagocytosis and Inflammatory stimuli induce GM-CSF mRNA in macrophages through posttranscriptionnal regulation. Cell 1987; 48:671–679.

171. Tocci MJ, Matkovich DA, Collier KA, et al. The immunosuppressant FK506 selectively inhibits expression of early T cell activation genes. J Immunol 1989; 143:718–726.

172. Bickel M, Tsuda H, Amstad P, et al. Differential regulation of colony-stimulating factors and interleukin 2 production by cyclosporing A. Proc Natl Acad Sci USA 1987; 84:3274–3277.

173. Rolfe FG, Hughes JM, Armour CL, et al. Inhibition of Interleukin-5 gene expression by dexamethasone. Immunology 1992; 77:494–499.

174. Wodnar-Filipowicz A, Heusser CH, Moroni C. Production of the haemopoietic growth factors GM-CSF and interleukin-3 by mast cells in response to IgE receptor-mediated activation. Nature 1989; 339:150–152.

175. Shaw G, Karmen. A conserved AU sequence from the 3' untranslated region of GM-CSF mRNA mediates selective mRNA degradation. Cell 1986; 46:659–667.

176. Schuler GD, Cole MD. GM-CSF and oncogene mRNA stabilities are independently regulated in trans in a mouse monocytic tumor. Cell 1988; 55:1115–1122.

177. Campbell HD, Sanderson CJ, Wang Y, et al. Isolation, structure and expression of cDNA and genomic clones for murine eosinophil differentiation factor. Eur J Biochem 1988; 174:345–352.

178. Chan JY, Slamon DJ, Nimer SD, et al. Regulation of expression of human granulocyte-macrophage colony stimulating factor. Proc Natl Acad Sci USA 1986; 83:8669–8673.

179. Nimer SD, Morita EA, Martis MJ, et al. Characterization of the human granulocyte-macrophage colony-stimulating factor promoter region by genetic analysis: correlation with DNase I footprinting. Mol Cell Biol 1988; 8:1979–1984.

180. Nimer SD, Gates MJ, Koeffler HP, et al. Multiple mechanisms control the expression of granulocyte-macrophage colony-stimulating factor by human fibroblasts. J Immunol 1989; 143:2374–2377.

181. Shannon MF, Gamble JR, Vadas MA. Nuclear proteins interacting with the promoter region of the human granulocyte-macrophage colony stimulating factor gene. Proc Natl Acad Sci USA 1988; 85:674–678.

182. Shannon MF, Pell LM, Leonardo MJ, et al. A novel tumour necrosis factor-responsive transcription factor which recognizes a regulatory element in hemopoietic growth factor genes. Mol Cell Biol 1990; 10:2950–2959.

183. Yokota T, Arai N, deVries J, et al. Molecular biology of interleukin 4 and interleukin 5 genes and biology of their products that stimulate B cells, T cells and hemopoietic cells. Immunol Rev 1988; 102:137–187.

184. Kaushansky K. Control of granulocyte-macrophage colony-stimulating factor production in normal endothelial cells by positive and negative regulatory elements. J Immunol 1989; 143:2525–2529.

185. Miyatake S, Seiki M, DeWaal Malefijt R, et al. Activation of T cell-derived lymphokine genes in T cells and fibroblasts: effects of Human T cell leukemia virus type 1 p40x protein and bovine papilloma virus encoded E2 protein. Nucleic Acids Res 1988; 16:6547–6566.

186. Miyatake S, Seiki M, Yoshida M, et al. T-cell activation signals and human T-cell leukemia virus type I-encoded p40x protein activate the mouse granulocyte-

macrophage colony-stimulating factor gene through a common DNA element. Mol Cell Biol 1988; 8:5581–5587.

187. Sugimoto K, Tsuboi A, Miyatake S, et al. Inducible and non-inducible factors cooperatively activate the GM-CSF promoter by interacting with two adjacent DNA motifs. Int Immunol 1990; 2:787–794.

188. Tsuboi A, Sugimoto K, Yodoi J, et al. A nuclear factor NF-GM2 that interacts with a regulatory region of the GM-CSF gene essential for its induction in response to T-cell leukemia line Jurkat cells and similarity to FN-κB. Int Immunol 1991; 3:807–817.

189. Miyatake S, Shlomai J, Arai K-I, et al. Characterization of the mouse granulocyte-macrophage colony-stimulating factor (GM-CSF) gene promoter: nuclear factors that interact with an element shared by three lymphokine genes—those for GM-CSF, interleukin-4 (IL-4) and IL-5. Mol Cell Biol 1991; 11:5894–5901.

190. Nishida J, Yoshida M, Arai K, et al. Definition of a GC-rich motif as regulatory sequence of the human IL-3 gene: coordinate regulation of the IL-3 gene by CLE2/GC box of the GM-CSF gene in T cell activation. Int Immunol 1991; 3:245–254.

191. Heike T, Miyatake S, Yoshida M, et al. Bovine papilloma virus encoded E2 protein activates lymphokine genes through DNA elements, distinct from the consensus motif, in the long control region of its own genome. EMBO J 1989; 8:1411–1417.

192. Staynov DZ, Cousins DJ, Richards D, et al. Transcriptional regulation of IL-5 gene expression in human T cells. FASEB J 1994; 8:A472.

193. Todd MD, Grusby MJ, Lederer JA, et al. Transcription of the IL-4 gene is regulated by multiple promoter elements. J Exp Med 1993; 177:1663–1674.

194. Abe E, de Waal Malefyt R, Matsuda I, et al. An 11 base pair DNA sequence motif apparently unique to the human IL-4 gene confers responsiveness to T cell activation signals. Proc Natl Acad Sci 1992; 89:2864–2868.

195. Szabo SJ, Gold JS, Murphy TL, et al. Identification of cis acting regulatory elements controlling IL-4 gene expression in T cells: roles for NF-Y and NF-ATc. Mol Cell Biol 1993; 8:4793–4805.

196. Li-Weber M, Krafft-Czepa H, Krammer PH, et al. A novel enhancer element in the human IL-4 promoter is suppressed by a position-independent silencer. J Immunol 1993; 151:1371–1382.

197. Li-Weber M, eder A, Krafft-Czepa H, et al. T cell specific negative regulation of transcription of the human cytokine IL-4. J Immunol 1992; 148:1913–1918.

198. Tokumitsu H, Masuda ES, Tsuboi A, et al. Purification of the 120kDa component of the human nuclear factor of activated T cells (NF-AT). Biochem Biophys Res Commun 1993; 196:737–744.

199. Wu C, Fargeas C, Nakajima T, Delespesse G. glucocorticoids suppress the production of interleukin 4 by human lymphocytes. Eur J Immunol 1191; 21:2645–2647.

200. Naora H, van Leeuwen BH, Bourke PF, Young IG. Functional role and signal-induced modulation of proteins recognizing the conserved TCATTT-containing

promoter elements in the murine IL-5 and GM-CSF genes in T lymphocytes. J Immunol 1994; 153:3466–3475.

201. Staynov DZ, Cousins DJ, Lee TH. A regulatory element in the promoter of the humangranulocyte-macrophage colony stimulating factor gene that has related sequences in other T-cell-expressed cytokine genes. Proc Natl Acad Sci USA 1995; 92:3606–3610.

202. Northrop JP, Ho SN, Chen L, et al. NF-AT components define a family of transcription factors targeted in T-cell activation. Nature 1994; 369:497–502.

Part Three

GLUCOCORTICOID ACTIVITY AND SELECTIVITY AT THE AIRWAY LEVEL

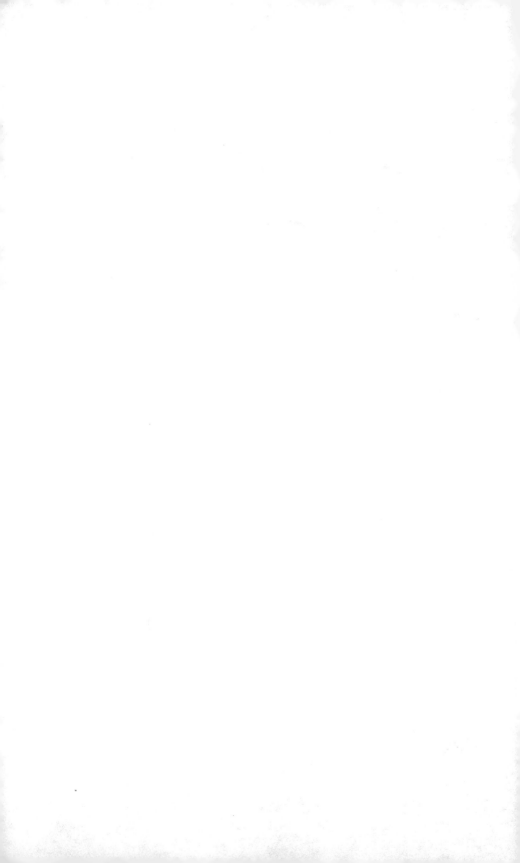

15

Basis of Airway Selectivity of Inhaled Glucocorticoids

RALPH BRATTSAND and BENGT I. AXELSSON

Astra Draco AB
Lund, Sweden

I. Development of Current Glucocorticoids with Airway Selectivity

Because the glucocorticosteroid receptor (GR) seems to be uniform in the body (1–3), there are small chances to differentiate the various GR actions at the receptor level (the alternatively spliced receptor form does not seem to be functionally active [4]. However, by exploiting the prospects of local-topical therapy, it has been possible to reach some differentiation of the various steroid actions. The major medical aim with that approach has been to reduce the well-known systemic adverse effects of glucocorticoids, but there has been also a hope to enhance the desired anti-inflammatory–immunosuppressive actions at the site of the local-topical application. Although that approach was successfully exploited for topical dermatological therapy already, within a few years after steroid therapy introduction in the early 1950s (5–7), it took two further decades of empirical development before success could be reached within the topical respiratory field (8–11). Description of the basis and current status of the latter development is the emphasis of this chapter.

By modifying the basic corticosteroid structure (starting from hydrocortisone), it appeared possible to modify the following functions.

Specific bindings (12–15): raising the affinity for the GR, reducing the affinity for the mineralocorticoid receptor, and reducing the affinity for corticosteroid-binding globulin, (CBG, or transcortin)

Biotransformation (12,14,15): modulating the metabolism via oxido-reductive or hydrolytic pathways

Other physicochemical aspects (12,14,15): uptake, tissue binding and systemic disposition.

When these options were gradually unraveled in the 1950s and 1960s, they led glucocorticoid drug development into two main directions—glucocorticoids with enhanced biostability for systemic therapy (5,14,15) and lipophilic steroids of high potency for topical dermatological use (6,7,16). This drug evolution was governed mainly by empiricism. In fact, still in the 1990s, we lack precise answers for the functional basis of topical selectivity:

1. Which are the key cells to be modulated by the steroid, and do these cells differ in topical and systemic steroid treatment, respectively?
2. What steroid concentration is required at that target?
3. For how long should this concentration last?

The development of topical steroids for respiratory diseases can to a great extent be characterized as a spin-off to the topical dermatological field. The major failures and successes of the exploitation by inhalation are illustrated in Figure 1 by the generic names of the key compounds. Today, we know that the 11-keto compounds cortisone and prednisone are prodrugs, which have to be reduced (mainly in the liver) to the corresponding 11-OH steroids (hydrocortisone and prednisolone) for triggering the GR (14,15). Thus, there is no rationale for using the 11-keto compounds by the topical route. Hydrocortisone and prednisolone work in systemic as well as in topical dermatological treatment (16), but it was shown early that they lack or have just weak antiasthmatic activity by inhalation (17). There seems to be two major reasons to their failing activity: First, the great dilution on the vast airway surface argues for using much more potent steroids. Second, and possibly more important, is the inactivation of these 11-OH compounds through the enzyme 11β-hydroxysteroid dehydrogenase into inactive cortisone and prednisone, respectively. This enzyme is prevalent in lung and airway tissues (18), and Schleimer (19) demonstrated an efficient in vitro inactivation of hydrocortisone. The enzyme can be blocked by, for example, the partly steroid-like glycyrrhetinic acid, and this may explain the anti-inflammatory effects of the latter compound by a potentiation of endogenous glucocorticoids (19,20). Still, we do not know whether an inhibition of 11β-hydroxysteroid dehydrogenase locally in airways-lung might potentiate the endogenous hydrocortisone sufficiently for attaining clinically useful

Step 1 *1950-1970:* *Failures!*

- ▸ Nonefficacious (cortisone, hydrocortisone, prednisolone)
- ▸ Nonselective (dexamethasone)

Step 2 *1970-1975: Spinoff from topical skin GCS*

- ▸ Betamethasone 17α valerate, beclomethasone 17α, 21-dipropionate, triamcinolone 16α, 17α-acetonide

Step 3 *1975-1990: Optimization of hepatic first-pass inactivation (but primary selection still in non-airway-lung models)*

- ▸ Budesonide, flunisolide, fluticasone 17α-propionate

Step 4 *1990- : Primary selection in airway-lung models to optimize local factors*

Figure 1 Scheme over major steps in the development of glucocorticoids for inhalation.

antiasthmatic efficacy. If so, this will be a novel approach for reaching a topical selectivity without adding exogenous steroid (20).

Oral steroid therapy is based on prednisolone, prednisone, or methylprednisolone (14,15,21,22), the structures of which are given in Figure 2. Their functional preferences over hydrocortisone depend on (1) an enhanced affinity for the glucocorticoids but a relatively reduced affinity for the mineralocorticoid receptor (14,15); (2) a reduced binding to CBG (methylprednisolone [13]; and (3) an increased metabolic stability (14,15). Compared with hydrocortisone, prednisolone has a 10-fold higher GR affinity, whereas its clearance is halved, leading to an oral bioavailability of approximately 80% (23). The 6α-methyl substitution in methylprednisolone contributes to a further reduction of the binding to the mineralocorticoid receptor (14,15) and to CBG (13). The latter compound is also better disposed into tissue including lung (24,25) owing to its higher volume of distribution.

The next chemical step was halogenation of the 6α and/or 9α positions of the B ring (see Fig. 2), introduced in triamcinolone, betamethasone, and dexamethasone. This modification enhances the oral potency due to combining a further rise of the GR affinity (12), a lack of CBG binding (13), and a high metabolic stability (14,15). However, these potent steroids do not provoke fewer adverse effects. Owing to its high receptor affinity and activity, dexamethasone has antiasthmatic activity by inhalation, but this is combined with as much systemic adverse effect as when it is given as tablets (26,27). This high systemic activity by inhalation depends on its high biostability (15)—the large frac-

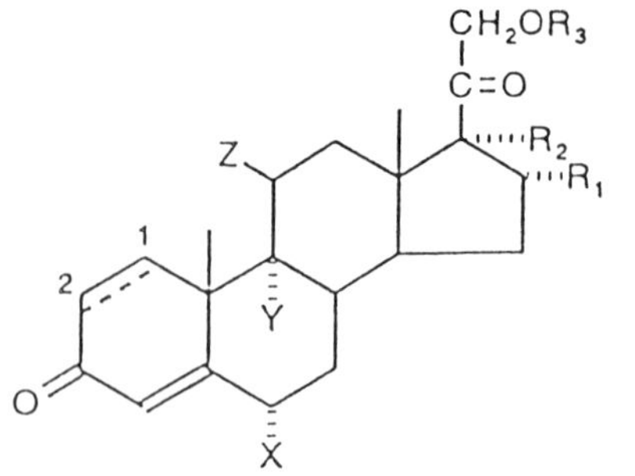

GCS	1-2	X	Y	Z	R₁	R₂	R₃
Cortisone	sat	H	H	O	H	α-OH	H
Hydrocortisone	"	"	"	β-OH	"	"	"
Prednisolone	unsat	"	"	"	"	"	"
Prednisone	"	"	"	O	"	"	"
6-methylpred-nisolone	"	α-Me	H	β-OH	"	"	"
Dexamethasone	"	H	α-F	"	α- Me	"	"
Betamethasone	"	"	α-F	"	β – Me	"	"
Triamcinolone	"	"	α-F	"	α-OH	"	"

Figure 2 Basic glucocorticoid structure and substances used in systemic therapy. Explanation of position numbers in the steroid skeleton. $x = 6$, $y = 9$, $z = 11$; $R_1 = 16$, $R_2 = 17$, $R_3 = 21$; M = methyl. (From Ref. 11.)

tion deposited in oropharynx will subsequently be swallowed and intestinally absorbed and having just a small hepatic first-pass inactivation (23,28). In addition, the airway-lung–derived fraction will have a long plasma half-life for the same reason.

A. First Generation of Glucocorticoids with Airway Selectivity

In spite of their high oral activity, triamcinolone and betamethasone had a surprisingly poor topical potency on skin (5–7). The chemical aim of the further development was making the triamcinolone and betamethasone types of steroids more lipophilic by introducing lipophilic substituents in the 16α and 17α positions of the D ring (see Fig. 2). Two different substituents were used depending on the D-ring structure: acetalization of the 16α,17α OH groups leading to acetals like triamcinolone acetonide (TAc, Fig. 3); or esterification of the 17α OH group giving a series of potent esters (7,29) like betamethasone valerate (BV) and beclomethasone dipropionate (BDP), which is esterified also in the 21-position (see Fig. 3). The dermatological development was very successful—giving the first topical preparations also ameliorating psoriasis and stubborn eczema. This drug development was aimed at reaching as high topical potency as possible (6,7), and very little attention was paid to the biotransformation routes and rates of these compounds (6,7,16)—substantiated by the small importance of adverse systemic actions in restricted topical skin therapy.

In the late 1960s and early 1970s, it was shown that inhaled BV and BDP ameliorated asthmatic and rhinitic symptoms (17,30–32). The therapeutic efficacy was awaited (cf. earlier findings with dexamethasone) (26,27), but the lack of concomitant systemic glucocorticoid actions was very surprising (17,28,30–33). The work of Martin et al. (34) elucidated that an efficient hepatic metabolism explained the low extent of systemic adverse effects: BDP exerted strong systemic activity when given intravenously, whereas its actions were weak when ingested or inhaled. The high hepatic first-pass metabolism of BV and BDP was a serendipitous finding as both are close and very potent derivatives of the very biostable betamethasone and dexamethasone (see above). A series of clinical trials demonstrated that the inhaled BDP, 400 μ/day, can substitute an oral prednisolone dose of 5–10 mg regarding antiasthmatic efficacy (35,36), whereas its systemic activity (measured as depression of morning HPA-axis function) was strongly reduced. However later on with more sensitive methods, especially in children, slight systemic actions can be also demonstrated with low doses (overnight HPA-axis function [37,38], short-term kneemometry [39]).

B. Second Generation of Glucocorticoids with Airway Selectivity

As stated above, BV and BDP had not been preselected and optimized for hepatic first-pass metabolism. However, in the late 1960s (before any results with BV and BDP inhalation were published), structure-activity work was started aimed at optimizing the local to systemic activity ratio of the 16α,17α acetal type of topical steroids (40). Pharmacological in vivo studies (41,42) and metabolic work (43) showed that it was possible to design new topical glucocorticoids with an even more rapid hepatic metabolism than that of earlier acetonides and 17α esters. This work (44) resulted in the inhalational glucocorticoid budesonide (see Fig. 3), introduced in most European countries in the mid 1980s. During the same period, flunisolide was documented as a 16α,17α

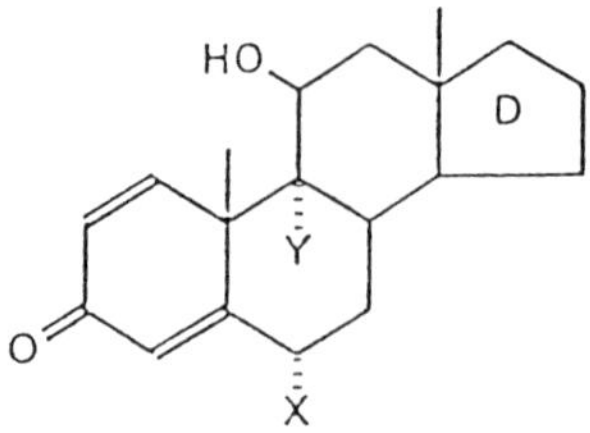

GCS	X	Y	D
Beclomethasone dipropionate	H	Cl	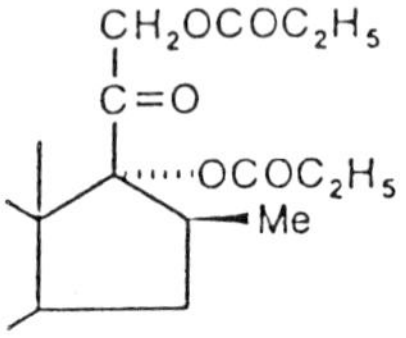 $CH_2OCOC_2H_5$ / $C=O$ / ····$OCOC_2H_5$ / Me
Budesonide	H	H	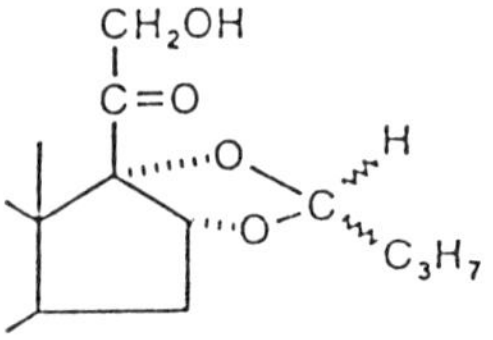 CH_2OH / $C=O$ / O, O–C–H, C_3H_7
Flunisolide	F	H	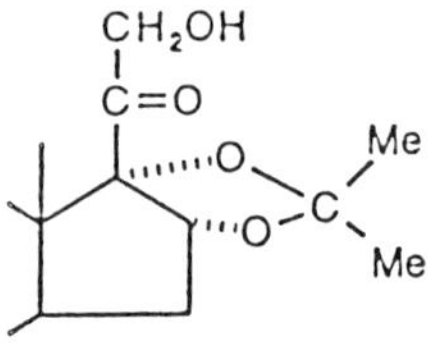 CH_2OH / $C=O$ / O, O–C, Me, Me
Triamcinolone acetonide	H	F	— '' —
Fluticasone propionate	F	F	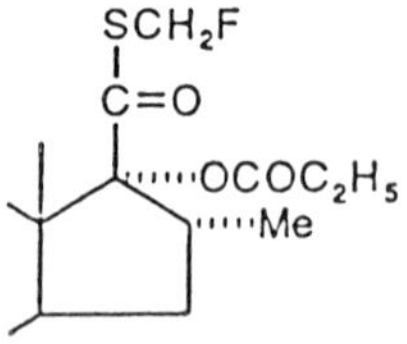 SCH_2F / $C=O$ / ····$OCOC_2H_5$ / ····Me

Figure 3 Structure of glucocorticoids in current use by inhalation. For explanation of position numbers see Figure 2. (From Ref. 11.)

acetonide glucocorticoid with a more efficient hepatic metabolism (45) than that of the pioneering acetonide TAc. Both these acetonides (see Fig. 3) have been documented (46–48) and introduced as inhalational formulations for North American and some European markets. Fluticasone propionate (FP, see Fig. 3) represents another structural line—androstane 17β-carboxylates (7)—leading to a glucocorticoids with a very high hepatic first-pass metabolism. It was selected in animal and human models (49,50) owing to its high ratio between topical and systemic glucocorticoid activities. FP is a carbothioate ester, where the 17β chain can be efficiently cleaved by liver cytochrome P450 enzymes but not by plasma or tissue esterases.

II. Basis of Airway Selectivity

As stated above, lipophilic substituents in the 17α or 16α,17α positions (and sometimes in the side chain too) conform the topical selectivity. When this substitution is properly designed, it can at one stroke add three crucial properties, which all seems necessary for gaining topical anti-inflammatory activity on mucous membranes: (1) a high affinity for and intrinsic activity at the GR, (2) a high uptake and binding into airway tissue, and (3) an efficient hepatic first-pass inactivation (Fig. 4). These key properties are discussed below.

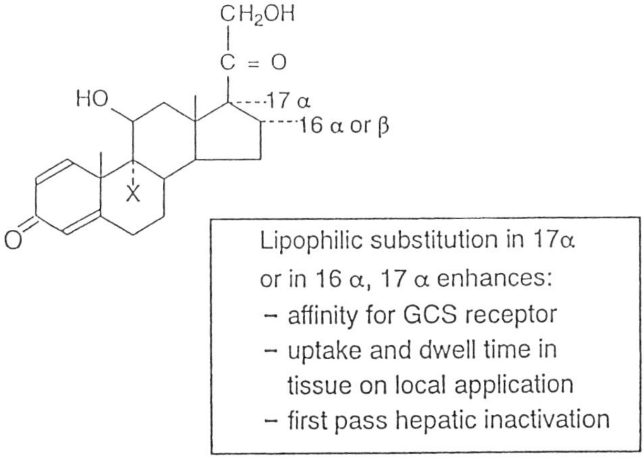

Figure 4 Chemical basis of topical activity and selectivity by inhalation. Lipophilic substitution is introduced in the 17α position as esters (e.g., beclomethasone dipropionate, fluticasone propionate) or in 16α, 17α positions as acetal (budesonide) or acetonides (triamcinolone acetonide, flunisolide).

A. High Affinity for and Intrinsic Activity at the GR

Empirically it has been found that only steroids with a high relative binding affinity (RBA) for the GR are active by inhalation (9). Based on the hitherto published data on antiasthmatic efficacy of inhaled steroids (reported from clinical use or from clinical trials), the minimum level of RBA seems to be about 20 times that of hydrocortisone. This level corresponds to the affinity of dexamethasone, and it is 5–10 times lower than that of the inhaled steroids in current clinical use (Table 1). One obvious reason for the need of a high RBA is the strong dilution occurring on the vast airway-lung surface. A substantial RBA must also be coupled to a metabolic stability in the airway lumen and wall (both extracellularly and intracellularly). That is one reason why several steroids fulfilling the affinity threshold with good margin have shown a too low topical antiasthmatic efficacy (53). However, for steroid agonists having metabolic stability at target, there is a correlation between RBA and topical anti-inflammatory potency (Fig. 5). Under such conditions, RBA can be used as a rough estimate of topical in vivo potential.

Of the three key properties discussed, the requirement of a high affinity-agonistic activity on the GR has the closest demands for proper structural specificity (7,12,55). For triggering a full glucocorticoid activity an agonist needs a configuration that mediates the necessary sequence: liganding the receptor and by that start the proper conformational change allowing the dimer formation, subsequent coupling of the dimer to GREs and to selected transcription factors

Table 1   Basic Properties of GCS

GCS	Water solubility (μg/ml)	Relative lipophilicity (log K'[0])	RBA rat tissue	RBA human lung	Blanching potency (human)
Oral					
hydrocortisone	290	2.8	0.01	–	<0.001
prednisolone	200	2.4	0.06	–	<0.001
dexamethasone	100	2.6	0.2	0.1	0.001
Inhaled					
budesonide	14	3.7	1	1	1
BDP/BMP	0.1/10	4.9/4.4	0.3/2.0	0.1/1.4	0.6/0.5
triamcinolone acetonide	40	3.3	0.5	0.4	0.3
flunisolide	95	3.3	–	0.2	0.3
fluticasone propionate	0.1	4.5	2.3	1.9	1.0

Source: Based on data in files of Astra Draco AB and on Rohdewald et al.

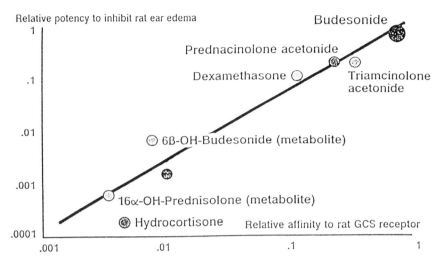

Figure 5 Correlation between the relative binding affinity (RBA) to rat GR (determined in cytosolic preparations) and the topical anti-inflammatory potency in the rat ear edema model (determined in vivo). (Adapted from Ref. 54.)

(2,3). Comparing low and high affinity GCS (see Table 1), there is a good correlation between RBA and lipophilicity (the latter measured as chromatographic capacity factor—log k'0). This supports that, when based on proper substituents, lipophilicity reinforces the potency (6,7,52). Some correlation can be found also within the group of inhalational steroids (see Table 1). The exception is BDP having a top lipophilicity but poor RBA, which however depends on its 21-ester configuration. As stated above, BDP is partly a prodrug, which on hydrolysis is converted into BMP with a free 21-OH, and this potent metabolite fits into the correlation (51,56). However, there is an optimum of lipophilicity for agonistic activity. In a series of nonsymmetrical 16α,17α acetals with successive elongation of the acetal chain (55), there is a progressive rise in RBA, whereas the agonistic activity peaks at the propyl substitution (same length as in budesonide). It can be speculated that a too high affinity does not lead to the proper conformational change of the GR complex for its proper subsequent functions.

It is underlined that a high-affinity–prolonged turnover time at the receptor does not singly lead to selectivity on mucous membranes (as has been proposed recently [58]). Because the receptor is uniform in the body, a strong agonistic potency—good for the local activity—will show up also as a negative factor for the systemic activity. For the orally absorbed fraction, the latter problem is to a very great extent abolished by the hepatic first-pass inactivation (Fig. 6).

In vivo pharmacokinetics

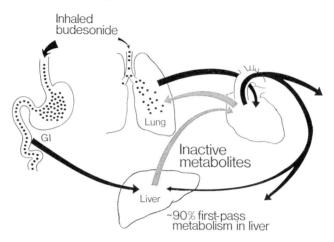

Figure 6 Pharmacokinetic properties of inhaled budesonide in humans: a schematic overview. (From Ref. 57.)

However, hepatic metabolism has a much more minor impact on the bioavailability of the dominating airway-lung absorbed fraction (Fig. 6, and see below). A high value of RBA depends mainly on a slow dissociation rate from the GR, and that will probably prolong the turnover time of the steroid at the receptor (58). Thus, there may be a higher risk of accumulation of systemic steroid actions on repeated administration of very potent glucocorticoids (with very high RBA).

III. Topical Uptake and Binding in Airway-Lung Tissue

Inhalation of 1600 μg of budesonide (BUD) led to lung parenchymal levels of approximately 10 nmol/L 1.5–4.0 hr later (59). The corresponding plasma level was 1 nmol/L, showing that inhalation favors high steroid concentrations even in peripheral lung. For estimating how much higher concentrations are obtained at the airway levels, we have to refer to rat experiments where tritiated glucocorticoids were administered by inhalation, intratracheal installation, or topical superfusion (53,60,61). Figure 7 illustrates uptake and retention of five glucocorticoids after topical superfusion for 10 min over the rat trachea. The concentration range chosen for superfusion (0.1–1.0 μmol/L) was based on functional efficacy in a corresponding leakage model (62). In this model, there is a rather close correlation between the superfused concentration and its uptake

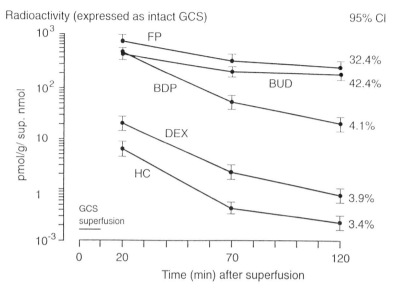

Figure 7 Tissue radioactivity in a locally superfused section of trachea (62) expressed as concentration of intact steroid pmol/g tissue and related to 1 nmol of superfused steroid (N = 3–5). Geometrical means with 95% CI. The figures express the ratio (%) of radioactivity at 120 min to that at 20 min. (From Ref. 61.)

into the tracheal tissue (data not shown). When normalized to superfused concentration, the inhalational glucocorticoids (FP, BUD, and BDP) demonstrate an at least 25 times higher uptake (based on tissue content 10 min after the initial superfusion) than attained by the dexamethasone (DEX) and hydrocortisone (HC). For BUD, the tracheal level at that early time was 100 times higher than in plasma (53). On the other hand, when the superfused dose level instead was injected subcutaneously, the tracheal and plasma levels approached each other and the tracheal concentration was then 100 times lower than after superfusion (60). These experiments show clearly that the preference of topical treatment works also on the highly vascularized airway mucosal surface.

After topical superfusion, the absolute concentrations of the inhalational steroids in tracheal tissue was 0.1–1.0 μmol/L (data in the files of Astra Draco AB). This high concentration, as well as the fact that the uptake was not saturable, show that such lipophilic steroids will bind to more sites than just to the specific receptors (which have a K_d of approximately 1 nmol/L) when applied locally in high concentrations. The character of this high-capacity but probably low-affinity binding has not been elucidated, but it may well be accumulation in cellular and subcellular membranes.

The steroid retention in airway tissues was determined as the percentage remaining in tissue at 120 min (based on the 20-min value, which was put to 100%). For BUD and FP 42, and 32% stayed over this period, whereas the figure was nearly 10 times lower for BDP, DEX, and HC (see Fig. 7). The identity of the released substances was checked in an ex vivo assay, and it was verified that the trachea released intact BUD and fluticasone (61). BDP was metabolized, and in this rat tissue, it was released to a great extent as the final hydrolysis product beclomethasone (data in the files of Astra Draco AB). Because the latter is much less lipophilic than BDP and BMP (52), this explains the poor retention of the BDP complex in rat tracheal tissue (there may be a greater retention in human tissue; see below).

This combination of high uptake and protracted local binding seems to be a hallmark for attaining topical selectivity on a mucous membrane. Such prolonged local binding is much more essential in airways than on skin, where the dermal stratum corneum barrier allows just a minute but nearly continuous uptake (16). This explains why the poorly tissue-bound DEX is topically selective when applied to restricted skin areas but not when deposited in the nose or in the bronchi (26,27). The strong tissue binding may be the major mechanism for retarding glucocorticoids within airway tissue. The retardation might be further improved by choosing glucocorticoids of low solubility or selecting a formulation with slow release properties (see final section). However, just a prolonged deposition of a poorly water-soluble particle in airway lumen will probably not singly lead to selectivity on ciliated airways (where particles may be transported away via mucociliary clearance). Ideally, the retardation process should combine a proper release from the formulation and a strong tissue binding of the glucocorticoid liberated, where the latter may be the more important for the airway levels.

Several key questions are still unanswered about this tissue binding to application site. Among them the following issues are central: (1) How are the steroids bound, and in what cellular and extracellular compartments?, (2) When slowly released from these compartments, will steroids then be available for receptor binding or will they be transported/disposed along other routes? (3) How do the inhalational steroids differ in this regard? This leads to the very basic question: What minimum concentration of active steroid is required in airway wall for inducing antiasthmatic efficacy, and what is the minimum contact time for that? These questions can yet be just vaguely answered, and then more on indirect evidences. An exact answer needs experiments with coupled functional and pharmacokinetic analyses at a defined airway level, and here we are still lacking good models and analytical procedures for that.

In a model based on adherent cell growth in 96 well-plates (where culture medium change plus subsequent intense washing can be performed, partly mimicking drainage via the circulation), we have estimated the minimum period of initial incubation giving the full response 24 hr later (data in the files of A. Draco). This model mimics in mechanistic terms the glucocorticoid mediated inhibition an AP-1–controlled gene (3). On continuous incubation over 24 hr, budesonide reaches its full inhibitory activity at a few nanomoles per liter, which roughly corresponds to its K_d in vitro (54). The results obtained with shorter initial incubation periods and at higher budesonide levels are summarized in Figure 8. For inducing a marked inhibition at 1 nmol/L (which level is reported in plasma for a period after BUD inhalation [59,63], a coincubation period of well over 6 hr was necessary. At levels found in peripheral lung a couple of hours after a high BUD dose (about 10 nmol/L), a few hours of initial coincubation were needed for remaining full activity 20 hr later. At 0.1–1.0 µmol/L, which seems relevant for airway lumen shortly after inhalation, an initial pulse period of 30–60 min induced a full agonism lasting at least 24 hr. Chemical analyses of the latter cells showed that a substantial budesonide fraction (10% or more) remained within the cells after the intense washing (data in the files of A. Draco), explaining the prolonged effect of this short pulse.

Owing to similar retention properties of budesonide in the cell and the rat models (61), these functional cell results may well be roughly extrapolated to

Method
- ► In vitro study in rat fibroblast line with transfected reporter gene
- ► GCS mechanism: inhibition of AP-1-mediated pathway
- ► Tested preincubation periods before intense washing: 30 min - 6 hr

Results
- ► Required preincubation periods for full activity

BUD	10^{-9}	mol/L	>6 hr
	10^{-8}	mol/L	2-4 hr
	10^{-7}	mol/L	1 hr
	10^{-6}	mol/L	30 min

Conclusion
- ► For BUD 10^{-7}- 10^{-6} mol/L, it is sufficient with a pulse of 30-60 min for reaching full and long-lasting activity

Figure 8 Time-response study in a cell model with a steroid-sensitive receptor gene. The cells were incubated with budesonide 10^{-9} to 10^{-6} mol/L and washed intensively after different treatment periods. Resulting inhibition determined after 24 hr. (In the files of Astra Draco and with courtesy to Eva-Lena Delander, Liv Severinsson, and Elisabet Wieslander.)

the airway-lung conditions for more than 6 hr. This explains why a protracted duration is achieved after an initial pulse for 0.1–1.0 μmol/L. Such a pulse seems to be efficiently taken up, bound to local tissue, and then slowly releases active budesonide. This may explain why budesonide has also demonstrated antiasthmatic efficacy in mild asthma on a once daily inhalation regimen (11).

IV. Efficient Hepatic First-Pass Metabolism

The current glucocorticoids are all inactivated by hepatic biotransformation (23) into metabolites of just low glucocorticoid potency (RBA in the magnitude of hydrocortisone or less) (11,49,50,54). BUD undergoes acetal splitting and 6β-hydroxylation (64), whereas TAc (23) and flunisolide (23) are inactivated mainly by the latter route. BDP is partly a prodrug (51), having just a modest affinity itself (see Table 1). Tissue esterases (prevalent in lung but more questionably in bronchial secretions [51,56] split the 21-propionate and release the potent monopropionate (see Table 1). In human lung (34,51,56), there is little further metabolism, and after systemic distribution, BMP is biotransformed in the liver via hydrolytic and oxidative pathways (34). According to a recent pharmacokinetic study based on mass spectrometric analyses, beclomethasone circulates with a plasma half-life of 6 hr (65). The carbothioates side chain of FP is split by the liver, forming a steroidal carboxylic acid of very low RBA, and this seems to be the only metabolic route for this compound (49,50).

The profound hepatic first pass of these steroids can be measured as a high-clearance (Cl) as well as a low oral bioavailability (11,23). Prednisolone and dexamethasone have a Cl of just 0.3 L/min, which is desirable, because they are designed for oral treatment and should then pass the liver largely unmetabolized (14,15). This means, on the other hand, that such compounds are unsuitable for a selective topical treatment. For the best topical compounds, BUD and FP, Cl reaches 1.2 L/min or above (11,23), which is close to the theoretically maximal level for hepatic clearance (1.5 L/min) corresponding to the liver blood flow). This high clearance explains the low oral bioavailability, which for BUD is just 10% (63) and for FP even lower (50).

Andersson et al. (66) recently clarified that cytochrome P450IIIA exerts the major metabolic transformations of budesonide deacetalization and 6β-hydroxylation). Pilot studies suggest that this key and ubiquitous cytochrome is central in the inactivation of also other inhalational steroids (P. H. Andersson, personal communication). A physiological function of this enzyme is 6β-hydroxylation of endogenous steroids, and its structural specificity has been partly characterized. One central property is its preference for lipophilic steroids and that it can accept also bulky substituents. This more moderate demand of structural specificity makes it possible to reach the profile required. Obviously, a properly selected lipophilic substituent can simultaneously fulfil three key properties: (1) raising RBA and intrinsic activity at receptor, (2) enhancing the local tissue binding, and (3) increasing affinity to and biotransformation by cytochrome P450IIIA.

V. Prospects for Further Improvement of Airway Selectivity

The systemic bioavailability of inhaled steroids is predominantly derived from the airway-lung–derived fraction (see Fig. 9 and Chapter 16). Thus, there seems to be no medical advantage in developing glucocorticoids with a still higher hepatic first pass than the approximately 90% valid for, for example, BUD. FP reaches a level closer to 100% (50), but there is currently no clear support that FP attains a better safety margin by inhalation than that of BUD. Instead, in studies in volunteers, there are evidences for a higher cumulation of systemic actions (67,68) on repeated administration, potentially depending on the slower turnover (58) of this very potent compound on GRs in the circulation (cf. above discussion) and/or its high volume of distribution (23) leading to a delayed inactivation.

The options for a further improvement of airway selectivity (53) seems to be:

1. Adding an extrahepatic metabolism (which in this therapy can be utilized as "presystemic"). If working, this may inactivate the steroid partially already during absorption and especially during its systemic disposition. If so, the high systemic availability of the airway-lung–derived fraction might be markedly reduced (cf. Figs. 6 and 9).

2. Prolonging the luminal deposition and the local tissue binding may enhance both local efficacy and retard the systemic absorption. If the latter could be slowed down strongly, the resulting plasma levels might come below the threshold for triggering systemic actions. A retardation may be especially important for steroid reaching peripheral lung, where this fraction otherwise will be rapidly absorbed via pulmonary circulation and contribute poorly to efficacy in airways.

These two options are discussed below.

A. Extrahepatic Metabolism

The overwhelming systemic bioavailability of an inhaled glucocorticoids with mainly hepatic inactivation comes from the airway-lung–deposited fraction rather than from the orally swallowed fraction (see Fig. 9). Therefore, it would be advantageous to introduce a structure in the glucocorticoid, making a rapid inactivation of the molecule possible during its systemic distribution, especially

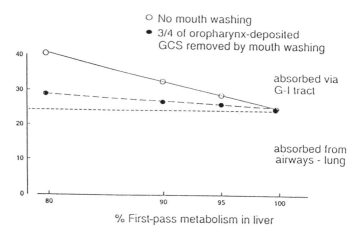

Assumption: Of the dose reaching the patient 1/4 is deposited
in airways and lung and 3/4 in oropharynx

Figure 9   Total systemic availability of inhaled glucocorticoid as a function of first pass metabolism in liver and mouth washing. (From Ref. 53.). Assumption: of the dose reaching the patient, one-quarter is deposited in airways and lung and three-quarters in oropharynx.

in blood. This presupposes that other inactivation routes than the mainly liver-based cytochrome P450 system have to be utilized. The routes tested have been via plasma and tissue esterases and via S-methyltransferases.

A leading compound in this regard has been fluocortin butylester (FCB), which is a 20-keto, 21-oic acid ester (69). This compound is inactivated to its corresponding 20-keto, 21-oic acid in both lung tissue and blood (70; data in the files of A. Draco) and the carboxylic acid lacks glucocorticoid activity (70). Inhalation of high doses of FCB does not induce adrenal suppression in the dog and human (71,72). However, inhaled FCB demonstrates no or low therapeutic efficacy in asthma (73,74). Inhalation of high doses of FCB has, however, shown a protective effect and a good safety profile in rhinitis (75,76). It is not known why FCB failed as an antiasthma drug, and answers to that question can only be speculative. The most probable explanations are a too poor intrinsic activity (the affinity of FCB to the GR is just similar to that of hydrocortisone [data on file at Astra Draco AB]), in combination with a local inactivation. Even though FCB showed insufficient antiasthmatic effect, it represents a class of compounds that might be improved. However, one can assume that a very much higher affinity for the GR is necessary for such substances as a compensation for the risk of a partial inactivation of the steroid in target tissue.

The critical question is what rate of inactivation can be accepted in the airway-lung tissue compared with the high blood clearance? A glucocorticoid that inactivates too rapidly locally, gives low systemic effect but also a too low local effect. On the other hand, a too slow hydrolysis of the glucocorticoid causes a high local potency, but then the risk of unwanted systemic effects may be more evident. Careful structure-activity studies, where rate of airway and blood inactivation as well as intrinsic activity of active and inactive metabolites are determined, have to answer whether it is possible to generate safer glucocorticoids based on plasma- and tissue-based hydrolytic pathways. Even if working, a steroid of that kind may have to be administered more often than twice a day.

The 21-thiol ester, burtixocort propionate ([53] JO 1222), has a partial extrahepatic metabolism via thiol esterases and S-methyltransferases (77). There are no publications available demonstrating sufficient clinical effectiveness. Tipredane is a double-thiol ether having a very high receptor affinity in vitro (three times that of budesonide [53]). However, its just modest clinical effectiveness in rhinitis and asthma (Fison, company information [78]) suggests that the steroid lacks either a sufficient metabolic stability in airways or the lipophilicity required for the prolonged local tissue binding.

B. Prolonged Deposition-Retention Time in Airways-Lung

Figure 9 shows that the overwhelming systemic bioavailability of inhaled steroid derives from the airways-lung deposited fraction. Initially, there is a rapid uptake of a bulk fraction, especially of the part that is peripherally deposited (53). By prolonging the uptake of that fraction and thereby increasing the retention time of the steroid in the airways-lung tissue, it might be possible to improve the local anti-inflammatory effect as well as to lower the undesired systemic effects. Even if the airways-lung–derived fraction will still be bioavailable once absorbed, the plasma level is reduced and over a very prolonged absorption period, the level may be below the threshold level for triggering systemic adverse effects.

One way to increase the time of retention would be to use suitable slow-release formulations. One type of vehicle used for that purpose is liposomes. They are membrane-like vesicles consisting of a series of phospholipid bilayers alternating with hydrophilic compartments.

A substitution with lipophilic acyl chains in the 21-OH position of glucocorticoids must be done in order to enhance further their lipophilic character, since the underivatized steroids are poorly incorporated into liposomes and are poorly retained in the vesicles (79). However, esterification of a glucocorticoid with fatty acids causes a decrease in the receptor affinity. Budesonide 21-palmitate (Fig. 10) binds to the receptor with an affinity which is at least 100

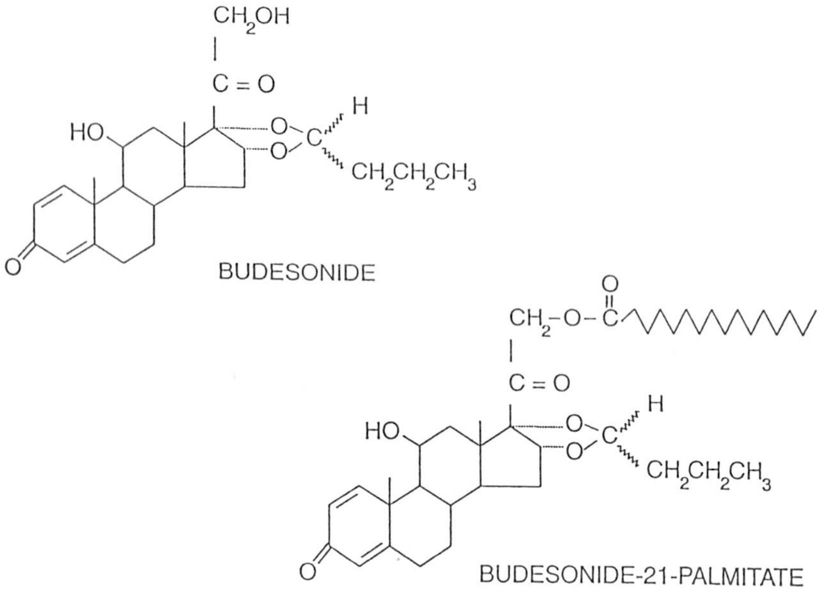

Figure 10 Structure of budesonide and budesonide-21-palmitate.

times lower than that of budesonide, which indicates that budesonide-21 palmitate is a prodrug. Relative binding affinity (RBA) for the GR in rat cytosolic preparations were performed according to Dahlberg et al. (54). Nonadrenal-ectomized animals were used. [^{3}H]Dexamethasone was used as radioactively labeled ligand, and the 50% specific binding level for each competitor was normalized by comparison with budesonide, which was assigned a relative binding affinity (RBA) of 1.

Steroid	RBA
Budesonide	1
Budesonide-palmitate	<0.01
Hydrocortisone	0.01

A prolonged time of retention in peripheral lung is obtained for bude-sonide-21-palmitate in liposomes compared with budesonide. Two hours after intratracheal instillation of budesonide, only a limited fraction of the steroid is found in peripheral lung, whereas the half-life time in the lung of budesonide-21-palmitate in liposomes is more than 6 hr (53). It should be emphasized, however, that this determination is based on peripherally deposited glucocorticoid. No retention studies, where liposomes encapsulated glucocorticoid ester has been administered more specifically in the central airway, have yet been reported.

The functional importance of a retention of this kind has been tested in the Sephadex-induced lung edema model—a rat model of bronchiolitis and alveolitis (Fig. 11). In one variant of the test, a local administration of glucocorticoid in only the left lung lobe makes it possible to determine the "local" (inhibition in the left lung lobe) and the systemic (inhibition in the right lung lobe) anti-inflammatory effect, respectively. First of all, budesonide-21-palmitate in liposomes shows an enhanced local anti-inflammatory effect compared with budesonide (Fig. 12). Second, and more important, the lipophilic ester reaches a markedly better local/systemic relationship (Fig. 12) owing to its lower effect in the nontreated right lung lobe (as well as in thymus) compared with its high efficacy in the left lung lobe, where the glucocorticoid was applied.

A different anti-inflammatory profile of budesonide-21-palmitate in liposomes is reached when the steroid is given locally to airways-lung compared with when it is administered intravenously or orally. The liposomal steroid formulation given locally (intratracheally) to the respiratory tract mediates a higher anti-inflammatory potency than after systemic administration (intravenously or orally) (Fig. 13). Furthermore, the glucocorticoid effects seen in other organs were more pronounced after intravenous and oral administration than after intratracheal instillation when equal pulmonary anti-inflammatory efficacy is compared (results exemplified with thymus [Fig. 13]).

Intratracheal administration of Sephadex causes an influx of inflammatory cells to the lung. An increase of the number of macrophages, eosinophils, and neutrophils is observed 20 hr after Sephadex administration (Fig. 14). Local treatment with liposome-encapsulated budesonide-21-palmitate or with plain budesonide causes an inhibition of the influx of inflammatory cells. The number of macrophages can be normalized by the use of both steroid formulations,

---

Intratracheal instillation of Sephadex beads (crosslinked dextran) to both lung halves leads to

- ► Bronchiolitis with infiltration of WBC (esp. eosinophils), peribronchial/perivascular edema
- ► Alveolitis with granuloma (incl. giant cell formation) and interstitial edema
- ► Impaired ventilation
- ► Bronchial hyperresponsiveness

Figure 11 Sephadex-induced bronchiolitis and alveolitis in the rat (80–82).

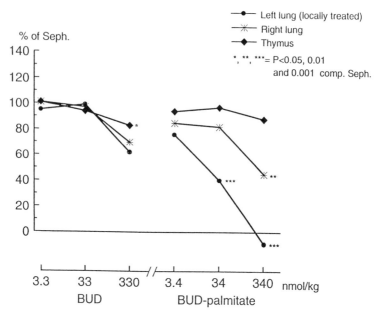

Figure 12 Effect of budesonide and budesonide-21-palmitate (the latter in liposomes) on Sephadex-induced lung edema. The local anti-inflammatory effects were measured as inhibition of lung weight increase 1 day after Sephadex administration by intratracheal instillation (glucocorticoid was administered 2 hr before Sephadex administration only in the left lung lobe). 100% indicates lung weight of Sephadex-treated animals without glucocorticoid treatment.

but a 10 times higher dose must be used with plain budesonide. The same pattern is true for eosinophils. The number of neutrophils is also reduced but to a lesser extent than for eosinophils and macrophages. For both budesonide and budesonide-21-palmitate in liposomes, there was a correlation between antiedema activity and inhibition of cell infiltration (Fig. 14).

VI. Summary

The glucocorticoids currently used by inhalation seem to reach their airway selectivity by a combination of a high and prolonged binding to local airway tissues and a very efficient hepatic first-pass inactivation. Both these properties are enhanced by introducing lipophilic substituents in the 17α or 16α,17α

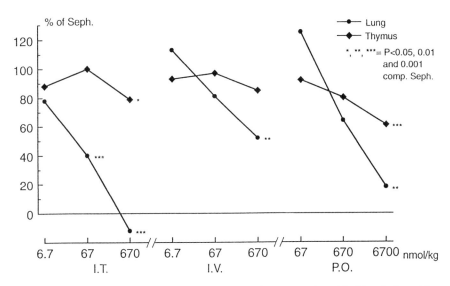

Figure 13 Local and systemic effects of budesonide and budesonide-21-palmitate (the latter in liposomes) after intratracheal (i.t.), intravenous (i.v.), and per oral (p.o.) administration of glucocorticoid. Glucocorticoid was administered 2 hr before Sephadex administration. The local anti-inflammatory effect was measured as inhibition of lung weight increase one day after Sephadex administration and systemic effects as decrease of thymus, spleen, and adrenal weights. 100% indicates lung, thymus, spleen, and adrenal weights of Sephadex-treated animals without glucocorticoid treatment.

positions. Even if none of these glucocorticoids have been primarily selected in airways–lung models, this developmental line may well have attained its optimum also for inhalation use. In parallel to this chemical work, the airway selectivity has been enhanced by new powder inhalers and spacers, markedly reinforcing airway deposition as well as reducing oral uptake.

The bioavailability and by that systemic activity of these steroids is derived predominantly from the airways-lung absorbed fraction. A better inactivation/reduction of that big fraction is necessary for a further, substantial improvement of airway selectivity. Under the assumption that airways are the major target, a development of this kind would lead to an improved safety margin also at high dose levels of inhaled steroid. Currently, there is no firm evidence that it is possible to attain airway efficacy and selectivity in humans by adding an extrahepatic (here exploited as presystemic) inactivation to the

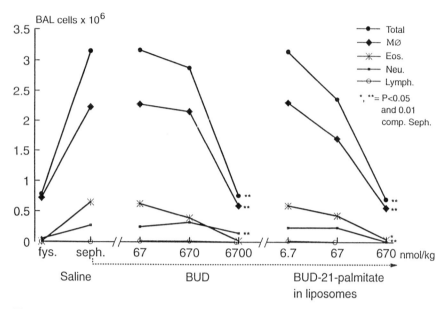

Figure 14   Effect of budesonide and budesonide-21-palmitate (the latter in liposomes) on Sephadex-induced cell influx into the lung. Sephadex was instilled intratracheally and bronchoalveolar lavage was performed 20 hr later. Control animals received 0.9% NaCl only. Glucocorticoid was administered 3 hr prior to Sephadex administration by intratracheal administration.

hepatic one. The other option tested—prodrugs with a strongly protracted absorption rate—is supported by a better topical selectivity in a rat model of pulmonary inflammation. However, it remains to be demonstrated whether improved topical selectivity is also reached in human alveolitis as well as in more central airway diseases like human asthma.

Acknowledgment

We thank our colleagues at Astra Draco AB at the departments of Pharmacology, Kinetics, and Metabolism and Medicinal Chemistry for joint work over the years on topical steroids for airway diseases.

Discussion

DR. O'BYRNE: There are a number of glucocorticoids which are esterase sensitive and rapidly metabolized. These have not been clinically effective. Are they topically active?

DR. BRATTSAND: Some steroids with a rapid inactivation via plasma and tissue esterases have recently been developed, but they have failed in clinical asthma. The probable reason is that the inactivating esterases are also prevalent in the target cells. We have found topical efficacy and selectivity (even better than for the hepatically inactivated drugs) in our animal lung models when we can give a sufficiently high dose by tracheal instillation. Under clinical conditions by inhalation, it is obviously not possible to give doses high enough. The option would be to develop biolabile steroids with even higher receptor affinity, formulate them in some slow-delivery system, and by that possibly improve local efficacy.

DR. McFADDEN: (1) What determines the movement of budesonide from the lumen of the airway to the mucosa? Does an inflammatory infiltrate or plasma exudation act as a barrier? (2) Can an inhaled steroid recirculate from the bronchus to the trachea and back?

DR. BRATTSAND: (1) The inhaled glucocorticoids are taken up by free diffusion—not due to inactive uptake. In the model with topical superfusion, the second highest concentration (after trachea itself) was the underlying esophagus, supporting its good penetration possibilities.

DR. PERSSON: (1) An exudative airway inflammation process and epithelial derangements may not impede the penetration of airway glucocorticoids such as budesonide into the airway tissue. The lipophilic budesonide molecule will rapidly be taken up by airway tissue and will, therefore, not be removed from the site of mucosal deposition by mucociliary clearance mechanisms. Even a lavage carried out already 10–20 min after budesonide application will not remove the drug, because it has penetrated and is bound to the tissue. (2) If we shut off the perfusion through tracheobronchial arteries and inject tracers into the pulmonary artery, they will be moved all along the airways up to the lower portion of the trachea.

DR. BARNES: Have you studied the localization of [^{3}H]budesonide to particular cell types in the trachea after local application using autoradiography? I am interested in whether there is any preferential localization in airway epithelial cells.

DR. BRATTSAND: Autoradiography performed 2 hr after administration of [^{3}H]budesonide shows the highest concentration in the mucosal and serosal compartments of the tracheal wall. The high serosal level probably depends on the shortcuts between the mucosal and serosal circulations. We have performed no microautoradiographic study, so I can not tell the distribution at the cellular level.

DR. LIU: Does inflammation affect local steroid binding or metabolism?

DR. BRATTSAND: Budesonide is fully inactivated first in the liver, and therefore metabolism would not affect local efficacy. The question is instead whether inflammation reduces its absorption and tissue binding. According to animal models, where we induced a strong plasma exudation in the tracheal model, there was no major inhibition of its uptake.

DR. EEDSBACKER: Data on inhaled budesonide in healthy subjects and patients with moderate asthma show that plasma concentrations are the same, implying that inflammation per se does not affect the pharmacokinetics of this drug.

DR. SCHLEIMER: For systemic (e.g., oral) steroids having a recovery period by using a single daily dose instead of divided doses may reduce side effects. Are you concerned that using lipophilic vehicles, for example, liposomes, to prolong the duration of local steroid action might enhance local side effects?

DR. BRATTSAND: According to the inhalation toxicity studies performed hitherto (3-month duration with such vehicles), we have seen no signs of local atrophy or other signs of local adverse effects.

DR. O'BYRNE: Do you know which airway vessels the corticosteroids diffuse into to be systemically available?

DR. BRATTSAND: To my knowledge, there is no precise information on how much of the total systemic absorption comes from the most peripheral lung area (which we do not consider a target in asthma and where the absorption is most rapid). The strategy to be tested is to slow down the absorption rate from both central and peripheral levels by reducing the uptake rate and enhancing the local tissue binding. What needs to be evaluated is whether reducing the uptake rate from the target tissue might both enhance antiasthmatic efficacy and reduce systemic adverse actions.

DR. LAITINEN: (1) Would it be possible based on the results of animal models that the local effects are too strong? For example, does decreasing the number of eosinophils have a negative effect on other cells like fibroblasts or matrix proteins? (2) At the cellular level, is there any explanation for the long-lasting carryover effect which inhaled corticosteroids often have?

DR. BRATTSAND: The speculation that too strong a reduction of tissue eosinophils in our inflammatory locus would enhance fibrosis is speculative. There are, on the other hand, in vitro findings (Hernäs, JB Särnstrand, P Lindroth, et al. Eosinophilic cationic protein alters proteoglycan metabolism in human lung fibroblast cultures. Eur J Cell Biol 1992; 59:352–363) showing that eosinophilic granule protein enhances the intracellular content of proteoglycan material (heparin and dermatan sulfate chains) in human lung fibroblast cultures. The increase depends on inhibited degradation of the glycosaminoglycans, which promotes a fibrotic response. Furthermore, it is still difficult in severe asthma to achieve a full inhibition of eosinophil recruitment and activation by steroid treatment.

DR. SMALDONE: The questions raised regarding unknown local pulmonary toxicities also reflect on our lack of understanding regarding the desired response.

References

1. Feldman D, Funder J, Loose D. Is the glucocorticoid receptor identical in various organs? J Steroid Biochem 1978; 9:141–145.
2. LaPointe MC, Baxter JD. Molecular biology of the glucocorticoid hormone action. In: Schleimer RP, Claman HN, Oronsky A, eds. Anti-inflammatory Steroid Action. Basic and Clinical Aspects. San Diego: Academic Press, 1989;3–29.
3. See Chapter 1.
4. Strasser-Wozak EM, Hattmanstorfer R, Hala M, et al. Splice site mutation in the glucocorticoid receptor gene causes resistance to glucocorticoid-induced apoptosis in a human acute leukemic cell line. Cancer Res 1995; 55:348–353.
5. Sarrett LH, Patchett AA, Steelman SL. The effect of structural alteration on the anti-inflammatory properties of hydrocortisone. In: Jucker E, ed. Progress in Drug Research. Basel: Birkhäuser Verlag, 1963; 5:13–153.
6. Popper TL, Watnick AS. Anti-inflammatory steroids. In: Scherrer RA, Whitehouse MW, eds. Anti-inflammatory Agents. Vol. I. New York: Academic Press, 1974:245–294.
7. Phillips GH. Locally active corticosteroids; structure-activity relationship. In: Wilson L, Marks R, eds. Mechanisms of Topical Corticosteroid Activity. Edinburgh: Churchill Livingstone, 1976:1–18.
8. Mygind N, Clark TJH. Topical Steroid Treatment for Asthma and Rhinitis. London: Baillière Tindall, 1980.
9. Clark TJH, Mygind N, Selroos O. Corticosteroid treatment in allergic airway diseases. Eur J Respir Dis 1982; 63(Suppl. 122):9–278.
10. Check WA, Kaliner M. Pharmacology and Pharmacokinetics of topical corticosteroid derivatives used for asthma therapy. Am Rev Respir Dis 1990; 141(No. 2, part 2):S44–S58.
11. Brattsand R, Selroos O. Glucocorticosteroids. In: Page CP, Metzer WJ, eds. Drugs and the Lung. New York: Raven Press, 1994:101–220.
12. Wolff ME. Structure-activity relationship in glucocorticoids. In: Baxter JD, Rousseau GG, eds. Glucocorticoid Hormone Action. Berlin: Springer Verlag, 1979:97–108.
13. Ballard PL. Delivery and transport of glucocorticoids to target cells. In: Baxter JD, Rousseau GG, eds. Glucocorticoid Hormone Action. Berlin, Springer Verlag, 1979:25–48.
14. Haynes RC. Adrenocorticotropic hormone: adrenocortical steroids and their syn-

thetic analogs; inhibitors of the synthesis and actions of adrenocortical hormones. In: Goodman Gilman A, Rall TW, Nies AS, Taylor P, eds. The Pharmacological Basis of Therapeutics. 8th ed. New York: Pergamon Press, 1990:1431–1462.

15. Szefler SJ. General pharmacology of glucocorticoids. In: Schleimer RP, Claman HN, Oronsky A, eds. Anti-inflammatory Steroid Action. Basic and Clinical Aspects. San Diego: Academic Press, 1989:353–376.

16. Robertson DB, Maibach HJ. Topical glucocorticoids. In: Schleimer RP, Claman HN, Oronsky A, eds. Anti-inflammatory Steroid Action. Basic and Clinical Aspects. San Diego: Academic Press, 1989:494–524.

17. Morrow-Brown H. The introduction and early development of inhaled steroid therapy. In: Mygind N, Clark TJH, eds. Topical Steroid Treatment for Asthma and Rhinitis. London: Baillière Tindall, 1980:66–76.

18. Abramovitz M, Branchand CL, Murphy BEP. Cortisol-corticosterone interconversion in human fetal lung: contrasting results using explant and monolayer culture suggest 11β-hydroxysteroid dehydrogenase (EC.1.1.1.146) comprises two ernzymes. J Clin Endocrinol Metals 1982; 54:563–568.

19. Schleimer RP. Potential regulation of inflammation in the lung by local metabolism of hydrocortisone. Am J Respir Cell Mol Biol 1991; 4:166–173.

20. Schleimer RP, Kato M. Regulation of lung inflammation by local glucocorticoid metabolism: an hypothesis. J Asthma 1992; 29:303–317.

21. Toogood JH. Bronchial asthma and glucocorticoids. In: Schleimer RP, Claman HN, Oronsky A, eds. Anti-inflammatory Steroid Action. Basic and Clinical Aspects. San Diego: Academic Press, 1989; 494–524.

22. See Chapter 18.

23. See Chapter 16.

24. Braude AS, Rebuck AS. Prednisolone and methyl-prednisolone disposition in the lung. Lancet 1983; 2:995–997.

25. Greos LS, Vichyanond P, Bloedow DC et al. Methylprednisolone achieves greater concentrations in the lung than prednisolone. A pharmacokinetic analysis. Am Rev Respir Dis 1991; 144:586–592.

26. Linder WR. Adrenal suppression by steroid inhalation. Arch Intern Med 1964; 113:655–656.

27. Toogood JH, Lefcoe NM. Dexamethasone aerosol for the treatment of steroid dependent chronic bronchial asthmatic patients. J Allergy 1965; 36:321–332.

28. Sparkes GS. Plasma cortisol levels in normal subjects after inhaled corticosteroids. Postgrad Med J 1974; 50(Suppl. 4):9–11.

29. McKenzie AW, Atkinson RM. Topical activities of betamethasone esters in man. Arch Dermatol 1964; 89:741–746.

30. Czarny D, Brostoff J. Effect of intranasal betamethasone 17-valerate on perennial rhinitis and adrenal function. Lancet 1968; 2:188–190.

31. Brostoff J, Czarny D. Effects of intranasal betamethasone 17-valerate on allergic rhinitis and adrenal function. J Allergy 1969; 44:77–81.

32. Harris DM, Postgrad Med J 1975; 51(Suppl. 4):20–25.

33. Harris DM, Martin LE, Harrison C, Jack D. The effect of intra-nasal beclomethasone dipropionate on adrenal function. Clin Allergy 1974; 4:291–294.

34. Martin LE, Tanner RJN, Clark TJH, Cochrane GM. Absorption and metabolism of orally administered beclomethasone dipropionate. Clin Pharm Ther 1974; 15:267–275.
35. Clark TJH. Beclomethasone Dipropionate Treatment of Asthma in Adults. London: Baillière Tindall, 1980:94–106.
36. Toogood JH, Lefcoe NM, Haines DSM et al. A graded dose assessment of the efficacy of beclomethasone dipropionate aerosol for severe chronic asthma. J Allergy Clin Immunol 1977; 59:298–308.
37. Law CM, Honour JW, Marchant JL, Preeze MA, Warner JO. Nocturnal suppression in asthmatic children taking inhaled beclomethasone dipropionate. Lancet 1986; 1:321–323.
38. Phillip M, Aviram M, Leiberman E, et al. Integrated plasma cortisol concentration in children with asthma receiving long-term inhaled corticosteroids. Pediatr Pulmon 1992; 12:84–89.
39. Pedersen S. Safety aspects of corticosteroids in children. Eur Respir Rev 1994; 4:33–43.
40. Brattsand R, Thuresson af Ekenstam B, Claesson KG, Thalén A. Steroids, processes for their manufacture and preparations containing some. US patent 3.929.768.
41. Thalén A, Brattsand R. Synthesis and anti-inflammatory properties of budesonide, a new nonhalogenated glucocorticoid with high local activity. Arzneim Forsch 1979; 29:1687–1690.
42. Brattsand R, Thalén A, Roempke K, et al. Influence of $16\alpha,17\alpha$-acetal substitution and steroid nucleus fluorination on the topical to systemic activity ratio of glucocorticoids. J Steroid Biochem 1982; 16:779–786.
43. Anderson P, Edsbäcker S, Ryrfeldt Å, von Bahr C. In vitro biotransformation of glucocorticoids in liver and skin homogenate fraction from man, rat and hairless mouse. J Steroid Biochem 1982; 16:787–796.
44. Brattsand R, Thalén A, Roempke K, et al. Development of new glucocorticosteroids with a very high ratio between topical and systemic activities. Eur J Respir Dis 1982; 63(Suppl. 122):62–73.
45. Chaplin M, Rooks W, Swensson E et al. Flunisolide metabolism and dynamics of a metabolite. Clin Pharmacol Ther 1980; 27:402–413.
46. Slavin RG, Izu AE, Bernstein et al. Multicenter study of flunisolide aerosol in adult patients with steroid-dependent asthma. J Allergy Clin Immunol 1980; 66:379–385.
47. Zaborny BA, Lukacsko P, Barinov-Colligon I, Ziemniak JA. Inhaled corticosteroids in asthma: a dose-proportionality studhy with triamcinolone acetonide aerosol. J Clin Pharmacol 1992; 32:463–469.
48. Altman LC, Findlay SR, Lopez M, et al. Adrenal function in adult asthmatics during long-term daily treatment with 800, 1200 and 1600 µg triamcinolone acetonide: multicenter study. Chest 1992; 101:1250–1256.
49. Phillips GH. Structure-activity relationship of topically active steroids: the selection of flutcasone propionate. Respir Med 1990; 84(Suppl. A):19–23.
50. Harding S. The human pharmacology of fluticasone propionate. Respir Med 1990; 84(Suppl A):25–29.

51. Würthwein G, Rohdewald P. Activation of beclomethasone dipropionate by hydrolysis to beclomethasone 17-monopropionate. Biopharm Drug Dispos 1990; 11:381–394.
52. Würthwein G, Rehder S, Rohdewald P. Lipophilie und Rreceptoraffinität von glucocortidoiden. Pharm Ztg Wiss 1992; 137(4/5):2–8.
53. Brattsand R, Axelsson B. New inhaled glucocorticosteroids. In: Barnes PJ, ed. New Drugs for Asthma. London: IBC Techn Serv, 1992:192–207.
54. Dahlberg E, Thalén A, Brattsand R, et al. Correlation between chemical structure, receptor binding and biological activity of some novel, highly active $16\alpha,17\alpha$-acetal substituted glucocorticoids. Mol Pharmacol 1984; 25:70–78.
55. Thalén A, Brattsand R, Gruvstad E. Synthesis and pharmacological properties of some $16\alpha,17\alpha$-acetals of 16α-hydroxyhyrocortisone, 16α-hydroxy-prednisolone and fluorinated 16α-hydroxyprednisolones. Acta Pharm Suec 1984; 21:109–124.
56. Rohdewald P, von Eift M, Würthwein G. Aktivierung von Beclometasondipropionat im Bronchialsekret sowie Receptoraffinität und Löslichkeit inhalativ angewandter Glukokortikoide. Atemw Lungenkrkh 1990; 16:79–84.
57. Brattsand R, Pipkorn U. Glucocorticoids: experimental approaches. In: Kaliner M, Barnes PJ, Persson CGA, eds. Asthma, Its Pathology and Treatment. New York: Marcel Dekker, 1991:667–710.
58. Högger P, Rohdewald P. Binding kinetics of flurticasone propionate to the human glucocorticoid receptor. Steroids 1994; 59:597–602.
59. van den Bosch JMM, Westmann CJJ, Aumann J, et al. Relationship between lung tissue and blood plasma concentrations of inhaled budesonide. Biopharm Drug Dispos 1993; 14:455–459.
60. Brattsand R, Miller-Larsson A, Nilsson M. Uptake and retention of the topical glucocorticoids budesonide in rat trachea and lung as influenced by the mode of administration and by inflammation (abstr.). Am Rev Respir Dis 1993; 147(4):A178.
61. Miller-Larsson A, Mattsson H, Ohlsson S, et al. Prolonged release from the airway tissue of glucocorticoids budesonide and fluticasone propionate as compared to beclomethasone dipropionate and hydrocortisone (abstr.). Am J Respir Crit Care Med 1994; 149(4 Pt 2):A466.
62. Miller-Larsson A, Brattsand R. Topical anti-inflammatory activity of the glucocorticoid budesonide on airway mucosa. Evidence for a "hit and run" type of activity. Agents Actions 1990; 29½:127–129.
63. Ryrfeldt Å, Andersson P, Edsbäcker S, et al. Pharmacokinetics and metabolism of budesonide, a selective glucocorticoid. Eur J Respir Dis 1982; 63(Suppl. 122):86–95.
64. Edsbäcker S, Jönsson S, Lindberg , et al. Metabolic pathways of the topical glucocorticoid budesonide in man. Drug Metab Dispos 1983; 11:590–596.
65. Riedel DJ, Harrison LI, Machacek JH, et al. Pharmacokinetics of beclomethasone from beclomethasone dipropionate in an HFA-134a (A) CFC-free propellant system (abstr.). J Aerosol Med 1995; 8(1):P97.
66. Jönsson G, Åström A, Andersson PH. Budesonide is metabolized by cytochrome P 45 3A (CYP3A) enzymes in human liver. Drug Metab Dispos 1995; 23:137–142.

67. Grahnén A, Eckernäs S-Å, Brundin RM, Ling-Andersson. An asssessment of the systemic activity of single doses of inhaled fluticasone propionate in healthy volunteers. Br J Clin Pharm 1994; 38:521–525.

68. Grahnén A, Ling-Andersson A, Brundin RM, Eckernäs S-Å. Suppressive effects of therapeutic doses of fluticasone propionate on the HPA-axis in healthy volunteers. Thorax 1995; 50(4):444P.

69. Brattsand R. Glucocorticosteroids for inhalation. In: PJ Barnes, ed. New Drugs for Asthma. London: IBC Techn Serv 1989:117–130.

70. Mützel W. Pharmakokinetic und Biotransformation von Fluocortin butylester beim Menschen. Arzneim Forsch/Drug Res 1977; 27 II:2230–2233.

71. Bhargava AS, Staben P, Siegmund F, Schöbel C, Günzel P. Effect of fluocortin butylester and beclomethasone dipropionate on adrenal gland in Beagle dogs. Arzneim Forsch 1978; 28:1638–1641.

72. Vlasses PH, Ferguson RK, Koplin JR, Clementi RA, Green PJ. Adrenocortical function after chronic inhalation of flucortinbutyl and beclomethasone dipropionate. Clin Pharmacol Ther 1981; 29:643–649.

73. Burge PS, Efthimiou J, Turner-Warwick M, et al. Double-blind trial of inhaled beclomethasone dipropionate and flucortin butylester in allergen induced immediate and late asthmatic reaction. Clin Allergy 1982; 12:523–531.

74. Wüthrich B, Chen Walden H. Evaluation of FCB, BDP and DSCG in allergen inhalation challenge test. Int J Clin Pharmacol Ther Toxicol 1982; 20:595–599.

75. Arbesman C, Bernstein IL, Bierman CW, Bocles JS, Katz R, Lieberman PL, Mattucci K, Meltzer Eo, Middleton E Jr, Noyes J, Pearlman DS, Pence HL, Slavin RG, Spector SL. Multi-center double-blind, placebo-controlled trial of fluocortinbutyl in perennial rhinitis. J Allergy Clin Immunol 1983; 71:597–603.

76. Orgel HA, Meltzer EO, Biermann CW, Bronsky E, Connell JT, Lieberman PL, Nathan R, Pearlman DS, Pence HL, Slavin RG, Naadimuthu A. Intranasal fluocortinbutyl in patients with perennial rhinitis: A 12-month efficacy study and safety study including nasal biopsy. J Allergy Clin Immunol 1991; 88:257–264.

77. Chanoine F, Grenot C, Heidmann P, Junien JL. Pharmacokinetics of butixocort 21-propionate, budesonide and beclomethasone dipropionate in the rat after intratracheal, intravenous and oral treatments. Drug Metab Dispos 1991; 19:546–553.

78. In Brief: Fisons' tipredane. Pink Sheet 1993; April 12, T & G18.

79. Shaw IH, Knight CH, Dingle JT. Liposomal retention of a modified anti-inflammatory steroid. Biochem J 1976; 158:473–476.

80. Brattsand R, Johansson U, Källström L. Sephadex-induced inflammation in the rat. I. Model description and protective action by drugs (abstr.) Int J Microcirc Clin Exp 1986; 5:263.

81. Willén H, Carlén B, Brattsand R. Sephadex-induced inflammation in the rat lung II Light and electron microscopic studies (abstr.) Int J Microcirc Clin Exp 1986; 5:263.

82. Bjermer L, Sandström T, Särnstrand B, Brattsand R. Sephadex-induced granulomatous alveolitis in rat-effect of antigen manipulation. Am J Industr Med 1994; 25:73–78.

16

Glucocorticoid Pharmacokinetics
Principles and Clinical Applications

STAFFAN EDSBÄCKER

Astra Draco AB
Lund, Sweden

STANLEY J. SZEFLER

National Jewish Center for Immunology
and Respiratory Medicine
Denver, Colorado

I. Introduction

Glucocorticoids represent a group of extremely potent anti-inflammatory agents. They are administered in the oral and parenteral forms as supplementary or rescue therapy for patients with severe, chronic asthma or acute exacerbations. At the present time, they are also highlighted as first-line therapy for patients with less severe forms of persistent asthma. This section focuses on information related to glucocorticoid pharmacokinetics and pharmacodynamics including both systemic and inhaled routes of administration.

Severe acute asthma, status asthmaticus, is treated with high-dose systemic glucocorticoids combined with frequent administration of inhaled β-adrenergic bronchodilator agents. Glucocorticoids can be administered by the parenteral route (methylprednisolone sodium succinate, hydrocortisone sodium succinate) or alternatively by the oral route (prednisone, methylprednisolone) either of which provides a rapid onset of action and systemic effects. Methylprednisolone sodium succinate may be administered in a dose of approximately 1 mg/kg IV every 6 hr (1,2). Following resolution of severe obstruction, the steroid dose is reduced and administered by the oral route. The duration of treatment and tapering doses are dependent on the patient's response and past history.

Glucocorticoids are also recommended for the treatment of impending episodes of severe asthma when bronchodilator therapy is inadequate (3,4). Prednisone, approximately 1–2 mg/kg per day, is administered orally once daily or in two or three divided doses for 3–7 days. There are no studies to date that compare the relative benefits of once daily administration versus divided doses. The dose and duration of treatment is based on the patient's response and past history.

In patients with poorly controlled chronic asthma, oral glucocorticoids may be administered in a dosing schedule similar to that previously described to maximize pulmonary function. Once this goal is achieved, the prednisone dose is tapered and may be supplemented and eventually replaced by inhaled glucocorticoids (1,5–7).

Recent emphasis has been placed on the development of inhaled glucocorticoids and the important property is topical potency. The biological response to steroids is related to modification of the basic structure of the steroid molecule. Structural modifications have successfully separated the mineralocorticoid from the metabolic and anti-inflammatory effects; however, it has not been possible to remove the metabolic effects and isolate the desired anti-inflammatory properties. The glucocorticoids available for inhalation in the United States, beclomethasone dipropionate, triamcinolone acetonide, and flunisolide, appear to have similar topical to systemic potency ratios; however, more clinical studies are needed to clarify issues around comparative efficacy and toxicity. All three are administered by a metered-dose inhaler. Two other inhaled glucocorticoids, budesonide and fluticasone propionate, which are available outside the United States, will likely be approved in the near future. Both have favorable properties of high topical potency, low oral bioavailability, and rapid systemic elimination. Budesonide is also available outside the United States in a suspension suitable for nebulized administration. Availability of the latter preparation provide means for glucocorticoid administration to infants.

With the increased awareness of asthma as an inflammatory disease, it is anticipated that the application of glucocorticoid therapy will be initiated at an earlier stage, will be used earlier in the disease process, and used for an extended period of time, and will continue to be placed as the cornerstone of an asthma treatment regimen. An appreciation of pharmacokinetic principles will continue to play a role in the optimization of medication selection and individualization of dose. The following sections will provide a detailed synopsis of the pharmacokinetic variables influencing drug response.

II. Overall Conditions Influencing Response to Glucocorticoids: Beneficial and Adverse

The most significant determinant for response to glucocorticoid therapy is the structural components of the administered agent. Although certain features are essential for pharmacological effect, additional structural modifications may increase the potency and duration of effect.

Another important determinant of response to glucocorticoid therapy relates to the systemic disposition of the individual compounds. This is integrally related to the structure, since this will affect the rate of elimination and distribution of the steroid. Glucocorticoid pharmacokinetics are also complicated by some unique features. The first factor to consider is the protein binding characteristics. Certain glucocorticoids are bound to both transcortin, a high-affinity–low-capacity glucocorticoid binding globulin, and albumin, a plasma protein with low affinity and high capacity. Second, certain glucocorticoids, such as prednisone and cortisone, are inactive and must undergo a conversion reaction to form the active component.

The time of onset and intensity of pharmacological effect is related to the specific glucocorticoid and its disposition parameters. It is likely that the cellular onset of action is immediate. However, the intricate mechanisms necessary to attain the desired physiological effect results in a lag time for the observed beneficial effect. Prolonged exposure to glucocorticoid therapy while maintaining the desired response may contribute to the development of adverse effects.

Certain pharmacokinetic factors such as impairment of glucocorticoid elimination may contribute to the development of adverse effects. A poor response to a standard regimen may be due to a number of factors, such as poor drug delivery or rapid elimination.

The efficacy and risk for adverse effects to inhaled glucocorticoids are related to the dose and frequency of administration, the specific glucocorticoid, and the systemic availability of the glucocorticoid. Very little is known regarding pulmonary distribution, retention, and metabolism of the inhaled glucocorticoids under clinical conditions. The systemic availability of the inhaled steroids can be influenced by the method of delivery, absorption from the lung and the intestinal tract, and metabolism both in the lung and in the body.

III. Structure-Activity Relationships

The basic chemical structure of the glucocorticoids consists of 21 carbon atoms with a total of four rings, three six-carbon rings (A, B, and C), and a five-carbon ring (D). Most of the anti-inflammatory glucocorticoids have a two-carbon chain at the 17 position and methyl groups at carbons 10 and 13. Other essential features of the anti-inflammatory corticosteroids consist of the following: (1) a ketone oxygen at C-3, (2) an unsaturated bond between C-4 and C-5, (3) a hydroxyl group at C-11, and (4) a ketone oxygen at C-20. Fluticasone has a carbothioic acid in the 17 position, but has otherwise the same structural features as other glucocorticoids.

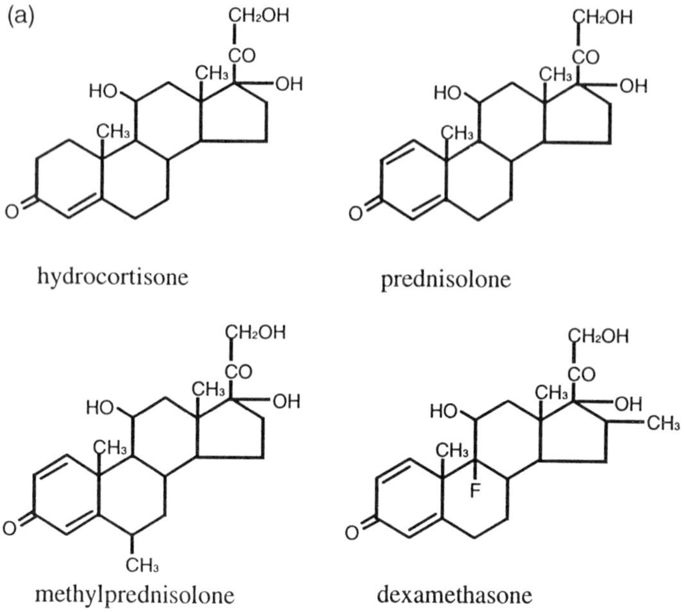

Figure 1   (a) Structure of systemic glucocorticoids. (b) Structure of inhaled gluco-corticoids.

Modifications of this basic structure aim at enhancing anti-inflammatory activity and reducing mineralocorticoid activity as compared with cortisol (Fig. 1). The introduction of an unsaturated double bond between C-1 and C-2 on cortisol provides the structure for prednisolone, which has a fourfold enhancement of glucocorticoid activity and less mineralocorticoid activity as compared with cortisol. Cortisone and the synthetic derivative prednisone are 11-keto compounds and lack anti-inflammatory activity until converted into the 11-β-hydroxyl compounds cortisol and prednisolone.

The addition of a methyl group at the 6α position of prednisolone forms methylprednisolone. Methylprednisolone is slightly more potent in glucocorticoid activity than prednisolone with less mineralocorticoid activity. Although this may seem like a minor structural modification, there is a significant difference between methylprednisolone and prednisolone with regard to protein binding and susceptibility to inhibition or induction of metabolism.

Dexamethasone is a synthetic analogue with a 25-fold increase in glucocorticoid potency and minimal mineralocorticoid effect. It is a modification of prednisolone with a fluorine atom at the 9α position (enhanced glucocorticoid activity) and a methyl group at the C-16α position (decreased mineralocorticoid

(b)

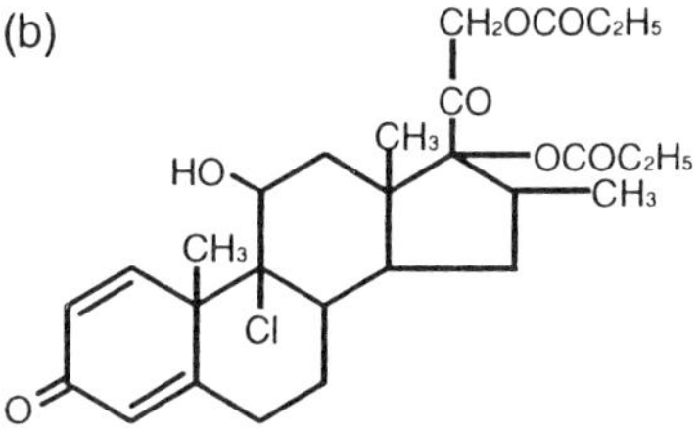

beclomethasone dipropionate

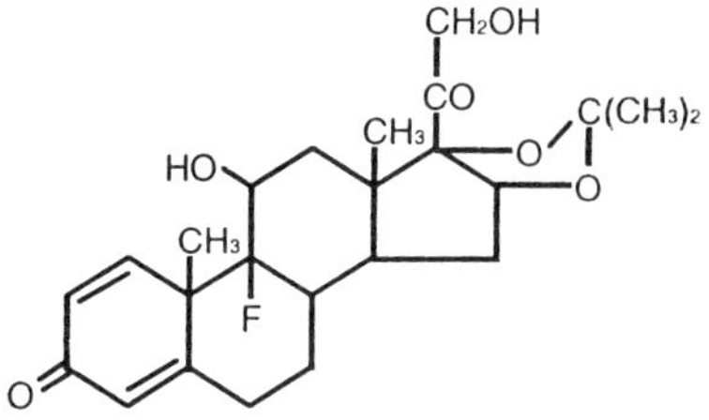

triamcinolone acetonide

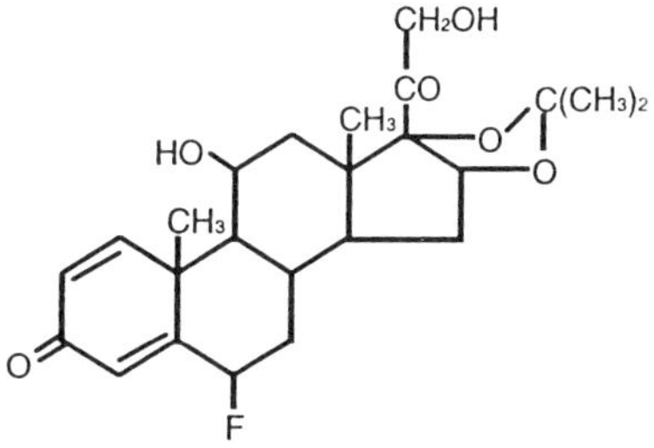

flunisolide

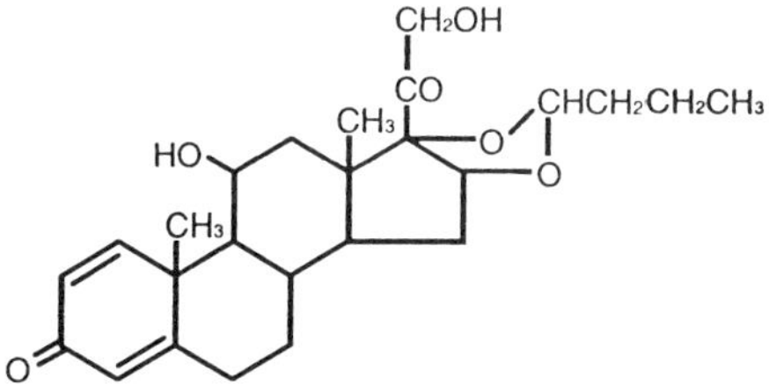

budesonide

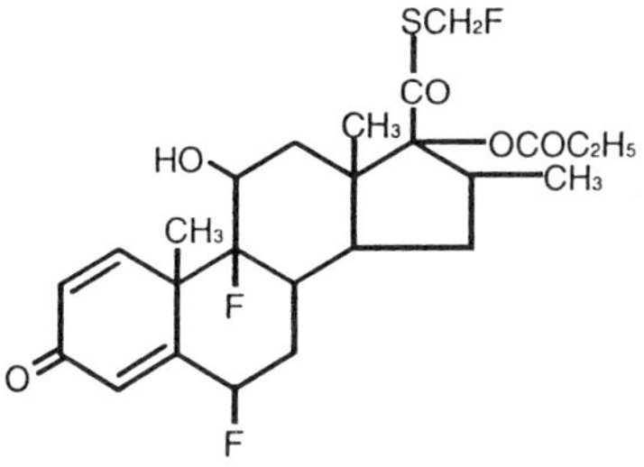

fluticasone propionate

Figure 1 Continued.

activity). The biological half-life of dexamethasone is increased to 36–54 hr. Betamethasone differs form dexamethasone only in the C-16 position, where betamethasone has a C-16β methyl group, whereas the methyl group is at the C-16α position for dexamethasone. The anti-inflammatory potency and duration of action for the two steroids are similar.

Fludrocortisone (9α-fluorocortisol) is a minor modification of cortisol with 10-fold anti-inflammatory activity as compared with cortisol. Since it has markedly increased mineralocorticoid activity, 125 times that of cortisol, it is used primarily for that purpose.

Most glucocorticoids are poorly water soluble so as to pass cell membranes easily, but some are conjugated to improve water solubility and extent of absorption. Conjugation also affects the rate of absorption and the duration of action. The phosphate and hemisuccinate conjugates at C-21 increase water solubility of glucocorticoids such as prednisolone, hydrocortisone, and methylprednisolone, providing a means for parenteral administration. Another conjugate, an acetate form of cortisone, results in slow absorption and delayed onset of action.

Further alterations at the C-17 and C-21 positions result in corticosteroids with high topical activity and minimal systemic adverse effects (Fig. 1b). Aerosol administration results in a potent topical effect on the lung with subsequent systemic absorption and metabolism to inactive or almost inactive metabolites.

IV. Pharmacokinetics

While pharmadynamics are characterized as the action of a drug on the organism, pharmacokinetics deal with the fate of the drug. However, a more operational description of pharmacokinetics includes all the process that determine the concentration of the active substance at the receptor site. By this definition, the essential pharmacodynamic link becomes more apparent.

The unifying concept is to explain and predict drug action in the human body, and it is based on the measurement of concentrations of the parent compound and its metabolites, most often by establishing plasma concentration time curves. Therefore, the value of such studies is heavily dependent on analytical assays that require a high degree of sensitivity, reproducibility, and specificity (see p. 400).

The intrinsic kinetic properties of a glucocorticoid is described by its volume of distribution (V), clearance (CL), and half-life ($t_{1/2}$) (Table 1). For a specific glucocorticoid, bioavailability (F) is often calculated. These pharmacokinetic parameters give an indication of the relative tissue uptake (V), the elimination capacity (CL), the time to attain and decay from steady-state conditions ($t_{1/2}$), and the rate and extent of body exposure (F) (Table 2). These properties can be described in physiological terms as the absorption, distribution, metabolism,and excretion (ADME) properties of the glucocorticoids.

A. Absorption

Intravenous

Rescue medication with high-dose glucocorticoids generally requires parenteral dosing as a bolus or as an infusion. To increase solubility, the glucocorticoid alcohols are often esterified. Phosphate and hemisuccinate esters promptly and

Table 1   Definition of Pharmacokinetic Parameters

Volume of distribution (V) is a measure of the apparent body space available to contain the drug and relates the amount of drug in the body to its concentration in blood or plasma. Vβ represents the apparent distribution space during the terminal log-linear elimination β phase, and Vss represents the volume in which the drug would appear to be distributed in at steady state if its concentration were the same as in the analyzed fluid (blood or plasma).

Clearance (CL) is the rate of elimination by all routes relative to the concentration in a biological fluid (plasma or blood). The clearance in an individual patient will determine the correct dosing rate and in a group of subjects will indicate the efficiency by which the body can eliminate the drug.

Half-life ($t_{1/2}$) is an expression of the relationship between volume of distribution and clearance. Measured in blood, plasma, or urine, it reflects the rate of elimination of the drug from the systemic circulation. It specificaly indicates the time required to reduce the amount of drug in the body by one-half.

Bioavailability (F), in strict terms, reflects the amount of drug absorbed systemically. Since the estimate of bioavailability more often is based on plasma or blood concentrations, *systemic availability* is a more appropriate term particulary for drugs which are administered locally and exert a local effect. The extent of systemic availability is generally expressed in percentage of a reference formulation. Absolute systemic availability implies intravenous dosing as the reference.

quantitatively release the pharmacologically active free alcohol and are therefore suitable for such formulations. Dexamethasone sulfate is an example of an ester which is almost inert and not suitable for intravenous treatment (46). Methylprednisolone hemisuccinate (29) and dexamethasone phosphate (35), having "robust" kinetics over a wide dose interval, are commonly used in emergency situations of, for example, status asthmaticus.

Oral

Price, long-term safety, and compliance influence the choice of the oral glucocorticoid regimen. Prednisolone and prednisone are by far the most commonly prescribed oral glucocorticoids; primarily for cost reasons. Prednisone, inactive in itself, has the disadvantage of requiring interconversion to prednisolone to exert its effect. This interconversion, however, occurs very efficiently in the liver and other organs by 11β-hydroxysteroid dehydrogenase and the systemic availability of prednisolone, using intravenous prednisolone as reference, is the same (>70%) irrespective of the mode of administration as oral prednisone or as oral prednisolone (47).

Table 2 Intravenous Pharmacokinetics of Glucocorticoids in Humans

Compound	Dose	Subjects	$t_{1/2}$ (hr)	V (L/kg)	CL (L/min)	Comments[a]	Reference
Hydrocortisone	100 mg	4F	1.8	1.42	—	Morning values. Phychiatric patients on maintenance therapy with haloperidol	8
	5, 10, 20, 40 mg[c]	6M	1.6	0.4	0.4	Dose dependent kinetics[b]	9
	Tracer	8F, 4M	1.07	0.24	0.22	Primarily convulsive patient	10
Prednisolone	50–500 mg	20	1.9	1	—		11
	5 mg	5M	2.8	0.49[c]	0.14		12
	0.075, 1.5 mg/kg	44M, 4F	–	0.67[c]	0.20	Dose dependent kinetics[b]	13
	40 mg	8M, 5F	3.2	0.82[c]	0.20		14
	20–80mg	3F	2.6	0.91[d]	0.23	Asthmatic patients[b]	15
	20 mg	3F, 4M	3.7	0.24	0.07	Tuberculosis patients	16
	Tracer, 0.15, 0.30 mg/kg	10	3.3	0.44	0.11	Four normal subjects and 6 osteoarthritic patients	17
	40 mg	8M	3.4	0.86	0.20		18
	0.8 mg/kg	10F	–	0.64[c]	0.17		19
	16.3 mg/kg	4M, 3F	2.6	1.1[c]	0.18	Bowel disease patients	20
	40 mg/1.73 m²IV	16	2.5	48[c,e]	0.21	Asthmatic children aged 6–17 years	21
Prednisone	10 mg	10	3.3	0.97	0.26		22
	81 mg IV[b]	8M	2.7	2.5[c]	0.2		23
	60 mg oral						

Drug	Dose	Subjects				Comments	Ref
Methylprednisolone	1mg/kg or 40 mg[g]	4F, 6M	2.5	1.13[c]	0.41	Severe asthmatics	24
	1 and 1.5 g[g,h]	4F	2.4	0.88	0.25	Rheumatoid patients	25
	10 mg/kg, 63 mg[h,i]	6F, 11M	3.3	1.12[d]	0.31	Dose dependent kinetics[b]	26
	2 mg	5F, 8M	2.8	0.87	0.27		27
	40 mg	14M	2.4	0.84[c]	0.27		28
	40 mg/1.73 m^2 IV[g]	9	2.3	80[e]	0.38	Asthmatic children aged 9–18 years	21
	16, 31, 63, 125, 250, 500 and 1000 mg IV[f]	12M	2.2–3.4	54–85[c,j]	0.31–0.39	Range of mean data listed	29
	20, 40, 80 mg IV[b,g] 20 mg oral	4M, 1F	1.9	1.5[c]	0.49	Dose linearity	30
Dexamethasone	6.7 mg[f,h]	6F, 6M	2.9	0.77[c]	0.25		31
	1 mg[f,h]	2M	2.8	1.45[d]	0.46		32
	4 mg[f,h]	8M	4.5	1.08[c]	-0.21		18
	0.5 or 1.5 mg	4F, 5M	4.2	0.61[m]	0.20[m]	Three hirsute, one epileptic and one peptic ulcer patients	33
	5, 10, or 20[f]	6F, 8M	3.0	1.15	0.4	Patients during neurosurgery	34
	15, 1.5 mg/kg[f,h,p]	13M, 6F	3.5	0.39[d]	0.09	Kinetic parameters were almost identical at the high dose	35
Betamethasone	8 mg[f,h]	6F, 2M	5.6	1.35[d]	0.18		36
Deflazacort[o]	50 mg	3M	2.9	–	0.14	Values based on total radioactivity	37
Fluocortolone		5M	1.3	0.84	0.45		12
Fluocortinbutyl-ester	1 mg	2M	2.5	–	–		38
Flunisolide	1.0 mg	12M	1.6	1.8[d]	0.96	Data based on whole blood levels	39

(continued)

Table 2 Continued

Compound	Dose	Subjects	$t_{1/2}$ (hr)	V (L/kg)	CL (L/min)	Comments[a]	Reference
Triaminolone acetonide	80 mg, 10 mg/kg[f,h]	8	1.5	1.88[d]	0.96	Dose dependent kinetics[b]	40
Budesonide	0.5 mg,	6M	2.8	4.3[d]	1.4		41
	0.1 mg	4M	2.5	2.8[d]	0.92		42
	0.5 mg	6M	1.5	4.0	1.5	Children 10–13 years	43
	0.5 mg	12M, 12F	2.3	2.7[c]	1.3		44
Fluticasone	2.0 mg IV	6	3.1	3.7	0.87		45
	0.25 mg, 0.5 mg 1.0 mg	12M	7.8	318[c]	1.1	Parameters were averaged from the two highest doses to increase robustness	178a
	20 µg	6M, 6F	14.4	594[c]	1.3		178

[a] Included subjects were healthy and "normal" unless otherwise stated.
[b] Values refer to mean in the investigated dosage interval.
[c] Apparent volume of distribution calculated using moment analysis.
[d] Apparent volume of distribution calculated using terminal rate constant.
[e] L/1.73 m².
[f] Administration as the phosphate ester.
[g] Administration as the sodium succinate ester.
[h] Dose based on the free alcohol.
[i] Administration as the hemisuccinate ester.
[j] V × body weight.
[m] Two compartment data; V = volume of outer pool (V_2) and CL_p-metabolic clearance rate = V_1*K_2.
[o] Oral data.
[p] Data given for low dose.

Prednisone and prednisolone have higher potency and longer duration of action than hydrocortisone. With methylprednisolone, dexamethasone, and betamethasone, other commonly prescribed oral glucocorticoids, potency and duration are increased even further (48).

In general, the systemic availability of the oral glucocorticoid formulations are high (Table 3) and are limited by first-pass liver metabolism rather than by incomplete absorption.

Very little information is available on the optimization of release profiles of oral glucocorticoid formulations. Sustained-release formulations of prednisolone have been developed, but only to reduce the possible peptic ulcer–promoting properties of the drug (59). Some of the sustained-release formulations have the disadvantage of erratic absorption, larger interindividual variability, and decreased efficacy (51,60).

Table 3 Systemic Availability (F) of Glucocorticoids After Oral Administration in Humans

Drug	F (%)	Reference
Hydrocortisone	40–71	9
Prednisolone	69–101	49
	73–89	12
	99	50
	106	51
	60–66	52
	75–84	18
	82	53
Methylprednisolone	49–58	25
	99	26
Dexamethasone	78–83	54
	53	55
	62	32
	62–64	18
Flurocortolone	78–89	12
Flunisolide	21	56
Beclomethasone dipropionate	Unknown	
Budesonide	11	41
	10	57
	6	58
Fluticasone	"virtually zero"	45

Inhalation

The rationale for administration of glucocorticoids by inhalation is that delivery of the drug directly to the lungs may reduce the dose needed for clinical efficacy, which in turn should decrease the incidence of systemic side effects.

Since the therapeutic effect of inhaled glucocorticoids appears to be local (61–63), efficient pulmonary deposition is essential. Another important aspect of inhalation therapy is the relative contributions of absorption from the lung and gastrointestinal tract of an inhaled dose to the overall systemic exposure. Although the desired therapeutic effect results from pulmonary deposited drug, the unwanted systemic side effects are a result of the systemically available drug. For drugs with a high oral availability, the relative contribution from the swallowed fraction to the overall systemic exposure is considerable (Fig. 2). For drugs with low oral availabilities, the swallowed fraction constitutes only a small part of the systemic exposure. Mouth rinsing may reduce the oral contribution, but it cannot be abolished all together. This is a major reason why low oral availability has been one of the goals of the recent and ongoing development of inhalation steroids with improved therapeutic ratios (see Table 3).

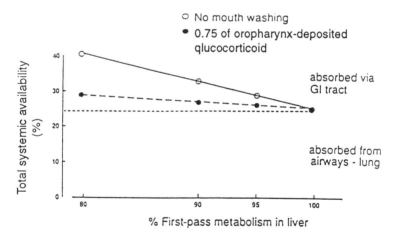

Figure 2 Systemic availability of an inhaled glucocorticosteroid. Total systemic availability is shown on the y-axis as the percentage of the dose reaching the patient. The systemic availability is made up of the fraction deposited in the lower respiratory tract (airways and lung), which is considered to be fully available, and the fraction deposited in the oropharynx, which is swallowed and absorbed from the gastrointestinal tract and subject to first-pass hepatic metabolism. The effect on mouthwashing is also shown. The figure is based on a theoretical calculation, but is supported by data from Thorsson et al. (44). (From ref. 64.)

Four modes of inhalation therapy are currently in use: the pressurized metered-dose inhaler (pMDI), spacer devices connected to the pMDIs, dry powder inhalers (DPIs), and nebulizers. The pMDIs are currently the most widely used. Average lung deposition for different pMDI formulations range from 9 to 33% of the metered dose (65,66). The dose delivered to the patient is high with these devices, in the order of 85–90%, but a major fraction of the delivered dose is swallowed. The swallowed fraction can be diminished by adding a spacer to the pMDI. The spacer reduces the need for coordination between firing and inhalation. In addition, by allowing time for evaporation, it reduces aerosol droplet size, thereby increasing the respirable fraction (particles less than 5–10 µm in diameter). Finally, larger particles which otherwise would have been swallowed will deposit in the spacer. Drawbacks include the size of the device and the problem of electrostatic charging, which may significantly reduce the delivered dose (67).

Dry powder inhalers are the most recently developed group of inhalation devices. They deliver micronized substances in pure form or mixed with lactose. Lung deposition and effect differ between different brands of DPIs. While fluticasone propionate inhaled via Diskhaler shows equal efficacy and safety as the same nominal dose inhaled via pMDI (68), effect and lung deposition of β-agonists and lung deposition of glucocorticoids is approximately doubled after inhalation via Turbuhaler as compared with pMDI (44,69).

Glucocorticoid respules intended for nebulization are available on many markets. Many brands of nebulizers are available, and the performance of these when used with different glucocorticoid formulations is often unknown. The amount of glucocorticoid delivered to the patient may differ threefold between different nebulizer systems (70). Added to this interproduct variability is the intraindividual differences related to technique, which may be considerable. To minimize the risk of adverse effects of poor treatment outcome following nebulized glucocorticoids, recommendations on which brand to be used and/or thorough documentation on different brands should be supplied by the pharmaceutical firms. This is of particular importance, since the nebulizer mode of administration is preferred in infants and children and during acute exacerbations in adults, where administration via pMDI or inhalation drive DPIs may be difficult to perform.

B. Distribution

Protein Binding

Cortisol and prednisolone compete for the same binding sites on two serum proteins: to albumin with a high binding capacity but with low affinity and to transcortin, or corticosteroid binding globulin (CBG), with high affinity but low capacity (71). Transcortin has a binding capacity of only 0.7 µmol (250 µg) cortisol per liter serum (72). Hence, at low concentrations, approximately 90% of prednisolone and hydrocortisone is plasma protein bound, but at higher plasma concentrations of these glucocorticoids, transcortin binding becomes saturated. The nonlinear binding also affects total clearance, which increases with increasing doses (9,15,73,74). In addition, reduced serum albumin levels may increase the frequency of steroid-related side effects (75). Prednisolone does not bind to α_1-acid-glycoprotein (orosmucoid) (20).

Serum or plasma protein binding of synthetic glucocorticoids, other than prednisolone, seems to be confined primarily to albumin (71,76,77). Consequently, the binding is independent of concentration at plasma levels normally obtained after therapeutic doses. Methylprednisolone plasma protein binding was 77% and linear with the dose range of 5–40 mg intravenously (78). Dexamethasone and betamethasone bind to plasma proteins to 77 and 63%, respectively, over a wide dose range (77). The plasma binding of triamcinolone was approximately 40% and mainly to albumin (76). Plasma protein binding of the more lipophilic inhaled steroids seems to be more extensive. For budesonide, it is about 90% (41) and for fluticasone about 99% (Astra Draco AB, unpublished data).

Tissue Distribution

Plasma protein binding affects tissue distribution, so that an increased free fraction increases volume of distribution. For albumin-bound drugs, knowing plasma protein binding and volume of distribution (V), the free fraction of tissues may be calculated (79). A glucocorticoid with a comparatively high free fraction in plasma (Fu) and a less extensive V (such as betamethasone) will have a high free tissue fraction (12% assuming V = 100 L and Fu = 0.4). For the more lipophilic topical glucocorticoids, V is larger and Fu approaches zero, resulting in free fractions in tissue of 1% or less. The pharmacodynamic implications of high tissue binding for a glucocorticoid has not been studied in great detail, although it may be speculated that it should favor targeted delivery but result in more heterogeneous uptake in different tissues and a longer elimination half-life.

Tissue distribution of radiolabeled methylprednisone and methylprednisolone was studied in the rabbit after infusion of single doses (80). Infusion of these compounds and subsequent analysis of concentration-time profiles permit analysis of the rate of formation of methylprednisone from methylprednisolone and the reverse process. Elimination parameters for each steroid can be calculated, as well as distribution parameters. These studies indicate that traditional pharmacokinetic analysis tends to underestimate true metabolic clearance by approximately 30%. The steady-state volumes of distribution are overestimated by 10% for methylprednisone and 61% for methylprednisolone. This is largely related to the interconversion phenomenon. Because of the continual recycling of glucocorticoid in this reaction, the systemic availability of a given dose of methylprednisone approximates 150%. Therefore, methylprednisolone serves as a storage pool for the glucocorticoid.

Tissue uptake varies in different tissues, as studied in the rabbit after continuous intravenous infusion of prednisolone (81). Intestines, liver, lung, heart, and kidney exhibited a comparatively high uptake. Fat and brain show a relatively low tissue uptake. After intravenous bolus dosing of [^{3}H]-budesonide in the mouse, an extensive uptake of radioactivity was noted in the liver, kidney, lung, and lymphatic tissues. Low uptake was noted in the brain (82).

The in vitro binding of different steroids to human lung tissue was determined by Högger et al. (83). Binding seemed to correlate with the lipophilicity of the glucocorticoid and was most pronounced for fluticasone and beclomethasone dipropionate (BDP) followed by beclomethasone monopropionate (BMP), budesonide, flunisolide, and hydrocortisone. However, after local superfusion of rat trachea with glucocorticoids, budesonide and fluticasone were similarly retained and both were more retained than BDP. The subsequent release was slower for budesonide than any of the tested glucocorticoids, including fluticasone (83a).

Similarly, there was a good correlation between lipophilicity and receptor affinity of glucocorticoids having a free C-21 hydroxyl group. Steroid esterified in the C-21 group were, irrespective of their lipophilicity, not or only weak binders to the receptor (84).

Bronchoalveolar lavage (BAL)/serum concentration ratios were assessed after intravenous injection of various water-soluble glucocorticoids. Equilibrium was achieved after about 10 min and lasted for at least 1 hr. During this time period, the BAL/serum concentration ratio of prednisolone was the highest (1.3) followed by dexamethasone (1.1), methylprednisolone (0.7), and triamcinolone acetonide (0.4) (85). Braude and Rebuck (86) showed a strong correlation and an approximately 1:1 relation between plasma levels and lung epithelial lining concentrations of hydrocortisone after intravenous dosing. Two studies have been performed on the lung uptake of prednisolone and methylprednisolone in the rabbit. After an intravenous bolus dose of prednisolone and methylprednisolone to rabbits, Greos et al. (87) found that the lung epithelial lining fluid (ELF)/plasma ratio was 3.6 for methylprednisolone and 1.7 for prednisolone. After continuous infusion, the penetration of prednisolone increased linearly with dose, but the penetration of methylprednisolone increased exponentially at higher infusion doses (88). Budesonide concentrations in lung biopsies and plasma after inhalation via a pMDI with a spacer were shown to differ by a factor of about 9 (89). The estimated partition coefficient (the ratio between tissue concentration and unbound concentration in plasma) was estimated to be

87. The corresponding value for prednisolone during constant infusion in the rabbit was 3 (81). The difference in antiasthma potency between inhaled budesonide and oral prednisolone (33 times according to Toogood [90]) was similar to the difference in tissue uptake (about 30 times), indicating that glucocorticoid potency and lung concentrations are interrelated.

C. Metabolism and Excretion

By 1965, the pathways of hydrocortisone metabolism were in large part elucidated (91), and by 1977, Monder and Bradlow (92–974), completed the picture by their work on corticoid and cortienic acid metabolites of cortisol. 11-Oxidoreduction, A-ring reduction, and 17β side chain oxidations are the major metabolic events for cortisol (Fig. 3). Hydroxylation in the 6α and 6β position also occur to a minor extent, with 6β-hydroxy cortisol being the major unconjugated cortisol metabolite in human urine (95,96). More than 90% of urinary radioactivity after an intravenous dose of radioactive hydrocortisone consists of conjugated metabolites, with the major fraction (~90%) being glucuronic acid conjugates (97,98).

Hydrocortisone catabolism is located mainly in the liver, although other organs such as the kidney, placenta, lung, muscle, and skin may contribute to the metabolism of endogenous and synthetic glucocorticoids (99–107). High 11β-hydroxysteroid dehydrogenase activity is present in kidney (108). The

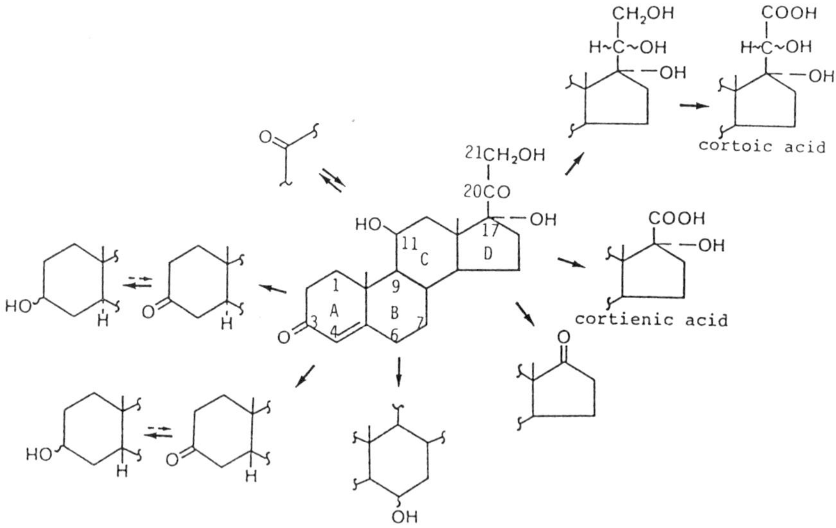

Figure 3   Major metabolic pathways of cortisol.

importance of intestinal microrganisms in the biotransformation of C_{21} steroids is unclear (109).

The metabolic pathways of synthetic glucocorticoids are summarized in Table 4.

Metabolism and Excretion of Synthetic Glucocorticoids

Cortisone and prednisone are converted to their active forms cortisol and prednisolone by reduction of the ketone group at C-11. The reaction between cortisone and cortisol and also between prednisone and prednisolone is reversible, and thus there is a continuous interconversion reaction. The enzyme responsible for the interconversion reaction, 11β-hydroxysteroid dehydrogenase (EC 1.1.1.146) comprises two enzymes (134). Methylprednisolone, which is administered orally as the active form, also undergoes conversion to methylprednisone (24).

The interconversion reaction takes place primarily in the liver but has also been demonstrated in other tissues, including the kidney (100). The rate of conversion of cortisone to cortisol and prednisone to prednisolone can be slower in patients with liver disease. The slower conversion in these patients combined with impaired elimination results in comparable bioavailability of cortisone and prednisone to that of normal volunteers (135,136). Although it is conceivable that genetic abnormalities could be present in either of the two components of 11β-hydroxysteroid dehydrogenase and thereby alter the conversion reaction, clinically significant deficiencies in humans have not been identified.

Potentiation of glucocorticoid activity may partly be achieved by slowing down the rate of elimination, and this was the ultimate purpose of the initial research in this area (137). The introduction of a Δ^1 double bond in cortisol to give prednisolone resulted in a lower rate of metabolism owing to less extensive reduction of the Δ^4-3-one group (110). 9α-Fluorination of cortisol (to triamcinolone) completely blocks 11-dehydrogenation as well as A-ring reduction. Main metabolic pathways of triamcinolone include 6β-hydroxylation and 20β-reduction (138).

Metabolic pathways of synthetic glucocorticoids were reviewed in 1972 (130). Table 4 mainly summarizes later work. 6β-Hydroxylation is an important metabolic pathway for many of the synthetic glucocorticoids. In general, A-ring reduction is less abundant than for hydrocortisone, chiefly due to the Δ^1 double bond (see above). Oxidation at C_{21} to the corresponding acid has been reported for a few of the synthetic glucocorticoids and complete degradation of the C_{20}–C_{21} side chain giving 17-keto-C_{19} steroids has also been reported. Reduction of the 20-keto group may be sterically hindered by substituents in 16, 17, and 21-positions (123,132). Esterase activity is high in many tissues in the body (140,141), and hydrolysis is generally the primary metabolic event. Data concerning phase II reactions with synthetic glucocorticoids are scarce and

Table 4 Metabolic Pathways of Synthetic Glucocorticoids in Humans and Various Animals

Metabolic pathway	Compound	Investigated species	Reference
11-oxidoreduction	Prednisone, prednisone	Human	110
	Prednisolone	Rat, human	111,112
	Prednisone	Mouse, dog, monkey	113
	Prednisolone, dexamethasone, and betamethasone	Human	103
	Dexamethasone	Human	108
	Betamethasone	Human	114
	Deflazacort	Cynomolgus monkey	115
	Methylprednisolone	Rabbit	80
	Methylprednisolone-21-acetate	Dog	116
6β-Hydroxylation	Prednisone, prednisolone	Human	52
	Dexamethasone	Horse	117
	Dexamethasone valerate	Rat	118
	Desoxymethasone	Rat, dog	119
	Deflazacort	Rat, dog, human	120
	Flucortolone	Human	121
	Halcinonide	Dog	122
	Triamcinolone	Dog	123
	Triamcinolone acetonide-21-phosphate	Dog, monkey, rat	124
	Triamcinolone acetonide	Rabbit, dog, monkey, rat	125
	Betamethasone	Human	121
	Betamethasone-17-benzoate	Rat	126
	Flunisolide	Mouse	127
	Flunisolide	Human	128
	Budesonide	Human, mouse, rat	129
	Fluticasone	Dog	130
	Tipredane	Human, rat	131
6α-Hydroxylation	Deflazacort	Cynomolgus monkey	115
	Flucortolone	Ram	132
6-Keto formation	Flunisolide	Mouse	127
7α-Hydroxylation	Desoxymethasone	Rat, dog	119
B-ring dehydrogenation	Deflazacort	Rat, dog, human	120
	Triamcinolone acetonide	Rabbit, dog, rat, monkey	125
	Flunisolide	Mouse	127
	Budesonide	Human, mouse, rat	133

21-Oxidation	Prednisolone	Hamster	133a
	Desoxymethasone	Rat, dog	119
	Flucocortolone	Human	121
	Halcinonide	Dog	122
	Triamcinolone acetonide	Rabbit, dog, monkey, rat	125
	Beclomethasone-17α,21-dipropionate	Rat	133b
17β-Side chain cleavage	Dexamethasone	Horse	133c
	Betamethasone	Human	114
	Betamethasone-17-benzoate	Rat	126
Acetal oxidation	Budesonide	Man, mouse, rat	133,149
A-ring reduction	Prednisone, prednisolone	Human	110
	Prednisolone	Rat, human	111,112
	Flucocortolone	Ram	132
	Delfazacort	Rat, dog, human	120
	Budesonide	Human, mouse, rat	133
20-Reduction	Prednisone, prednisolone	Human	110
	Prednisone	Human, rat	111,112
	Prednisone	Mouse, dog, monkey	113
	Methylprednisolone-21-acetate	Dog	116
	9αF-cortisol	Rat	133d
	Dexamethasone	Horse	117
	Dexamethasone	Rat	133e
	Dexamethasone valerate	Rat	133f
	Beclomethasone-17α,21-dipropionate	Rat	133b
	Betamethasone-17-benzoate	Rat	126
	Deflazacort	Cynomolgus monkey	115
	Flucocortolon	Human	121
Ester hydrolysis	Flucocortinbutylester	Human	133g
	Difluocortolonvaleriat	Rat, guinea pig, human	133h
	Beclomethasone-17,21-dipropionate	Human	133i
	Beclomethasone-17,21-dipropionate and cyclomethasone	Human, rat	133k,133l
	Beclomethasone-17,21-dipropionate	Rat	133m
	Flucocortinbutylester	Human	133g
	Various water-soluble glucocorticoid esters	Human	133n
	Methylprednisolone acetate and betamethasone-17, 21-dipropioante	Human	133o
	Fluticasone	Man, rat, dog	130
C_{21} Decarboxylation	Flucocortinbutylester	Human	133g

incomplete, but the conjugated fraction of urinary metabolites is generally less than that for cortisol (39,112,114,132,142–146).

Of the clinically more important systemic glucocorticoids, prednisone and dexamethasone are excreted in the urine mainly as its 6β-hydroxy metabolite, whereas the authentic drug and the 20-hydroxy metabolite are present in minor amounts (147). Bethamethasone appears in human urine mainly unchanged with a small amount of the 11-keto metabolite, the 20-hydroxy metabolite, and the 6β-hydroxy metabolite (148).

The symmetrical 16α,17α-isopropylidene substituent, present in many topical glucocorticoids, is metabolically stable (124,129,145). Two major metabolic pathways of budesonide involve the nonsymmetrical 16α,17α-acetal group; the acetal side chain hydroxylation giving 23-hydroxybudesonide (133) and the acetal side chain cleavage giving 16α-hydroxyprednisolone (133,149). 16α-Hydroxyprednisolone was formed only from (22R)-budesonide. The 16α,17α substituent in budesonide and in deflazacort (120) inhibits biotransformation of both the 11-hydroxy and the C_{20}–C_{21} groups, although hydrolysis to the active metabolite 21-hydroxydeflazacort occurs in humans (150). Flunisolide and triamcinolone acetonide are chiefly 6β-hydroxylated (125,127, 128), and BDP and fluticasone are primarily hydrolyzed (130,133k,173). However, the hydrolysis of BDP to B-17-MP is an activation pathway, and further hydrolysis to the free alcohol is required for reduced activity.

D.   Pharmacokinetics of Selected Glucocorticoids

Bioanalytical Assays

The basic pharmacokinetic properties of clinically utilized and investigational glucocorticoids are given in Table 2. Generally, sensitive and selective assays for the quantification of glucocorticoids in plasma and blood have been included using high-pressure liquid chromatography (HPLC) (151), radioimmunoassay (152), gas chromatography–mass spectroscopy (GC-MS) (153), and HPLC-MS (154,155). Early reports describe the pharmacokinetics of total radioactivity following the administration of tritium-labeled or carbon 14–labeled drug. Since metabolism of glucocorticoids often is extensive, the kinetic parameters derived from such studies is of no or poor value for the estimation of extent and duration of action and the prediction of optimal dosing regimens.

HPLC assays have been used for the quantitation of dexamethasone and its phosphate ester, and hydrocortisone, triamcinolone, triamcinalone acetonide (TAAc), and its phosphate ester (151). Limits of quantitation were about 100 ng/ml. Prednisolone assays with sensitivities down to 5 ng/ml have been developed (23).

For the inhaled glucocorticoids, more sensitive assays are required, because of the low doses used. Radioimmunoassay (RIA) methods for the quantitation of beclomethasone dipropionate (BDP) and the active metabolite beclomethasone monopropionate (BMP) were developed by Jenner and Kirkham (156). The limit of quantitation in plasma was 0.1 ng/ml; still not sufficient to follow the parent compound and the active metabolite for more than 90 min after intravenous dosing. A sensitive RIA assay was developed for flunisolide (157) and applied in the pharmacokinetic documentation of the drug (39). Assay sensitivity was 0.1–0.2 ng/ml. The RIA method for TAAc allowed quantitation down to 0.06 ng/ml (158). The budesonide epimers have been quantitated in plasma with a combined HPLC (separation) and RIA (quantitation) assay with a sensitivity of 0.1 ng/ml for each epimer of the drug (43). A more recent method for the analysis of budesonide (sum of both epimers) in plasma utilizes HPLC and thermospray mass spectrometry with higher sensitivity (0.04 ng/ml) and capacity (154). For fluticasone, a combination of solid-phase extraction and RIA gave an assay sensitivity of 0.05 ng/ml (159).

Systemically Active Glucocorticoids

Cortisone and later hydrocortisone were the first glucocorticoids to be used pharmacologically (160). Because of low anti-inflammatory potency and high mineralocorticoid activity, the current use of these glucocorticoids is fairly limited. Studies of the pharmacokinetics of cortisone and hydrocortisone are hampered by the high endogenous concentrations, which either need to be suppressed by exogenous steroids or require radioactively labeled analogues. Both compounds are extensively metabolized in the most part in the liver. Plasma $t_{1/2}$ is short, less than 2 hr, but the variation in reported data on volume of distribution, clearance, and systemic availability (see Table 2) is noteworthy.

The pharmacokinetics of prednisone and prednisolone has been thoroughly investigated and reviewed (49,73,161). Prednisolone pharmacokinetics are characterized by a lower clearance and a more extensive tissue distribution than hydrocortisone. Plasma $t_{1/2}$ is between 2 and 4 hr. Plasma concentrations of prednisone are about one-sixth to one-eighth of those of prednisolone, irrespective of mode of administration (as prednisone or as prednisolone) (47). The pharmacokinetics of total prednisolone is not linear with dose, and 20 and 40 mg orally gives very similar plasma concentrations (162). The lack of dose linearity is not as apparent when free prednisolone concentrations are studied. Also, the conversion of prednisolone to prednisone shows nonlinear changes with increasing dose (163). Reported systemic availabilities of prednisolone after oral dosing range from 60 to 100%.

In low doses, methylprednisolone exhibits similar pharmacokinetics to prednisolone and, like prednisolone, is partly converted to its inactive dehydrogenated form, methylprednisone. After intravenous dosing of its phosphate ester, kinetics were linear in the investigated dose range (16–1000 mg) (29).

However, following intravenous dosing of its hemisuccinate ester, 63 mg and 10 mg/kg, a slight nonlinearity was found (26). Reported oral availabilities of methylprednisolone versus intravenous dosing as its sodium or hemisuccinate ester range from 50 to 100%.

In contrast to methylprednisolone, prednisolone, and triamcinolone acetonide, dexamethasone shows no dose-dependent pharmacokinetics in the high-dose range that is used for emergency therapy (35). Dexamethasone phosphate rather than the sulfate should then be used, since the former is efficiently hydrolyzed to its free alcohol but the latter is virtually inert (46).

Betamethasone, differing structurally from dexamethasone only by the stereochemistry at the 16-methyl moiety, seems to have similar volume of distribution but a lower clearance and longer half-life than its 16α-methyl analogue (see Table 2). This has been confirmed in a study where the drug was given orally (164) and should result in longer duration of action. No data are available on the dose linearity, but plasma protein binding is constant within a wide dose range (77).

Deflazacort is an investigational glucocorticoid with a pharmacological potency similar to that of prednisone but with less effect on bone metabolism and carbohydrate metabolism. It has been successfully tried in rheumatoid arthritis and systemic lupus erythematosus (165) and lung inflammation (166). The pharmacokinetic properties of deflazacort have not been elucidated in great detail, and its oral availability has not been determined. Kinetically, deflazacort appears to resemble prednisolone (37).

Topically Active Glucocorticoids

The pharmacokinetic data of the topically active glucocorticoids administered by inhalation are summarized in Table 5.

Beclomethasone dipropionate was the first glucocorticoid successfully employed for local treatment of asthma. It became clinically available in the early 1970s when its pharmacokinetic properties and the rationale for topical efficacy and safety were also revealed (171,172). The drug is metabolized in the lung to the monopropionate (BMP) and the free steroid. Martin et al. (171) suggested that the therapeutic effect is derived from a combination of BDP and BMP. Later work indicates that the major effect emanates from beclomethasone-17-monopropionate, since the glucocorticoid receptor affinity (GRA) of B-17-MP is 25 times higher than that of BDP (relative affinity was 1345 versus 53, when dexamethasone was given a value of 100) (84). Based on the amount of radioactivity recovered in feces after oral dosing of [^{3}H]BDP as a microfine suspension or as a capsule, the drug seems to be readily absorbed after oral dosing. After intravenous dosing of [^{3}H]BDP in humans, plasma levels of radioactivity followed a biphasic curve with a rapid initial fall representing tis-

Table 5 Pharmacokinetics of Inhaled Glucocorticoids in Humans

Compound	Inhalation device	Nominal dose (µg)	C_{max} (ng/ml)	T_{max} (hr)	Systemic availability (% of metered dose)	Comments	Reference
Triamcinolone acetonide	pMDI	400 800 1600	0.5 1.0 2.0	2.3 2.4 3.7	— — —	$t_{1/2}$ was 1.8, 2.3, and 2.2 hr, respectively	158
Triamincolone actonide	pMDI	400	0.3	4.0	—	$t_{1/2}$ was 2.3 hr	167
Beclomethasone dipropionate	pMDI	400 800 1600	0.06 0.1 0.2	3.2 3.6 3.9	— — —	$t_{1/2}$ was 5.9, 5.4, and 4.9 hr, respectively. All data were on beclomethasone alcohol	168
Flunisolide	pMDI	1000	2.8	<30 min	39 (32 with mouthwash)[a]		56
Budesonide	Turbuhaler pMDI	1000 1000	3.5 2.3	0.3 0.5	38 26	Pulmonary availability was 32 and 15% for TBH and pMDI, respectively	44
Budesonide	Turbuhaler	400 800 1600	0.7 1.5 2.7	0.3 0.4 0.3	— — —	Single doses in asthmatic patients	169
Budesonide	pMDI + spacer nebulizer	1000 1000	— —	— —	28[1] 15[1]	Asthmatic children 10–13 years	170
Fluticasone	Diskhaler	1000	0.5	1.4	—	C_{max} and T_{max} given after a single dose	178
Fluticasone	pMDI	1000	0.5	1.0	—	Data in one subject	159

TBH, Turbuhaler; C_{max} = maximum concentration; T_{max} = time of C_{max}.
[a] % of nominal dose.

sue distribution and then a slow terminal phase with a $t_{1/2}$ of about 15 hr. For the first 3 hr, plasma radioactivity represented unchanged drug (173). In one subject using a RIA assay, unchanged BDP and BMP could be followed for 60 and 90 min, respectively (156). Based on these preliminary data, plasma half-life (up to 60 min after dosing), plasma clearance and volume of distribution ($V\beta$) of BDP were estimated to be 30 min, 3.8 L/min, and 167 L. The high systemic clearance value indicates substantial extrahepatic elimination. Apart from these data, the basic pharmacokinetic parameters of BDP and B-17-MP have not been elucidated. Oral availability seems, however, to be higher than that of budesonide, as BDP results in two to four times higher systemic potency than budesonide following doses which are topically equipotent (174).

Flunisolide has been studied in more depth than BDP concerning its pharmacokinetic properties in healthy subjects (39,56). After intravenous dosing, mean flunisolide $t_{1/2}$ in plasma was estimated to be 1.6 hr, systemic clearance at 0.96 L/min, and volume of distribution at 1.8 L/kg. After oral dosing, absorption was prompt and the slope of the terminal phase of the plasma concentration time curve was the same as after intravenous dosing. Systemic availability after oral dosing was between 13 and 60% in three volunteers (average 20%). After inhalation of 1 mg flunisolide via a nebulizer, the absorption was very rapid, with levels reaching peak between 2 and 30 min after dosing. Systemic availability was 39% without mouthwashing and 32% with mouthwashing (56).

Triamcinolone acetonide (TAAc) has been studied pharmacokinetically after intravenous dosing of high doses of the phosphate ester (40), after oral dosing of the free alcohol (175) and the diacetate (176), and after inhalation of the free alcohol via pMDI (158). Plasma $t_{1/2}$ after 80 mg intravenously was 1.5 hr, plasma clearance was 1.2 L/min, and volume of distribution ($V\beta$) was 2.2 L/kg. At higher doses (10 mg/kg), clearance and volume of distribution decreased to 0.8 L/min and 1.5 L/kg, respectively (40). After oral dosing of TAAc or its diacetate, the pharmacokinetics of the free alcohol was similar. The mean systemic availability after oral dosing of the free alcohol is similar to that after oral flunisolide, around 20% (H. Derendorf, 1994, personal communication). Triamcinolone acetonide inhaled via pMDI shows dose proportional pharmacokinetics in the dose range of 400–1600 µg (158).

Budesonide, which is in clinical use in many countries except in the United States where it is yet only approved as a nasal inhaler, has been pharmacokinetically characterized in humans after intravenous (42,177) and oral dosing (41,57) and after inhalation (43,44,169). After intravenous dosing, oral dosing of a capsule and oral inhalation via pMDI with a tube spacer (Inhalet) attached, plasma $t_{1/2}$ was similar for the three routes of administration. After intravenous dosing, plasma $t_{1/2}$ was about 2 hr, plasma clearance 1.0–1.4 L/min, and volume of distribution ($V\beta$) 3–4 L/kg (41,42). In children with asthma, plasma $t_{1/2}$ was shorter (about 1.5 hr) than in adults (43). Absorption was prompt both after oral dosing (T_{max} was 2.7 hr) and after inhalation (T_{max} was 0.2 hr) (41). Mean systemic availability (in three subjects) was estimated to be 11% after oral dosing. Later studies have given similar values on the systemic availability after oral dosing (mean values of 6 and 10% have been published [57,58]). In spite of the low oral availability, absorption is probably complete, since the same fraction of recovered radioactivity was found in urine (60% of totally recovered radioactivity) after oral dosing (41) as after intravenous dosing (63%, Edsbäcker et al., unpublished data).

Budesonide is a mixture of two pharmacologically active epimers having different pharmacokinetic properties. Plasma clearance and volume of distribution are about twice as high for the more lipophilic 22R epimer than for the 22S epimer (solubility in water is 8 and 14 µg/ml, respectively). Plasma $t_{1/2}$ is, however, almost identical for the two epimers (177). In vitro, the more lipophilic 22R epimer has a higher glucocorticoid receptor affinity and is taken up in the guinea pig lung to a larger extent (1.4 times) than the 22S epimer (177a).

The systemic availability of budesonide after inhalation via a pMDI and Turbuhaler, a dry powder inhaler, was 26 and 38% after inhalation in 24 healthy subjects (44). Lung deposition, determined in the same study, was 15 and 32%, respectively. After inhalation via Turbuhaler, budesonide shows dose linear kinetics in the dose range of 400–1600 µg b.i.d. (169).

Fluticasone (Flutide, Flovent) is the most recent inhaled glucocorticoid in clinical use. Like the other inhalation glucocorticoid has a large V (3.7 L/kg) and a high systemic clearance (0.9 L/min) (45). In two recent studies (178,178a), elimination half-life was reported to be 14.4 hr and about 7.8 hr, respectively. In the latter study,the pharmacokinetics after intravenous dosing was linear in the 250- to 1000-µg dose range. In both studies, the plasma concentration time curves were best described by three exponentials.

After oral dosing of fluticasone in a dose range of 5–40 mg, absorption was reported to be saturable and bimodal, with the main site of absorption being the large intestine (179). Very low peak concentrations, 0.42 ng/ml, were obtained after the 40-mg dose. Probably, incomplete absorption of this lipophilic glucocorticoid may explain the findings.

The pharmacokinetics of fluticasone after inhalation have been studied in one subject after inhalation of 1 mg (nominal dose) via a metered-dose inhaler (159). C_{max} and T_{max} were 0.5 µg/ml and 1 hr, respectively. In the study by Thorsson et al., in 12 healthy subjects, the rate of systemic absorption after inhalation of 1 mg via Diskhaler was rapid as compared with the rate of elimination (178). C_{max} and T_{max} were similar to that other pMDI (159). The systemic availability was estimated to be 16% of the nominal dose. This figure (16%) should also equal the lung deposition, since the swallowed fraction is absorbed unchanged to a negligible extent (45). After treatment for one week (1 mg b.i.d.), plasma concentrations increased by 1.7 times, indicating systemic accumulation (178).

Investigational Glucocorticoids

The limited pharmacokinetic data available on fluocortolone and fluocortinbutyl ester are depicted in Table 2. Other investigational glucocorticoids include triamcinolone acetonide-21-oic acid methyl ester, mometasone (Schering Plough, Kenilworth, USA), tipredane (Fisons, Loughborough, England), cyclesonide (Elmu SA, Madrid, Spain), butixocort propionate (Jouveinal), and cloprendol (Syntex, Maidenhead, England). The pharmacokinetic and pharmacodynamic properties of these compounds are not yet available.

E. Factors Regulating the Disposition and Metabolic Inactivation of Glucocorticoids

Drug Interactions

The enzymes primarily responsible for oxidative biotransformation of glucocorticoids, are in the cytochrome P450 IIIA superfamily. These enzymes are not subject to any quantitatively important genetic polymorphism regarding steroid metabolism. They are, however, both inducible and inhibitive. Cytochrome P450 IIIA catalyses hydroxylations (e.g., steroid 6β-hydroxylations), N-oxygenations, aromatizations, sulfoxidations, and dealkylations and is involved in many clinically important interactions with glucocorticoids, some of which are listed in Table 6.

Phenytoin, phenobarbital, rifampin, primidone, ephedrine, phenylbutazone, and thyroxine are examples of compounds which alter glucocorticoid disposition by inducing liver metabolic capacity (10,16,27,33,49,53,181–192).

Table 6 Selected Inhibitors and Inducers of Cytochrome P450 3A (180)

Inhibitors of 3A	Inducers of 3A
17α-Estradiol	Dexamethasone
17α-Ethynylestradiol	Rifampicin
Testosterone	Phenobarbital
Cyclosporine	Phenytoin
Terfenadine	
Ketoconazole	
Troleandomycin	
Cimetidine	
Erythromycin	

The metabolism of synthetic glucocorticoids may furthermore be accelerated after long-term treatment (142), and specific forms of rat liver cytochrome P450 are in fact induced by glucocorticoids (193).

The changes in the pharmacokinetic parameters of prednisolone caused by rifampin reached a near maximum 1.5- to 2-fold plateau effect at about 14 days after coadministration or discontinuation of rifampin. The half-maximal change was found within 5 days (194).

Prednisolone and methylprednisolone CL was increased and $t_{1/2}$ decreased in children receiving anticonvulsant therapy (either phenobarbital, carbamazepine, or phenytoin) (21). Methylprednisolone was more susceptible to increased elimination (e.g., a 350% increase in methylprednisolone CL as compared with an 80% increase of prednisolone CL). Also, volume of distribution of prednisolone and methylprednisolone increased (about 30% for both drugs) in children treated with anticonvulsants. Enzyme induction and displacement from binding proteins may explain the findings.

Of more concern in topical glucocorticoid therapy may be agents that slow down the systemic elimination of steroid drugs, thereby increasing the risk for glucocorticoid side effects. Sex hormones and anabolic steroids (181) as well as oral contraceptives (14,19,195,196) may have this effect on glucocorticoid disposition.

Macrolide antibiotics, specifically troleandomycin and erythromycin, are associated with impaired methylprednisolone elimination (24,197). At full therapeutic doses, the macrolide antibiotics reduce the elimination of methylprednisolone by 60%; but the magnitude of effect of troleandomycin on the inhibition of methylprednisolone elimination is related to the dose and time of administration of troleandomycin (198). The macrolide antibiotics form a metabolite that is capable of binding to cytochrome P450 to produce a hypoactive cytochrome complex (199,200). Troleandomycin can also reduce methylprednisolone elimination in the presence of potent enzyme-inducing agents such as phenobarbital and phenytoin (201).

Troleandomycin has a "steroid-sparing" effect on methylprednisolone but not on prednisolone, possibly due to selective inhibition of methylprednisolone metabolism (24,202). Dapsone seems to have a steroid-sparing effect on prednisone (203), but an effect on prednisolone metabolism has not been identified. Cyclosporine inhibits prednisolone metabolism in kidney transplanted patients (204,205) and may contribute to its observed "steroid-sparing" effect.

A number of studies in oral contraceptive users have reported marked changes in prednisolone distribution (which is decreased because of increased corticosteroid binding globulin levels) and clearance (which is increased because of inhibition of metabolism) (14,19,163,196). Legler and Benet (163) proposed careful monitoring of women taking oral contraceptive steroids who were concurrently undergoing prednisolone therapy.

Ketoconazole inhibits methylprednisolone clearance by approximately 50% and augments the effect of methylprednisolone on cortisol AUC (area under the curve) (206). The comparatively slight effect on cortisol AUC may be partly explained by the antagonistic effect of ketoconazole on the glucocorticoid receptor (207). Regarding ketoconazole and prednisolone interactions, there seems to be a controversy. A lack of kinetic and dynamic interaction between ketoconazole and prednisolone was reported by Yamashita et al. (208). Zurcher et al. (209) reported significant reduction of prednisolone clearance, volume of distribution, and 6β-hydroxylase activity during concomitant ketoconazole treatment.

The minor alterations seen in prednisolone (210) and budesonide (57) pharmacokinetics during concomitant cimetidine dosing were judged to have little clinical significance regarding effect and side effects. An interesting clinical implications of a metabolic interaction was postulated by Schleimer and Kato (211). Glycyrrhethinic acid and carbenoxolone are potent inhibitors of 11β-hycroxysteroid dehydrogenase (11β-HSD), which catalyzes the transformation of hydrocortisone to inactive cortisone. Schleimer postulated that the known anti-inflammatory actions of glycyrrhethinic acid and carbenoxolene derives from this inhibition and therefore could be useful as inhalation treatment in asthma (212). However, the kidneys are an important organ for cortisol metabolism and seem to be the major source of 11β-HSD (213). It has been suggested that congenital deficiency in renal 11β-HSD may be associated with essential hypertension (214).

Effect of Glucocorticoids on the Kinetics of Other Drugs

Dexamethasone seems significantly to induce the elimination of phenytoin (215,216). Inhibitive effects of dexamethasone on phenytoin elimination have also been reported (217). Triamcinolone acetonide, but not budesonide, inhibits testosterone oxidation in vitro (218). Testosterone reduction was unaffected. Triamcinolone acetonide may affect its own metabolism: Clearance increased considerably between days 1 and 6 of chronic treatment in a patient with lung fibrosis. During this time $t_{1/2}$ decreased from 2 hr to less than 30 min (40).

Effect of Disease State

Asthma does not seem to influence prednisolone pharmacokinetics following oral dosage (15). Clearance of methylprednisolone was increased in a patient with cystic fibrosis (219), but further studies are warranted to estimate the clinical relevance of this finding. Impaired renal and adrenal function have been reported to influence the metabolic clearance rate of glucocorticoids (185,220–222), but the reasons for this remain unclear. Thyroid disease affects glucocorticoid disposition, such that hyperthyroidism accelerates and hypothyroidism slows down the clearance of cortisol (223,224). Also, the nonrenal clearance was increased for prednisolone and the volume of distribution and immunosuppressive activity was reduced in hyperthyroidism (225). The effect of thyroid disease on the metabolism of methylprednisolone was variable (226).

Liver disease, including cirrhosis, may decrease the rate of glucocorticoid elimination (11,185,227–233) and induce side effects (195,234). Altered serum protein binding following liver disease may also affect drug disposition (234,235). Impaired liver function seems not greatly to affect total and unbound prednisolone plasma concentrations after oral prednisone (233). The slightly impaired conversion of prednisone into prednisolone was counterbalanced by a decreased nonrenal clearance of prednisolone. Oxidative metabolism, assessed by the formation of 6β-hydroxyprednisolone, was most affected, whereas the formation of other metabolites seemed to be preserved (233). Methylpredniso-lone pharmacokinetics was not altered in middle-aged patients with chronic liver disease as compared with six younger healthy subjects after intravenous dos-ing of its prodrug hemisuccinate (236).

Little is known on the effect of impaired liver function on the kinetics of the inhaled glucocorticoids. Being more prone to hepatic elimination in general and oxidative metabolism in particular, the inhaled glucocorticoids may be more affected by liver impairment. Data with intravenous and oral budesonide in patients with biopsy-verified liver cirrhosis and healthy subjects show a longer plasma $t_{1/2}$ after intravenous dosing (4.6 vs 3.6 hr) and a significantly higher oral availability (19% vs 7%) (Astra Draco, unpublished observations). Oral availability correlated closely to the suppression of plasma cortisol levels as well as exhaled ^{14}C-dimethylantipyrine (DMA) after intravenous ^{14}C-DMA.

Sex and Age

Few pharmacokinetic studies on glucocorticoids have specifically addressed gender differences. The activity of the P450 isoform CYP3A, which catalyzes many of the oxidations involved in glucocorticoid biotransformation, seems to be higher in women (237). The finding of Lew et al. (238) of a higher clear-ance of methylprednisolone in women than in men (0.45 vs 0.29 L/hr/kg) is therefore not surprising. However, women were more sensitive to the effects of methylprednisolone on cortisol suppression and may be more sensitive with respect to basophils and T lymphocytes as well. Still, Lew et al (238) suggests that men and women should receive the same dose normalized to ideal body weight, because even though women eliminate the drug faster, they seem to have a greater response to the same concentration of the drug. Similar phar-macokinetic differences between men and women were shown for prednisolone (13).

The exposure of total and unbound prednisolone in 12 elderly subjects (aged 65–89 years) was higher than in 19 young subjects (23–34 years) given the same dose (239). Both renal and nonrenal clearance was lower in the elderly. 6β-Hydroxylase activity decreased linearly with the metabolic clearance of prednisolone. The systemic availability of unbound prednisolone after oral prednisone and the apparent interconversion between prednisolone into prednisone and vice versa (reflecting 11β-hydroxysteroid dehydrogenase activity) were, however, independent of age. Despite increased prednisolone exposure, endogenous cortisol concentrations were less suppressed in the elderly (239).

The pharmacokinetics of prednisolone, methylprednisolone, and dexamethasone do not seem to differ to any large extent between children (21,240) and adults, although in newborns, plasma concentrations may be elevated (240). For budesonide, clearance seems to be higher and $t_{1/2}$ shorter in children than in adults, possibly as a result of the higher relative liver blood flow per kilogram body weight noted in children (43).

Other Factors

Racial differences have been noted in the pharmacokinetics of glucocorticoids. Clearance was about twice as high in white than in African-American renal transplant patients (241). Mean half-life was 3.4 hr in the African-American patients and 2.1 hr in the white patients.

Pharmacokinetic polymorphism (242), altered hepatic blood flow (243), food intake (181,244,245), body weight (33,246–248), and extrahepatic metabolism (246) may theoretically influence glucocorticoids pharmacokinetics. Smoking seems not to affect the pharmacokinetics of glucocorticoids (18), although a stimulation of cortisol secretion has been shown in humans (249). Circadian variations in hepatic drug metabolism have been suggested (250,251), and this could possibly be one factor explaining the diurnal variations in plasma disappearance rate of prednisolone (13,252) and cortisol (8,253). Surgery and stress depress hepatic inactivation of glucocorticoids (254).

V. Influence of Pharmacokinetics on Pharmacodynamics

A. Cellular Distribution and Response

Glucocorticoids exert their effect by binding to a specific receptor localized in the cytosol in target cells. On activation by the glucocorticoid, the receptor moves into the nucleus and interacts with glucocorticoid-responsive elements on the DNA, which either inhibit or stimulate transcription in steroid-responsive target genes. Glucocorticoids inhibit the transcription of many cytokines that are relevant in asthma, including interleukin-1 (IL-1), tumor necrosis factor α (TNF-α), granulocyte-macrophage colony-stimulating factor (GM-CSF), IL-3, IL-4, IL-6, and IL-8 (255). In addition, steroids inhibit the synthesis of cytokine receptors (256) and induce the breakdown of cytokine mRNA (257).

Glucocortioids increase the expression of neutral endopeptidase (258) and inhibit the inducible form of nitric oxide synthase (259), which result in reduced plasma exudation and airway blood flow. Other effects include the induction of lipocortin synthesis. This protein has nonspecific anti-inflammatory effects via inhibition of proinflammatory eicosanoids.

These molecular events initiate an array of events important for the treatment of asthma. Via cytokine inhibition, glucocorticoids inhibit the migration of inflammatory cells, such as lymphocytes and eosinophils, to the lung and the release of inflammatory cell mediators and cytotoxic agents from migratory and epithelial cells. They inhibit mucus production and reduce airway hyper-responsiveness. The pharmacological and clinical effects of glucocorticoids are extensively covered in other chapters of this book.

The pharmacological potency of a certain glucocorticoid is affected by the affinity to the glucocorticoid receptor and the physicochemical properties of the compound. The glucocorticoid receptor affinity value is calculated from the ratio between dissociation and association constants. Generally, the dissociation constant is the major determinant of receptor affinity with the association constant being similar between different glucocorticoids (260). Whether a high-affinity steroid bound to the receptor interacts with more than one mRNA binding site before dissociation or if increased binding merely increases the chance for a single interaction is not known.

The receptor affinity of the most important glucocorticoids are depicted in Table 7. Lipophilicity and relative binding affinity (RBA) are interrelated, as lipophilic glucocorticoids generally are those that show the highest RBA values. In many cases, the receptor affinity correlates with the pharmacological potency (262), although exceptions are known. Tipredane has a RBA value

Table 7 Relative Binding Affinity to the Glucocorticoid
Receptor (64,261)

Cortisol	0.04
Dexamethasone	1.0
Prednisolone	1.6
Methylprednisolone	4.2
Flunisolide	1.9
Triamcinolone acetonide	2.3
Beclomethasone	0.75
Beclomethasone dipropionate	0.5
Beclomethasone 21-monopropionate	0.0
Beclomethasone 17-monopropionate	13.0
Budesonide	9.4
Fluticasone	22.0
Tipredane	27.0

three times that of budesonide (64) but a very small effect in vasoconstrictor assay (263). In clinical trials, the therapeutic effect of inhaled tipredane in asthma was too weak to motivate a new drug application.

Onset of Clinical Effect

Many of the effects seen after a single dose of a glucocorticoid are compatible with the nuclear pathway of GC action described above. Several factors can influence the onset and extent of the response (Fig. 4), and a common feature is the time delay from drug dosing to drug effect (264). Numerous effects of glucocorticoids appear, however, to be compatible with a direct pathway, the mechanism being as yet poorly understood (264). Such effects include changes in plasma cortisol concentration, circulating amounts of various leukocytes, and changed activity or amounts of enzymes and inflammatory markers in blood and lung tissue.

Glucocorticoids already can be detected in BAL 10 min after intravenous injection, and for at least 1 hr a constant relation exists between blood and BAL concentrations (265,266). In patients with nonspecific hyperreactivity of airways and asthma, this was accompanied by improved airway resistance as early as 15 min after intravenous injection (266). The effect reached a maximum after 4 hr. Patients with chronic obstructive lung disease and emphysema showed no change in resistance, but symptoms were reduced beginning 20–30 min after injection.

Within 12 hr after a single dose of oral and inhaled glucocorticoid, lung function is improved (Fig. 5) (267). At 3 hours after glucocorticoid inhalation, an effect already can be demonstrated (268). The maximum effect of a single dose of an inhaled glucocorticoid appears 1–3 hr earlier than after oral gluco-

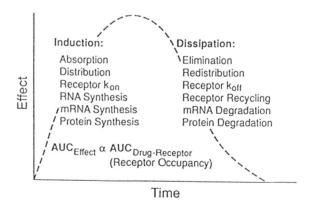

Figure 4 Schematic depiction of major determinants of the time course of onset and dissipation of corticosteroid effects as well as the overall area-under-the-curve (AUC) of effect. (From Ref. 264.)

corticoid and seems to lose its effect somewhat sooner. The slower rate of uptake following oral dosing may explain at least part of these findings.

In the clinical situation, a significant pharmacological effect of a glucocorticoid is thus expected within a few days, but continuous treatment for several weeks is generally required to attain maximum therapeutic benefit (269,270). In acute asthma, a high single dose of intravenous or oral glucocorticoid is generally efficacious and without severe side effects, and this regimen has been associated with reduced morbidity and need for hospital care (271). The onset of clinical effect after intravenous glucocorticoid is apparent in about 2 hr and maximum effect reached in about 6 hr (272).

The effect of antiasthma drugs may be tested by assessing lung function after allergen challenge. In this model, an immediate (within 10–15 min after provocation) and a late (within 4–6 hr) bronchial reaction evolves, leading to a reduction in lung function parameters. Although the immediate reaction is characterized by the release of spasmogenic mediators, the late reaction is characterized by inflammatory edema and cellular infiltration (273). The late allergic reaction is generally inhibited by single doses of glucocorticoids, but

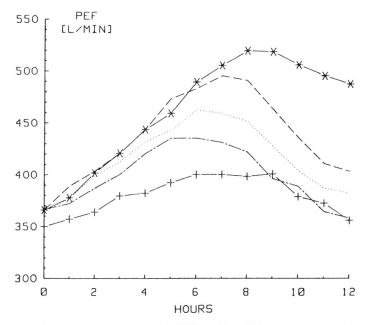

Figure 5 Time course of response in PEFR to five different treatments with single doses of corticosteroids (mean values for 12 patients with chronic asthma). Prednisolone 40 mg PO (*-*-*); budesonide 1600 μg inhalation (----); budesonide 400 μg inhalation (·····); budesonide 100 μg inhalation (-··--); budesonide 1600 μg PO (-+-+-). (From Ref. 267g.)

the early reaction requires several days of glucocorticoid treatment to become apparent and several weeks to reach its full effect (Fig. 6) (274).

Dose-Response Relationship

Increased systemic exposure of glucocorticoids generally leads to proportional increases in systemic effects. With increasing doses of glucocorticoid, linear or log-linear increases in effects on basal (275,276) and ACTH-stimulated plasma cortisol (277,278), on androgens and markers of bone formation (275), and on short term growth (279,280) have been shown for oral and inhaled glucocorticoids. The sensitivity toward glucocorticoid treatment of selected systemic variables as well as the sensitivity and variability of the assay used in the assessment generally determines whether a dose-response can be shown rather than a nonlinear response per se.

In spite of the fact that most systemic and inhaled glucocorticoids show dose linearity in pharmacokinetics and systemic effects, few studies have convincingly shown a dose response in clinical efficacy. In a review on systemic glucocorticoid therapy in acute severe asthma, only 2 of 10 studies were able to show a dose-response effect, and then only at comparatively low doses (281). Whether this is a result of wrong dose ranges being selected or some intrinsic property of glucocorticoids remain to be elucidated. The large interindividual variability in the sensitivity toward glucocorticoids with some patients needing very small doses to achieve maximum benefit and some being completely steroid resistant, most certainly contributes to the weak dose response seen in clinical trials.

In parallel group clinical trials with inhaled glucocorticoids, large groups have been required to show dose response. In a large Pulmicort Turbuhaler trial (473 patients with moderate to severe asthma), a significant dose response in peak expiratory velocity (PEF) and forced expiratory velocity in 1 sec (FEV_1) could be discerned in the dose range of 200–1600 μg daily (282). Similarly, in 672 patients with moderate asthma, dose response regarding morning and evening peak expiratory flow (PEF) and reduction in β-agonist use was shown for fluticasone administered 100–800 μg daily via pressurized metered-dose inhaler (pMDI) (283). In other studies with these drugs using approximately the same dose range but other study designs, no clear dose response has been shown (283a).

In crossover studies, dose-response effects have been shown in smaller patient groups. In a comparison of the potency of budesonide and prednisone, a clear dose-response relationship for both drugs was obtained (284). Doubling the doses of inhaled BDP from 200 to 1600 μg daily every 2 weeks for 8 weeks gave a steep dose-related improvement in several parameters of lung function, symptom scores, and bronchodilator requirements (285). Single doses of inhaled budesonide from 100 to 1600 μg demonstrated a significant dose-response ef-

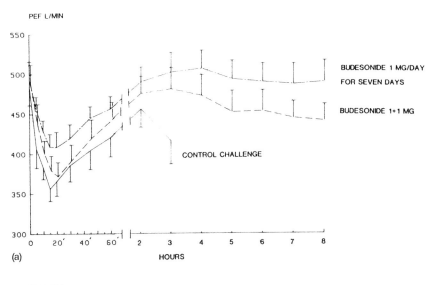

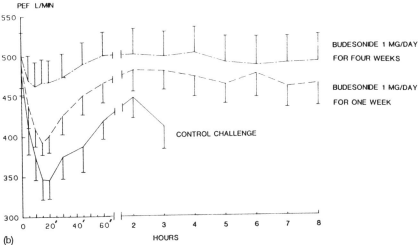

Figure 6 (A) Mean PEF ± SEM (L/min) from 0 to 8 hr after control challenge and after pretreatment with budesonide for 12 hr and 1 week. (From ref. 274.) (B) Mean PEF ± SEM (L/min) from 0 to 8 hours after challenge and after pretreatment with budesonide for 1 and 4 weeks. (From ref. 274.)

fect on PEF, where the lowest dose also gave a therapeutic effect different from that of 1.6 mg orally administered (286).

In an interesting study utilizing an allergen provocation model, the topical to systemic ratio of three different inhaled glucocorticoid aerosols (flunisolide, TAAc, and BDP) were assessed after a 1-week treatment period (287). The decrease in obstruction after allergen challenge and the decrease in circulating eosinophils were used as indices of topical and systemic effect, respectively. The ratio was similar for the three compounds, and from this the authors deduced that none of the aerosol glucocorticoids showed a clear advantage in the risk-benefit ratio when compared on a weight basis. Another recent study suggested that exercise-induced challenge can be used to demonstrate a dose-response effect, whereas other measures of pulmonary function were inadequate (288).

Effect of Dosing Frequency on Response

Attempts have been made to improve the risk-benefit ratio by optimizing the time of the day of dose intake and the dosing frequency. Prednisolone given at 0600, 1200, 1800, and 0000 hr clearly showed a significant diurnal variation in kinetics of this drug (252). C_{max} and AUC were the highest following the noon dose and the lowest following the 1800 dose. The higher plasma concentrations found after a morning versus an evening dose of prednisolone was, however, not followed by similar differences in the effects of blood cell count and blood glucose (162).

Methylprednisolone clearance was significantly greater in the afternoon (4 PM) than in the morning (8 AM) (289). Similar to prednisone, the different plasma concentrations obtained between the two regimens were not accompanied by different net effects on blood histamine, blood T lymphocytes, and plasma cortisol, again illustrating the difficulty in making accurate predictions of the expected effect time relationships. There was, however, a tendency for the circadian rhythm to be better preserved following the morning dosing (289,290). Also, after a single 40-mg IV dose of methylprednisolone at 3 AM, 3 PM, and 7 PM in asthmatic children, improvement in peak expiratory flow was greater following the 3 PM dose (291).

The time of administration had only weak effects on the pharmacokinetics of dexamethasone (292), but it did affect the systemic response: Oral dexamethasone (0.5 mg) given in the morning caused adrenal suppression lasting for 10 hr. The same dose given at midnight resulted in a 24-hr suppression of adrenal function (293). Similarly, for inhaled doses of glucocorticoids, evening dosing seems to accentuate the effect on adrenal function as compared with the same dose given in the morning (294).

Severe asthma often requires frequent dosing, and then morning or, if required, morning and early afternoon dosing seems best to preserve the clinical efficacy compromising normal diurnal cortisol secretion as little as possible (295,296). A "steroid-sparing effect" was noted after splitting of the dose of methylprednisolone from 40 mg at 8 AM to 20 mg at 8 AM and 5 mg at 4 PM (296). In addition, the data suggested less risk of adverse effects following the split-dose regimen.

A similar principle was proposed by Reinberg et al. (297) using a specially designed glucocorticoid preparation. A double-blind, randomized, crossover, placebo-controlled study compared two methods of steroid dosing and the consequent effect on pulmonary function. A preparation called Dutimelan 8-15 (DTM 8-15, Hoechst, Italy) was administered for 8 days according to the following regimen: at 8 AM, the patients received a tablet with 7 mg prednisolone acetate and 4 mg prednisolone alcohol; at 3 PM, a tablet with 15 mg cortisone acetate and 3 mg prednisolone alcohol; and at 8 PM, a placebo. On the alternate 8 days they received placebo at 8 AM; at 3 PM, a tablet consisting of 15 mg cortisone acetate and 3 mg prednisolone alcohol; and at 8 PM, another tablet with 7 mg prednisolone acetate and 4 mg prednisolone alcohol, a treatment labeled Rx 15-20. The 24-hr peak mean expiratory flow (based on five measures per day for 8 days) and the morning pulmonary function were approximately 15% higher for the DTM 8-15 regimen as compared with the Rx 15-20 regimen. The investigators concluded that the steroid regimen at 8 AM and 3 PM, DTM 8-15, was more effective in the control of asthma than the steroid regimen administered at 3 and 8 PM. Unfortunately, the study did not compare DTM 8-15 to conventional therapy administered at 8 AM in a single dose. One of the disadvantages of DTM 8-15 is the fixed dose that limits individualization of treatment.

In chronic asthmatics, halving the frequency of the same total daily dose of inhaled budesonide (from four to two times per day) caused significant falls in PEF values (298). It was also clearly shown that Malo et al. (299) that a four times a day regimen of budesonide offers better control of asthma symptoms in moderate to severe asthma than the twice-a-day regimen. The risk of achieving oropharyngeal candidiasis after pMDI without spacer is, however, less when reducing the dosing frequency from four to two times per day (300).

Because of assumed increased compliance, once daily dosing is being increasingly advocated. Studies with the new potent inhaled glucocorticoids in mild to moderate asthmatics have indeed indicated preserved therapeutic efficacy after halving the frequency from two or four times a day to single doses of the same daily dose (277,301,302). Selecting morning or evening dose depends on the stability and symptom pattern of each patient, but individual consideration has to be taken to the increased risk of HPA effects following evening dosing (294).

Originally proposed for prednisone by Harter et al. (303), the alternate-day regimen is commonly advocated to optimize the clinical efficacy and reduce the adverse effects on, for example, the HPA axis. With this regimen, there is, however, ample evidence that both wanted (272) and unwanted (303) effects diminish when an alternate-regimen is prescribed in lieu of a daily regimen of the same total dose. It has been disputed whether lower body exposure to prednisolone at higher doses due to nonlinear pharmacokinetics may explain part of these findings (304,305).

So far, alternate-day treatment with inhaled glucocorticoids has not been clinically documented. Possibly, this regimen may lead to improved risk-benefit ratio in steroid-sensitive patients having mild asthma. However, for a majority of patients having mild asthma, the inhaled glucocorticoid dose required for asthma control causes no or negligible systemic side effects irrespective of dosing frequency.

Physiological Drug Interactions

β-Adrenergic Agonists

There is no clear evidence of any pharmacokinetic interactions between glucocorticoids and β-agonists. There is, however, profound dynamic interactions; glucocorticoids increase the expression of β-adrenoreceptors (but not α-adrenoreceptors) (306), probably by increasing gene transcription (307). Some of the effects of β-agonists associated with cardiovascular symptoms (e.g., hypokalemia and increased heart rate) are augmented by concomitant oral glucocorticoids (308,309). Fenoterol may be more potent than other β-agonists in this respect (308). In addition, β-agonists have been shown to reduce the binding of the GR to glucocorticoid-responsive elements within the nucleus by activating a transcription factor (CREB) which interacts with the GR (310).

There is strong evidence to suggest a therapeutic advantage of combining glucocorticoids and β_2-agonists in the treatment of acute severe asthma (311). Intravenous glucocorticoids in combination with intravenous terbutaline improved lung function (FEV_1) significantly more than either drug given separately. The bronchodilatory effect seems to be additive rather than synergistic in nature (274). However, although bronchial responsiveness to inhaled methacholine was significantly reduced in asthmatic children receiving inhaled budesonide for 6 months, a slight increase was seen in asthmatic children receiving terbualine (312). In fact, β-agonists may negate the beneficial effects of budesonide therapy on lung function and protection against the early response to antigen (313). In another study, the reduced bronchial reactivity to histamine and adenosine monophosphate following inhaled budesonide was not negated by concomitant terbutaline (314).

Sex Hormones

Eosinophils are believed to play an important role in the pathogenesis of asthma and hay fever, and the cytokine IL-5 is an important regulator of eosinophilic homeostasis. Testosterone and progesterone induce IL-5 gene expression in T cells, but this induction is completely blocked by dexamethasone (315), implying an important physiological interaction between sex hormones and glucocorticoids.

Ethinyl estradiol inhibits the enzymatic degradation of prednisolone (163). Although estrogen and ethinyl estradiol elevate endogenous cortisol levels

(316,317), the effect is comparatively minor. In addition, the feedback regulation of the HPA axis during estrogen treatment seems to be normal as assessed by the dexamethasone test (318).

Testosterone suppression may occur in a variety of respiratory conditions. Hypoxia has been suggested to suppress the hypothalamic-pituitary-testicular axis (319), but also treatment with glucocorticoids may have this effect (320,321). Glucocorticoids may act directly on testicular biosynthesis (321) and/ or on hepatic elimination (218).

VI. Clinical Applications of Pharmacokinetics: Optimizing Efficacy, Overcoming Apparent Steroid Resistance, and Minimizing the Risk of Adverse Effects

Glucocorticoid therapy may be used as replacement for adrenal insufficiency syndromes, used in the treatment of inflammatory disorders, or suprapharmacologically for the prevention of transplant rejection or management of shock. In each case, the glucocorticoid dose must be appropriately initiated and properly titrated to maximize beneficial effects and minimize undesirable effects.

A. Route of Administration

A number of glucocorticoid formulations are available and may be selected based on the specific application. Parenteral forms, such as hydrocortisone and methylprednisolone sodium succinate are prodrugs and must be converted to the parent compound. This conversion is very rapid and assures rapid attainment of systemic availability (322). Other parenteral forms, such as cortisone acetate and methylprednisolone acetate suspension, are designed for prolonged absorption in order to sustain the availability of glucocorticoid concentrations. These preparations are useful as intra-articular injections and in the treatment of adrenocortical insufficiency disorders.

Oral preparations are the most commonly used forms of glucocorticoid therapy. It is important to select preparations that have demonstrated complete or almost complete uptake (323). The most significant development in glucocorticoid therapy is the introduction of topical preparations. These are designed to provide maximal concentrations of potent glucocorticoid at the site of action; for example, dermatological preparations for skin disorders and aerosol formulations for the treatment of asthma.

B. Patient Variables Influencing Response

Besides the previously described determinants of response to glucocorticoid therapy, other conditions must be considered. Of obvious importance is the patient's compliance for the prescribed regimen. With the severity of adverse effects related to prolonged high-dose systemic glucocorticoid therapy, especially those affecting physical appearance, the clinician must carefully assess the patient's attitude toward self-care. Attempts should be made to minimize glucocorticoid exposure by using alternative forms of treatment and topical corticosteroid preparations if feasible.

Initial treatment of severe life-threatening illness requires high-dose glucocorticoid therapy. The dose and duration of treatment is related to the specific disease, severity, and prognosis. High-dose glucocorticoid therapy for short periods of time (less than 2 weeks) has a minimal risk of adverse effects, and the glucocorticoid dose can be discontinued abruptly. More prolonged treatment courses require a careful dosage reduction to avoid complications of adrenal insufficiency secondary to HPA suppression. For chronic glucocorticoid therapy, attempts should be made to convert the patient to an alternate-day regimen or to an inhaled glucocorticoid. If possible, all doses should be administered in the morning to minimize HPA suppression.

C. Apparent Steroid Resistance

Most patients respond promptly to a carefully structured course of glucocorticoid therapy; certain patients, however, appear refractory. Following a careful review of the treatment regimens, as well as the patient's compliance, several factors may be considered in determining the possible refractoriness to glucocorticoid therapy.

The severity of the disease may require more aggressive treatment regimens. In addition, the presence of other clinical disorders, such as renal disease or hyperthyroidism, or concomitant medications, specifically anticonvulsants or rifampin, may be associated with increased glucocorticoid elimination. The availability of techniques to assess glucocorticoid disposition in patients may readily assist in the identification of those patients with unusually rapid elimination (324).

Another factor to consider is the possibility of an abnormality at the level of the GR. Chrousos and colleagues (325) described a familial disorder of apparent cortisol resistance consisting of high 24-hr mean plasma cortisol levels with the absence of the stigmata of Cushing's syndrome. Plasma ACTH levels were high, and the patients were resistant to adrenal suppression by dexamethasone. The GR as measured in peripheral leukocytes and fibroblasts had decreased binding affinity for dexamethasone. A reduced number of cytosolic GRs receptors was also observed. The implication of this phenomenon for response to glucocorticoid therapy was not evaluated.

In addition, Carmichael et al. (326) identified a population of patients with chronic asthma with apparent glucocorticoid resistance. These patients demonstrated poor response to glucocorticoid therapy as determined by pulmonary function tests following a course of daily high-dose glucocorticoid therapy for

7 days. These patients more frequently had a family history of asthma and a longer duration of symptoms as compared with the glucocorticoid-responsive patients. The resistant patients had a relatively lower peak expiratory flow rate in the morning compared with that measured later in the day, as well as a greater degree of bronchial reactivity to methacholine. These investigators subsequently demonstrated a defect in the expression and mobilization of complement receptors on the monocyte cell membrane (327) and cellular response to glucocorticoid (328).

Recently, Sher et al. (329) described glucocorticoid receptor abnormalities in patients with severe steroid-resistant asthma. Some patients had reduced GR binding affinity (type 1) and others had reduced GR number (type 2). Kam et al. (330) demonstrated that the type 1 defect could be induced in normal peripheral blood mononuclear cells with the coincubation of cells with IL-2 and IL-4, suggesting that this abnormality is related to proinflammatory cytokines. Spahn et al. (331) demonstrated that the type 1 abnormality could be reversed with high-dose glucocorticoid therapy. Therefore, it appears that persistent inflammation can attenuate the response to glucocorticoid therapy.

VII. Future Directions

Although recent advances have contributed to the safe and effective use of glucocorticoids in severe life-threatening disorders, chronic glucocorticoid therapy is associated with significant risk for adverse effects. The development of topical formulations has reduced the systemic availability of glucocorticoids while providing an equivalent therapeutic response. An area of intensive investigation is the development of site-specific glucocorticoid derivatives. Identification of a glucocorticoid derivative selective for cells involved in the pathogenesis of inflammatory disorders, such as asthma, could provide beneficial effects while minimizing adverse effects secondary to systemic exposure.

Until such advances are made, it is necessary to continue to identify conditions that may alter the response to glucocorticoid therapy. Similar to the observations of accelerated or impaired glucocorticoid elimination in the presence of concomitant anticonvulsant or macrolide antibiotic therapy, it is important to evaluate the effect of other medications on the disposition of glucocorticoids. Significant advances in the identification of conditions influencing medications such as theophylline, anticonvulsants, and anticoagulants were facilitated by the application of methods to measure plasma concentrations of the medication. Methods to measure glucocorticoid concentrations are available, although they are labor intensive and require the assessment of a series of concentrations to analyze disposition. This technique has been applied to evaluate specific patients, and the results have been beneficial (324,332).

Monitoring of glucocorticoid concentrations can be useful in evaluating compliance, as well as the adequacy of absorption, conversion of prednisone to prednisolone, and rate of elimination. Additional insight could be provided by the development of techniques to measure the glucocorticoid response, especially if this could be used to alter dosage regimens.

Pharmacodynamic modeling of glucocorticoid effects are being increasingly used to optimize dosing strategies. However, pharmacokinetic-pharmacodynamic (PK/PD) modeling of glucocorticoids have been focused on systemic effects, including helper T cells in blood (290), the OKT3 and OKT4 lymphocyte subsets in blood (333), whole blood histamine (334), fasting blood sugar (335), plasma cortisol (336), and hepatic tyrosine aminotransferase (337,338). However, in anti-inflammatory asthma treatment, the local events are probably of more importance for the therapeutic effect. Today, glucocorticoid concentrations in tissues have been assessed in a few studies (89), but such data have been connected neither with local dynamic events, nor with kinetic or dynamic events in the systemic circulation, nor with events in side effect compartments.

In an interesting report by Hochhaus and co-workers (339), PK/PD models for targeted delivery to the lungs were elucidated using relatively simple two-compartment and E_{max} models (339). From these simulations, pronounced targeting was predicted for drugs with large systemic distribution volumes, slow absorption, and rapid systemic elimination. The biggest difference between systemic and pulmonary drug levels will be observed for drugs with a pronounced difference between rates of systemic absorption and systemic elimination and between the pulmonary and systemic volume of distribution. The most pronounced lung targeting was also observed with frequent application of small doses, and this points to the existence of optimal dosing regimens for inhalational therapy.

Hopefully, future developments of tissue assays of total, free, and receptor-bound glucocorticoids as well as migratory cells and inflammatory mediators will more accurately reflect the therapeutic outcome. Possibly microdialysis and positron emission techniques will have a role in such investigations together with the more conventional biopsy, BAL, scintography, and pharmacokinetic techniques. Together with the dynamic modeling of systemic effects, such data will aid in developing future generations of glucocorticoids by optimizing lung deposition (either central or peripheral), tissue and cellular targeting (Is a tissue depot achievable and desirable?) and elimination (Can this be achieved already in the target organ without losing the therapeutic response?).

Discussion

DR. DURHAM: How is systemic bioavailability measured? Is all of the deposited lung dose of topical corticosteroid absorbed?

DR. EDSBACKER: The systemic availability of inhaled glucocorticoids is obtained as the ratio between plasma concentrations after inhalation and after intravenous dosing. Lung bioavailability can be derived from scintigraphic studies using a technitium-labeled compound and from plasma concentration measurements compensating for oral availability. Systemic available drug comprises the combined lung and gastrointestinal contribution. It is important to emphasize that the lung contribution constitutes a dominant fraction of the systemic exposure. All of that which is deposited in the lungs is also systemically absorbed as active drug.

DR. BARNES: Patients may show differences in susceptibility to systemic side affects of inhaled glucocorticoids. Can any of this variability be explained by differences in pharmacokinetics?

DR. SZEFLER: There appears to be a wide spectrum of beneficial and adverse effects to a given steroid dose among patients. This variation is not easily explained with one answer. It probably reflects disease severity and receptor sensitivity and other conditions, such as receptor binding, diet, body habitus, and other unexplained cellular mechanisms.

DR. PEDERSEN: (1) When systemic effects of an inhaled steroid are studied, is it then sufficient just to evelute total bioavailability or is the absorption profile also important; that is, rapid absorption with high peaks of drug concentration or slow, more prolonged absorption? (2) A high first-pass metabolism is important. However, the drug being absorbed through the gastrointestinal tract may exert adverse local effects; for example, on calcium metabolism. Is there any data on this aspect?

DR. SZEFLER: Theoretically, a low bioavailability should reduce the risk of adverse effects. However, localized adverse effects could occur with prolonged localized tissue exposure; for example, in the gastrointestinal tract. This would be a concern for drugs that are poorly absorbed but remain at high concentrations at the site of absorption.

DR. EDSBACKER: To address specifically the two questions raised by Dr. Pedersen: (1) There might be a connection between peak concentrations of the glucocorticoids and systemic side effects. Data in our laboratory suggest however, that AUC and cortisol suppression are very closely correlated. (2) The experience with oral budesonide for inflammatory bowel disease indicates that the extent and array of systemic effects are similar and related to the systemic exposure. However, a report on oral BDP indicates a local intestinal effect on calcium uptake.

DR. BRATTSAND: I want to stress that the low systemic availability depends on hepatic first-pass metabolism. In the bowel wall, budesonide and BDP are fully active. Thus, when choosing between inhaled formulations, the one giving the least oral deposition would be preferable.

DR. LEUNG: Severe side effects to systemic glucocorticoids can be seen in some but not all patients. This subset of patients frequently has normal glucocorticoid pharmacokinetics. What are the potential mechanisms at a cellular or molecular level for increased susceptibility to side effects from glucocorticoids?

DR. EDSBACKER: Literature data are scarce. A study by Lew has shown that women have greater sensitivity than men toward methylprednisolone, but clearance in women is higher, implying no need for dose adjustments. The molecular mechanisms behind this increased sensitivity are not known. (Lew K, Ludwig E, Milad M, et al. Gender based effects on methylprednisolone pharmacokinetics and pharmacodynamics. Clin Pharmacol Ther 1993; 54:403–414.)

DR. SZEFLER: As discussed in the answer to Dr. Barnes' question, there is no single explanation for the differences in adverse effects among various patients. This may be related to individual patient or tissue binding, availability of the medication to specific tissue sites, or other confounding features, such as tissue susceptibility related to diet or body habitus. (Jusko WJ, Ludwig EA. Corticosteroids. In: Evans WE, Schentag JJ, Jusko WJ, eds. Applied Pharmacokinetics: Principles of Therapeutic Drug Monitoring. Applied Therapeutics, Vancouver, WA, 1992: 27-1–27-34.)

DR. LANE: Could you expand on pharmacokinetic polymorphism and how it may relate to reduced responsiveness to glucocorticoid treatment?

DR. SZEFLER: There are well-described population differences for certain drugs, especially those where metabolism involves cytochrome P450, but these have not been specifically described for glucocorticoids. This may be relevant for the inhaled glucocorticoids where it is not possible to obtain specific pharmacokinetic evaluations, as we can do with prednisolone and methylprednisolone.

DR. DURHAM: Are the pharmacokinetics for steroid-resistant patients different than those for steroid-responsive patients?

DR. SZEFLER: Rapid metabolism or poor absorption is not the only explanation for a poor response to steroid therapy. It does occur in some patients. Therefore, the evaluation of steroid absorption and elimination is important in patients who fail to respond to high-dose steroid therapy. Once identified, treatment can be improved by selecting an alternative steroid, by discontinuing a medication that induces steroid metabolism or by changing the dosing schedule, for example, using a split-dosing regimen. Dr. Leung will review our observations regarding other reasons for apparent steroid resistance.

DR. HARGREAVE: Are you sure you are not missing poor compliance in your patients who do not have expected side effects from glucocorticoids?

DR. SZEFLER: Compliance is always a concern in patients who are receiving high-dose therapy and is still difficult to control. The absence of adverse effects should raise questions about compliance. This can be evaluated by prescription refills, morning plasma cortisol, or measurement of the specific steroid in a plasma sample several hours after the time of the administered dose.

References

1. Hargreave FE, Dolovich J, Newhouse MT. The assessment and treatment of asthma: a conference report. J Allergy Clin Immunol 1990; 85:1098–1111.
2. Haskell RJ, Wong BM, Hansen JE. A double-blind, randomized clinical trial of methylprednisolone in status asthmaticus. Arch Intern Med 1983; 143:1324–1327.
3. Harris JB, Weinberger MM, Nassif E, Smith G, Milavetz G, Stillerman A. Early intervention with short courses of prednisone to prevent progression of asthma in ambulatory patients incompletely responsive to bronchodilators. J Pediatr 1987; 110:627–633.
4. Tal A, Levy N, Bearmen JE. Methylprednisolone therapy for acute asthma in infants and toddlers. A controlled clinical trial. Pediatrics 1990; 86:350–356.
5. Woolcock AJ. Use of corticosteroids in treatment of patients with asthma. J Allergy Clin Immunol 1989; 84:975–978.
6. Toogood JH. Bronchial asthma and glucocorticoids. In: Schleimer RP, Claman HN, Oronsky A, eds. Anti-inflammatory Steroid Action: Basic and Clinical Aspects. Academic Press: San Diego, 1989:423–468.
7. Brenner M. Use of steroids in pediatric asthma. Pediatr Ann 1989; 18:810–818.
8. Morselli PL, Marc V, Garathini S, Zaccala M. Metabolism of exogenous cortisol in humans. I Diurnal variations in plasma disappearance rate. Biochem Pharmacol 1970; 19:1643–1647.
9. Toothaker RD, Craig WA, Welling PC. Effect of dose size on the pharmacokinetics of oral hydrocortisone suspension. J Pharm Sci 1982; 71:1182–1185.
10. Choi Y, Thrasher K, Werk EE, Sholiton LJ, Olinger C. Effect of diphenylhydantoin on cortisol in humans. J Pharmacol Exp Ther 1971; 176:27–34.
11. Petersen RE, Wyngaarden JB, Guerra SL, Brodie BB, Bunim JJ. The physiological disposition and metabolic fate of hydrocortisone in man. J Clin Invest 1955; 34:1779–1794.
12. Täuber U, Haack D, Nieuweboer B, Kloss G, Vecsei P, Wendt H. The pharmacokinetics of fluocortolone and prednisolone after intravenous and oral administration. Int J Clin Pharmacol Ther Toxicol 1984; 22:48–55.
13. Meffin PJ, Brooks PM, Sallustio BC. Alterations in prednisolone disposition as a result of time of administration, gender and dose. Br J Clin Pharmacol 1984; 17:395–404.
14. Boeckenoogen SJ, Szefler SJ, Jusko WJ. Prednisolone disposition and protein binding in oral contraceptive users. J Clin Endocrinol Metabol. 1983; 56:702–709.
15. McAllister WAC, Winfield CR, Collins JU. Pharmacokinetics of prednisolone in normal and asthmatic subjects in relation to dose. Eur J Clin Pharmacol 1981; 20:141–145.
16. Bergrem H, Refvem OK. Changes in prednisolone pharmacokinetics and protein binding during treatment with rifampicin. Proc EDTA 1982; 19:552–557.

17. Pickup ME, Lowe JR, Leatham PA, Rhind VM, Wright V, Downie WW. Dose dependent pharmacokinetics of prednisolone. Eur J Clin Pharmacol 1977; 12:213–219.
18. Rose JQ, Yarchak AM, Meikle M, Jusko WJ. Effect of smoking on prednisone, prednisolone and dexamethasone pharmacokinetics. J Pharmacokin Biopharm 1981; 9:1–14.
19. Frey BM, Schaad HJ, Frey FJ. Pharmacokinetic interaction of contraceptive steroids with prednisone and prednisolone. Eur J Clin Pharmacol 1984; 26:505–511.
20. Milsap RL, George DE, Szefler SJ, Murray KA, Lebenthal E, Jusko WJ. Effect of inflammatory bowel disease on absorption and disposition of prednisolone. Dig Dis Sci 1983; 28:161–168.
21. Bartoszek M, Brenner AM, Szefler SJ. Prednisolone and methylprednisolone kinetics in children receiving anticonvulsant therapy. Clin Pharmacol Ther 1987; 42:424–432.
22. Schalm SW, Summerskill WHJ, Go VLW. Prednisone for chronic active liver disease: pharmacokinetics, including conversion to prednisolone. Gastroenterology 1977; 72:910–913.
23. Lee K-H. Bioavailability of oral prednisolone. Seoul J Med 1991; 32:131–137.
24. Szefler SJ, Rose JQ, Ellis EF, Spector SL, Green AW, Jusko WJ. The effect of troleandomycin on methylprednisolone elimination. J Allergy Clin Immunol 1980; 66:447–451.
25. Narang PK, Wilder R, Chatterji DC, Yeager RL, Gallelli JF. Systemic bioavailability and pharmacokinetics of methylprednisolone in patients with rheumatoid arthritis following 'high-dose' pulse administration. Biopharm Drug Dispos 1983; 4:233–248.
26. Derendorf H, Möllman H, Rohdewald P, Rehder J, Schmidt EW. Kinetics of methylprednisolone and its hemisuccinate ester. Clin Pharmacol Ther 1985; 37:502–507.
27. Stjernholm MR, Katz FH. Effects of diphenylhydantoin, phenobarbital, and diazepam on the metabolism of methylprednisolone and of its sodium succinate. J Clin Endocrinol Metab 1975; 41:887–893.
28. Antal EJ, Wright CE, Gillespie WR, Albert KS. Influence of route of administration on the pharmacokinetics of methylprednisolone. J Pharmacokinet Biopharm 1983; 11:561–576.
29. Möllman H, Rohdewald P, Barth J, Verho M, Derendorf H. Pharmacokinetics and dose linearity of methylprednisolone phosphate. Biopharm Drug Dispos 1989; 10:453–464.
30. Al-Habet SM, Rogers HJ. Methylprednisolone pharmacokinetics after intravenous and oral administration. Br J Clin Pharmacol 1989; 27:285–290.
31. Tsuei SE, Moore RG, Ashley JJ, McBride WG. Disposition of synthetic glucocorticoids: pharmacokinetics of dexamethasone in healthy adults. J Pharmacokinet Biopharm 1979; 7:249–264.
32. Kasuya Y, Althaus JR, Freeman JP, Mitchum RK, Skelly JP. Quantiative determination of dexamethasone in human plasma by stable isotope dilution mass spectrometry. J Pharm Sci 1984; 73:446–451.
33. Haque N, Thrasher K, Werk EE Jr, Knowles HC Jr, Sholiton LT. Studies on

dexamethasone metabolism in man: Effect of diphenylhydantoin. J Clin Endocr Metab 1972; 34:44–50.

34. McCafferty J, Brophy TROR, Yelland JD, Chan BE, Bochner F, Eadie MJ. Intraoperative pharmacokinetics of dexamethasone. Br J Clin Pharmacol Toxicol 1977; 17:511–527.

35. Rohdewald P, Möllman H, Barth J, Rehder J, Derendorf H. Pharmacokinetics of dexamethasone and its phosphate ester. Biopharmac Drug Dispos 1987; 8:205–212.

36. Petersen MC, Nation RL, McBride WG, Ashley JJ, Moore RG. Pharmacokinetics of betamethasone in healthy adults after intravenous administration. Eur J Clin Pharmacol 1983; 25:643–650.

37. Alessandro A, Antonio P, Guiseppe B, Valeria P. Disposition of a new steroidal anti-inflammatory agent, deflazacort, in rat, dog and man. Eur J Drug Metab Pharmacokinet 1980; 5:207–215.

38. Mützel W. Pharmakokinetik und Biotransformation von Fluo-cortin-bulytester beim Menschen. Arzneim-Forsch/Drug Res 1977; 27:2230–2233.

39. Chaplin MD, Rocks II W, Swenson EW, Cooper WC, Nerenberg C, Chu NI. Flunisolide metabolism and dynamics of a metabolite. Clin Pharmacol Ther 1980; 27:402–413.

40. Möllman H, Rohdewald P, Schmidt EW, Salomon V, Derendorf H. Pharmacokinetics of triamcinolone acetonide and its phosphate ester. Eur J Clin Pharmacol 1985; 29:85–89.

41. Ryrfeldt Å, Andersson P, Edsbäcker S, Tönnesson M, Davies D, Pauwels R. Pharmacokinetics and metabolism of budesonide, a selective glucocorticoid. Eur J Respir Dis 1982; 63(Suppl 122):86–95.

42. Edsbäcker S, Andersson KE, Ryrfelt Å. Nasal bioavailability and systemic effects of the glucocorticoid budesonide in man. Eur J Clin Pharmacol 1985; 29:477–481.

43. Pedersen S, Steffensen G, Ekman I, Tönnesson M, Borgå O. Bioavailability of inhaled budesonide in children with asthma. Eur J Clin Pharmacol 1987; 31:579–582.

44. Thorsson L, Edsbäcker S, Conradson T-B. Lung deposition of budesonide from Turbuhaler is twice that from a pressurized metered dose inhaler pMDI. Eur Respir J 1994; 7:1839–1844.

45. Harding SM. The human pharmacology of fluticasone propionate. Respir Med 1990; 84:A25–A29.

46. Miyabo S, Nakamura T, Kuwazima S, Kishida S. A comparison of the bioavailability and potency of dexamethasone phosphate and sulphate in man. Eur J Clin Pharmacol 1981; 20:277–282.

47. Ferry JJ, Horvath AM, Bekersky I, Heath EC, Ryan CF, Colburn WA. Relative and absolute bioavailability of prednisone and prednisolone after separate oral and intravenous doses. J Clin Pharmacol 1988; 28:81–87.

48. Swartz SL, Dluhy RG. Corticosteroids. Clinical pharmacology and therapeutic use. Drugs 1978; 16:238–255.

49. Gambertoglio JG, Amend WJ, Benet LZ. Pharmacokinetics and bioavailability of prednisone and prednisolone in healthy volunteers and patients. J Pharmacokinet Biopharm 1980; 8:1–52.

50. Tanner A, Bochner F, Caffin J, Halliday J, Powell L. Dose-dependent prednisolone kinetics. Clin Pharmacol Ther 1979; 25:571–578.

51. Al-Habet SM, Rogers HJ. Pharmacokinetics of intravenous and oral prednisolone. Br J Clin Pharmacol 1980; 10:503–508.

52. Frey BM, Brandenberger AW, Frey FJ, Widmer HR. Systemishe Verfügbarkeit von Prednisolon nach oral verabreichtem Prednison. Pharm Acta Helv 1984; 59:301–309.

53. Petereit LB, Meikle AW. Effectiveness of prednisolone during phenytoin therapy. Clin Pharmacol Ther 1977; 22:912–916.

54. Duggan DE, Yeh KC, Matalia N, Ditzler CA, McMahon FG. Bioavailability of oral dexamethasone. Clin Pharmacol Ther 1975; 18:205–209.

55. Brophy TROR, McCafferty J, Tyrer JH, Eadie MJ. Bioavailability of oral dexamethasone during high dose steroid therapy in neurological patients. Eur J Clin Pharmacol 1983; 24:103–108.

56. Chaplin MD, Cooper WC, Segre EJ, Oren J, Jones RE, Nerenberg C. Correlation of flunisolide plasma to eosinopenic response in humans. J Allergy Clin Immunol 1980; 65:445–453.

57. Edsbäcker S, Ryrfeldt Å, Tönneson M. Does cimetidine influence budesonide kinetics? Acta Pharmacol Toxicol 1986; 59:97A.

58. Dahlström K, Edsbäcker S, Källén A. Rectal pharmacokinetics of budesonide. Eur J Clin Pharmacol 1996; 49:293–298.

59. Piper JM, Wayne AR, Dauherty JJR, Griffin MR. Corticosteroid use and peptic ulcer disease: role of nonsteroidal antiinflammatory drugs. Ann Intern Med 1991; 114:735–740.

60. Thomas P, Richards D, Richards A, et al. Absorption of delayed-release prednisolone in ulcerative colitis and Crohn's disease. J Pharm Pharmacol 1985; 37:757–758.

61. Kwaselow A, Mc Lean J, Busse W, et al A comparison of intranasal and oral flunisolide in the therapy of allergic rhinitis. Evidence for a topical effect. Allergy 1985; 40:363–367.

62. Norman PS, Winkenwender W, Murgatroyd G, Parson J. Evidence for the local action of intranasal dexamethasone aerosols in the suppression of hay fever symptoms. J Allergy 1966; 38:93–97.

63. Toogood JH, Frankish CW, Jennings BH, et al. A study of the mechanism of the antiasthmatic action of inhaled budesonide. J Allergy Clin Immunol 1990; 85:872–880.

64. Brattsand R, Axelsson BI. New inhaled glucocorticoids. In: Barnes PJ, ed. New Drugs for Asthma. Vol. 2, London, 1992:193–208.

65. Newman SP, Pavia D, Morén F, Sheathan NF, Clarke SW. Deposition of pressurized aerosols in the human respiratory tract. Thorax 1981; 36:52–55.

66. Köhler D, Fleischer W, Matthys H. New method for labelling of beta$_2$-agonists in the metered dose inhaler with technetium 99m. Respiration 1988; 53:65–73.

67. Barry PW, O'Callaghan C. Poor output of salbutamol from a spacer device. The effect of spacer static charge and multiple actuations. Thorax 1994; 49:402P.

68. Dahl R. The safety and efficacy of fluticasone propionate 200µg daily given via the Diskhaler Inhaler as compared with the pressurized metered dose inhaler for asthma. Clin Exp Allergy 1993; 23(suppl):81A.

69. Derom E, Wåhlin-Boll E, Borgström L, Pauwels R. Pulmonary deposition and effect of terbutaline administered by metered dose inhaler or Turbuhaler. Thorax 1994; 49:402P.

70. Denyer J, Dyche T. Improving the efficiency of gas power nebulizers. Eur Respir J. 1993; 6(suppl 17):148s.

71. Ballard PL. Delivery and transport of glucocorticoids to target cells. Monogr Endocrinol 1975; 12:25–48.

72. Brien TG. Human corticosteroid binding globulin. Clin Endocrinol 1981; 14:193–212.

73. Pickup ME. Clinical pharmacokinetics of prednisolone and prednisone. Clin Pharmacokinet 1979; 4:111–128.

74. Rose JQ, Yurchak AM, Jusko WJ: Dose dependent pharmacokinetics of prednisone and prednisolone in man. J Pharmcokinet Biopharm 1981; 9:389–417.

75. Lewis GP, Jusko WJ, Burke CW, Graves L. Prednisone side-effects and serum protein levels. Lancet 1971; 2:778–781.

76. Florini JR, Buyske DA. Plasma protein binding of triamcinolone-^{3}H and hydrocortisone-4-^{14}C. J Biol Chem 1961; 236:247–251.

77. Peets EA, Staub M, Synchowicz S. Plasma binding of betamethasone-^{3}H, dexamethasone-^{3}H, and cortisol-^{14}C—a comparative study. Biochem Pharmacol 1969; 18:1655–1663.

78. Szefler SJ, Ebling WF, Georgitis JW, Jusko WJ. Methylprednisolone versus prednisolone pharmacokinetics in relation to dose in adults. Eur J Clin Pharmacol 1986; 30:323–329.

79. Öje S, Tozer TN. Effect of altered plasma protein binding on apparent volume of distribution. J Pharm Sci 1979; 68:1203–1205.

80. Ebling WF, Szefler SJ, Jusko WJ. Methylprednisolone disposition in rabbits: analysis, prodrug conversion, reversible metabolism, and comparison with man. Drug Metab Dispos 1985; 13:296–304.

81. Khalafallah N, Jusko WJ. Tissue distribution of prednisolone in the rabbit. J Pharmacol Exp Ther 1984; 229:719–725.

82. Andersson P, Appelgren LE, Ryrfelt Å. Tissue distribution and fate of budesonide in the mouse. Acta Pharmacol Toxicol 1986; 59:392–402.

83. Högger P, Rawert I, Rohdewald P. Dissolution, tissue binding, and kinetics of receptor binding of inhaled glucocorticoids. Eur Respir J 1993; 6(suppl 17):584s.

83a. Miller-Larsson A, Mattson H, Ohlsson D, et al. Prolonged release from the airway tissue of glucocorticoids budesonide and fluticasone propionate as compared to beclomethasone dipropionate and hydrocortisone. Am J Respir Crit Care Med 1994; 149(suppl 4, part 2):A466.

84. Würtwein G, Rehder S, Rohdewald P. Lipophilicity and receptor affinity of glucocorticoids. Pz Wiss 1992; 137:161–167.

85. Barth J, Möllman H, Schmidt EW, Rehder J, Rohdewald P. Concentration of glucocorticoids in serum and broncheoalveolar lavage (BAL) fluid. Atemwegs-Lungenkrankh 1986; 12:89–92.

86. Braude AC, Rebuck AS. Pulmonary disposition of cortisol. Ann Intern Med 1982; 97:59–60.

87. Greos LS, Vichyanond P, Bloedow DC, et al. Methylprednisolone achieves

greater concentrations in the lung than prednisolone. Am Rev Respir Dis 1991; 144:586–592.
88. Vichyanond P, Irvin CG, Larsen GL, Szefler SJ, Hill MR. Penetration of corticosteroids into the lung: evidence for a difference between methylprednisolone and prednisolone. J Allergy Clin Immunol 1989; 84:867–873.
89. van den Bosch JMM, Edbäcker S, Westermann CJ, Aumann J, Tönnesson M, Selroos O. Relationship between lung tissue and blood plasma concentrations of inhaled budesonide. Biopharm Drug Dispos 1993; 14:455–459.
90. Toogood JH. Comparisons between inhaled and oral corticosteroids in patients with chronic asthma. In: Ellul-Micaleff R, Lam WK, Toogood JH, eds. Advances in the Use of Inhaled Corticosteroids, Proceedings of an International Symposium in Hong Kong. Amsterdam: Excerpta Medica, 1987:159–169.
91. Dorfman RI, Ungar F. Catabolic reactions of the steroids. In: Metabolism of Steroid Hormones. New York: Academic Press, 1965; 289–381.
92. Monder C, Bradlow HL. Carboxylic acid metabolites of steroids. General review. J Steroid Biochem 1977; 8:897–908.
93. Monder C, Bradlow HL. Cortoic acids. Explorations at the frontier of corticosteroid metabolism. Rec Progr Horm Res 1980; 36:345–400.
94. Bradlow HL, Monder C. Steroid carboxylic acids. In: Hobkirk R, ed. Steroid Biochemistry. CRC Press, Boca Raton, FL, 1979:29–82.
95. Frantz AG, Katz FH, Jailer JW. 6β-Hydroxycortisol and other polar corticosteroids: measurements and significance in human urine. J Clin Endocrinol Metab 1961; 21:1290–1303.
96. Pal SB. 6-Hydroxylation of cortisol and urinary 6β-hydroxycortisol. Metabolism 1978; 27:1003–1011.
97. Kornel L, Satio Z. Studies on steroid conjugates. VIII. Isolation and characterization of glucuronide-conjugated metabolites of cortisol in human urine. J Steroid Biochem 1974; 6:1267–1284.
98. Gower DB. Catabolism and excretion of steroids. In: Makin HLJ, ed. Biochemistry of Steroid Hormones. London: Blackwell, 1975:149–185.
99. Reach G, Nakane H, Nakane Y, Auzan C, Corvol P. Cortisol metabolism and excretion in the isolated perfused rat kidney. Steroids 1977; 30:605–619.
100. Rocci ML, Szefler SJ, Acara MA, Jusko WJ. Prednisolone metabolism and excretion in the isolated perfused rat kidney. Drug Metab Dispos 1981; 9:177–182.
101. Hierholzer K, Lichtenstein I, Siebe H, Tsiakriras D, Witt I. Renal metabolism of corticosteroid hormones. Klin Wochenschr 1982; 60:1127–1135.
102. Levitz M, Jansen V, Dancis J. The transfer and metabolism of corticosteroids in the perfused human placenta. Am J Obstet Gynecol 1978; 132:363–366.
103. Blanford AT, Pearson M. In vitro metabolism of prednisolone, dexamethasone, betamethasone and cortisol by the human placenta. Am J Obstet Gynecol 1977; 127:264–267.
104. Kolanowski J, Corcelle-Cerf F, Lammerant J. Cortisol uptake, release and conversion into cortisone by the heart muscle in dogs. J Steroid Biochem 1981; 14:773–781.
105. Hartiala J. Steroid metabolism in adult lung. Agents Actions 1976; 6:522–526.

106. Nicholas TH, Lugg MA. The physiological significance of 11β-hydroxysteroid dehydrogenase in the lung. J Steroid Biochem 1982; 17:113–118.

107. Hisa SL. Steriod metabolism in human skin. In: Borrie P, ed. Modern Trends in Dermatology. Butterworh, London: 1971:69–88.

108. Siebe H, Baude G, Lichtenstein I, Wang D, Bühler H, Hoyer GA, Hierholzer K. Metabolism of dexamethasone: sites and activity in mammalian tissues. Renal Physiol Biochem 1993; 16:79–88.

109. Gustafsson JÅ, Rafter J, Gustafsson B. Kost-tarmfloracancer bakteriernas roll vid omsättningen av endogena och exogena ämnen. Läkartidningen 1984; 81:4015–4021.

110. Gray CH, Green MAS, Holness NJ, Lunnon JB. Urinary metabolic products of prednisone and prednisolone. J Endocrinol 1956; 14:146–154.

111. Vermeulen A, Caspi E. The metabolism of prednisolone by homogenates of rat liver. J Biol Chem 1958; 233:54–56.

112. Vermeulen A. The metabolism of 4-^{14}C prednisolone. J Endocrinol 1959; 18:278–291.

113. ElDareer SM, Struck RF, White VM, Mellett LB, Hill DL. Distribution and metabolism of prednisolone in mice, dogs and monkeys. Cancer Treat Resp 1977; 61:1279–1289.

114. Butler J, Gray CH. The metabolism of betamethasone. J Endocrinol 1970; 46:379–390.

115. Assandri A, Ferrari P, Perazzi A, Ripamonti A, Tuan G, Zerilli L. Disposition and metabolism of a new steroidal anti-inflammatory agent, deflazacort in cynomolgus monkeys. Xenobiotica 1983; 13:185–196.

116. Buhler DR, Thomas RC, Schlagel CA. Absorption, metabolism and excretion of 6α-methylprednisolone-^{3}H, 21-acetate following oral and intramuscular administrations in the dog. Endocrinology 1965; 76:852–864.

117. Dumasia MC, Houghton E, Moss MS, Chakraborty J. Metabolism of dexamethasone in the horse. Proceedings of the 3rd International Symposium on Equine Medication Control. Lexington, KY, 1979:247–252.

118. Esumi Y, Ohtsuki T, Alsumi K, et al. Studies on the metabolic fate of dexamethasone-17-valerate III. Metabolites in rat. Iyakuhin kenkuy 1982; 13:1037–1045.

119. Hornke I, Cavagna F, Christ O, Felhhaber H-W, Kellner H-M, Sandow J. Pharmakokinetik und metabolismus von Desoximetason. Arzneim-Forsch/Drug Res 1980; 30:47–54.

120. Martinelli M, Ferrari P, Ripamonti A, Tuan G, Perazzi A, Assandri A. Metabolism of deflazacort in the rat, dog, and man. Drug Metab Dispos 1979; 7:335–339.

121. Gerhads E, Neuweboer B, Schultz G, Gibian H, Hecker W. Stoffwechsel von 6α-fluoro-16α-methylpregna-1,4-dien-11, 21-diol-3, 21-dion (fluocortolon) beim Menschen. Acta Endocrinol 1971; 68:98–126.

122. Kripalani KJ, Zern El-Abdin A, Dean AV, Cohen AI. Biotransformation of halcinonide in the dog. Pharmacology 1977; 19:168A.

123. Florini JR, Smith LI, Buyske DA. Metabolic fate of a synthetic corticosteroid (triamcinolone) in the dog. J Biol Chem 1961; 236:1038–1042.

124. Kripalani KJ, Cohen AI, Weliky I, Schreiber EC. Metabolism of triamcinolone acetonide 21-phosphate in dogs, monkeys, and rats. J Pharm Sci 1975; 64:1351–1359.
125. Gordon S, Morrison J. The metabolic fate of trimcinolone acetonide in laboratory animals. Steroids 1978; 32:2272–2284.
126. Tan K, Kumakura M, Kobari T, Watanabe S, Kobayashi H, Namekawa H. Pharmacometrics (Sendai) 1976; 12:351–362.
127. Teitelbaum PJ, Chu NI, Cho D, et al. Mechanism for the oxidative defluorination of flunisolide. J Pharmacol Exp Ther 1981; 218:16–22.
128. Tökes L, Cho D, Maddox ML, Chaplin MC, Chu NI. Isolation and identification of an oxidatively defluorinated metabolite of flunisolide in man. Drug Metab Dispos 1981; 9:485–486.
129. Edsbäcker S, Jönsson, Lindberg C, Ryrfelt Å, Thalén A. Metabolic pathways of the topical glucocorticoid budesonide in man. Drug Metab Dispos 1983; 11:590–596.
130. Daniel MJ, Ayres DW, MacLean AV, Shenoy EV, Ayrton J. Pharmacokinetics and metabolism of fluticasone propionate in rat, dog and man. Abstract at European Academy of Allergology, Clinical Immunology, Glasgow, 1990.
131. Lan SJ, Scanlan LM, Weinstein SH, et al. Biotransformation of tipredane, a novel topical steroid, in mouse, rat, and human liver homogenates. Drug Metab Dispos 1989; 17:532–541.
132. Lambe R, Hudson S, O'Kelly D, Darragh A. The metabolism of fluocortolone in the ram. Ir J Med Sci 1978; 147:393–403.
133. Edsbäcker S, Andersson P, Lindberg C, Ryrfelt Å, Thalén A. Liver metabolism of budesonide in rat, mouse, and man. Drug Metab Dispos 1987; 15:403–411.
133a. Lee HJ. Acidic metabolite of prednisolone. Experentia 1977; 33:253–254.
133b. Oishi T, Deguchi T, Marumo H. Metabolic fate of beclomethasone 17,21-dipropionate. Oyo Yakori 1981; 22:717–727.
133c. Skrabalak DS, Maylin GA. Dexamethasone metabolism in the horse. Steroids 1982; 39:233–244.
133d. Rafestin-Oblin ME, Michaud A, Claire M, Nakane H, Corvol P. Tritiated 9α-fluorocortisol metabolism and binding in rat kidney. Steroids 1977; 30:605–619.
133e. English J, Chakraborty J, Marks V. The metabolism of dexamethasone in the rat: effect of phenytoin. J Steroid Biochem 1975; 6:65–68.
133f. Esumi Y, Ohtsuki T, Alsumi K, Katami Y, Kato T, Yokoshima T, Takahara Y. Studies on the metabolic fate of dexamethasone-17-valerate. III. Metabolites in rat. Iyakuhin Kenkyu 1982; 13:1037–1045; Chem Abstr 98:47157 v.
133g. Mützel W. Pharmakokinetik und Biotransformation von Fluocortinbulytester beim Menschen. Arzneim-Forsch/Drug Res 1977; 27:2230–2233.
133h. Täuber U, Toda T. Biotransformation von Diflucortolonvaleriat in der Haut von Ratte, Meerschweinchen und Mensch. Arzneim Forsch/Drug Res 1976; 26:1484–1498.
133i. Andersson P, Ryrfeldt Å. Biotransformation of the topical clucocorticoids budesonide and beclomethasone 17α, 21-dipropionate in human liver and lung homogenate. J Pharmacol 1984; 36:763–765.
133k. Ronca-Testoni S, Rotondara L. Absorption and metabolism of cyclomethasone. Drugs Exp Clin Res 1983; 9:73–76.

133l. Ronca-Testoni S. Hydrolysis of cyclomethasone by the human lung. Int J Clin Parm Res 1983; 3:17–20.

133m. Nakano M, Nishiuchi M, Takeuchi M, Yamada H. Correlation between metabolism of betamethasone 17,21-dipropionate and adrenal hypertrophy in rat fetuses. Steroids 1981; 37:511–525.

133n. Miyabo S, Hisada T, Kishida S, Asato T. Metabolism of synthetic corticosteroid esters in man. Folia Endocrinol Jpn 1976; 52:997–1007.

133o. Myers C, Lockridge O, LaDu BN. Hydrolysis of methylprednisolone acetate by human serum cholinesterase. Drug Metab Dispos 1982; 10:279–280.

134. Abramovitz M, Branchaud CL, Murphy BEP. Cortisol-cortisone interconversion in human fetal lung: contrasting results using explant and monolayer cultures suggest that 11β-hydroxysteroid dehydrogenase (EC 1.1.1.146) comprises two enzymes. J Clin Endocrinol Metab 1982; 54:563–568.

135. Jenkins JS, Sampson PA. Conversion of cortisone to cortisol and prednisone to prednisolone. Br Med J 1967; 2:205–207.

136. Powell LW, Axelsen E. Corticosteroids in liver disease: Studies on the biological conversion of prednisolone and plasma protein binding. Gut 1972; 13:690–696.

137. Glenn EM, Stafford RO, Lyster SC, Fowman BJ. Relation between biological activity of hydrocortisone analogues and their rates of inactivation by rat liver enzyme systems. Endocrinology 1957; 61:128–142.

138. Able SM. Cortisol metabolism by human liver in vitro. IV. metabolism of 9α fluorocortisol by human liver microzones and cytosol. J Steroid Biochem Mol Biol 1993; 46:833–839.

139. Fotherby L, James F. Metabolism of synthetic glucocorticoids. In: Briggs MH, Christie GA, eds. Advances in Steroid Biochemistry and Pharmacology. Vol. 3. New York: Academic Press, 1972:67–165.

140. Junge W. Human microsomal carboxylesterase (EC 3.1.1.1). Enzymes in Health and Disease. Inaugural Scientific Meeting of the International Society Clinical Enzymology, London, 1977:37–58.

141. Williams FM. Clinical significance of esterases in man. Clin Pharmacokinet 1985; 10:392–403.

142. Araki Y, Yokota O, Kato T, Kashima M, Miyazaki T. Dynamics of synthetic corticosteroids in man. In: Pincus G, Nakao T, Tait JF, eds. Steroid Dynamics. New York: Academic Press, 1966:462–480.

143. Rice MJ, Tredger JM, Chakraborty J, Parke D.V. The metabolism of dexamethasone in the rat. Biochem Soc Trans 1974; 2:107–109.

144. Tredger JM, Chakraborty J, Parke DV. A comparative study of the excretion of corticosterone and betamethasone in the rat. Biochem Soc Trans 1973; 1:998–999.

145. Chu NI, Amos BA, Tökés L, et al. Disposition of flunisolide in the rat, mouse, dog, rhesus monkey and cynomolgus monkey. Drug Metab Dispos 1979; 7:81–89.

146. Miyabo S, Hisada T, Kishida S, Asato T. Metabolism of synthetic corticosteroid esters in man. Folia Endocrinol Jpn 1976; 52:997–1007.

147. Rodchenkov GM, Uralets VP, Semenov VA, Leclerq PA. Analysis for dexamethasone, triamcinolone, and their metabolites in human urine by microcolumn liquid and capillary gas chromatography mass spectrometry. J High Resolut Chromatogr Commun 1988; 11:283–288.

434 *Edsbäcker and Szefler*

148. Rodchenkov GM, Uralets VP, Semenov VA. Gas chromatographic and mass spectral study of betamethasone synthetic corticosteroid metabolism. J Chromatogr 1988; 432:283–289.
149. Edsbäcker S, Andersson P, Lindberg C, Ryrfelt Å, Thalén A. Metabolic acetal splitting of budesonide. A novel inactivation pathway for topical glucocorticoids. J Pharmacol Exp Ther 1987; 15:412–417.
150. Santos-Mondes A, Gonzalo-Lumbreras R, Gasco-Lopez AI, Izquierdo-Hornillos R. Extraction and HPLC of deflazacort and its metabolite 21-hydroxydeflazacort. J Chromatogr Biomed Appl 657. 1984;248–253.
151. Derendorf H, Rohdewald P, Hochhaus G, Möllman H. HPLC determination of glucocorticoid alcohols, their phosphates and hydrocortisone in aqueous solutions and biological fluids. J Pharmacol Biomed Anal 1986; 4:197–206.
152. Haack D, Vecsei P, Lichtwald K, Klee HR, Gless KH, Weber M. Some experiences on radioimmunoassays of synthetic glucocorticoids. Allergologie 1980; 3:259–267.
153. Midgley JM, Watson DG, Healy T. The quantification of synthetic corticosteroids using isotope dilution gas chromatography negative chemical ionization mass spectrometry. Biomed Environ Mass Spectrom 1988; 15:479–483.
154. Lindberg C, Paulson J, Blomqvist A. Evaluation of an automated thermospray liquid chromatography–mass spectrometry system for quantitative use in bioanalytical chemistry. J Chromatogr 1991; 554:215–226.
155. Girault J, Istin B, Malgouyat JM. Simultaneous determination of beclomethasone, beclomethasone monopropionate and beclomethasone dipropionate in biological fluids using a particle beam interface for combining liquid chromatography with negative ion chemical ionization mass spectrometry. J Chromatogr 1991; 564:43–53.
156. Jenner WN, Kirkham DJ. Immunoassay of beclomethasone 17, 21-dipropionate and metabolites. In: Reid E, Robinson JD, Wilson ID, eds. Bioanalysis of Drugs and Metabolites. New York: Plenum Press, 1988; 77–86.
157. Nerenberg C, Martin SB. Radioimmunoassay of flunisolide in human plasma. J Pharm Sci 1981; 70:900–904.
158. Zaborny BA, Lukacsko P, Barinov-Colligon I, Ziemniak JA. Inhaled corticosteroids in asthma: a dose-proportionality study with triamcinolone acetonide aerosol. J Clin Pharmacol 1992; 32:463–469.
159. Bain BM, Harrison G, Jenkins KD, Pateman AJ, Shenoy EV. A sensitive radioimmunoassay, incorporating solid-phase extraction, for fluticasone 17-propionate in plasma. J Pharm Biomed Anal 1993; 11:557–561.
160. Hench PS, Kendall EC, Slocumb CH, Polley HF. The effect of a hormone of the adrenal cortex (17-hydroxy-11-dehydrocorticosterone: compound E) and of pituitary adrenocorticotropic hormone on rheumatoid arthritis: preliminary report. Staff Meet Mayo Clinic, 1949; 24:181–197.
161. Frey BM, Frey FJ. Clinical pharmacokinetics of prednisone and prednisolone. Clin Pharmacokinet 1990; 19:126–146.
162. Barth J, Damoiseaux M, Möllman H, Bradis K.-H, Hochhaus G, Derendorf H. Pharmacokinetics and pharmacodynamics of prednisolone after intravenous and oral administration. Int J Clin Pharmacol Ther Toxicol 1992; 30:317–324.

163. Legler UF, Benet LZ. Marked alterations in dose-dependent prednisolone kinetics in women taking oral contraceptives. Clin Pharmacol Ther 1986; 39(4):425–429.
164. Loo JCK, McGilveray IJ, Jordan N, Brien R. Pharmacokinetic evaluation of betamethasone and its water soluble phosphate ester in humans. Biopharm Drug Dispos 1981; 2:265–272.
165. Inimbo B, Tuzi T, Porzio F, Schiavetti L. Clinical equivalence of a new glucocorticoid, deflazacort and prednisone, in rheumatoid arthritis and systemic lupus erythematosus (SLE) patients. Adv Exp Med Biol 1984; 171:241–256.
166. Richards IM, Shields SK, Griffin RL, Fidler SF, Dunn CJ. Novel steroid-based inhibitors of lung inflammation. Clin Exp Allergy 1992; 22:432–439.
167. Blauert-Cousounis SP, Ziemniak JA, McMahon SC, Grebow PE. The pharmacokinetics of triamcinolone acetonide after intranasal, oral inhalation and intramuscular administration. J Allergy Clin Immunol 1989; 83:221A.
168. Riedel DJ, Harrison LI, Machacek JH, Chang SF, Cline AC, Kanniainen CM. Pharmacokinetics of beclomethasone (B) from beclomethasone dipropionate in an HFA-134a (A) CFC-free propellant system. J Aerosol Med 1995; 8:97.
169. Kaiser HH, Edsbäcker S. The Pulmicort Turbuhaler Study Group. Dose-proportional pharmacokinetics (PK) of inhaled budesonide (Pulmicort Turbuhaler) in patients with mild asthma. Am J Respir Crit Care Med 1994; 149(Suppl 4 pt 2):A467.
170. Pedersen S, Steffensen G, Ohlsson SV. The influence of orally deposited budesonide on the systemic availability of budesonide after inhalation from a Tubuhaler. Br J Clin Pharmacol 1993; 36:211–214.
171. Martin PD, Gebbie T, Salmond CE. A controlled trial of beclomethasone dipropionate by aerosol in chronic asthmatics. NZ Med J 1974; 79:773–776.
172. Martin LE, Tanner RJ, Harrison C. Metabolism of beclomethasone dipropionate by animals and man. Postgrad Med J 1975; 51(suppl 4):11–20.
173. Martin LE, Tanner RJN, Clark TJH, Cochrane GM. Absorption and metabolism of orally administered beclomethasone dipropionate. Clin Pharm Ther 1973; 15:267–265.
174. Johansson SA, Andersson KE, Brattsand R, Gruvstad E, Hedner P. Topical and systemic glucocorticoid potencies of budesonide and beclomethasone dipropionate in man. Eur J Clin Pharmacol 1982; 22:523–529.
175. Pörtner M, Möllman H, Barth J, Rohdewald p. Pharmacokinetics of triamcinolone following oral application. Arzneim-Forsch/Drug Res 1988; 38(II):12:1838–1840.
176. Hochhaus G, Pörtner M, Möllman H, Rohdewald P. Oral bioavailability of triamcinolone tablets and a triamcinolone diacetate suspension. Pharm Res 1990; 7:558–560.
177. Ryrfelt Å, Edsbäcker S, Pauwels R. Kinetics of the epimeric glucocorticoid budesonide. Clin Pharmacol Ther 1984; 35:525–530.
177a. Ryrfeldt Å, Persson G, Nilsson E. Pulmonary disposition of the potent glucocorticoid budesonide evaluated in an isolated perfused rat lung model. Biochem Pharmacol 1989; 38:17–22.
178. Thorsson L, Källén A, Wirén J-E, Paulson J. Pharmacokinetics and effect of

inhaled fluticasone propionate. Abstract presented at the American Thoracic Society, New Orleans, 1996.

178a. Mackie AE, Vewntresca P, Moss JA, Bye A. Pharmacokinetics of intravenous fluticasone propionate in healthy subjects. Br J Clin Pharmacol 1995; 40:198 P.

179. Ventresca GP, Mackie AE, Moss JA, McDowall JE, Bye A. Absorption of oral fluticasone propionate in healthy subjects. Am J Respir Crit Care Med 1994; 149(Suppl 4 pt 2):A 209.

180. Price Evans D. Genetic factors in drug therapy. In: Clinical and Molecular Pharmacogenetics. Cambridge, UK: Cambridge University Press, 1993;102–112.

181. Schriefers H. Factors regulating the metabolism of steroids. Vitam Horm 1967; 25:271–314.

182. Kupfer D, Partridge R. 6β-Hydroxylation of triamcinolone acetonide by a hepatic enzyme system. The effect of phenobarbital and 1-benzyl-2-thio-5,6-dihydrouracil. Arch Biochem Biophys 1970; 140:23–28.

183. Buffington GA, Dominquez JA, Piering WF, Herbert LA, Kauffman M, Lemann J. Interaction of rifampin and glucocorticoids. Adverse effect on renal allograft function. JAMA 1976; 236:1958–1960.

184. Jubiz W, Meikle AW, Levinson RA, Mizutani S, West CD, Tyler FH. Effect of diphenylhydantoin on the metabolism of dexamethasone N Engl J Med 1970; 283:11–14.

185. Kawai S, Ichikawa Y, Hommo M. Differences in metabolism properties among cortisol, prednisolone, and dexamethasone in liver and renal diseases. Accelerated metabolism of dexamethasone in renal failure. J Clin Metab 1985; 60:848–854.

186. Hancock KW, Level MJ. Primidone/dexamethasone interaction. Lancet 1978; 2:97–98.

187. Brooks SM, Werk EE, Ackerman SJ, Sullivan I, Thrasher K. Adverse effects of phenobarbital on corticosteroid metabolism in patients with bronchial asthma. N Engl J Med 1972; 286:1125–1128.

188. Brooks PM, Buchanan WW, Grove M, Downie WW. Effects of enzyme induction on metabolism of prenisolone. Ann Rheum Dis 1976; 35:339–343.

189. Brooks SM, Sholiton LJ, Werk EE Jr, Altenau P. The effects of ephedrine and theophylline on dexamethasone metabolism in bronchial asthma. J Clin Pharmacol 1977; 17:308–318.

190. Conney AH, Levin W, Jacobson M, Kuntzman R. Effects of drug and environmental chemicals on steroid metabolism. Clin Pharmacol Ther 1973; 14:727–741.

191. Kuntzman R, Jacobson M, Conney AH. Effect of phenylbutazone on cortisol metabolism in man. Pharmacologist 1966; 8:195A.

192. Al-Hadramy M, Zawawi T. Rifampicin-dexamethasone interaction. J Irish Coll Physic Surg 1994; 23:111–113.

193. Schuetz EG, Wrighton SA, Barwick JL, Guzelian PS. Induction of cytochrome P-450 by glucocorticoids in rat liver. I. Evidence that glucocorticoids and pregnenolone 16α-carbonitrile regulate *de novo* synthesis of a common form of cytochrome P-450 in cultures of adult rat hepatocytes and in the liver *in vivo*. J Biol Chem 1984; 259:1999–2006.

194. Lee KG, Shin JG, Chong WS, Lee JS, Jang IJ, Shin SG. Time course of the

changes in prednisolone pharmacokinetics after co-administration or discontinuation of rifampin. Eur J Clin Pharmacol 1993; 45:287-289.

195. Kozower M, Veatch I, Kaplan MM. Decreased clearance of prednisolone, a factor in the development of corticosteroid side effects. J Clin Endocrinol Metab 1974; 38:407-412.

196. Meffin PJ, Wing LMH, Sallustio BC, Brooks PM. Alterations in prednisolone disposition as a result of oral contraceptive use and dose. Br J Clin Pharmacol 1984; 17:655-664.

197. LaForce CF, Szefler SJ, Miller MF, Ebling W, Brenner M. Inhibition of methylprednisolone elimination in the presence of erythromycin therapy. J Allergy Clin Immunol 1983; 72:34-39.

198. Szefler SJ, Brenner M, Jusko WJ, Spector SL, Flesher K, Ellis EF. Dose and time-related effect of troleandomycin on methylprednisolone elimination. Clin Pharmacol Ther 1982; 32:166-171.

199. Pessayre D, Descatoire V, Konstantinova-Mitcheva M, et al. Self-induction by triacetyloleandomycin of its own transformation into a metabolite forming a stable 456 nm-absorbing complex with cytochrome P-450. Biochem Pharmacol 1981; 30:553-558.

200. Delaforge M, Jaquen M, Mansuy D. Dual effects of macrolide antibiotics on rat liver cytochrome P-450. Induction and formation of metabolite-complexes: a structure-activity relationship. Bioch Pharmacol 1983; 32:2309-2318.

201. Szefler SJ, Ellis EF, Brenner M, et al. Steroid-specific and anticonvulsant interaction aspects of troleandomycin-steroid therapy. J Allergy Clin Immunol 1982; 69:455-460.

202. Kamada AK, Hill MR, Iklé DN, Brenner AM, Szefler SJ. Efficacy and safety of low-dose troleandomycin therapy in children with severe steroid requiring asthma. J Allergy Clin Immunol 1993; 91:873-882.

203. Berlow BA, Liebhaber MI, Dyer Z, Spiegel TTM. The effect of dapsone in steroid-dependent asthma. J Allergy Clin Immunol 1991; 87:701-705.

204. Öst L. Effects of cyclosporine on prednisolone metabolism (letter). Lancet 1984; 1:451.

205. Langhoff E, Madsen S, Flachs H, Olgaard K, Ladefoged J, Hvidberg EF. Inhibition of prednisolone metabolism by cyclosporine in kidney-transplanted patients. Transplantation 1985; 39:107-109.

206. Kandrotas RJ, Slaughter RL, Brass C, Jusko WJ. Ketoconazole effects on methylprednisolone disposition and their joint suppression of endogenous cortisol. Clin Pharmacol Ther 1987; 42:465-470.

207. Loose DS, Stoner DP, Feldman D. Ketoconazole binds to glucocorticoid receptors and exhibits glucocorticoid antagonist effect activity in cultured cells. J Clin Invest 1983; 72:404-408.

208. Yamashita SK, Ludwig EA, Middleton E, Jusko WJ. Lack of pharmacokinetic and pharmacodynamic interactions between ketoconazole and prednisolone. Clin Pharmacol Ther 1991; 49:558-570.

209. Zurcher RM, Frey BM, Frey FJ. Impact of ketoconazole on the metabolism of prednisolone. Clin Pharmacol Ther 1989; 45:366-372.

210. Sirgo MA, Rocci ML, Ferguson RK, Eshleman FN, Vlasses PH. Effects of cimetidine and ranitidine on the conversion of prednisone to prednisolone. Clin Pharmacol Ther 1985; 37:534–538.
211. Schleimer RP, Kato M. Regulation of lung inflammation by local glucocorticoid metabolism; an hypothesis. J Asthma 1992; 29:303–317.
212. Schleimer RP. Potential regulation of inflammation in the lung by local metabolism by hydrocortisone. Am J Respir Cell Mol Biol 1991; 4:166–173.
213. Withworth JA, Stewart PM, Atherden SM, Burt D, Edwards CRW. The kidney is the major site of cortisone production in man. Clin Endocrinol 1989; 31:355–361.
214. Stewart PM, Edwards CW. The cortisol-cortisone shuttle and hypertension. J Steroid Biochem Molec Biol 1991; 40:501–509.
215. Wong DD, Longenecker RG, Liepman M, Baker S, Lavergne M. Phenytoin-dexamethasone: A possible drug-drug interaction. JAMA 1985; 254:2062–2063.
216. Lackner TE. Interaction of dexamethasone with phenytoin. Pharmacotherapy 1991; 11:344–347.
217. Lawson I, Blouin R, Smith et al. Phenytoin-dexamethasone interaction. A previously unreported observation. Surg Neurol 1981; 16:23–24.
218. Edwards, RJ, Freeling AB, Watson D, Davies FS. The effect of budesonide and triamcinolone acetonide on hepatic microsomal testosterone metabolism in the rat. Biochem Pharmacol 1992; 43:271–282.
219. Green CG, Kraus CK, Lemanske RF, Farrell PM, Jusko WJ. Rapid methylprednisolone clearance in a patient with cystic fibrosis. Drug Intell Clin Pharm 1988; 22:876–878.
220. Papen CV, Benker G, Hackenberg K, Reinwein D. Pharmakokinetic von Prednisolon bei Neberennierreninsuffizienz. Klin Wochenschr 1982; 60:681–686.
221. Gatti G, Perucca E, Frigo GM, Notarangelo LD, Barberis L, Martini A. Pharmacokinetics of prednisone and its metabolite prednisolone in children with nephrotic syndrome during the active phase and in remission. Br J Clin Pharmacol 1984; 17:423–431.
222. Bergrem H, Jervell J, Flatmark A. Prednisolone pharmacokinetics in cushingoid an non-cushingoid kidney transplant patients. Kidney Int 1985; 27:459–464.
223. Beisel WR, Col LT, Di Raimondo VC, Forshamn PH. Cortisol transport and disappearance. Ann Intern Med 1964; 60:641–652.
224. Jubiz W, Meikle AW. Alterations of glucocorticoid actions by other drugs and disease states. Drugs 1979; 18:113–121.
225. Frey FJ, Horber FF, Frey BM. Altered metabolism and decreased efficacy of prednisolone and prednisone in patients with hyperthyroidism. Clin Pharmacol Ther 1988; 44:510–521.
226. Lavins B, Vaughan R, Szefler S, Weber R, Nelson H. Effect of thyroid disease on metabolism of theophylline and methylprednisolone. Ann Allergy 1988; 60:184A.
227. Brown H, Williardson DG, Samuels LT, Tyler FH. 17-Hydroxycorticosteroid metabolism in liver disease. J Clin Invest 1954; 33:1524–1532.
228. Peterson RE. Adrenocorticoid steroid metabolism and adrenal cortical function in liver disease. J Clin Invest 1960; 39:320–331.

229. Zumoff B, Bradlow L, Gallagher TF, Hellman L. Cortisol metabolism in cirrhosis. J Clin Invest 1967; 46:1735–1743.

230. Davies M, Williams R, Chakraborty J, et al. Prednisone or prednisolone for the treatment of chronic active liver disease. Gastroenterology 1977; 72:1143A.

231. Uribe M, Go VLW. Research review. Corticosteroid pharmacokinetics in liver disease. Clin Pharmacokinet 1978; 4:233–240.

232. Miyachi Y, Yorsumoto H, Kano T, Mizuchi A, Muto T, Yanagibashi K. Blood levels of synthetic glucocorticoids after administration by various routes. Endocrinology 1979; 82:149–157.

233. Renner E, Horber FF, Jost G, Frey B, Frey FJ. Effect of liver function on the metabolism of prednisolone in humans. Gastroenterology 1986; 90:819–828.

234. Uribe M, Summerskill WHJ, Go VLW. Why hyperbilirubinemia and hypoalbuminemia predispose to steroid side effects during treatment of chronic active liver disease. Gastroenterology 1977; 72:1143A.

235. Blaschket TF. Protein binding and kinetics of drugs in liver diseases. Clin Pharmacokinet 1977; 2:32–44.

236. Ludwig EA, Kong AN, Camara DS, Jusko WJ. Pharmacokinetics of methylprednisolone hemisuccinate and methylprednisolone in chronic liver disease. J Clin Pharmacol 1993; 33:805–810.

237. Hunt CM, Westerkam WR, Stave GM. Effect of age and gender on the activity of human hepatic CYP3A. Biochem Pharmacol 1992; 44:275–283.

238. Lew KH, Ludwig EA, Milad MA, et al. Gender-based effects on methylprednisolone pharmacokinetics and pharmacodynamics. Clin Pharmacol Ther 1993; 54:402–414.

239. Stuck AE, Frey BM, Frey FJ. Kinetics of prednisolone and endogenous cortisol concentrations in the elderly. Clin Pharmacol Ther 1988; 43:354–361.

240. Richter O, Ern B, Reinhardt D, Becker B. Pharmacokinetics of dexamethasone in children. Pediatr Pharmacol 1983; 3:329–337.

241. Tornatore KM, Reed KA, Venuto RC. Racial differences in the pharmacokinetics of methylprednisolone in black and white renal transplant recipients. Pharmacotherapy 1993; 13:481–4863

242. Eichelbaum M. Defective oxidation of drugs. Pharmacokinetic and therapeutic implications. Clin Pharmacokinet 1982; 7:1–22.

243. Gillette JR. Factors affecting drug metabolism. Ann NY Acad Sci 1971; 179:43–66.

244. Quigley ME, Yen SSC. A mid-day surge in cortisol levels. J Clin Endocrinol Metab 1979; 49:945–946.

245. Barbahaiya RH, Welling PG. Influence of food on the absorption of hydrocortisone from the gastrointestinal tract. Drug-Nutrient Interactions 1982; 1:103–112.

246. Tsuei SE, Petersen MC, Ashley JJ, McBride WG, Moore RG. Disposition of synthetic glucocorticoids. II. Dexamethasone in parturient women. Clin Pharmacol Ther 1980; 28:88–98.

247. Milsap RL, Plaisance KI, Jusko WJ. Prednisolone disposition in obese men. Clin Pharmacol Ther 1984; 36:824–831.

248. Dunn TE, Ludwig EA, Slaughter RL, Camara DS, Jusko WJ. Pharmacokinetics

and pharmacodynamics of methyprednisolone in obese and non-obese men. Clin Pharmacol Ther 1991; 49:536–549.
249. Kershbaum A, Pappajohn DJ, Bellet S, Hirabyashi M, Shafiiha H. Effect of smoking and nicotine on adrenocortical secretion. JAMA 1968; 203:275–278.
250. Radzialowski FM, Bousquet WF. Circadian rhythm in hepatic drug metabolism activity in the rat. Life Sci 1967; 6:2545–2548.
251. Jori A, Di Salle E, Santini V. Daily rhythmic variation and liver drug metabolism in rats. Biochem Pharmacol 1971; 20:2965–2969.
252. English J, Dunne M, Marks V. Diurnal variation in prednisolone kinetics. Clin Pharmacol Ther 1983; 33:381–385.
253. DeLacerda L, Kowarski A, Migeon CJ. Diurnal variations of the metabolic clearance rate of cortisol. Effect on measurement of cortisol production rate. J Clin Endocrinol Metab 1973; 36:1043–1049.
254. Ganong WF. Circulation through special regions. In: Review of Medical Physiology. 10th ed. Los Altos, CA: Lange, 1981:476.
255. Barnes PJ, Pedersen S. Efficacy and safety of inhaled corticosteroids in asthma. Am Rev Respir Dis 1993; 148:S1–S26.
256. Grabstein K, Dower S, Gillis S, Urdal V, Larsen A. Expression of interleukin-2, interferon-γ, and the IL-2 receptor by human peripheral blood lymphocytes. J Immunol 1986; 136:4503–4508.
257. Shaw G, Kamen R. A conserved AU sequence from the 3' untranslated region of GM-CSF on RNA mediates selective mRNA degradation. Cell 1986; 46:659–667.
258. Borson DB, Jew S, Gruenert DC. Glucocorticoids induce neutral endopeptidase in transformed human trachea epithelial cells. Am J Physiol 1991; 260:L83–L89.
259. DiRosa, Radomski M, Carnuccio R, Moncada S. Glucocorticoids inhibit the induction of nitric oxide synthase in macrophages. Biochem Biophys Res Commun 1990; 172:1246–1252.
260. Baxter JD, Rousseau GG. Glucocorticoid hormone action: An overview. In: Baxter JD, Rousseau DG, eds. Glucocorticoid Hormone Action. Berlin: Springer-Verlag, 1979:1–24.
261. Reed CE. Glucocorticoids in asthma. Immunol Allergy Clin North Am 1993; 13:903–915.
262. Dahlbertg E, Thalén A, Brattsand R, et al. Correlation between chemical structure, receptor binding, and biological activity of some novel, highly active, 16α, 17α-acetal substituted glucocorticoids. Mol Pharmacol 1984; 25:70–78.
263. Lutsky BN, Millonig RC, Wojnar RJ, et al. Androstene-17-thioketals. 2nd Communication: Pharmacological profiles of tipredane and (11 beta,17 alpha)-17-(ethylthio)-9 alpha-fluoro-17-(2-fluoroethyl)thio)-11 beta-hydroxyl-androsta-1,4-dien-3-one, structurally novel 20-thiasteroids possessing potent and selective topical antiinflammatory activity. Arzneimittelforschung 1986; 36(12):1787–1795.
264. Jusko WJ. Corticosteroid pharmacodynamics: models for a broad array of receptor-mediated pharmacologic effects. J Clin Pharmacol 1990; 30:303–310.
265. Barth J, Möllman HW, Schmidt EW, Rohdewald P, Rehder J. Measurement of synthetic glucocorticosteroids in the lung after intravenous administration. Nachweis intravenös applizierter synthetischer Glukokortikoide. In: der Lunge. Atemwegs-Lungenkrankh 1984; 10:410–413.

266. Barth J, Möllman HW, Rohdewald P, Marek W, Schmidt EW, Kowalski J. Onset of glucocorticoid action after intravenous injection in acute airway obstruction. Bull Eur Physiopathol Respir 1986; 22(Suppl 8):46.

267. Ellul-Micallef R. The acute effects of corticosteroids in bronchial asthma. Eur J Respir Dis 1982; 63(Suppl 122):118–125.

268. Engel T, Dirksen A, Heinig JH, Nielson NH, Weeke B, Johansson SÖ. Single dose inhaled budesonide in subjects with chronic asthma. Allergy 1991; 46:547–553.

269. LaForce C, Chervinsky P, Selner J, et al. Onset of action of inhaled corticosteroids in asthma. J Allergy Clin Immunol 1993; 91:223A.

270. Haahtela T, Järvinen M, Kavat T, et al. Comparison of a beta$_2$-agonist, terbutaline, with an inhaled corticosteroid, budesonide, in newly detected asthma. N Engl J Med 1991; 325:388–392.

271. Storr J, Barry W, Barrell E, Lenney W, Hatcher G. Effect of a single oral dose of prednisolone in acute childhood asthma. Lancet 1987; 1:879–882.

272. Klaustermeyer WB, Hale FC. The physiologic effect of an intravenous glucocorticoid in bronchial asthma. Ann Allergy 1976; 37:80–86.

273. Dahl R. Glucocorticoids and immediate and late allergic reaction. In: Hogg JC, Ellul-Micallef R, Brattsand R, eds. Glucocorticosteroids, Inflammation, and Bronchial Hyperactivity. Amsterdam: Excerpta Medica, 1985:86–90.

274. Dahl R, Johansson S-Å. Importance of duration of treatment with inhaled budesonide on the immediate and late bronchial reaction. Eur J Respir Dis 1982; 63(Suppl 122):167–175.

275. Jennings BH, Andersson KE, Johansson SÅ. Assessment of systemic effects of inhaled glucocorticosteroids. Comparison of the effects of inhaled budesonide and oral prednisolone on adrenal function and markers of bone turnover. Eur J Clin Pharmacol 1991; 40:77–82.

276. Grahnén A, Eckernäs SÅ, Brundin RM, Ling-Andersson A. An assessment of the systemic activity of single doses of inhaled fluticasone propionate in healthy volunteers. Br J Clin Pharmacol 1994; 38:521–525.

277. Aaronson D, Kaiser H, Dockhorn R, Findlay S, Korenblat P. Pharmacodynamic effects of inhaled budesonide (Pulmicort Turbuhaler) on HPA-axis in patients with mild asthma. J Allergy Clin Immunol 1994; 93(suppl 1, pt 2):259.

278. Feiss G, Morris R, Rom D, et al. A comparative study of the effects of intranasal triamcinolone acetonide aerosol (TAA) and prednisone on adrenocortical function. J Allergy Clin Immunol 1992; 89:1151–1156.

279. Wolthers OD, Pedersen S. Short term growth treatment with inhaled fluticasone propionate and beclomethasone dipropionate. Arch Dis Child 1993; 68:673–676.

280. Wolthers OD, Pedersen S. Growth of asthmatic children during treatment with budesonide: a double blind trial. Br Med J 1991; 303:163–165.

281. Engel T, Heinig JH. Glucocorticosteroid therapy in acute severe asthma—a critical review. Eur Respir J 1991; 4:881–889.

282. Busse W. Dose-related efficacy of Pulmicort® (budesonide) Tubuhaler® in moderate to severe asthma. J Allergy Clin Immunol 1994; 93:186A.

283. Dahl R, Lundbäck B, Malo JM, et al. A dose-ranging study of fluticasone propionate in adult patients with moderate asthma. Chest 1993; 104:1352–1358.

283a. Boe J, Rosenhall L, Alton M, et al. Comparison of dose-response effects of inhaled beclomethasone dipropionate and budesonide in the management of asthma. Allergy 1989; 44:349–355.

284. Toogood JH, Baskerville JC, Jennings B, Lefcoe NM, Johansson SÅ. Bioequivalent doses of budesonide and prednisone in moderate and severe asthma. J Allergy Clin Immunol 1989; 84:668–700.

285. Toogood JH, Lefcoe NM, Haines DS, et al. A graded dose assessment of the efficacy of beclomethasone dipropionate aerosol for severe chronic asthma. J Allergy Clin Immunol 1977; 59:298–308.

286. Ellul-Micallef R, Johansson SÅ. Acute dose-response studies in bronchial asthma with a new corticosteroid, budesonide. Br J Clin Pharmacol 1983; 15:419–422.

287. McCubbin MM, Milavetz G, Grandegeorge S, et al. A bioassay for topical and systemic effect of three inhaled corticosteroids. Clin Pharmacol Ther 1995; 57:455–460.

288. Pedersen S, Ramsgaard-Hansen O. Budesonide treatment of moderate and severe asthma in children: a dose-response study. J Allergy Clin Immunol 1995; 95:29–33.

289. Fisher LE, Ludwig EA, Wald JA, Sloan RR, Middleton E, Jusko WJ. Pharmacokinetics and pharmacodynamics of methylprednisolone when administered at 8 AM vs 4 PM. Clin Pharmacol Ther 1992; 512:677–688.

290. Fisher LE, Ludwig EA, Jusko WJ. Pharmacoimmunodynamics of methylprednisolone: trafficking of helper T lymphocytes. J Pharmacokinet Biopharm 1992; 20(No 4):319–331.

291. Reinberg A, Helberg F, Falliers CJ. Circadian timing of methylprednisolone effects in asthmatic boys. Chronobiologia 1974; 1:333–347.

292. Lamiable D, Vistelle R, Fay R, Millart H, Caron J, Choisy H Chronopharmacokinetics of dexamethasone in young subjects. Therapie 1991; 46:405–407.

293. Nichols T, Nugent CA, Tyler FH. Diurnal variation in suppression of adrenal function by glucocorticoids. J Clin Endocrinol 1965; 25:343–349.

294. Andersson N, Dahl L. Effect of inhaled budesonide on the HPA axis with different dosing regimens. Abstract at the 5th International Conference of Chronopharmacology (Biological Rhythms and Medications), Amelia Island, FL, July 12–16, 1992.

295. Reinberg A, Smolensky MH, D'Alonzo GE, McGovern JP. Chronobiology and asthma. III. Timing corticotherapy to biological rhythms to optimize treatment goals. J Asthma 1988; 25:219–248.

296. Reiss WG, Slaughter RL, Ludwig EA, Middleton E Jr, Jusko WJ. Steroid dose sparing: pharmacodynamic responses to single versus divided doses of methyprednisolone in man. J Allergy Clin Immunol 1990; 85:1058–1066.

297. Reinberg A, Gervais P, Chaussade M, Fraboulet G, Durburque B. Circadian changes in effectiveness of corticosteroids in eight patients with allergic asthma. J Allergy Clin Immunol 1983; 71:425–433.

298. Toogood JH, Baskerville JC, Jennings B, Lefcoe NM, Johansson SÅ. Influence of dosing frequency and schedule on the response of chronic asthmatics to the aerosol steroid, budesonide. J Allergy Clin Immunol 1982; 70:288–298.

299. Malo JL, Cartier A, Merland N, et al. Four-times-a-day dosing frequency is better than a twice-a-day regimen in subjects requiring a high-dose inhaled steroid, budesonide, to control moderate to sever asthma. Am Rev Respir Dis 1989; 140:624–628.

300. Toogood JH, Jennings B, Baskerville J, Anderson J, Johansson SÅ. Dosing regimen of budesonide and occurrence of oropharyngeal complications. Eur J Respir Dis 1984; 65:35–44.

301. Jones AH, Langdon CG, Lee PS, et al. Pulmicort Turbuhaler once daily as initial prophylactic therapy for asthma. Respir Med 1994; 88:283–289.

302. Stiksa G, Glennow C. Once daily inhalation of budesonide in the treatment of chronic asthma: A clinical comparison. Ann Allergy 1985; 55:49–51.

303. Harter JG, Reddy WJ, Thorn GW. Studies on an intermittent corticosteroid dosage regimen. N Engl J Med 1963; 269:591–596.

304. Greenberger PA, Chow MJ, Atkinson AJ Jr, Ambre JJ, Patterson R. Comparison of prednisolone kinetics in patients receiving daily or alternate-day prednisone for asthma. Clin Pharmacol Ther 1986; 39:163–168.

305. Frey FJ, Rüegsegger MK, Frey BM. The dose-dependent systemic availability of prednisone: one reason for the reduced biological effect of alternate-day prednisone. Br J Clin Pharmacol 1986; 21:183–189.

306. Reinhart D, Bcker B, Nagel-Hiemke M, Schiffer R, Zehmisch T. Influence of beta-receptor-agonists and glucocorticoids on alpha- and beta-adrenoreceptors of isolated blood cells from asthmatic children. Pediatr Pharmacol 1983; 3:293–302.

307. Mak JCW, Adcock I, Barnes PJ. Dexamethasone increases β_2-receptor gene expression in human lung. Am Rev Respir Dis 1992; 145:834A.

308. Taylor DR, Wilkins GT, Herbison GP, Flannery EM. Interaction between corticosteroid and beta-agonist drugs: biochemical and cardiovascular effects in normal subjects. Chest 1992; 102:519–524.

309. Spätling L, Staisch KJ, Huch R, Huch A. Effect of ritordine and betamethasone on metabolism, respiration and circulation. Am J Perinatol 1986; 3:41–46.

310. Peters MJ, Adcock IM, Brown CR, Barnes PJ. β-agonist inhibition of steroid-receptor DNA binding activity in human lung. Am Rev Respir Dis 1993; 147:772A.

311. Arnaud A, Charpin J. Interaction between corticosteroids and beta$_2$-agonists in acute asthma. Eur J Respir Dis 1982; 63(Suppl 122):126–131.

312. Kerrebijn KF, van Essen-Zandvliet EEM, Neijens HJ. Effect of long-term treatment with glucocorticosteroids and beta-agonists on bronchial responsiveness in asthmatic children. In: Hogg JC, Ellul-Micallef R, Brattsand R, eds. Glucocorticosteroids, Inflammation and Bronchial Hyperreactivity. Amsterdam: Excerpta Medica; 1985:104–109.

313. Wong CS, Wahedna I, Pavord ID, Tattersfield AE. Effect of regular terbutaline and budesonide on bronchial reactivity to allergen challenge. Am J Respir Crit Care Med 1994; 150:1268–1273.

314. Wilding PJ, Clark MM, Oborne J, Thompson Coon JS, Bennett JA, Tattersfield AE. The effect of the addition of terbutaline therapy on the airway response to inhaled budesonide. Am J Respir Crit Care Med 1994; 149(Suppl 4, pt 2):209A.

315. Wang Y, Campbell HD, Young IG. Sex hormones and dexamethasone modulate interleukin-5 gene expression in T lymphocytes. J Ster Biochem Mol Biol 1993; 44:203–210.

316. Lindholm J, Schultz-Möler N. Plasma and urinary cortisol in pregnancy and during estrogen-gestagen treatment. Scand J Clin Lab Invest 1973; 31:119–122.

317. Pauwels R, Lamont H, Hidinger K, van der Straeten M. Influence of an extension tube on the bronchodilator efficacy of terbutaline derived from a metered dose inhaler. Respiration 1984; 45:61–66.

318. Baumann G. Estrogens and the hypothalamo-pituitary-adrenal axis in man: Evidence for normal feedback regulation by corticosteroids. J Clin Endocrinol Metab 1983; 57:1193–1197.

319. Semple P, Beastall GH, Watson WS, Hume R. Hypothalamic-pituitary dysfunction in respiratory hypoxia. Thorax 1981; 36:605–609.

320. Reid IR, Ibbertson HK, France JT, Pubys J. Plasma testostrone concentrations in asthmatic men treated with glucocorticoids. Br Med J 1985; 291:574.

321. Schaison G, Durand F, Mowszowicz I. Effect of glucocorticoids on plasma testosterone in men. Acta Endocrinol 1978; 89:126–131.

322. Ebling WF, Szefler SJ, Jusko WJ. Analysis of cortisol, methylprednisolone, and methylprednisolone sodium succinate: Absence of effects of troleandomycin on ester hydrolysis. J Chromatogr Biomed 1984; 305:271–280.

323. Sugita ET, Niebergall PJ. Prednisone. J Am Pharm Assoc 1975; 15:529–532.

324. Hill MR, Szefler SJ, Ball BD, Bartoszek M, Brenner M. Monitoring glucocorticoid therapy: A pharmacokinetic approach. Clin Pharmacol Ther 1990; 48:390–398.

325. Chrousos GP, Vingerhoeds A, Brandon D, et al. Primary cortisol resistance in man: A glucocorticoid receptor-mediated disease. J Clin Invest 1982; 69:1261–1269.

326. Carmichael J, Paterson IC, Diaz P, Crompton GK, Kay AB, Grant IWB. Corticosteroid resistance in chronic asthma. Brit Med J 1982; 282:1419–1422.

327. Kay AB, Diaz P, Carmichael J, Grant IWB. Corticosteroid-resistant chronic asthma and monocyte complement receptor. Clin Exp Immunol 1981; 44:576–580.

328. Poznansky MC, Gordon ACH, Douglas JG, Krajewski AS, Wylie AH, Grant IWB. Resistance to methylprednisolone in cultures of blood monoclear cells from glucocorticoid-resistant asthmatic patients. Clin Sci 1984; 67:639–645.

329. Sher ER, Leung DYM, Surs W, et al. Steroid resistant asthma: cellular mechanisms contributing to inadequate response to glucocorticoid therapy. J Clin Invest 1994; 93;33–39.

330. Kam J, Szefler SJ, Surs W, Sher ER, Leung DYM. Combination IL-2 and IL-4 reduces glucocorticoid receptor-binding affinity and T cell response to glucocorticoids. J Immunol 1993; 151:3460–3466.

331. Spahn JD, Leung DYM, Surs W, Harbeck RJ, Nimmagadda S, Szefler SJ. Reduced glucocorticoid binding affinity in asthma is related to ongoing allergic inflammation. Am J Respir Crit Care Med 1995; 151:1709–1714.

332. Spahn J, Leung DYM, Szefler SJ. Difficult to control asthma: new insights and

implications for management. In: Szefler SJ, Leung DYM, eds. Severe Asthma: Pathogenesis and Clinical Management. Lung Biology in Health and Diseases Series. New York: Marcel Dekker, 1995:497–535.

333. Oosterhuis B, Ten Berge JM, Peter T, Schellekens A, Koopman RP, van Boxtel CJ. Prednisolone concentration-effect relations in humans and the influence of plasma hydrocortisone. J Pharm Exp Ther 1986; 239:919–939.

334. Wald AJ, Salazar DE, Cheng H, Jusko WJ. Two-compartment basophil cell trafficking model for methylprednisolone pharmacodynamics. J Pharm Biopharm 1991; 19:521–537.

335. Derendorf H, Möllman H, Krieg M, et al. The pharmacodynamics of methylprednisolone phosphate after single intravenous administration to healthy volunteers. Pharm Res 1991; 8:263–268.

336. Lew KH, Jusko WJ. Pharmacodynamic modeling of cortisol suppression from flucortolone. Eur J Clin Pharmacol 1993; 45:581–583.

337. Boudinot FD, Ambrosio R, Jusko WJ. Receptor-mediated pharmacodynamics of prednisolone in the rat. J Pharmacokinet Biopharm 1986; 14:469–493.

338. Jusko WJ, Ludwig EA. Corticosteroids: In: Evans WE, Schentag JJ, Jusko WJ, eds. Applied Pharmacokinetics: Principles and Therapeutic Drug Monitoring. 3rd ed. Vancouver, WA: Applied Therapeutics, 1992; 27.1–27.34.

339. Hochhaus G, Derendorf H. Dose optimization based on pharmacokinetic-pharmacodynamic modelling. In: H. Derendorf, ed. Handbook of Pharmacokinetic/Pharmacodynamic Correlation. Boca Raton, FL: CRC Press, 1995:528.

17

Determinants of Dose and Response to Inhaled Therapeutic Agents in Asthma

GERALD C. SMALDONE

State University of New York at Stony Brook
Stony Brook, New York

I. Introduction

The treatment of asthma with aerosolized bronchodilators has provided the major stimulus to research for aerosolized drug delivery in clinical medicine. However, novel therapies for relatively uncommon diseases such as aerosolized pentamidine in acquired immunodeficiency syndrome (AIDS) and DNase in cystic fibrosis have provoked investigators to ask new questions regarding techniques of inhalational therapy. The purpose of this chapter is to outline the basic principles of the delivery of aerosols to the respiratory tract. In developing the topics summarized below, it will often be necessary to refer to drugs other than steroids, owing to the newness of this field and lack of specific data regarding steroid preparations for certain delivery systems.

Although topical therapy to the airway has long been recognized as a theoretically useful route for therapy of pulmonary disease, as well as a possible entrance way to the body for systemic therapy, modern therapeutic agents can be less forgiving than their bronchodilator counterparts. Bronchodilator therapy is essentially a "titration" in which the patient inhales increasing doses of an aerosolized agent and can assess the response within minutes by sensing a reduction in symptoms or with an objective measure of peak flow or FEV_1

(forced expiratory volume in 1 sec). This process can be carried out empirically until there is either a suitable therapeutic effect or the development of a
side effect that precludes further treatment (i.e., tremor or tachycardia). Newer
drugs, such as aerosolized steroids, do not exhibit an instantaneous therapeutic response. Moreover, the therapeutic response may not even be well defined
at the time of the clinical trial. Further, although possibly significant, "side
effects" may be subtle and difficult to detect. The importance of the balance
between the anti-inflammatory effects and significant and, to some extent,
poorly defined toxicities makes the measurement and control of the "dose" of
prime importance. The concept of the "dose versus response" relationship in
aerosol therapy is relatively new in clinical trials. Although our understanding
of aerosol physics is reasonable, the application of basic aerosol science to
therapeutic modalities in lung disease remains in its infancy. Further, there is
some lag between the acquisition of new knowledge and its incorporation into
the regulatory process as drugs become approved. The increased costs of newer,
sophisticated aerosolized agents, environmental forces, and the desire for ease
of drug delivery and increased patient compliance have led to a proliferation
of new devices which may or may not have an impact on the dose-response
relationship to a given drug.

   Although somewhat daunting, there is increasing recognition of these
issues among clinicians and scientists that has led to rapid advances in the
sophistication of aerosol studies over the last 5–10 years.

II. The Aerosol

An aerosol is a suspension of particles in a gas. It is important to consider the
gas as well as the aerosol particles when describing its properties (1), and, in
general, the deposition of particles within the lung can be thought of as the
result of an interaction between forces intrinsic to the aerosol itself versus the
specific effects of lung physiology and pathophysiology on those forces. In
predicting the behavior of an aerosol, physiologists lay heavy emphasis on the
aerodynamic behavior of the particles. For an aerosol that exhibits a log normal particle distribution, the aerodynamic behavior of the particles can be defined in terms of the mass median aerodynamic diameter (MMAD) and the
geometrical standard deviation σg (2).

A. Cascade Impaction, Breathing Pattern, and Particle Inertia

Although there are several ways to measure the aerodynamic behavior of a
given particle distribution, the common mode of analysis is cascade impaction.
This procedure serves as a useful example to describe the behavior of aerosols
in terms of particle size, as well as to point out the strength and weaknesses

of confining deposition predictions to simply the characteristics of the aerosol itself. A cascade impactor consists of a series of stages with different sized orifices which fix local linear velocities of the carrier gas of the aerosol as it passes through the device. (Fig. 1). The flow through the impactor is rigidly controlled, and then the linear velocity in each orifice can be predicted and the ability of a particle to negotiate the baffles downstream from each orifice is a function of its aerodynamic particle diameter. The cascade impactor affords the investigator several advantages. First, it gives a reasonable estimate of aerodynamic behavior of a aerosol sample. Second, analysis of the particles which impact on the stages can confirm the distribution of the active agent to be delivered by the aerosol, such as a drug or a radiolabel, which is used to trace the aerosol's path in the lung. The technical aspects of techniques for radiolabeling and their use in human studies have been detailed elsewhere (3). The inertia of the particles in the cascade impactor is rigidly controlled by the impactor geometry coupled with the control of the volumetric rate of flow through

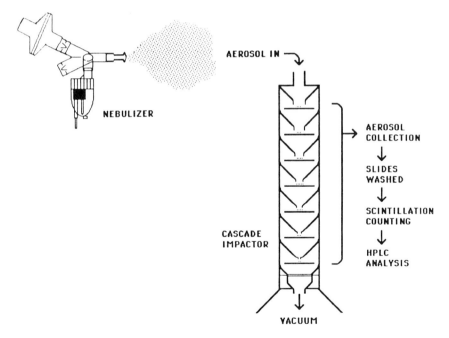

Figure 1 Sketch of a cascade impactor. The particles enter the top and are drawn through via controlled suction from below. Local velocities through each stage are precisely determined by the orifice diameter of the stage and the volumetric flow. Particles impact on the various stages as a function of their aerodynamic diameter. The stages can be removed for analysis of drug activity.

the device. However, when particles are inhaled by a patient, their behavior can be heavily influenced by the local flows within the lung, or the aerosol generator, and aerodynamic behavior cannot be rigidly predicted simply by the MMAD. A better prediction is obtained by consideration of particle inertia during inhalation, which is estimated by the Stokes number. This dimensionless number (eq. 1) is defined by local velocity (U), the "relaxation time" (τ) and a geometrical factor (i.e., tube diameter [d]).

$$\text{Stokes number} = \tau U/d \qquad (1)$$

where

$$\tau = \frac{2\rho_p a^2 C}{9\eta} \qquad (2)$$

and ρ_p is the particle density, a is the particle diameter, C the slip correction factor, and η is the viscosity of the gas. The importance of particle inertia has been shown on the bench in constricted tubes (4) as well as in human studies (3,5-7). Figure 2 illustrates a series of images from human subjects following the deposition of a radiolabeled aerosol described by cascade impaction to have a MMAD of 1.5 μm and a σg of 1.2. On the upper left is a typical deposition image from a normal subject following quiet breathing. On the upper right is the image from the same individual after a rapid inhalation. The deposition pattern is very different with significant visualization of central airways (3). A similar picture (Fig. 2, lower right) was obtained from a patient with severe obstructive lung disease, who inhaled the same particles during quiet breathing. Again, the central airways are the major focus for deposition (6,7). On the lower left of Figure 2 is the deposition pattern from a normal subject following the inhalation of the same particles with a quiet inspiration but followed by a rapid *exhalation* (5). A simplified prediction of particle behavior based only on aerodynamic particle diameter in these subjects would have assumed that they would all follow the same path and deposit in similar airways. In reality, local flows influence the particle's inertia and patterns of deposition. In the normal subject (Fig. 2, upper left), deposition was in small airways and alveoli and can be well described by mechanisms of gravitational settling (8). In the next image in Figure 2, central deposition was affected by the inspiratory flow imparting significant inertia to the same particles, which cannot negotiate the central airway bifurcations (*inspiratory* impaction). *Expiratory* impaction at similar sites has been described in normal subjects (5) and patients with airway disease (6,7). Marked changes in local geometry, due to dynamic compression of central airways induced by emphysematous lung disease and voluntary forced expiration, cause local acceleration of particles during expiration; either forced (normal subject, lower left) or with tidal breathing (obstructed patient, Fig. 2, lower

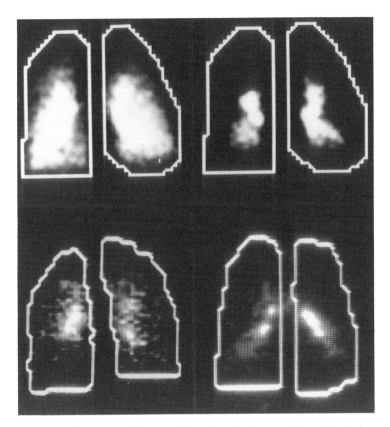

Figure 2 Deposition images following inhalation of 1.5-μm particles. Clockwise, upper left, normal subject quiet tidal breathing; normal subject rapid inhalation; patient with severe chronic obstructive pulmonary disease (COPD) quiet tidal breathing; normal subject quiet tidal inspiration; rapid exhalation. The lung outlines were drawn around a xenon equilibrium scan (3,5-7).

right). Thus, a better predictor of the deposition patterns illustrated in Figure 2 would be knowledge of the local inertia of the particles contained in the inhaled aerosol.

Particle inertia resulting from the aerosol generator itself can be an important determinant of sites of deposition. Figure 3 (left) illustrates a pattern of deposition that reflects inhalation of an aerosol generated by a metered-dose inhalation (9). A significant number of the particles has been deposited in the pharynx and larynx owing to the increased inertia of particles as they are sprayed out of the device. In the cascade impactor, the MMAD has been described as being 2 μm (10), and one might expect the particles to bypass the

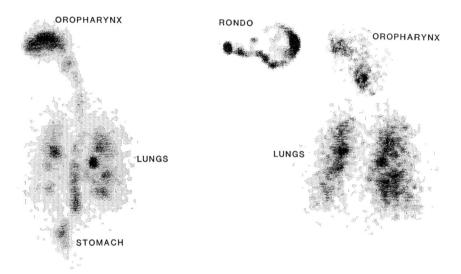

Figure 3 Influence of intrinsic particle inertia on deposition pattern. On the left, a patient inhaling particles generated by a MDI without a spacer. On the right, the same patient inhaling the same aerosol but after modification by a Rondo (Leiras, Finland) spacer device. (From ref. 9.)

upper airway. However, it is particle inertia that causes upper airway deposition. On the right of Figure 3, laryngeal deposition is reduced by utilizing a metered-dose inhaler (MDI) plus a spacer (9). Particles leaving the spacer have a lower inertia, because their velocity is primarily a reflection of the tidal breath of the patient rather than the explosive generation of the aerosol when the metered-dose inhaler is triggered. Figure 4 shows an image from a patient who inhaled nebulized DNase (Pulmozyme, Genentech, USA). This patient was inhaling tidal breaths from a nebulizer which the cascade impactor indicated had an MMAD of 3 μm. Approximately 50% of the deposited radioactivity was detected in the patient's larynx and stomach (both of which essentially represent "upper airway deposition," G. Smaldone, unpublished observations). The increased particle size, even with quiet breathing, resulted in a similar pattern to that seen in Figure 3 (left). These examples demonstrate that particle inertia defines the pattern of deposition in human subjects and it results from a combination of factors; aerodynamic diameter and local properties of the carrier gas (see eqs. 1 and 2).

Aerosolized drug particles can be solid spheres, water droplets containing dissolved agonists, particles consisting of two phases (e.g., suspensions), as well as droplets from organic materials such as propylene glycol or alcohol

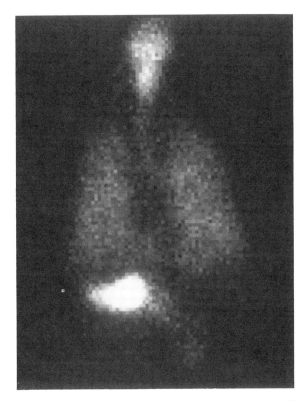

Figure 4 Deposition image during quiet tidal breathing in a young girl inhaling recombinant DNase. The MMAD was 3 μm. There is significant upper airway deposition (approximately 50%) as reflected by combined laryngeal and stomach activity.

(11). The predictive ability of the cascade impactor and other devices in determining aerodynamic behavior and deposition has not been well studied for many types of particles that can change size during inhalation. There are studies that describe the hygroscopic growth of particles under controlled conditions, such as dried sodium chloride particles (12); but each drug and solvent-solute combination can have its own dynamics in the human body, and this particular aspect of deposition has not been well studied. Further, the atmosphere surrounding inhaled particles is ever changing. Although changing humidity is a classic example, the atmosphere of Freon from an MDI or the changing atmosphere of an organic solvent may also affect particle behavior. In addition, the solubility of the material in the droplets can change as the liquid is concentrated in a delivery system such as a nebulizer (for example, the supersaturated precipitation of pentamidine during nebulization. However, cascade impaction data do have some predictive value, as illustrated above from practical clinical studies in patients. It has been our policy to study delivery systems on the bench and, combined with some knowledge of lung physiology, the gross behavior of particles can be estimated in advance. In all cases, it has been a principle in our laboratory to confirm these estimates with in vivo human studies.

B. Aerosol Generator

Most drugs are packaged as liquids or solids. To bring these materials into the gas phase suitable for inhalation, some form of energy is transferred to the solid or liquid and the material is suspended in the carrier gas. Three commonly used delivery systems are illustrated in Figure 5. The MDI consists of a pressurized metal canister that contains a mixture of Freons which, when in equilibrium, are both in liquid and gaseous form at room temperature (13). Suspended in the liquid, the agonist usually consists of solid particles, which have been milled into an aerodynamically respirable distribution of diameters. This two-phase suspension is evenly distributed by shaking and than a "metered dose" is released into the atmosphere via the valving system when the canister is compressed and triggered. The metering valve carefully controls the volume of liquid released into the atmosphere. At that point, the Freon instantly evaporates, imparting a relatively high kinetic energy to the solid particles. Thus, the metering valve provides precise control of the triggered amount of drug, but the high kinetic energy of the aerosolized particles affects their behavior when inhaled, as described above.

Environmental pressures have led to the development of aerosol dispensers that are free of fluorocarbons. The dry powder devices (e.g., Turbuhaler (Astra Draco, Sweden); see Fig. 5 [14]) store the drug as a solid mass, or as a premeasured quantity of powder (Diskhaler, Rotahaler, Glaxo, UK). To create an aerosol, two maneuvers are necessary. First, a measured quantity of drug must be separated from the storage cake or capsule. This is accomplished in the Turbuhaler by scraping a quantity of material from the main source by rotating a blade across the surface, in the Diskhaler by puncturing the disk, and in devices such as the Rotahaler by opening a capsule manually. To suspend the powder in air, the required energy is provided by the patient. This is usually accomplished via a rapid inhalation through the device and turbulence, cre-

---

Figure 5   Commonly used delivery devices: (top) MDI, which uses a phase change of Freon to deliver the solid particles; (lower left) Turbuhaler, a dry powder inhaler which utilizes the patient's own inspiratory flow to generate the aerosol; (lower right) a nebulizer (AeroTech II, CIS-US, USA), which incorporates energy from a gas jet to generate the aerosol which is inhaled during tidal breathing.

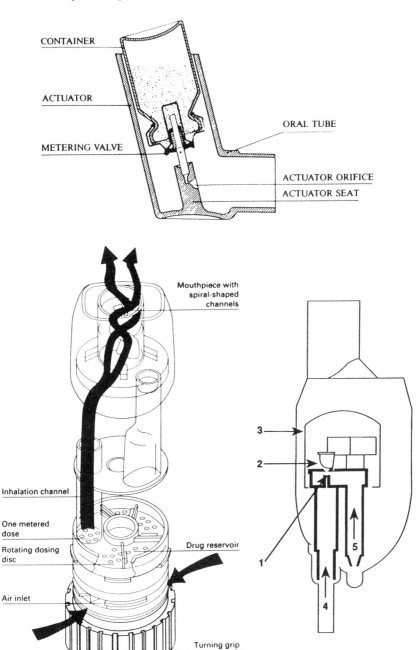

CONTAINER

ACTUATOR

METERING VALVE

ORAL TUBE

ACTUATOR ORIFICE

ACTUATOR SEAT

Mouthpiece with spiral-shaped channels

Inhalation channel

One metered dose

Rotating dosing disc

Air inlet

Drug reservoir

Turning grip

3

2

1

4

5

ated by a series a baffles, blends the powder into a respirable distribution, which is inhaled from the device. By modifying the design features, there is precise control of the released dose, but these systems are flow dependent to a varying degree and, in a manner similar to the MDI, the inhaled material of necessity leaves the device at relatively high velocity.

Nebulizers generate aerosols usually from liquids (see Fig. 5 [15]). Energy can be transferred to the liquid surface by either a jet, as the liquid phase is forced through a narrow orifice at high velocity, or by sheer forces at the surface generated by ultrasonic waves. Usually, the agonist is dissolved in the solvent, but it is possible to nebulize suspensions, although there are few studies of two-phase nebulization systems. In terms of the basics of aerosol generation, the major difference between nebulizers and the metered systems (MDIs and dry powder inhalers) is that the velocity of particles leaving the generator is really a function of the patient's method of breathing. Commonly, a patient quietly breathing through a nebulizer will inhale particles whose inertia is a function of the aerodynamic diameter and the local convective flows of the physiological situation, defined by the breathing pattern, rather than the rapid evaporation of Freon in the MDI, or the high flow rates necessary via rapid inhalation in a dry powder device. Therefore, even though particles may have the same aerodynamic characteristics as described by cascade impaction, the nature of the aerosol generator significantly influences the actual aerosol that is inhaled (aerosol being defined as the distribution of particles and the carrier gas, with the carrier gas imparting its own velocity to the particles), and the subsequent deposition patterns are, as described above, significantly affected.

C. Modifiers of Aerosol Generators

Recognition of the differences described above has led to attempts to modify the behavior of the aerosol as it is generated. This particularly applies to devices which produce particles of respirable diameters, but high inertia, such as MDIs and dry-powder devices. For the MDIs in particular, the spacer device (Fig. 6) has had a significant influence on drug delivery. As shown in the deposition study of Figure 3, the spacer device (instead of the pharynx and larynx) absorbs those particles that have high inertia, and the resulting pattern of distribution within the body more closely simulates that found using aerosol-delivery systems that follow the patient's own oropharyngeal convective flow (e.g., nebulizer). Significant losses occur in the spacer, as particles impact on the walls, but the available data in human studies indicate that the parenchymal deposition of drug within the lung is similar with and without the spacer, resulting in decreased exposure of the larynx and pharynx to the inhaled agonist (9). Spacer devices also provide coordination control for the patient. Rather than relying on the patient to inhale at the instant of MDI triggering, the spacer

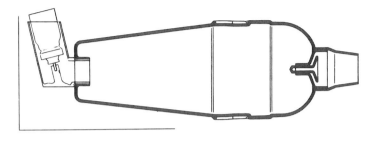

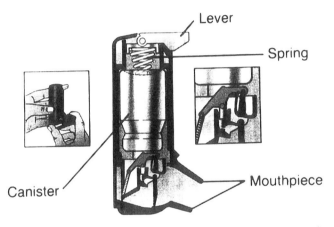

Figure 6 MDI with spacer Nebuhaler, Astra Draco, Sweden) (upper panel): coordinated inspiratory triggering device (Autohaler) (lower panel).

serves as a reservoir from which the particles, which remain in the gas phase, can be inhaled more conveniently. The presence of one-way valves within some spacer devices also facilitates this maneuver. The dry-powder inhalers, because they require the patient's own rapid inhalation to generate the aerosol, are by definition coordinated to the patient's breathing.

The Autohaler (3M, USA) (Fig. 6) is another form of automatic device in which the MDI is triggered by the patient during inhalation, much as a dry-powder inhaler. The trigger is controlled by a spring-loaded system which can be energized electively by the patient using a lever. Therefore, patients with problems of digital manipulation (e.g., arthritis) can use a MDI more conveniently.

MDIs and powder inhalers are approved for use by regulatory agencies in concert with the drug, and therefore are highly regulated. There is much more variability and nonuniformity in the manufacture of nebulizers. Aerosols emitted from nebulizers are primarily modified by baffling systems that are either internal or external to the device and nebulizer-delivery systems must be evaluated with the tubing and mouthpieces with which they are marketed. In addition, the nature of the nebulizer itself (e.g., jet vs ultrasonic) will affect the quantity of aerosol delivered in concert with the patient's breathing pattern. Although this field is largely undeveloped, it has been recognized that significant enhancements are possible, in terms of drug delivery, by coordinating nebulization with inspiration and recycling impacted material within nebulizer baffles back into the nebulizing chamber. Further examples of these principles are illustrated below.

III. Dose to the Patient

A. Inhaled Mass (Bench Experiments)

Equation 3 is a simplified version of the concept that the actual dose of a drug has little to do with the "nominal" dose filling a delivery system (e.g., the amount in a nebulizer or in the metering chamber of an MDI).

$$\text{Deposition} = [\text{Drug Nebulized and Inhaled}] - \text{Drug Exhaled} \qquad (3)$$

$$[\text{Drug Nebulized and Inhaled}] = \text{Inhaled Mass} \qquad (4)$$

$$\text{Deposition Fraction} = \text{Deposition/Inhaled Mass} \qquad (5)$$

$$\text{Deposition} = (\text{Inhaled Mass}) \times (\text{DF}) \qquad (6)$$

The actual amount of drug remaining in a patient after a treatment is expressed as "deposition." The factors determining deposition are divided into two main components, the "inhaled mass" (eq. 4), which reflects the characteristics of the specific delivery system (16), and the DF (eq. 5), the deposition fraction, which is simply a measure of the fraction inhaled that actually deposits (17). The reason for this separation of terms is that the inhaled mass is a strong function of the type of delivery system utilized and this term can often be modified by in vitro bench experiments. The DF is affected primarily by the physiology of the patient's respiratory tract and, for a given patient group, requires in vivo measurement. Failure to make a distinction between differences in drug-delivery systems versus variation in human pathophysiology (i.e., eq. 6) can lead to inappropriate conclusions regarding factors that ultimately determine the deposited dose in the lung. Depending on the device, and the disease, both the inhaled mass and the DF can be affected by the breathing pattern. Thus, breathing pattern is a common link between measurement of both factors and it should be taken into account in bench testing as well as physiologic deposition experiments.

Federal regulation of aerosol "doses" varies with devices. The MDI depicted in Figure 5 utilizes a metering valve which is highly regulated and functionally precise. However, as illustrated in the above paragraphs because of the high particle inertia inherent in the aerosol plume, coordination issues with respect to the patient and the necessity for particles to negotiate the upper respiratory tract, the lung dose has very little to do with the metered dose. MDI/spacer combinations modify the behavior of particles as well as assist in patient coordination and therefore, can reduce variability in inhaled mass but at the same time reduce inhaled mass dramatically. Although beneficial effects of reduced variability of inhaled mass and decreased deposition in the upper airway have been described (18) agency regulation of the dose, at this time, is much less for MDI/spacer than MDI alone. The Turbuhaler is also highly regulated, assuring precision of manufacture and aerosol presentation to the patient. However, because it is sensitive to breathing pattern and the particles leave with high velocity, prediction of the inhaled mass from the regulated dose is difficult.

Nebulizers as drug delivery systems are essentially unregulated. Early studies which led to the concept of inhaled mass (16,19) demonstrated that the quantity of drug placed in a nebulizer (nebulizer charge) often had little to do with the actual quantity of aerosolized particles inhaled by the patient. Figure 7 represents data for delivery systems originally used for aerosolized pentamidine prophylaxis in patients with AIDS. Over time, twice as much drug is inhaled by a patient breathing with a standardized breathing pattern with the AeroTech II versus the Respirgard II (Marquest, USA). From equation 6, a patient with a given DF would receive a dose twice as large from the AeroTech II versus the Respirgard if both nebulizers had been filled with the same "nebulizer charge." Failure to appreciate this concept could lead to overdosing or underdosing, depending on the thresholds for efficacy and toxicity of a given drug. Historically, the lack of recognition of this issue has not led to significant problems, because the major drugs nebulized in the clinical arena have been bronchodilators. Treatment of patients with these agents has been essentially a "titration" of acute bronchodilation versus acute side effects such as tachycardia and tremor, and therapy has been empirically tailored to the patient. Obviously, this situation does not apply to agents with delayed effects such as aerosolized steroids. Further, as the costs of newer agents mount, the efficiency of delivery systems becomes important.

The first drug studied quantitatively, utilizing the concepts outlined above, was aerosolized pentamidine (NebuPent, Fujisawa, USA). Bench testing revealed differences between commonly used nebulizers, as illustrated in Figure 7, and subsequent in vivo experiments measured DF in a group of patients receiving therapy (19). Although DF varied considerably from patient to pa-

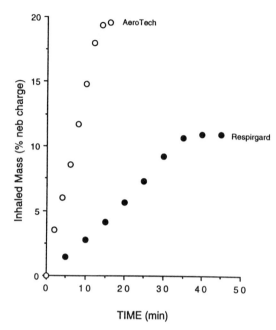

Figure 7 Inhaled mass (percentage of nebulizer charge actually inhaled by a patient) as a function of delivery device; upper curve. AeroTech II; lower curve, Respirgard II. (Modified from 19.)

tient, variability in nebulizer delivery was the dominant factor influencing differences in lung dose. This is because nebulizer variability extended over a range approximating an order of magnitude. This degree of variability usually exceeds that found for DF in patients with similar pathology (19). Further, variability in nebulizer delivery not only is a function of the type and manufacture of a given device but also in quality control between samples of the same device, which are not as regulated as MDIs and powder-delivery systems. Nebulizers often exhibit significant variability in drug delivery when measured on the bench (19–21). For example, in Figure 8, are illustrated data from the original study measuring pentamidine deposition in patients (19). When studied on the bench, 10 examples of Respirgard II and AeroTech II nebulizers demonstrated significant variability in both slope and plateau of the relationships measured in Figure 7. This variability differed between devices and between the components of the overall inhaled mass curve. From these data for pentamidine, we have since modified our aerosol delivery practices such that we utilize AeroTech II nebulizers, generally run to dryness, because of the reduced variability of that device's plateau.

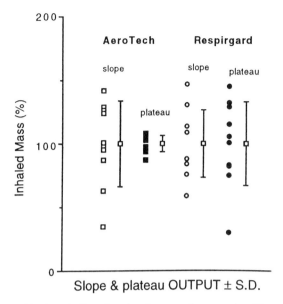

Figure 8 Variability in nebulizer function from random samples. Data are represented as averages of the slope and plateau of the inhaled mass versus time relationship as depicted in Figure 7. Both the AeroTech II and Respirgard II nebulizers exhibit similar variability in the slope of the relationship, but the plateau (i.e., the quantity of material delivered if the nebulizer is run to dryness) is significantly less variable for the AeroTech II. (From ref. 19.)

It is important to recognize that the tubing and baffles are often critical in determining a device's overall performance as well as the inhaled particle distribution. The proper measurement of inhaled mass requires that the bench set-up duplicate the clinical situation as closely as possible. Figure 9 demonstrates this effect. Two particle distributions from an ultrasonic nebulizer (the Fisoneb, Fisons, UK) which has also been utilized for the delivery of aerosolized pentamidine are shown. That nebulizer produces 5-μm polydisperse droplets when it is simply turned on and particles are vented to the atmosphere. However, as shown in Figure 9, the particle distribution is significantly modified when a patient breathes through the nebulizer. That is, the mass median aerodynamic diameter is reduced from 5.0 to 2.5 μm. This degree of shift in particle distribution may be important ultimately in lung deposition and efficacy. Although the Fisoneb has been criticized for producing "large particles," in reality, the distribution of inhaled particles is much closer to that of a typical MDI. Because the Fisoneb's particles were inhaled quietly rather than being sprayed into the oropharynx, lung deposition utilizing that device has been quite

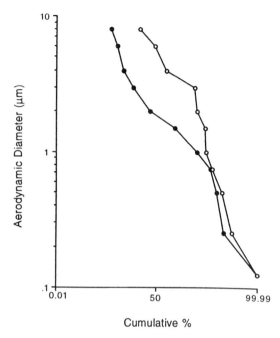

Figure 9 Variability of particle distribution from Fisoneb nebulizer as a function of air flow through the nebulizer; open circles, standing cloud; closed circles, simulated patient breathing. The MMAD decreases from approximately 5 to 2.5 μm (20).

reasonable, and with its enhanced efficiency patients have been successfully treated with much lower quantities of pentamidine in the nebulizer charge (22).

Most of the points illustrated above for pentamidine, like those for bronchodilators, have been measured after the fact with respect to their approval as therapeutic agents by regulatory agencies. Pentamidine is accumulated in lung tissues and does not readily enter the blood. Its local toxicity appears limited and, therefore, pentamidine has also led a "charmed life" similar to that of bronchodilators in terms of the ultimate dose versus response. That is, a nebulizer delivery system that delivers a low dose or high dose of drug probably would not have a significant influence on clinical efficacy, because an "underdosed" patient would eventually receive an adequate level of drug, because it would accumulate in the tissues and those patients who are "overdosed" would not experience significant toxicity, at least at the systemic level. The insensitivity of pentamidine efficacy to the lung dose has been shown in several studies (23,24). It is very unlikely that this situation will extend to aerosolized steroids, which are systemically absorbed to some degree and can have measurable toxicity, local and systemic.

Finally, the importance of bench testing cannot be overemphasized with respect to estimating drug delivery in advance of in vivo delivery studies. Here bronchodilators serve as examples. Early investigators in this field recognized that the nebulizer/tubing arrangements in patients on mechanical ventilation were more complex than delivery systems in spontaneously breathing subjects and questioned the ability of nebulizers to deliver adequate amounts of drug when compared with other delivery systems such as MDI/spacer devices incorporated into the respiratory tubing (25). They measured differences in drug deposition that suggested approximately a seven times difference in delivery efficiency between MDIs and nebulizers in terms of lung deposition measured in patients. Subsequent bench studies have determined that the major differences measured by those investigators were related to differences in inhaled mass between different nebulizer versus MDI/spacer combinations. In a series of studies incorporating bench measurements and human data, important factors for both MDIs and nebulizers have been assessed which markedly influence inhaled mass (21,26–28). Figure 10 illustrates the inhaled mass over time delivered by both an optimized nebulizer system and an optimized MDI/spacer system via mechanical ventilator. For both devices, the actual amount of bronchodilator (albuterol) delivered at the distal tip of the endotracheal tube in a standard mechanical ventilatory apparatus is very similar over time. In order to generate those relationships, the nebulizer circuit was modified by a series of experiments which demonstrated that humidification of ventilator circuitry and the brand of nebulizer were critical factors in terms of drug delivery (21,26,27). For the MDI/spacer combination, the efficiency of aerosol delivery was closely tied to synchronization of the MDI triggering to the beginning of inspiration as well as a 1-min pause between actuations (28). Failure to follow any of these protocol modifications would lead to significant decreases (72%) in drug delivery as estimated by measurement of inhaled mass (28) and ultimately to failure of therapy (29).

In the last 5–10 years, clinical and physiological studies have greatly enhanced our ability to gain a practical knowledge of drug delivery of aerosolized medications. Regulatory agencies are adjusting to these findings, but most regulations regarding devices relate to quality control testing by the manufacturer which does not always duplicate conditions of drug delivery. In vitro testing on the bench of delivery systems can be useful for all types of delivery devices and has been shown to influence our ability to reduce variability in deposition. We are reaching the point where these basic principles should be known by all physicians specializing in this area, not just those who are performing the basic studies. In parallel to clinical studies that are performed to determine the efficacy and safety of aerosolized drugs such as topical steroids, it is important that those health care professionals who will utilize the agents in different patient populations be educated as to the principles of drug delivery.

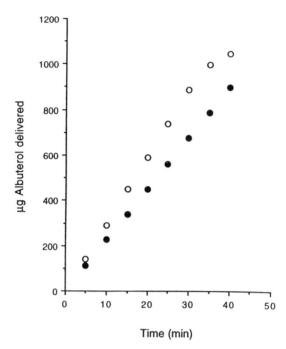

Figure 10 Drug activity (albuterol) delivered to the distal tip of an endotracheal tube in a model of mechanical ventilation for different delivery devices. The upper curve represents an AeroTech II nebulizer on an optimized ventilator circuit (27); the straight line, albuterol delivery from an MDI/spacer combination, synchronized actuation with inspiration, one minute pause (28).

B. Deposition Fraction and Breathing Pattern

During tidal breathing, it is generally well recognized that a variable fraction of inhaled particles is exhaled. Earlier studies were usually performed with monodisperse, nonhygroscopic particles, which may not duplicate the clinical delivery of aerosolized drugs. Further, those studies (30–32) were to a large extent carried out in normal subjects and were useful in defining normal parameters of airway geometry and the effects of the breathing pattern on deposition (31,32). Because of the sophisticated nature of those experiments the literature, even in normal subjects, is sparse with some uncertainty remaining as to the relative contributions of variation in airway geometry versus breathing pattern in predicting values of DF (33). Clinical data are even more limited. The availability of monodisperse nonhygroscopic particles has facilitated physiological studies with relatively straightforward techniques (light scattering) which are not available for polydisperse, nonhygroscopic particles. Of necessity, therefore, clinical studies have been carried out utilizing filters to determine the bulk mass of drug inhaled and subsequently exhaled during maneuvers simulating therapy with different aerosol delivery systems.

Equation 6, which describes deposition in terms of inhaled mass and DF, as described above, provides a separate determination of the efficiency of the delivery system (inhaled mass measurement) as well as physiological and pathophysiological influences on DF. The breathing pattern remains a critical factor that influences both terms. For example, the breathing pattern affects inhaled mass in various ways. For continuously operating nebulizers, duty cycle can be a direct determinant of inhaled mass (26). For the powder inhalers, the quantity of drug generated by the device can be a direct function of inspiratory flow (34). For all devices, once the particles are generated and inhaled, the breathing pattern influences DF, the fraction of aerosol inhaled that deposits, by the forces of inspiratory impaction and gravitational settling. For delivery systems that generate particles with high inertia (MDI, Turbuhaler, Rotahaler, Diskhaler), DF approximates 1 (35). The situation is very different for nebulizers. In normal human subjects, DF can be predicted for monodisperse nonhygroscopic particles in terms of the overall breathing pattern (32). Figure 11 (normal subjects, upper panel). demonstrates a relatively tight relationship between DF and patterns of breathing ranging from tidal breathing to exercise. On the lower panel are data from experiments in patients with human immunodeficiency virus (HIV) infection receiving aerosolized pentamidine (19). Those subjects were breathing tidally and the particles were polydisperse. However, the MMAD of both particle distributions between the two studies were similar. Obviously, for the patients, breathing pattern does not predict DF. On the other hand, the variability in DF in the patient studies was much less than overall variability in lung deposition (Fig. 12) which ranged over an order of magnitude. The data of Figure 12 demonstrates that the inhaled mass was the major determinant of deposition primarily because of differences in aerosol delivery systems (19,23). These observations suggest that assessment of the aerosol delivery system in advance of clinical studies can significantly reduce variability in lung deposition; that is, to the order of magnitude in DF itself.

IV. Regional Dose

A. Assessment of Regional Deposition; Analytic Techniques

In the earlier sections of this chapter, it was emphasized that the method of drug delivery and particle diameters in the aerosol can greatly influence the pattern of deposition in the human subject. Once the whole-body dose of the drug is determined (see eq. 6), the ultimate dose versus response relationship will re-

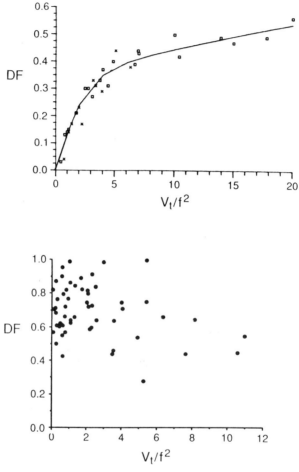

Figure 11 Relationship between deposition fraction (DF) and breathing pattern for normal subjects (32) (upper panel). DF versus breathing pattern in patients with AIDS receiving aerosolized pentamidine (19) (lower panel).

quire some assessment of the regional distribution of the drug within the patient. Because the lung is often the target organ, early studies have concentrated on regional analysis within that organ; but upper airway deposition, stomach activity, and other issues may be important depending on the agent in question. Radioisotope scanning is the most common method for analyzing regional drug deposition in the lung and upper airways. A typical analytical technique is outlined in Figure 13. To determine the overall lung outline, investigators often use an equilibrium xenon scan (^{133}Xe) which determines regional lung volume as well as the lung outline. Others use transmission images or perfusion

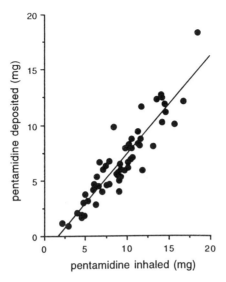

Figure 12 Lung deposition of aerosolized pentamidine versus inhaled mass ($r = 0.919$, $p < .001$). (Modified from ref. 19)

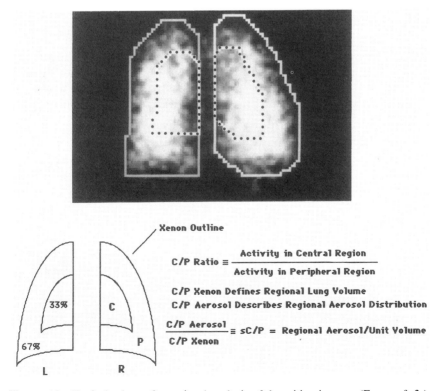

Figure 13 Typical scheme for regional analysis of deposition images. (From ref. 3.)

scans (3). Additional regions of interest can be superimposed over the anatomical lung outline which describe the distribution of deposited particles. Depending on the drug and delivery system, regional analysis can be emphasized over the upper airway and stomach, the central and peripheral airways, or upper and lower lobes. Figure 13 demonstrates a two-dimensional view obtained from a gamma camera. Three-dimensional analysis is also available (SPECT), and these techniques have been described in more detail in other reviews (3,36). To date, utilization of these techniques actually to determine the dose and/or response of inhaled drugs and the determination of efficacy in patients is at the earliest stages of development. However, because of the therapeutic/toxic issues regarding newer drugs, such as inhaled steroids, these techniques of analysis may prove to be critical in ultimately assessing therapeutic value.

The deposition image sketched in Figure 13 can be represented quantitatively by the central to peripheral ratio (C/P ratio), which has been determined from regional outlines based on the xenon equilibrium scan. This ratio, when normalized for regional lung volume (sC/P ratio), is a measurement of the quantity of particles deposited in a given lung region per unit volume. The sC/P ratio has allowed comparison of deposition between different subjects and, when coupled with a measure of whole-lung deposition, will give an estimate of regional dose of drug. Similar analyses can be carried out for upper and lower lung regions, stomach, and upper airways. It should be recognized that there are technical pitfalls in these measurements which are at present being quantitatively measured. By simply measuring regional lung counts and comparing with whole-body deposition as measured by filters, errors can be introduced primarily by geometrical effects and their influence on lung scanning (3).

V. Response to Therapy

Once the aerosol is characterized, delivered, and deposited in the patient, the most difficult challenge facing investigators is an assessment of efficacy. Although it is logical that a combination of whole-body dose and regional analysis would yield important information regarding local dose of drug with concomitant assessment of response, little data presently exist for aerosolized drugs. For example, Figure 14 represents a deposition image following inhalation of aerosolized cyclosporine in a patient with sarcoidosis, who had received a single lung transplant (left lung, left side of Fig. 14). This patient ultimately lost her transplant because of chronic rejection. Regional analysis of Figure 14 indicates that the transplanted lung received less drug than the native lung. The native lung maintained a high level of ventilation and, therefore, received a large quantity of aerosolized drug. The transplanted lung was affected by an obstructive process (obliterative bronchiolitis and chronic rejection) with reduced re-

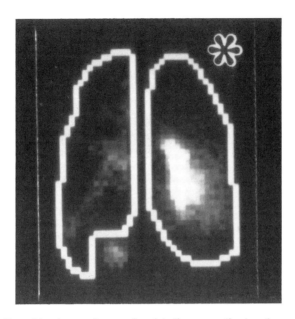

Figure 14 Deposition images from patient inhaling aerosolized cyclosporine. The left lung is a unilateral transplant with histological evidence of severe rejection and obliterative bronchiolitis, the right lung (asterisk, native lung) suffers from interstitial fibrosis due to sarcoidosis. As indicated, deposition predominates in the native lung.

gional ventilation and received a lower dose (6.9 mg left lung vs 15.8 mg right lung). Did this patient's transplant fail because the drug was inactive or was the dose inadequate? Evaluating this question is not easy. Although measuring the dose seems possible, deposition assessments occur only in a single instant of time. Further, quantitating the response to therapy is also difficult to assess. Ultimately there should be a dose-response relationship that would provide a minimum dose necessary for therapeutic success or a definitive statement the drug has failed. Often, a large number of clinical variables must be studied, because it is not known which specific entity is most reflective of the disease process. Similar problems to lung transplantation exist in asthma.

A. Aerosols and Airway Reactivity (Methacholine Bronchoprovocation)

The measurement of airway reactivity is an interesting technique for assessing clinical efficacy of drug therapy, because the test itself involves aerosols, and regional deposition of drug may be important in terms of both the delivery of the constricting agent as well as assessing the response. The nature of the increased reactivity seen in asthmatic airways is not well understood. However, a hallmark of asthma is the increased reactivity to agonists such as inhaled methacholine. How important is the local dose of deposited methacholine in assessing airway reactivity? Some investigators have proposed that different airways exhibit different levels of reactivity (37). However, most studies assessing reactivity of different pulmonary regions have perturbed methacholine delivery such that the test utilized in the specific investigation does not closely mimic the clinical measurement of airway reactivity to methacholine (i.e., rapid inhalation vs quiet tidal breathing). However, a few studies measuring methacholine deposition following protocols that match typical clinical determinations of airway reactivity, suggest that reactivity in asthma is not strongly related to the technique of methacholine delivery. Mass balance studies, using the filter technique to measure patient deposition of inhaled methacholine, did not detect a consistent difference in deposition between normal subjects and patients with asthma (38), and they indicated that the dose to the patient, therefore, was not a determining factor of reactivity. The regional deposition of inhaled methacholine has also been studied (39). Expressed as the sC/P ratio, the initial pattern of methacholine deposition in the lung during a standard methacholine inhalation is shown in Figure 15 between asthmatic patients and normal subjects. As methacholine was continuously inhaled, those patients with asthma developed a bronchoconstriction. At that point, repeat measurement of the pattern of deposition of the inhaled methacholine revealed a significant shift in deposition to the central airways. This observation has been made by several laboratories and suggests that the deposition of methacholine in central airways may be responsible for the enhanced reactivity to inhaled methacholine. However, in the normal subjects depicted in Figure 15, who did not exhibit significant bronchoconstriction, the same shift to central airways of inhaled methacholine was observed during the latter phases of the standard methacholine bronchoprovocation regimen. These findings indicate that the normal subjects had a similar constriction of their airways to those with asthma resulting in a shift of equal magnitude in the pattern of deposition, but only the asthmatic patients demonstrated a measurable drop in lung function. Although the clinical separation of asthmatics from normal individuals remains valid, the physiological basis of methacholine testing still remains obscure. But, it does not appear that the differences in measured reactivity between asthmatic patients and normal subjects are related to technical differences in either lung dose of methacholine nor the regional distribution of the deposited particles.

Serial measurement of airway reactivity may also have an important role in assessing response to therapeutic agents. Clinical studies have shown that as patients improve they appear to have a decrease in measured reactivity (40). The data described above suggest that technical variation in measurement of airway reactivity is not important in making the diagnosis of asthma, but the

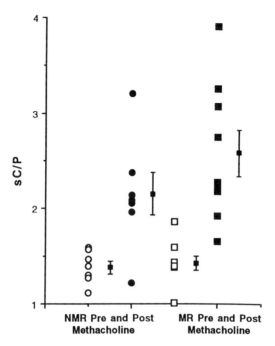

Figure 15 Distribution of deposited methacholine during aerosolized broncho-provocation testing in normal subjects and patients with asthma. MR, subjects achieving a PC_{20} (i.e., methacholine reactive): NMR, subjects not receiving a PC_{20}; sC/P_1, initial deposition pattern; sC/P_2, post-methacholine deposition pattern. Mean $\pm$ SE are also shown. sC/P ratios are not different at the beginning of methacholine inhalation. After methacholine inhalation, deposition in both normal subjects and asthmatic patients has shifted significantly to central airways. (From ref. 39.)

question remains, are there important differences in methacholine deposition that affect changes in reactivity following therapy? Most clinical estimates of airway reactivity do not measure the deposited dose nor the regional deposition of deposited methacholine. Although the definition of asthma may not be sensitive to methacholine dose, changes in reactivity due to a given therapeutic regimen may be affected by changes of site of deposition or the deposited dose. Almost all therapeutic entities thought to be successful in the treatment of asthma will result in improved airway function and diminished peripheral airways resistance. It is known that sites of particle deposition will likely become more peripheral under those circumstances and, in a given subject, this may result in a change in airway reactivity. Thus, the measured change in PC_{20} may reflect an amelioration of the disease process but not due to an intrinsic change in airway reactivity but to the physiological influences on the test itself.

B. Mucociliary Clearance

Bronchoalveolar lavage, airway epithelial biopsy, and analysis of expectorated sputum have been utilized to measure efficacy of both topical and systemic treatments for asthma. Aerosol techniques may be useful in providing additional modes for measuring response, without the need for invasive procedures. Because the deposition of particles is sensitive to local airway geometry, test aerosols can be used as probes of peripheral airway function independent of, and complementary to, standard pulmonary function testing. In a given patient, breathing with a standardized breathing pattern, a test aerosol may provide important insights as to changes in small airway function before and after a given therapeutic regimen. Besides the pattern of deposition, the clearance of radiolabeled test aerosols from the airways may also be an index of overall epithelial function, as assessed by the performance of the mucociliary apparatus. Mucociliary clearance has been shown to vary depending on the clinical state of patients with asthma (41). It is likely that this pathophysiological change is related, in some way, to inflammatory processes seen in airway epithelial biopsies. As shown in Figure 16, clearance measurements appear to differ between groups of patients with significant differences in clinical disease activity (42). In basic studies of drug efficacy, these techniques may serve to complement more invasive measurements.

Finally, besides the clearance of test aerosols from the airways, there are little data regarding the clearance of active drug from various regions of the respiratory tract. Although deposition sites of topical agents are intuitively thought to be important for the ultimate effect, it is conceivable that a deposited drug may move from one region of the lung to another via forms of airway clearance. The drug can pass into the bronchial circulation, for example, and regions of the lung may be exposed independent to the initial sites of aerosol delivery.

VI. Summary

Topical anti-inflammatory therapy in respiratory diseases, especially asthma, is an important therapeutic modality. Aerosolized therapy in asthma continues to serve as an important paradigm for inhalational therapy for all diseases. The search for improved treatments of asthma is a major stimulus for research in techniques of aerosolized drug delivery, as well as efforts to analyze regional deposition and ultimately determine an effective response. Table 1 presents an outline, which can be considered an algorithm, for the development and testing of aerosolized agents in clinical disease. The properties of the drug may be critical in determining which delivery system is most effective. Solubility, physical characteristics, and other factors should be considered at the earliest

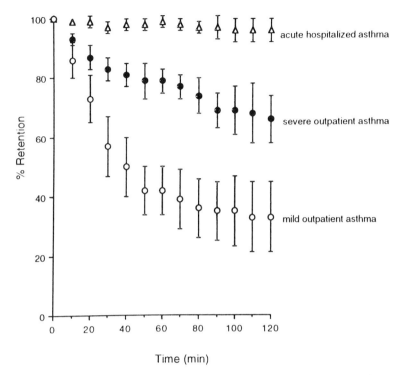

Figure 16 Mucociliary clearance from patients with asthma as assessed by radioaerosol techniques. Radioactivity measured in lung regions drawn in the same manner as in Figure 13 is decay corrected and plotted over time. The upper panel represents clearance from hospitalized patients with status asthmaticus (41), the middle curve ambulatory patients with sever chronic obstruction, and the lower, ambulatory patients with mild disease (42).

Table 1 Testing Schema for New Therapeutic Aerosols (prior to clinical trials)

Assess proposed patient population (e.g., obstructed vs restricted)
Estimate therapeutic goal (e.g., desired local drug levels)
Estimate delivery efficiency (e.g., determine nebulizer charge)
Examine drug properties ('solubility' testing and other physical properties)
Test delivery system on the bench mimicking the full range of clinical delivery situations (inhaled mass and particle distribution)
Particle deposition studies (measure dose and regional distribution of deposited drug)
Assess possible measures of response (directed biopsies, mucociliary clearance, pulmonary function testing, changes in reactivity)

stages. Delivery systems should be tested in advance of clinical studies, to confirm a reasonable inhaled mass, particle distribution, and complicating factors such as high particle inertia that may affect delivery to the lung. Most of these properties can be tested effectively on the bench and optimized beforehand. Our understanding of aerosol delivery systems is not complete enough to avoid practical testing before initiating clinical studies. Bench testing has been shown effectively to predict drug delivery, when utilized in a manner that accurately simulates the proposed clinical regimen. The next stage in development should include deposition studies; for example, utilizing radiolabeled particles to estimate the effectiveness of parenchymal delivery. Early knowledge of the lung dose and pattern of deposition of a given drug-delivery system may provide a preliminary assessment of response before large clinical trials.

Acknowledgments

I wish to thank Drs. Kurt Nikander and Patrice Diot for their helpful comments.

Discussion

DR. LIU: What is the distribution of particle sizes produced by MDIs versus nebulizers?

DR. SMALDONE: The measured particle distributions produced by MDIs and nebulizers vary depending on the particular drug and/or technique of measurement. In our laboratory, the particle distribution for nebulized bronchodilators is strongly dependent on the nebulizer and averages between 1 and 4 μm. For MDIs, we have measured average diameters of approximately 2 μm.

DR. HARGREAVE: A limited number of studies suggest that the overall distribution of deposited drug is similar between the MDI and Turbuhaler. I am aware of one study that measured lung deposition and found it to be higher than MDI. Mechanisms were not investigated, but I would speculate that a component of the difference is related to coordination differences in inspiration.

DR. HOWARTH: (1) It might be anticipated that the endobronchial circulation would distribute inhaled drugs throughout the lung. Is there any evidence that in some asthmatics in which there is predominantly a central airway deposition that corticosteroids get distributed to the peripheral airways? (2) The evidence suggests that it is the total dose of bronchodilator that reaches the lower airways that determines the physiological response rather than the site of deposition. Could the total dose going to the airways explain your different response between repeated application versus single application?

DR. SMALDONE: A very important issue. Unfortunately, there are no data to my knowledge that address this problem. I would speculate that the physical properties (e.g., solubility) of the drug will be key variables.

DR. BOCHNER: For some patients, the use of intranasal steroids appears to improve their lower airways function as well. Although it is presumed that this effect is due to improvement of the upper airways, I was just wondering whether any intranasal steroid aerosol actually gets deposited into the lower airways.

DR. SMALDONE: A direct effect is unlikely, because most nasal steroids are sprayed and deposited nasally rather than passing to the lung. However, a decrease in inflammation in the nasopharynx may moderate the clinical presentation of asthma and therefore affect lower airway function.

DR. PEDERSEN: It is feasible for drugs inspired through the nose to enter into the intrapulmonary airways. The most effective way to achieve this seems to be inhalation through a spacer, which is often used in young children, who can be given inhaled therapy through a spacer with a face mask while they are asleep and breathing through their nose. In addition, asthma during pollen season can be improved by inhalation through the nose from a nebuhaler. Inhalation through the nose, however, is very inefficient.

DR. SMALDONE: We would expect significant reductions in lung deposition with nasal breathing. But depending on mouth versus nasal breathing pattern and particle distribution, there could be unexpected results—more studies are needed especially in pediatrics.

References

1. Heyder J. Definition of an aerosol. J. Aerosol Med 1991; 4:217–221.
2. Ayer HE. Occupational air sampling strategies. In: Herring SV, ed. Air Sampling Instruments. 7th ed. Cincinnati: American Conference of Governmental Industrial Hygienists, 1989:21–31.
3. Smaldone GC, O'Riordan TG. Aerosol deposition and clearance. In: Wagner HN Jr. ed. Principles of Nuclear Medicine, 2nd ed. Philadelphia: Saunders, 1995:895–905.
4. Itoh H, Smaldone GC, Swift DL, Wagner HN Jr. Quantitative evaluation of aerosol deposition in constricted tubes. J Aerosol Sci 1985; 16:167–174.
5. Smaldone GC, Messina MS. Enhancement of particle deposition by flow-limiting segments in humans. J Appl Physiol 1985; 59:509–514.
6. Smaldone GC, Messina MS. Flow-limitation, cough, and patterns of aerosol deposition in humans. J Appl Physiol 1985; 59:515–520.
7. Itoh H, Ishii Y, Maeda H, Todo G, Torizuka K, Smaldone GC. Clinical observations of aerosol deposition in patients with airways obstruction. Chest 1981; 80(suppl): 837–839.

8. Heyder J. Gravitational deposition of aerosol particles within a system of randomly oriented tubes. J Aerosol Sci 1975; 6:133–137.
9. Newman SP, Talae N, Clarke SW. Pressurized aerosol in man with the Rondo spacer. Acta Ther 1991; 17:49–58.
10. Aug C, Perry RJ, Smaldone GC. Technetium 99m radiolabeling of aerosolized drug particles from metered dose inhalers. J. Aerosol Med 1991; 4:127–138.
11. O'Riordan TG, Duncan SR, Burchkart GJ, Griffith BP, Smaldone GC. Production of an aerosol of cyclosporine as a prelude to clinical studies. J Aerosol Med 1992; 5:171–177.
12. Blanchard JD, Willeke K. An Inhalation system for characterizing total lung deposition of ultrafine particles. Am Ind Hyg Assoc J 1983; 44:846–856.
13. Morén F. Aerosol dosage forms and formulations. In: Morén S, Dolovich MB, Newhouse MT, Newman SP, eds. Aerosols in Medicine. 2 ed. Amsterdam: Elsevier, 1993:329–336.
14. Morén F. Aerosol dosage forms and formulations. In: Morén S, Dolovich MB, Newhouse MT, Newman SP, eds. Aerosols in Medicine, 2nd ed. Amsterdam: Elsevier, 1993:324–329.
15. Nerbrink O, Dahlbäck M, Hansson H-C. Why do medical nebulizers differ in their output and particle size characteristics. J Aerosol Med 1994; 7:259–276.
16. Smaldone GC. Drug delivery via aerosol systems: concept of "aerosol inhaled." J Aerosol Med 1991; 4:229–235.
17. Bennett WD. Aerosolized drug delivery: fractional deposition of inhaled paticles. J Aerosol Med 1991; 4:223–229.
18. Toogood JH, Baskerville J, Jennings B, Lefcoe NM, Johansson S. Use of spacers to facilitate inhaled corticosteroid treatment of asthma. Am Rev Respir Dis 1984; 129:723–729.
19. Smaldone GC, Fuhrer J, Steigbigel RT, McPeck M. Factors determining pulmonary deposition of aerosolized pentamidine in patients with human immunodeficiency virus infection. Am Rev Respir Dis 1991; 143:727–737.
20. Smaldone GC, Perry RJ, and Deutsch DG. Characteristics of nebulizers used in the treatment of AIDS-related *Pneumocystis carinii* pneumonia. J Aerosol Med 1988; 1:113–126.
21. McPeck M, O'Riordan TG, Smaldone GC. Predicting aerosol delivery to intubated patients: influence of choice of mechanical ventilator on nebulizer efficiency. Respir Care 1993; 38:887–895.
22. Montaner J, Lawson L, Gervais A, Hyland RH, Chan CK, Falutz JM, et al. Aerosol pentamidine for secondary prophylaxis of AIDS-related *Pneumocystis carinii* pneumonia: a randomized, placebo-controlled study. Ann Intern Med 1991; 114:948–953.
23. Smaldone GC, Dickinson G, Marcial E, Young E, Seymour J. Deposition of aerosolized pentamidine and failure of *Pneumocystis* prophylaxis. Chest 1991; 101:82–87.
24. O'Riordan TG, Baughman RP, Dohn M, Shipley R, Buchsbaum JA, Frame PT, Smaldone GC. Lobar pentamidine levels and *Pneumocystis carinii* pneumonia following aerosolized pentamidine. Chest 1994; 105:53–56.
25. Fuller HD, Dolovich MB, Postmituck G, Wong Pack W, Newhouse MT. Pressur-

ized aerosol versus jet aerosol delivery to mechanically ventilated patients. Am Rev Respir Dis 1989; 141:440–444.

26. O'Riordan TG, Greco MJ, Smaldone GC. Nebulizer function during mechanical ventilation. Am Rev Respir Dis 1992; 145:1117–1122.

27. O'Riordan RG, Palmer L, Smaldone GC. Aerosol deposition In mechanically ventilated patients: optimizing nebulizer delivery. Am J Respir Crit Care Med 1994; 149:214–219.

28. Diot P, Morra L, Smaldone GC. Albuterol delivery in a model of mechanical ventilation: comparison of MDI and nebulizer efficiency. Am J Respir Crit Care Med 1995; 152:1391–1394.

29. Manthous CA, Hall JB, Schmidt GA, Wood LDH. Metered dose inhaler versus nebulized albuterol in mechanically ventilated patients. Am Rev Respir Dis 1993; 148:1567–1570.

30. Davies CN, Heyder J, Subba Ramu MC. Breathing of half-micron aerosols. 1 experimental. J Appl Physiol 1972; 32:591–600.

31. Heyder J, Armbruster L, Gebhart J, Grein E, Stahlhofen W. Total deposition of aerosol particles in the human respiratory tract for nose and mouth breathing. J Aerosol Sci 1975; 6:311–328.

32. Bennett WD, Smaldone GC. Human variation in peripheral air-space deposition of inhaled particles. J Appl Physiol 1987; 62:1603–1610.

33. Bennett WD, Editorial. Probing the lung with aerososl: the next generation. J Aerosol Med 1993; 6:149–150.

34. Clark AR, Hollingworth AM. The relationship between powder inhaler resistance and peak inspiratory conditions in healthy volunteers—implications for *in vitro* testing. J Aerosol Med 1993; 6:99–110.

35. Newman SP, Morén F, Pavia D, Little F, Clarke SW. Deposition of pressurized suspension aerosols inhaled through extension devices. Am Rev Respir Dis 1981; 124:317–320.

36. Chan HK. Use of single photon emission computed tomography in aerosol studies. J Aerosol Med 1993; 6:23–36.

37. Ruffin RE, Dolovich MB, Wolff RK, Newhouse MT. The effects of preferential deposition of histamine in the human airway. Am Rev Respir Dis 1978; 117:485–492.

38. Donna E, Danta I, Kim CS, Wanner A. Relationship between deposition of and responsiveness to inhaled methacholine in normal and asymptomatic subjects. J Allergy Clin Immunol 1989; 83:456–461.

39. O'Riordan TG, Walser L, Smaldone GC. Changing patterns of aerosol deposition during methacholine bronchoprovocation. Chest 1993; 103:1385–1389.

40. Cockcroft DW, Hargreave FE. Editorial. Airway hyperresponsiveness: relevance of random population data to clinical usefulness. Editorial: Am Rev Respir Dis 1990; 142:497–500.

41. Messina MS, O'Riordan TG, Smaldone GC. Changes in mucociliary clearance during acute exacerbations of asthma. Amer Rev Respir Dis 1991; 143:993–997.

42. O'Riordan TG, Zwang J, Smaldone GC. Mucociliary clearance in adult asthma. Amer Rev Respir Dis 1992; 146:598–603.

Part Four

CLINICAL ASPECTS

18

A Comparison of Inhaled Versus Oral Corticosteroids as Maintenance Therapy in Asthma

WILLIAM W. BUSSE

University of Wisconsin Medical School
Madison, Wisconsin

I. Introduction

Corticosteroids are potent anti-inflammatory compounds and form an important maintenance therapy for many patients with asthma. Fortunately for most patients with asthma, inhaled corticosteroids are sufficient to control symptoms, decrease the need for rescue treatment with β-agonists, and improve lung function. However, there are some individuals with asthma who have very severe disease and require prolonged use with oral corticosteroids. Although high-dose systemic corticosteroids are highly efficacious for acute asthma, there are the obvious safety concerns with long-term use of such an approach. In addition to the safety issues, there are questions as whether there are circumstances in which maintenance therapy with oral corticosteroids may be more effective than inhaled corticosteroids, or vice versa.

In the following discussion, the question of inhaled versus oral corticosteroids in the treatment of asthma will be examined in three areas. First, what are the findings of studies which have compared inhaled and oral corticosteroids as maintenance therapy of asthma? Second, are there circumstances in which oral and inhaled corticosteroids have been evaluated as to their ability either to prevent or control exacerbations of asthma? Finally, what is the effect of oral and inhaled corticosteroids on one characteristic of bronchial asthma; that is, airway hyperresponsiveness. From this discussion, it is hoped that some insight may be gained as to the relative roles of these forms of corticosteroid therapy in the treatment of asthma.

II. Comparison of Oral and Inhaled Corticosteroids

Bosman et al. (1) recently compared the effect of inhaled beclomethasone, 1000 µg twice per day, with oral prednisone, 10 mg daily, in the treatment of asthmatic patients. In this study, 17 patients were identified who had evidence of reversible airflow obstruction and active symptoms while on therapy with 800 µg per day of inhaled beclomethasone. In this study, baseline measurements of symptoms and pulmonary function were monitored for 2 weeks while on placebo therapy. Once a baseline level of disease activity was established, patients were then treated for 4 weeks with either 1000 µg of beclomethasone twice daily or placebo. Following this 4-week therapeutic regimen, there was a 4-week washout time; the patients were then crossed over to the second therapy, which consisted of 10 mg of prednisone per day and placebo inhaler. With this design, a number of significant observations were noted. First, no differences in FEV_1 (forced expiratory volume in 1 sec) values were found after treatment with either oral or inhaled corticosteroids. In contrast, however, morning peak flow rates were higher when the patients were taking the inhaled corticosteroids (Table 1). Third, airway responsiveness diminished in intensity on inhaled, but not oral, corticosteroids. Finally, there was no significant effect of either form of therapy on the basal cortisol level, although these values tended to be lower when the subjects took oral prednisone.

From these observations, it is apparent that oral and inhaled corticosteroids, in the doses administered, are equally efficacious when spirometry is the

Table 1 Mean ($\pm$SD) Lung Function After Treatment with Beclomethasone (BDP) and Prednisone

	BDP (1000 µg/day)		Prednisone (10 mg/day)		
	before	after	before	after	*P*
FEV_1 (% predicted)	85 $\pm$ 18	93 $\pm$ 18	86 $\pm$ 16	91 $\pm$ 15	NS
PEF (% predicted) AM	81 $\pm$ 18	92 $\pm$ 15	82 $\pm$ 15	86 $\pm$ 11	<0.05
PC_{20} histamine (geometric means)	0.28	0.76	0.27	0.43	0.06

Source: From ref. 1.

outcome variable. However, a number of other important parameters were more responsive to inhaled corticosteroids; these include early morning peak flow values and changes in airway responsiveness. Although it is possible to attribute the greater improvement in AM peak flow to timing the inhaled corticosteroid doses (doses administered twice a day), this does not fully answer the question. Since the AM peak flow value is a sensitive assessment of asthma control, improvement in this parameter may support an advantage for inhaled steroids. Furthermore, as will also become apparent in other studies, inhaled steroids are particularly effective on airway responsiveness.

In a study by Ilangovan and colleagues (2), the investigators identified 36 preschool children who were dependent on oral corticosteroids (minimum dose was 0.75 mg/kg/day prednisone on alternate days for at least 4 weeks) to control asthma symptoms. After the subjects were identified, the investigators had a "run-in" stabilization period during which the dose of prednisone was adjusted to achieve "minimum asthma symptom control." The subjects were then randomized to active treatment for 8 weeks with either budesonide, 1 mg twice a day be nebulizer, or placebo. During the 8 weeks of active treatment, the investigators attempted to reduce the oral corticosteroid dose by 25% per week if the subject was asymptomatic. Therapeutic efficacy was assessed by the reduction in oral corticosteroid dose and parental assessment of the children's health score. Because these children were small, pulmonary function measurements were not a practical outcome option. After 8 weeks of both placebo and inhaled budesonide, the investigators were able to reduce the corticosteroid dose, but the reduction was greater in those children receiving the active form of therapy; that is, inhaled budesonide. After the blinded portion of the study, the subjects, who received placebo therapy, were entered into an open label study and given inhaled corticosteroids. On the active medication, the patients were able to lower their dose of oral corticosteroids (Fig. 1).

The investigators (2) also found that health symptom scores improved significantly in those children on the active form of therapy. Higher health scores were also observed in placebo-treated children when they were switched to the nebulized budesonide. These studies in small children indicate that not only are large doses of inhaled corticosteroids effective replacement for systemic corticosteroids, but asthma symptom control was even better than on the systemic prednisone.

The study by Ilangovan et al. (2) does not address the question as to whether the systemic steroid effects of inhaled corticosteroids are dose dependent. In a study conducted by Hummel and Lehtonen and a large study group (3), a population of adult patients were identified who needed a prednisolone dose of 10–40 mg/day to control asthmatic symptoms. In their study, the identified subjects were first treated for 3 months with 300 µg/day of inhaled beclomethasone and an increasing dose of oral prednisolone to achieve asthma con-

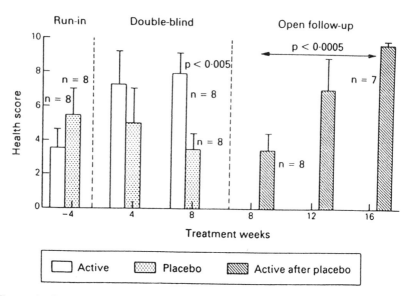

Figure 1   Dose of prednisolone by month (mg/kg/alternate day) showing a significant reduction for the group treated with budesonide during the double-blind period and the open follow-up period. Mean + SEM. (From ref. 2.)

trol. Asthma control was defined as peak expiratory flow rates greater than 60% predicted and less than 10 puffs per day of fenoterol. Following this run-in period, the subjects were randomized to either 1500 µg/day of inhaled beclomethasone or continuing on their present maintenance dose of 300 µg/day of beclomethasone for 6 months. The investigators found that treatment with either dose of inhaled corticosteroids was sufficient to allow the patients to lower their oral corticosteroid dose by an equivalent degree. Furthermore, the number of responders, defined as those having a greater than a 5 mg/day reduction in prednisone dose was the same. Similarly, the number of patients able to discontinue their oral prednisone altogether was equivalent.

These investigators (3) concluded that there does not appear to be an advantage, at least in this particular group of subjects, for high doses of inhaled corticosteroids to control asthmatic symptoms or reduce oral corticosteroids. These observations suggest that it is the inhaled dosing of corticosteroids rather than the dose of medications that determines efficacy. These observations also raise the possibility that some patients who require long-term oral corticosteroids may actually become refractory to larger doses of inhaled corticosteroids. Nonetheless, the collective observations of these investigators are further evidence that inhaled corticosteroids are effective in allowing patients to reduce systemic steroids without a loss of asthma control.

To extend such observations, Otolana and colleagues (4) identified 18 adult patients with stable asthma who required 7.5 mg/day of prednisolone. Conventional high-dose inhaled corticosteroid treatment had failed to decrease their oral corticosteroid requirements. Following an establishment of baseline measurements, the patients were given nebulized budesonide, beginning at 1 mg twice daily and progressing to 4 mg twice daily in an open-label study. These patients were then followed for a 12- to 18-month period of time. The investigators found FEV_1 values had a tendency to improve after therapy on the nebulized corticosteroids (1.9 $\pm$ 0.9 vs 2.2 $\pm$ 0.9 L). Furthermore, the need for hospital admissions (per year) decreased significantly, and the prednisolone dose was also reduced from a mean daily requirement of 17.8 $\pm$ 10 mg to 3.2 $\pm$ 6.7 mg (Table 2). These observations indicate that if sufficiently large doses of inhaled corticosteroids are administered, it is possible to maintain asthma control with inhaled corticosteroids, reduce systemic corticosteroids, and yet maintain equivalent levels of lung function.

Salmeron and colleagues (5) compared high doses of inhaled corticosteroids in patients with unstable but chronic asthma. In this study, 43 adult patients were identified and observed for 2 weeks to establish the level of disease activity. Oral corticosteroids were given for 2 weeks, at a dose of 0.5 mg/kg/day, to stabilize the patient's asthma. During the study period, which lasted 8 weeks, the patients were randomized to either placebo or beclomethasone, 1500 μg/day, if their disease was still active. The investigators noted that pulmonary functions improved following 2 weeks of oral corticosteroids. However, patients on placebo were unable to sustain improvement in pulmonary functions. In contrast, the patients receiving inhaled corticosteroids were able to maintain and stabilize asthmatic symptoms. Furthermore, the proportion of patients who were able to continue without worsening of asthma was also greater on beclomethasone treatment. Although not directly addressing the efficacy of oral versus inhaled corticosteroids, these observations suggest that inhaled corticos-

Table 2 Data Before and After Budesonide (( ) = P values))

FEV_1 (L)		Hospital Ad/Yr		Prednisolone (mg/day)	
before	after	before	after	before	after
1.9 $\pm$ 0.9	2.2 $\pm$ 0.9	1.5 $\pm$ 1.8	0.9 $\pm$ 1.1	17.8 $\pm$ 10.0	3.2 $\pm$ 6.7
	(0.06)		(0.05)		(0.00)

Source: From ref. 4.

teroids are sufficient to maintain control of asthma after this level of stabilization was achieved with oral corticosteroids. Such findings would indicate an
equal efficacy of 0.5 mg/kg/day with 1500 µg/day inhaled beclomethasone.

These cited studies provide valuable insights into the relative efficacy or
oral and systemic corticosteroids as maintenance therapy in asthma. First, in
most patients with stable asthma, it is possible to reduce systemic corticosteroids without a loss of asthma control. Second, there are components of asthma
that are more responsive to inhaled corticosteroids than systemic steroids, such
as airway responsiveness. Finally, maintenance therapy with inhaled corticosteroids may, in some individuals, give a better overall control of asthma (i.e.,
improved health score) than systemic steroid therapy.

III. Effect of Oral Versus Inhaled Corticosteroids in Preventing Infectious Exacerbations of Asthma

Respiratory infections are a significant cause of asthma exacerbations. A number
of studies have evaluated oral and inhaled corticosteroids for their ability to
prevent exacerbations of asthma with colds. These studies are meaningful for
our discussion, as they provide insight and evidence as to differences between
these two routes of corticosteroid administration on asthma.

Brunette and colleagues (6) studied children who had a history of asthmatic exacerbations with respiratory infections. In this study, 32 children were
identified who had experienced increased wheezing with respiratory infections
and had required two or more hospitalizations for these events. In this study,
the enrolled patients were divided into two groups. The first group received a
conventional form of therapy, primarily bronchodilators, and the other received
1 mg of prednisone per kilogram of body weight per day at the onset of virus-induced asthma. The relative effectiveness of prednisone intervention was
compared with events prior to enrollment into the blinded portion of study and
a conventional, nonsteroid, early intervention approach.

The investigators (6) found prednisone reduced the number of attacks of
asthma, days with wheezing, emergency room visits, number of hospitalizations,
and days of hospitalization (Table 3). Consequently, these investigators concluded that intervention with oral corticosteroids was effective in preventing
exacerbations of infectious symptoms of asthma.

Second, investigators addressed this question with another approach. Connett and Lenney (7) recruited children who wheezed with respiratory infections.
With the infectious wheezing, treatment was started with either budesonide 800
µg/day via nebuhaler or 600 µg/day via nebuhaler plus face mask. Treatment
was continued until the patients were symptom free. During another exacerbation with a respiratory infection, the patients were crossed over to placebo

Table 3 Effect of Prednisone Treatment on Virus-Induced Asthma

	Group I		Group II (prednisone/mg/kg/day)	
	(I)	(II)	(I)	(II)
Number of attacks	12.4 ± 2.0	12.3 ± 2.0	15.4 ± 3.5	6.6 ± 1.0
	(NS)		(P<.002)	
Number days with	89 ± 21	82 ± 18	65 ± 12	23 ± 6
wheezing	(NS)		(P<.001)	
Emergency room visits	9.1 ± 1.0	8.9 ± 0.6	9.3 ± 0.9	3.6 ± 0.6
	(NS)		(P<.001)	
Number of	5.8 ± 0.9	5.9 ± 0.7	7.6 ± 25	0.7 ± 0.2
hospitalizations	(NS)		(P<.001)	
Days of	25.1 ± 3.0	24.1 ± 2.5	23.4 ± 2.5	2.3 ± 0.8
hospitalization	(NS)		(P<.001)	

Source: From ref. 6.

therapy. The investigators did not find differences between the inhaled corticosteroid and placebo on daytime cough, nighttime cough or wheeze, or doses of terbutaline, or days of terbutaline. The only symptom showing any difference was a slight reduction in daytime wheeze. These observations would suggest that although initiation of inhaled corticosteroid can modify the severity of wheezing in children with asthma during a viral respiratory tract infection, the effects are modest.

In a subsequent study, Bisgaard and colleagues (8) examined the effect of inhaled budesonide on recurrent wheezing in early childhood. Seventy-seven children were recruited for study and all had recurrent wheezing. They ranged in age from 11 to 36 months. Although the causes of recurrent wheezing were not always identified, respiratory infections were felt to be a contributing factor in most situations. After recruitment, the 77 children were randomized to 12 weeks of treatment with either budesonide, 400 μg twice daily, or placebo. The investigators found a significant reduction in wheezy symptoms while on the active form of therapy. Furthermore, the percentage of days on oral corticosteroids was also less when the patients took the nebulized form of corticosteroid therapy. In this situation, the inhaled corticosteroids were capable of stabilizing the childhood symptoms of asthma and preventing exacerbations of asthma when a presumed viral illness occurred.

When asthma exacerbations follow respiratory infections, systemic corticosteroids appear to be more effective than inhaled forms. The reason for this is not clear but is an important clinical issue. These studies also suggest that an exacerbation of asthma by viral infections has a mechanism that is more responsive to corticosteroid effects that are achieved by systemic administration.

IV. Effects of Prednisone or Inhaled Corticosteroids on Airway Responsiveness

A cardinal feature of asthma is airway hyperresponsiveness. The intensity of airway hyperresponsiveness has been linked to airway inflammation. To evaluate the effectiveness of inhaled versus oral corticosteroids on bronchial responsiveness, Jenkins and Woolcock (9) identified 18 asthmatic patients who still had a significant degree of FEV_1 reversibility. Baseline measurements of airway responsiveness were obtained following a 3-week phase-in period. Following this, patients were treated in a double-blind fashion for 3 weeks with either inhaled budesonide (1200 µg/day) or oral prednisone (12.5 mg/day). Following treatment, airway responsiveness was reevaluated. Then the patients underwent another 3-week washout and were crossed over to the other form of treatment. Baseline lung functions improved on both the oral and inhaled corticosteroids. However, only inhaled corticosteroids improved airway responsiveness (Table 4). These observations suggest inhaled corticosteroids are more effective in reducing airway responsiveness and possibly airway inflammation.

In another study, Bhagat and Grustein (10) identified 10 children who ranged in age from 9 to 15 years of age. Methacholine challenges were done on three occasions: preenrollment, postplacebo therapy, and 1 week posttreatment with 60 mg of prednisone per day. The investigators found a significant decrease, or improvement, in airway responsiveness after 1 week of oral corticosteroids. Furthermore, they found a direct relationship with the percentage of improvement in airway responsiveness and the change in FEV_1 postbron-

Table 4 Comparison of BDP versus Prednisone on PD_{20} (µmol) to Histamine (Geometric Means)

Baseline		Oral steroid (prednisolone 12.5 mg/day)		Inhaled steroid (budesonide 1200 µg/day)	
Pre	Post	Pre	Post	Pre	Post
0.38	0.43	0.56	0.59	0.38	1.01
					(<0.01)

Source: From ref. 9.

chodilator. This raises the question, and possibility, that the efficacy of therapy may be directly related to the improvement in lung function.

V. Summary

Corticosteroids are highly effective forms of treatment in asthma. Although systemic steroids are essential for acute exacerbation of asthma, comparisons of maintenance treatment with oral or inhaled corticosteroids are less easy to identify. However, studies have indicated that inhaled steroids may be more effective than low-dose prednisone in the control of asthma. Furthermore, inhaled corticosteroids also appear to reduce airway responsiveness more effectively than oral products. These observations further underscore the importance of inhaled steroids in the treatment of asthma and the improved safety associated with their use.

Discussion

DR. SMALDONE: I have not been able to wean adult patients from daily chronic oral prednisone (i.e., 20 mg every day) by using high doses of aerosolized steroids. How long were your patients followed afterwards?

DR. BUSSE: In the study I referred to patients receiving inhaled budesonide were able to reduce the oral prednisone dose from a mean level of 19 mg/day to approximately 4 mg/day. However, not all individuals were able to reduce their oral steroid dose to that level. What determines the ability of patients to reduce their dose of prednisone is not clear.

DR. PEDERSEN: When you say high doses of inhaled steroids, what do you define as high and which steroids and inhaler (delivery systems) do you use to deliver these high doses?

DR. BUSSE: One milligram of flunisolide three to four times/day.

DR. HOWARTH: Perhaps with the United Kingdom where high-dose inhaled steroids have been available for a number of years, some anecdotal information may address your views that is difficult to get patients on oral steroids off treatment and that inhaled therapy is inadequate in asthma. We now see very few patients who require chronic therapy with oral as well as inhaled steroids, and this may relate to the early use of inhaled steroids. A recent study, which I am sure you will hear about from Paul O'Byrne, suggests that a delay in initiating inhaled steroids leads to a irreversible decline in the maximum achievable lung function.

DR. GLEICH: In a group of patients on optimal doses of topical glucocorticoids, after stopping the treatment how long does it take to see an exacerbation of symptoms? Do you have any data or impressions from your review of the literature?

DR. BUSSE: The protective or beneficial effect of inhaled corticosteroids on airway function is variable depending on the study. With a 1-year use of inhaled steroids in adults, the beneficial effects were beginning to be lost by 3 months. This can be seen in control of symptoms and airway responsiveness. Laitinen and colleagues have recently published observations on this question, and Dr. Laitinen can comment on their observations.

DR. LAITINEN: When we compared two groups of newly diagnosed asthmatics, one getting inhaled budesonide (*122* μg/day) and the other terbutaline (750 μg/day) for 2 years, inhaled corticosteroid treatment was superior in all parameters measured (Haahtela T, Järvineu M, Kava T, et al., Comparison of a B_2 agonist, terbutaline, with an inhaled corticosteroid, budesonide, in newly diagnosed asthma. N Engl J Med 1991; 352:388; and Haahtela T, Järvineu M, Kava T. Effects of reducing or discontinuing inhaled budesonide in patients with mild asthma. N Engl J Med 1994; 331:700.) We then divided the group receiving inhaled budesonide into two groups, one getting only placebo and the other a lower dose of budesonide (400 μg/day). In the group receiving the lower dose of budesonide, there was no change in lung function and bronchial reactivity. The group receiving placebo had decreased lung functions and increased bronchial reactivity after 1 year.

DR. HARGREAVE: Whether deterioration occurs when steroid treatment is reduced or stopped depends on whether the treatment is needed. In some studies in which steroid has been discontinued, there has been no deterioration. In short-term treatment which has improved airway responsiveness, stopping the treatment results in a return of responsiveness to baseline in 1 or 2 weeks. In the steroid reduction study of Gibson et al., an exacerbation of symptoms occurred between 7 and about 26 days. (Gibson PG, Wong BJO, Hepperle, MJE, et al. A research method to induce and examine a mild exacerbation of asthma by withdrawal of inhaled corticosteroid. Clin Exp Allergy 1992; 22:525–532.)

DR. SCHLEIMER: The literature indicates that oral steroids do not improve bronchial reactivity as well as inhaled steroids. What is your experience?

DR. BUSSE: We have not evaluated this question. There are observation from other groups.

DR. DURHAM: In our double-blind study of prednisolone, 40 mg/day for 2 weeks, we observed a marked improvement in airway methacholine responsiveness, compatible with that found by Dr. Woolcock following inhaled corticosteroid treatment. (Du Toit JI, Salome CM, Woolcock AJ. Inhaled corticosteroids reduce the severity of bronchial hyperresponsiveness in asthma but oral theophylline does not. Am Rev Respir Dis 1987; 136:1174–1178.) I think it is a question of dose and duration of treatment. (Robinson D, Hamid QQ, Ying S et al. Prednisolone treatment in asthma is associated with modulation of bronchoalveolar lavage cell IL-4, IL-5, and interferon-γ cytokine gene expression. Am Rev Respir Dis 1993; 148:401–406.)

DR. LEMANSKE: I would like to comment that with the inhaled corticosteroids currently available in the United States, it has been very difficulty to demonstrate a dose-response effect consistently. When a relationship can be shown, it is variable depending on the end point parameter one chooses to evaluate. For example, in a recent publication by Chervinsky et al., a dose-response effect of fluticasone could not be shown when FEV_1 was measured but could be shown with regard to drop out rates. (Chervinsky P, van As A, Bronsky EA, et al. Fluticasone propionate aerosol for the treatment of adults with mild to moderate asthma. J Allergy Clin Immunol 1994; 94:676–683.)

DR. ROCKLIN: A probable reason that the oral steroid-sparing study with budesonide did not show a dose response, whereas the dose-response study did relate to the range of doses employed in the two studies. The oral steroid-sparing study evaluated only a twofold difference in doses (800 and 1600 µg), whereas the dose-ranging study evaluated a eightfold range in doses (200 g–1600 µg).

DR. McFADDEN: Has the use of inhaled steroids in regular and/or high doses reduced the admission rates in asthma? Are such data available?

DR. PEDERSEN: In our long-term study, we find an 85% reduction in acute admissions in the children who received inhaled steroids. At present, we are evaluating our results in preschool children, and they seem to be very similar to those obtained in school children.

DR. HOWARTH: We have some information to address your question concerning asthma admissions. The Southampton health district has a population of 470,000. Asthma is largely managed within the community often with special asthma clinics and asthma nurses. The use of inhaled corticosteroids is high, with approximately 60–70% of patients receiving this mode of therapy. Last year we had just over 50 adult admissions for acute asthma. This figure is markedly down from admissions for adult asthma 10–20 years ago. I cannot comment on admissions for childhood asthma.

DR. SMALDONE: Is there a qualitative difference between oral and inhaled steroids for treating asthma?

DR. BUSSE: There have been previous comments that address this issue. Systemic corticosteroids appear to be more effective in acute, severe asthma. Furthermore, in some patients with more severe chronic disease, oral corticosteroids are needed to control the disease along with inhaled steroids. But whether there is a different site of action or different qualitative mechanisms of action between oral and inhaled is not established.

References

1. Bosman HG, vanUffelen R, Tamminga JJ, Paanakker LR. Comparison of inhaled beclomethasone dipropionate 1000 μg twice daily and oral prednisone 10 mg once daily in asthmatic patients. Thorax 1994; 49:37-40.
2. Ilangovan, P, Pedersen, S, Godfrey S, Nikander K, Noviski N, Warner JO. Treatment of severe steroid dependent preschool asthma with nebulised budesonide suspension. Arch Dis Child 1993; 68:356-359.
3. Hummel S, Lehtonen L, and Study Group. Comparison of oral-steroid sparing by high-dose and low-dose inhaled steroid in maintenance treatment of severe asthma. Lancet 1992; 340:1483-1487.
4. Otulana BA, Varma N, Bullock A, Higenbottam, T. High dose nebulized steroid in the treatment of chronic steroid-dependent asthma. Respir Med 1992; 86:105-108.
5. Salmeron S, Guerin J-C, Godard P, Renon D, Henry-Amar M, Duroux P, Taytard A. High doses of inhaled corticosteroids in unstable chronic asthma. Am Rev Respir Dis 1989; 140:167-171.
6. Brunette MG, Lands L, Thibodeau L-P. childhood asthma: Prevention of attacks with short-term corticosteroid treatment of upper respiratory tract infection. Pediatrics 1988; 81:624-629.
7. Connett G, Lenney W. Prevention of viral induced asthma attacks using inhaled budesonide. Arch Dis Child 1993; 68:85-87.
8. Bisgaard H, Munck SL, Nielsen JP, Petersen W, Ohlsson SV. Inhaled budesonide for treatment of recurrent wheezing in early childhood. Lancet 1990; 336:649-51.
9. Jenkins CR, Woolcock AJ. Effect of prednisone and beclomethasone diproprionate on airway responsiveness in asthma: a comparative study. Thorax 1988; 43:378-384.
10. Bhagat R, Grunstein MM. Effect of corticosteroids on bronchial responsiveness to methacholine in asthmatic children. Am Rev Respir Dis 1985; 131:902-906.

19

Inhaled Corticosteroids in Asthma: Importance of Early Intervention

PAUL M. O'BYRNE

McMaster University
Hamilton, Ontario, Canada

I. Introduction

Asthma is a disease characterized by the presence of symptoms such as dyspnea, wheezing, chest tightness, and cough. These symptoms are usually caused by airflow obstruction, which is characteristically variable. Asthmatics are also known to have airway hyperresponsiveness to a variety of chemical bronchoconstrictor stimuli and physical stimuli such as exercise and hyperventilation of cold dry air (1). This means that asthmatics require less of a bronchoconstrictor agonist to induce airway narrowing than normal individuals. In general, the severity of airway hyperresponsiveness is associated with the severity of asthma (2) and with the amount of treatment needed to optimally control symptoms of asthma (3). More recently, it has been recognized that asthmatic symptoms, variable airflow obstruction, and airway hyperresponsiveness occur as a consequence of a characteristic form of cellular inflammation and structural changes in the airway wall (4). The inflammation consists of the presence of activated eosinophils, lymphocytes, and an increased number of mast cells, which have been described both in bronchoalveolar lavage and airway biopsies from patients with mild stable asthma (5–8), as well as asthmatic patients with much more severe disease (9). Also, there are characteristic structural changes described in asthmatic airways, which appear to be characteristic of the disease and which are likely caused by persisting airway inflammation (9). These changes include patchy desquamation of the airway epithelium, thickening of the reticular collagen layer of the basement membrane (10), and airway smooth muscle hypertrophy.

For more than 100 years, airway inflammation has been known to be present in asthmatic airways (11); however, only recently has an emphasis been placed on treating airway inflammation (12) rather than the consequences of the inflammation, which is bronchoconstriction and asthmatic symptoms (13). The only antiasthma medications which have been demonstrated to improve airway inflammation (14,15), airway hyperresponsiveness (16,17), airflow obstruction, and symptoms (18) in asthmatics are corticosteroids. This evidence has been used as a rationale for using inhaled corticosteroids much earlier in the treatment of asthma then was previously the case, where they were suggested to be reserved as third or fourth line therapy for asthma, and only when bronchodilators were not providing control of asthma (13). This chapter considers the currently available evidence that inhaled corticosteroids should be used early in managing asthma as the initial regular treatment in patients with daily symptoms.

II. Objectives of Asthma Management

There have been several recent published consensus statements from a variety of countries on asthma management (12,19–21). These reports have been remarkably consistent in identifying the goals and objectives of asthma treatment. These are:

1. To minimize or eliminate asthma symptoms
2. To achieve the best possible lung function
3. To prevent asthma exacerbations
4. To do the above with the least possible medications
5. To educate the patient about the disease and the goals of management

One objective which is implied, but not explicitly stated, is the prevention of the decline in lung function and the development of fixed airflow obstruction which occurs in some asthmatic patients.

In addition to these goals and objectives, each of these reports has identified what is meant by the term *asthma control*. This includes the above objectives of minimal or no symptoms and best lung function, but it also includes minimizing the need for rescue medications, such as inhaled β_2-agonists to less than daily use, minimizing the variability of flow rates that is characteristic of asthma, as well as having normal activities of daily living. Achieving this level of asthma control should be an objective from the very first visit of the patient to the treating physician. Unfortunately, many studies suggest that this does not happen. This may be, in part, because the patient has learned to live with daily asthmatic symptoms and limitations in his or her daily activities and minimizes these to the physician. Alternatively, the idea of asthma control may not be widely accepted or understood by many physicians who see patients with asthma. This means that many (perhaps even most) patients with diagnosed asthma are not optimally controlled.

III. Reasons for Early Intervention with Inhaled Corticosteroids

Early intervention with inhaled corticosteroids in asthma means beginning this treatment as the first regular treatment used after a diagnosis is established. An argument for early intervention with inhaled corticosteroids could be made if one or more of the following conditions were met:

1. Inhaled corticosteroids were *more effective* than other regular treatment to achieve optimal asthma control and meet the other treatment objectives.
2. Inhaled corticosteroids prevented the decline in lung function over time that occurs in asthmatics.
3. Inhaled corticosteroids were safer than an *equally effective* treatment modality.
4. Inhaled corticosteroids were cost beneficial as an initial treatment of asthma, as measured by a benefit to the patient and/or to society by reducing the morbidity of asthma, which was not available by using any other medication.

Studies using inhaled corticosteroids have addressed all of these issues and these will be considered below.

IV. Efficacy of Early Intervention with Inhaled Corticosteroids

There is little debate in the literature that corticosteroids are the most effective treatment for asthma (22) and that the inhaled route is preferable to minimize unwanted effects. There is, however, considerable debate over the early use of inhaled corticosteroids in asthmatic patients considered to have mild asthma

(23). These patients are usually treated with regular inhaled β_2-agonists or oral theophylline or with drugs considered to be less clinically effective than inhaled corticosteroids, such as cromoglycate or nedocromil sodium. In a study of newly diagnosed asthmatics seen in speciality clinics, early intervention with the inhaled corticosteroid budesonide, was shown to be an effective first-line treatment when compared with an inhaled β_2-agonist, as indicated by reduced symptoms, improvements in lung function, and improvements in methacholine airway hyperresponsiveness (18). However, many patients considered to have mild asthma are not seen in speciality clinics but are managed in primary care practices. It is possible that these patients are, in fact, ideally controlled without the use of inhaled corticosteroids. To address this issue, we have recently examined the efficacy and cost-benefit of inhaled corticosteroids, supplemented with bronchodilators as needed, compared with bronchodilators alone as first-line treatment of asthma in primary care practice (24). The double-blind study compared budesonide, 400 μg/day, budesonide, 800 μg/day, and placebo in patients considered by their primary care physician to have such mild asthma that they would not derive any clinical benefit from inhaled corticosteroids. In this patient population in whom self-reported symptoms were mild at the start of the study, 40–60% of the patients were experiencing nocturnal or early-morning symptoms in the month before entering the study. These symptoms suggested that their asthma control was not optimal. The study demonstrated that inhaled budesonide, 400 μg/day, provided better asthma control and is cost beneficial when compared with bronchodilators alone in the management of these patients with mild asthma, and that no differences could be demonstrated between 400 and 800 μg/day of budesonide; however, the study could not detect differences between dosages had they been present. The percentages of patients experiencing daily symptoms fell to less than 10% over the course of the study in the budesonide treatment groups. Also, there was a mean 60–70 L/min increase in morning and evening peak expired flow rates and an elimination of exacerbations of asthma requiring emergency room management, indicating that a clinically useful improvement was achieved in this patient population with a dose of budesonide as low as 400 μg/day. This study supports the early intervention with inhaled corticosteroids for adult patients with regular daily symptoms of asthma, and suggests that low doses (budesonide, 400 μg/day or possibly less) are effective in the management of asthmatic patients with mild to moderate asthma. In addition, the study reinforces the need to strive for optimal control of asthma, and once control is achieved, to identify the minimum amounts of medication needed to maintain control. Last, this study has demonstrated that inhaled corticosteroid treatment are more cost beneficial than asthma therapy with bronchodilators alone.

V. Effects of Inhaled Corticosteroids on Lung Function over Time

Asthmatics lose lung function more rapidly than nonasthmatics, although less rapidly than cigarette smokers. In some asthmatics, this leads to severe, permanent, fixed airflow obstruction, with all of the attendant disability and handicap associated with this condition. A number of recent studies in both adults and children have demonstrated that inhaled steroids provide a protective effect against the deterioration in lung function seen with prolonged regular use of inhaled bronchodilator therapy alone. In one study, patients with asthma and patients with chronic obstructive pulmonary disease, previously treated with regular inhaled bronchodilators, were treated with inhaled beclomethasone, 800 μg/day, or placebo for 2 years (25). Prior to the addition of inhaled corticosteroids, the forced expired volume in 1 sec (FEV_1) had been declining at a rate of 160 ml/year. In the first 6 months of corticosteroid therapy, the FEV_1 *increased* by 460 ml and then continued to decline at a rate of 100 ml/year (significantly less than with bronchodilators alone). This protective effect of inhaled corticosteroids was most marked in the asthmatic patients, and it was associated with significant improvement in methacholine airway hyperresponsiveness in the asthmatic patients only and with decreased asthma symptoms and exacerbations.

A second, recently reported study, has addressed this issue in a different way (26). These investigators had previously reported that the treatment of newly diagnosed asthmatics with inhaled budesonide, 1200 μg/day for 2 years, improved asthma control as indicated by reduced symptoms, improvements in lung function, and improvements in methacholine airway hyperresponsiveness when compared with inhaled β_2-agonists (18). The patients receiving budesonide were subsequently randomly allocated to continuing for a third year on a lower dose of inhaled budesonide (400 μg/day) or placebo (26). The improvements in all parameters were maintained on the lower dose of budesonide but were lost on placebo. The patients who had previously been treated with inhaled β_2-agonists only were treated with the higher dose of inhaled budesonide for the third year, and although they improved in all parameters when compared with the first 2 years of treatment, the improvement in lung function or methacholine airway hyperresponsiveness was significantly less than that achieved by the subjects treated for the first year of the study with inhaled budesonide (Fig. 1). This suggests that these asthmatics had lost lung function which might have been preserved with the early use of inhaled corticosteroids.

A final study which supports these observations has been reported by Agertoft and Pedersen (27), who have studied two cohorts of asthmatic children for up to 7 years. One cohort had been treated with inhaled corticoster-

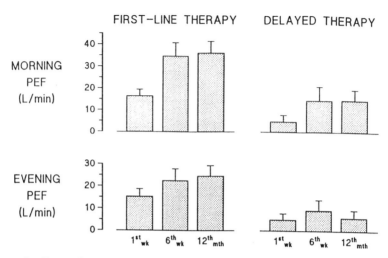

Figure 1 Comparison of the improvements in peak expired flow rates in patients with budesonide as first line therapy within one year of diagnosis of asthma and patients treated more than 2 years after diagnosis. (Redrawn and from ref. 26.)

oids shortly after diagnosis, whereas the other had received a variety of other antiasthma medications, including chromones, theophylline, and regular inhaled β_2-agonists but not inhaled corticosteroids. Some children in the second cohort were converted to inhaled corticosteroids, but on average 5 years after an initial diagnosis. These children in whom treatment with inhaled corticosteroids was started later did not achieve the level of lung function of the children treated early, even after 3 years of treatment with inhaled corticosteroids (Fig. 2). The study also measured growth velocity in these children and concluded that doses of inhaled budesonide up to 400 µg/day were not associated with a reduction in growth velocity. These studies, taken together, indicate that inhaled corticosteroids can diminish the decline in lung function that occurs in asthmatics, and suggests that early intervention with inhaled corticosteroids can optimize lung function in asthmatics.

VI. Safety of Early Intervention with Inhaled Corticosteroids

Inhaled corticosteroids are absorbed across the lung into the systemic circulation and do have effects beyond the lungs. Concerns about their systemic unwanted effects have greatly limited their use, especially in children. There are antiasthma medications, such as the chromones, which have no systemic unwanted effects. However, these drugs are, in general, not as effective in achiev-

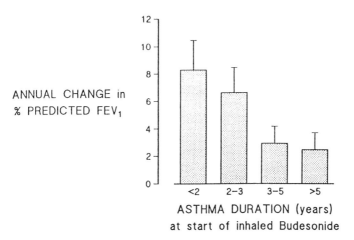

Figure 2 Influence of asthma duration at the start of inhaled budesonide upon the mean annual increase in FEV_1 seen after budesonide treatment. Mean values and 95% confidence intervals are shown. (Reproduced from ref. 27.)

ing optimal asthma control as are inhaled corticosteroids, nor have they been shown to prevent the decline in lung function in asthmatics. Another reason for recommending low doses of inhaled corticosteroids as first-line therapy for asthma is the recent concern about the safety of regular inhaled β_2-agonists. Sears et al. (28) have demonstrated deterioration in a number of parameters of asthma control and reduced the time to an asthma exacerbation (29) when the inhaled β_2-agonist fenoterol was used on a regular rather than intermittent basis. Also, retrospective studies have associated increased risk of asthma mortality with increased use of the β_2-agonist fenoterol (30,31) and salbutamol (31). Regular use of inhaled β_2-agonists has been demonstrated to increase airway responsiveness in asthmatics (32,33) and to result in loss of functional antagonism to the bronchoconstrictor effects of inhaled methacholine (34) and adenosine monophosphate (AMP) (35).

The unwanted effects of inhaled corticosteroids are dose related, with little or no evidence of clinically relevant unwanted effects at doses of < 400 μg/day of beclomethasone or budesonide in children and of < 1000 μg/day in adults (22). Fortunately, optimal asthma control can be achieved with these or lower doses in the majority of asthmatics. Indeed, the studies of Haahtela et al. (26), and Agertoft and Pedersen (27) have demonstrated that once optimal control is achieved by inhaled corticosteroids, it can be maintained by much lower doses. Therefore, drugs that are as effective as inhaled corticosteroids as first line therapy of asthma and have fewer unwanted effects do not currently exist.

VII. Cost-Benefit of Inhaled Corticosteroids

Until recently, few studies have examined the cost-benefit of early intervention with inhaled corticosteroids. However, several recent studies have demonstrated that inhaled corticosteroids are cost-beneficial when compared with other anti-asthma treatments. For example, Adelroth and Thompson (36) have shown that the costs to the Swedish health care system declined when patients were treated with inhaled corticosteroids because of a reduction in hospital utilization and physician visits when asthma control was optimized. Also, in the study by Cuddy et al. (24), a cost-effectiveness analysis of the use of inhaled corticosteroids in patients thought to have very mild asthma in primary care practice demonstrated an advantage with inhaled corticosteroids; again mainly by keeping patients out of hospital emergency rooms as asthma control is improved.

VIII. Summary

Inhaled corticosteroids are the most effective medications currently available to treat symptomatic asthma and are, fortunately, free of clinically relevant unwanted effects when used in the doses needed to provide optimal control in most asthmatics. Inhaled corticosteroids also improve the physiological abnormalities of variable airflow obstruction and airway hyperresponsiveness that characterize asthma as well as reducing the decline in lung function over time that occurs in asthmatics. Inhaled corticosteroids are also cost-beneficial when compared with other treatments even in patients with milder asthma treated in primary care. For these reasons, inhaled corticosteroids should be considered the first-line therapy for patients with regular, daily asthma symptoms, and they should be started early after a diagnosis is made rather than delaying until all other treatment options have been tried and not provided optimal control of asthma.

There are, however, several issues about the early intervention with inhaled corticosteroids that have not yet been resolved. One such issue is whether inhaled corticosteroids should be used in asthmatic patients who have very mild and infrequent symptoms or who develop symptoms only after being exposed to an inciting stimulus, such as exercise or cold air, and who have normal airway caliber most of the time. The current consensus statements do not recommend regular treatment in such patients, and this recommendation should be adhered to until more information is available about the natural history of asthma in such patients. These asthmatics do have evidence of airway inflammation and structural changes in airway biopsies (5–8); however, we do not yet know whether they lose lung functions more rapidly than nonasthmatics, or whether the morbidity of having very mild asthma warrants the use of regular treatment. Also, not enough is yet known about the long-term effects of even low doses of inhaled corticosteroids. Although the studies of Agertoft and Pedersen (27) has provided details of up to 7 years of treatment on some of the potential unwanted effects in children, these studies will need to be more prolonged before the concerns and fears of using inhaled corticosteroids very early in asthma will be allayed.

Discussion

Dr. Busse: Greening and colleagues (Greening AP, Ind, PW, Northfield, M, Shaw G. Added salmeterol versus higher-dose corticosteroids in asthma patients with symptoms on existing inhaled corticosteroids. Lancet 1994; 344:219–224) found that the addition of salmeterol to unstable asthma was more effective than an increased dose of inhaled corticosteroids. One interpretation of these data is that β-agonist can be protective against exacerbations of asthma. These studies also raise the question of why the long-acting β-agonists are capable of protective effects and precisely how this is accomplished.

Dr. O'Byrne: This study has demonstrated improvement in symptoms and peak flow rates in patients not optimally controlled on moderate doses of inhaled corticosteroids when treated with salmeterol with no increase in exacerbations.

Dr. Hargreave: There are two problems with the interpretation of Greening's study. First, if one is to compare the effect of a long-acting bronchodilator with a nonbronchodilator steroid, one needs also to examine the results in the latter group after bronchodilation has been produced by a short-acting bronchodilator. This was not done, and it is, therefore, is not surprising that the physiological measurements were higher in the salmeterol group. Second, if one wishes to examine the anti-inflammatory effects of a drug, one needs to measure whether inflammation is present or not. If it was not present in the steroid group, it would again not be surprising that this group would not show improvement. Indices of inflammation might be measured in future noninvasively by new methods of examination of sputum.

Dr. Busse: A good method to assess effectiveness of inhaled steroids is their action on exacerbation of disease. In some studies, inhaled steroids will prevent clinical exacerbations. In others, this protective effect is not noted and may relate to the intensity of the exacerbating stimulus; therefore, protective efficacy may be dose related. If the stimulus to disease is large, large doses of steroids would be necessary to provide protection.

DR. O'BYRNE: The clinical experience is that, for most asthmatics, the doses of inhaled corticosteroids can be reduced once optimal control is acheived. Therefore, there is little clinical evidence for receptor downregulation with regular use of inhaled corticosteroids.

DR. LAITINEN: Do asthmatics have to use inhaled corticosteroids for the rest of the their lives or would it be better to start as early as possible with a moderate dose and then introduce pauses in therapy? I refer to our recent study (26).

DR. O'BYRNE: I agree that this study and that of Agarloft and Pedersen (27) suggest that early intervention is useful and may protect against loss of lung functions. I am not aware of studies which have introduced passive therapy and looked at outcome.

DR. SZEFLER: Is there a significant difference between available inhaled glucocorticoids?

DR. O'BYRNE: There is little to choose between the various inhaled corticosteroids at low doses. At higher doses ($\geq$1000 µg/day), budesonide probably the slightly less risk of effects than BDP. Also, fluticasone is more potent microgram for microgram than either budesonide or BDP.

DR. BOCHNER: Are there studies available on the use of inhaled steroids in acute asthma?

DR. BUSSE: I am aware of one abstract which evaluated inhaled corticosteroids in acute asthma. The author found benefit from inhaled corticosteroids that were given in large doses and frequently. The concept is interesting but needs further evaluation.

References

1. Hargreave FE, Ryan G, Thomson NC, O'Byrne PM, Latimer K, Juniper EF, Dolovich J. Bronchial responsiveness to histamine or methacholine in asthma: measurement and clinical significance. J Allergy Clin Immunol 1981; 68:347–355.
2. Cockcroft DW, Killian DN, Mellon JJA, Hargreave FE. Bronchial reactivity of inhaled histamine: a method and clinical survey. Clin Allergy 1977; 7:235–243.
3. Juniper EF, Frith PA, Hargreave FE. Airway responsiveness to histamine and methacholine: relationship to minimum treatment to control symptoms of asthma. Thorax 1981; 36:575–579.
4. Djukanovic R, Roche WR, Wilson JW, Beasley CRW, Twentyman OP, Howarth PH, Holgate ST. State of the art: mucosal inflammation in asthma. Am Rev Respir Dis 1990; 142:434–457.
5. Kirby JG, Hargreave FE, Gleich GJ, O'Byrne PM. Bronchoalveolar cell profiles of asthmatic and nonasthmatic subject. Am Rev Respir Dis 1987; 136:379–383.

6. Beasley R, Roche WR, Roberts JA, Holgate ST. Cellular events in the bronchi in mild asthma and after bronchial provocation. Am Rev Respir Dis 1989; 139:806–817.

7. Jeffery PK, Wardlaw AJ, Nelson FC, Collins JV, Kay AB. Bronchial biopsies in asthma. An ultrastructural, quantitative study and correlation with hyperreactivity. Am Rev Respir Dis 1989; 140:1745–1753.

8. Kelly C, Ward C, Stenton CS, Bird G, Hendrick PJ, Walters EH. Number and activity of inflammatory cells in bronchoalveolar lavage fluid in asthma and their reaction to airway hyperresponsiveness. Thorax 1988; 43:684–692.

9. Dunnill MS, Massarell GR, Anderson JA. A comparison of the quantitative anatomy of the bronchi in normal subjects, in status asthmaticus, in chronic bronchitis and in emphysema. Thorax 1969; 24:176–179.

10. Roche WR, Beasley R, Williams JH, Holgate ST. Subepithelial fibrosls in the bronchi of mild asthmatics. Lancet 1989; 1:520–524.

11. Osler W. The Principals and Practice of Medicine. New York: Appleton, 1892:497.

12. National Heart, Lung, and Blood Institute, National Institutes of Health. Guidelines for the diagnosis and management of asthma. US Department of Health and Human Services Publication no. 91-3042, 1991.

13. Rebuck AS, Chapman KR. Asthma: 2. Trends in pharmacologic therapy. Can Med Assoc J 1987; 136:483–488.

14. Adelroth E, Rosenhall L, Johansson S-A, Linden M, Venge P. Inflammatory cells and eosinophil activity in asthmatics investigated by bronchoalveolar lavage. The effects of antiasthmatic treatment with budesonide or terbutaline. Am Rev Respir Dis 1990; 142:91–99.

15. Jeffery PK, Godfrey RW, Ädelroth E, Nelson F, Rogers A, Johansson S-Å. Effects of treatment on airway inflammation and thickening of the basement membrane reticular collagen in asthma. A quantitative light and electron microscopic study. Am Rev Respir Dis 1992; 145:890–899.

16. Juniper EF, Kline PA, Vanzieleghem MA, Ramsdale EH, O'Byrne PM, Hargreave FE. Effect of long-term treatment with inhaled corticosteroids on airway hyperresponsiveness and clinical asthma in nonsteroid dependent asthmatics. Am Rev Respir Dis 1990; 142:832–836.

17. Juniper E, Kline P, Vanzieleghem M, Hargreave F. Reduction of budesonide after a year of increased use: a randomized controlled trial to evaluate whether improvements in airway responsiveness and clinical asthma are maintained. J Allergy Clin Immunol 1991; 87:483–489.

18. Haahtela TH, Jarvinen M, Kava T, et al. Comparison of a β_2 agonist, terbutaline, with an inhaled corticosteroid, budesonide, in newly detected asthma. N Engl J Med 1991; 325:388–392.

19. Woolcock AJ, Rubinfeld A, Seale P, et al. The Australian asthma management plan. Med J Aust 1989; 151:650–653.

20. Hargreave FE, Dolovich J, Newhouse MT. The assessment and treatment of asthma: a conference report. J Allergy Clin Immunol 1990; 85:1098–1111.

21. British Thoracic Society, Research Unit of the Royal College of Physicians of London, King's Fund Center, National Asthma Campaign. Guidelines for management of asthma in adults: I—chronic persistent asthma. Br Med J 1990; 301:651–654.
22. Barnes PJ, Pedersen S. Efficacy and safety of inhaled corticosteroids in asthma. Am Rev Respir Dis 1993; 148:S1–S26.
23. Drazen J, Israel E. Treating mild asthma, when are inhaled steroids indicated? N Engl J Med 1994; 331:737–738.
24. Cuddy L, Taylor DW, Birch S, Morris J, Syrotuik J, O'Byrne PM. The clinical efficacy if inhaled corticosteroids as first line therapy for asthma in primary care practice. Am Rev Respir Dis 1992; 145:A420.
25. Dompeling E, Van Schayk CP, Van Grunsven PM, Van Herwaarden CLA, Akkermans R, Molema J, Folgering H, Van Weel C. Slowing the deterioration of asthma and chronic obstructive pulmonary disease during bronchodilator therapy by adding inhaled corticosteroids. Ann Intern Med 1993; 118:770–778.
26. Haahtela TH, Jarvinen M, Kava T, et al. Effects of reducing or discontinuing inhaled budesonide in patients with mild asthma. N Engl J Med 1994; 331:700–705.
27. Agertoft L, Pedersen S. Effects of long-term treatment with an inhaled corticosteroid on growth and pulmonary function in asthmatic children. Respir Med 1994; 88:373–381.
28. Sears MR, Taylor DR, Print CG, Lake DC, Li Q, Flannery EM, Yates DM, Lucas MK, Herbison GP. Regular inhaled beta-agonist treatment in bronchial asthma. Lancet 1990; 336:1391–1396.
29. Taylor DR, Sears MR, Herbison GP, Flannery EM, Print CG, Lake DC, Yates DM, Lucas MK, Li O. Regular inhaled β-agonists in asthma: effects on exacerbations and lung function. Thorax 1993; 48:134–138.
30. Crane J, Pearce N, Flatt A, Burgess C, Jackson R, Kwong T, Ball M, Beasley R. Prescribed fenoterol and death from asthma in New Zealand, 1981–83: case-control study. Lancet 1989; 1:917–922.
31. Spitzer WO, Suissa S, Ernst P, Horwitz RI, Habbick B, Cockcroft DW, et al. The use of β-agonists and the risk of death and near death from asthma. N Engl J Med 1992; 326:501–501.
32. Krahn J, Koeter, van der Mark TW, Sluiter HJ, de Vries K. Changes in bronchial hyperreactivity induced by 4 weeks of treatment with anti-asthmatic drugs in patients with asthma: a comparison between budesonide and terbutaline. J Allergy Clin Immunol 1985; 76: 628–636.
33. Vanthenen AS, Knox AJ, Higgins BG, Britton JR, Tattersfield AE. Rebound increase in bronchial responsiveness after treatment with inhaled terbutaline. Lancet 1988; 1:554–558.
34. Cheung D, Timmers MC, Zwinderman AH, Bel EH, Dijkman JH, Sterk PJ. Long-term effects of a long acting β_2-adrenoceptor agonist, salmeterol, on airway hyperresponsiveness in patients with mild asthma. N Engl J Med 1992; 327:1198–203.

35. O'Connor BJ, Aikman SL, Barnes PJ. Tolerance to the nonbronchodilator effects of inhaled β_2-agonists in asthma. N Engl J Med 1992; 327:1204–1208.
36. Adelroth E, Thompson S. Advantages of high dose budesonide (letter). Lancet 1988; 1:476.

20

Role of Glucocorticoids in the Therapy of Acute Asthma

E. R. McFADDEN, JR.

Case Western Reserve University School of Medicine
Cleveland, Ohio

I. Introduction

Asthma is a common disorder with immense medical and economical impacts. It is estimated that this disease affects 10–12 million people in the United States with costs in excess of 6 billion dollars per year (1). Most of the morbidity of asthma tends to be associated with acute exacerbations, and the treatment of these events accounts for the majority of expenditures in money and health care resources. Obviously, if one wishes to influence this situation in a favorable fashion, a critical evaluation of emergent care strategies and their outcomes would seem to be in order. One of the major difficulties with undertaking such a project is that the treatment of acute asthma has not been standardized, and although recommendations for the care of such patients have been published (2), they have little in the way of objective data to support their utility. No where is this lack of information more apparent than in the use of glucocorticoids. Despite 45 years of clinical experience which has produced a general consensus that these agents are of value in the therapy of acute asthma, such basic issues as to when to give them and the amounts to employ are still matters of considerable uncertainty.

II. General Considerations

Virtually every available glucocorticoid has been used systematically in the treatment of acute asthma, and there is little to suggest that one compound provides major therapeutic advantages over others at comparable doses (3–5). Thus, this issue is not an important pharmacological consideration. There are, however, differences in side effects and cost. Of the two injectable corticosteroids, methylprednisone and hydrocrotisone, the former has greater anti-inflammatory potency, lower mineralocorticoid activity, and is less expensive; hence, it should be the drug of choice for intravenous therapy. In the United States, prednisone is the most popular oral agent, whereas in other parts of the world, the use of prednisolone predominates. Compounds such as cortisone and prednisone need to be hydroxolated before they become active but, in the absence of severe liver disease, this is not a rate-limiting step. There are no data to indicate that these agents are any less effective than prednisolone or methylprednisolone, which do not need such conversion. Equally importantly, there is no evidence that chronic use leads to tachyphylaxis. There are no apparent differences in the manner in which steroid-dependent asthmatics, asthmatics naive to steroids and normal subjects bind, distribute, or metabolize glucocorticoids. Consequently, these factors need not be considerations in determining dosage.

III. Mechanisms of Action

The mechanisms by which steroids improve asthma are unknown. Those that are potentially important are a diminution in the numbers of circulating inflammatory cells, especially eosinophils, vasoconstriction of small vessels, and a reduction in the metabolism of arachidonic acid via the inhibition of phospholipase A_2 (6,7). Improving β-adrenergic function is often cited as a major activity, but there are few data in humans to support this position, and those that exist are contradictory (8–10). Irrespective of mechanisms, it is likely that the beneficial effects of glucocorticoids involve the synthesis of a new protein as a secondary messenger (see Chapter 1). Because of this, their onset of action is slow and does not develop until the requisite biological transformations occur.

It is important to keep in mind that glucocorticoids do not have any inherent bronchodilator properties and their administration does not decrease bronchial tone. Although several studies have implied that steroids in and of themselves can improve lung function in asthmatics over the course of several hours (11,12), these observations were only undertaken in a few asymptomatic individuals. Such effects have never been confirmed in symptomatic patients in any published series (3–5,9,13–19), and the available data overwhelmingly demonstrate that steroids do little to improve lung function rapidly in these circumstances. In fact, there is convincing evidence that glucocorticoids require a minimum of 6–12 hr to augment the action of bronchodilators and initiate significant improvements in pulmonary mechanics in patients experiencing acute exacerbations (4,5,9,13–15,18,19). This time delay fits well with the need to manufacture a new effector molecule via gene induction. This phenomenon in combination with the other pharmacological features discussed have several important clinical implications. First, the use of corticosteroids as single agents for the treatment of acute asthma is unacceptable. These drugs do not influence existing obstruction; rather they seem to prevent or limit new airway pathology from developing and, therefore, they will not ameliorate the patient's discomfort unless other agents are employed to reverse the airway narrowing already present. Second, steroids are slow working. For reasons to be discussed, they are not needed in the vast majority of patients who present for emergency care. In the minority where glucocorticoids may be important, one cannot rely on them as the prime drug. It is imperative to continue aggressive bronchodilator treatment until the steroids take effect. Since the airway narrowing of acute asthma is a process that is inherently reversible with bronchodilators, the most one sees with the addition of steroids is an improvement in the rate of recovery many hours after the initiation of therapy. An abrupt increase in lung function early in the course of treatment has never been found with any dose of corticosteroids despite being repetitively sought (4,5,9,13–20). Third, because of the existence of a secondary messenger system there is no correlation between glucocorticoid blood levels and the therapeutic response. Although it is likely that a minimum level is required before any beneficial effect is seen, there are no data as to how much this should be. It has been suggested that quantities of plasma cortisol greater than 100 µg/100 ml are necessary (13), but it is unclear where this value fits in terms of an overall dose-response effect.

IV. Influence of Glucocorticoids in the Resolution of Acute Asthma

Since 1956 until the present their have been 15 papers that have appeared in the English language that have explored the effects of glucocorticoids on the resolution of acute attacks of asthma (3,4,9,13–16,21–28). Only six of these studies have included a placebo arm (9,15,16,21,22,28). The remainder made the assumption that glucocorticoids were of proven worth and sought only to find differences between amounts of active drug. Of the placebo-controlled trials, two found steroids to add to the effects of bronchodilators (15,21) and four did not (9,16,21,22,28). The positive studies involved reasonably long periods of observation, employed appropriate comparison groups, used reliable and reproducible endpoints, and demonstrated that patients with acute obstruction respond favorably to glucocorticoids if followed for sufficient time. One effort is particularly important for the study design it employed eliminated many of the potentially confounding variables in other trials (15). Before randomization to hydrocortisone or placebo, this work first demonstrated that all of the participants where unresponsive to aggressive therapy with methylxanthines and sympathomimetics for 8 hr (15). In this study, the effect of glucocorticoids on pulmonary mechanics did not become manifest for 12 hours. At this point, the FEV_1 (forced expiratory volume in 1 sec) rose from a baseline of 25% to 40% of predicted. After 24 hr of hydrocortisone, it increased further to 55% of normal. The placebo group was also improving and had the study been carried out further, it is likely that both groups would have eventually coalesced (21).

In some of the negative trials (9,16), the quantity of steroids administered may have been too small and/or the subjects followed for insufficient periods to have shown a response (29). In other efforts, the results are clouded by the study design. For example, in one recent publication, intravenous doses of methylprednisolone equivalent to 60 and 300 mg/kg/24 hr of hydrocortisone did not perform any better than placebo (28). However, the investigators also gave undisclosed quantities of oral steroids to a significant portion of the participants in each of the three experimental arms (low and high methylprednisolone and placebo). By using this extra medication, they contaminated the study by changing the doses in the active arms and compromised the integrity of their controls. Such confounding factors materially limit the impact of the conclusions reached. Studies that avoided these irregularities have not found similar results (29).

Problems with experimental design are clearly not the only explanation for the negative findings in the literature. Luksza (22), in a well-controlled trial, which contrasted the effects of a high and low dose of hydrocortisone with placebo, concluded that steroids may not be effective in status asthmatics. He followed his subjects for an appropriate period, but his low-dose regimen would not have provided adequate treatment as judged by the findings of the MRC trial (21) and Fanta and associates (15). There is no ready explanation, however, as to why the high (1200 mg) dose of hydrocortisone did not have any effect. One possible reason may have been the severity of the obstruction in Luksza's patients. Four of the 10 individuals who received this dose required ventilatory assistance. The observed response may also have been influenced by the nature of the obstruction. We have data that suggests the airway narrowing in status asthmaticus is not due only to simple smooth muscle contraction. Other elements of inflammation such as plasma exudation, airway wall edema, and failure to eliminate an increased secretory load all play a role. Few of the current drugs, including steroids, work well in these circumstances. It seems that the inflammatory cascade leading to this state of affairs needs to be interrupted before the pathological end results can be eliminated. It may be that the early stages of inflammation are the most amenable to glucocorticoids.

V. Dose-Response Relationships

A current clinical approach is to treat acutely ill asthmatics with high doses of glucocorticoids to facilitate resolution. Although this approach is intuitively appealing, there are no data to support it. The literature demonstrates that dose-response relationships do not exist and that there is nothing to suggest that very high quantities of glucocorticoids are more efficacious than smaller ones. The 10 studies that have examined this question have used quantities of steroids ranging from 4 to 300 mg hydrocortisone/kg/24 hr (3,9,14,22–28), and only 1 study has found a relationship between medication amounts and clinical effect (14). Unfortunately, this work is flawed. Haskell and colleagues (14) gave 15, 40, and 125 mg of methylprednisolone at 6 hourly intervals and reported that lung function improved significantly in the high-dose group by the end of the first 24 hr, but that such changes did not develop in those given the medium dose until the middle of the second day. The low-dose group did not change significantly from its presteroid baseline over the 3-day period of observation. Reanalysis of these data, however, demonstrates that no statistical comparisons were made between doses using all of the data at each observation period, and it does not appear that any major differences existed among the various doses during the first day or between the high and medium quantities at any time. In the remaining trials in the literature, variations in medication amounts from 3- to 21-fold have not produced even a semblance of a dose-response effect (3,9,22–28).

What dose should one use in emergent situations? In composite, the published data indicate that 10–15 mg/kg/24 hr of hydrocortisone, or its equivalent, may be appropriate for acutely ill asthmatic adults. This translates into a total of approximately 600–900 mg of hydrocortisone, 150–225 mg of prednisone, or 120–180 mg of methylprednisolone per day for an average adult. All of these are very large amounts, and one cannot help but wonder if they are needed. Clinical experience suggests that smaller quantities may work; however, there are no objective data that demonstrate this to be the case. For maximum therapeutic benefit, treatment should be maintained for 36–48 hr depending on the patient's condition (3–5,14,15,20,24,25). Since the duration of action of glucocorticoids in acute asthma is unknown, either constant administration or periodic dosing over 24 hr is currently required in the acute phase. There are no data as to whether a continuous intravenous infusion or an intermittent bolus technique is more effective, but given that oral and parenteral administration have been shown to produce the same results (25–30), this is unlikely to be an important issue.

VI. Timing of Administration

The goal in treating acute asthma is to eliminate the patient's symptoms and improve lung function as quickly as possible with a minimum of side effects. For some, this means the early administration of glucocorticoids. In emergency departments, circles it is in vogue to give glucocorticoids as first-line treatment to all symptomatic asthmatics on presentation in an effort to reduce admissions (31,32) and/or to prevent relapse after discharge (33). Although this seems like a good idea, the data base supporting it is not very firm and is predicted on several unfounded assumptions that the pathogenesis of an asthmatic attack and recovery. There is nothing to suggest that the sequence of events that produces an acute episode of asthma continues to be operational after the attack is over, or that it unfavorably alters airway reactivity. If it did either, asthma morbidity would be an ever-expanding exponential function for anything that produced an attack would produce another and so forth. This simply does not happen. Finally, there are no data that steroids prevent acute exacerbation from occurring with any known precipitant. They may decrease airway reactivity and alter late reactions in the laboratory, but they do not block the development of acute obstruction. In this context, it seems appropriate to evaluate critically the literature that the first study purporting to show an advantageous effect of steroids on acute asthma morbidity and admission rates in adults was essentially uncontrolled. It did not standardize either the quantity or duration of care given in the emergency department and did not find any significant differences in pulmonary function between the steroid and control groups (30). A trial in children suggested that a single dose of prednisone would reduce the need for hospitalization (32), but here too the study design limited the confidence that one could place in the conclusions. Endpoints were not defined, nor was bronchodilator administration standardized. Although positive results were claimed in this work, there were no significant differences between the admission rates for the placebo- and steroid-treated groups as a whole. The investigators suggested that only the patients with the most severe disease benefitted from prednisone. This suggestion, if valid, is in stark contrast to the situation in adults (see below). When trials such as the above are undertaken with rigorous controls, the results are unrewarding (34).

Negative observations are not all that surprising. We know from serial studies using managed care paths in 529 acutely ill asthmatics in the emergency department and 120 inpatients with status asthmaticus that only 20% of patients with acute asthma will require admission to hospital and that the remainder can be discharged within 2 hr of initiating treatment with β_2-agonists (35). Thus, glucocorticoids are unnecessary in the vast majority of cases, and even if they given immediately on entrance into the emergency department, their slow onset of action would preclude them from playing any role in facilitating resolution if adequate amounts of bronchodilators are used.

What of the remaining 20%? Will steroids help them with any degree of immediacy? Here too, the answer appears to be negative. These patients responded poorly in the emergency department to nebulized sympathomimetics, methylxanthines, and parasympatholytics and by definition had status asthmaticus which required inpatient care to resolve. Intravenous steroids did not have any appreciable influence on their emergency department stay or rate of improvement. More importantly, despite very aggressive use of all available bronchodilators in combination with high-dose glucocorticoids, these patients required on average hospital stay of 4+ days to ameliorate their symptoms. In this group, rapid resolution was not forthcoming with any combination of drugs.

VII. Prevention of Recurrences

The issue as to whether steroids will prevent or minimize acute episodes of asthma from recurring is also not clear. In our studies, patients must meet well-defined criteria before they can be released from the emergency department. In these circumstances, we experience a 2% return rate within 24 hr and an additional 1% over the next 6 days (35). Clearly the first are recurrences and we have been able to trace them, in the main, to protocol violations. The reason for the late resolutions are far less obvious. The prevalence of recurrences following acute therapy in the emergency department in the general asthmatic population is unknown; however, even if it is far more common than we see, the impact of glucocorticoids given prior to release is at best questionable. Again, the study designs of the works recommending such an approach are not optimal (36,37). In one study, no objective assessments of patient improvement or lung function were presented (36), and in the other study, the emergency department treatment was not standardized and a significant portion of the study population was lost to follow-up (37). Others have concluded that steroids work in this capacity, but again analysis of the measured parameters in these trials does not confirm much benefit (38,39). Some of these deficits were corrected in a recent report when patients were carefully followed for 2 weeks with serial pulmonary function measurements and symptom diaries (33). The investigators concluded that an 8-day course of prednisone significantly reduced the rate of recurrence during the first 2 days following the emergency visit. Analysis of these data, however, show a curious pattern. The differences in relapse rates were most marked between days 4 and 10, and there were no significant differences between groups after this time, or perhaps, before it.

VIII. Summary

Few would doubt that glucocorticoids are an important part of the therapeutic armamentarium for asthma. Their use in acute situations has a long history, but much of the fundamental pharmacology still remains poorly defined. Dose-response relationships have been sought in numerous studies but have not been found. Hence, the minimum effective dose is unknown as are the factors that modulate the response. The use of steroids in emergent situations to reduce admissions and/or the frequency of recurrences, although popular, still remains controversial. Unfortunately, much of the confusion surrounding the role of glucocorticoids in the treatment of asthma will remain until the acute care for this disease is standardized so that the effects of various interventions can be isolated and studied individually.

Acknowledgments

Supported in part by Specialized Center of Research Grant (SCOR) HL-37117 from the National Heart, Lung and Blood Institute and General Clinical Research Center Grant MO1 RR00-80 from the National Center for Research Resources.

Discussion

DR. BARNES: There is a striking contrast between the good response of moderate exacerbations to a course of oral steroids given at home, yet glucocorticoids have little or no effect in the acute severe exacerbations in hospital despite the fact that these patients are likely to have a severe inflammation. It is possible that high doses of β-agonists given in hospital induce a resistance to the anti-inflammatory action of steroid, and this requires further study.

DR. McFADDEN: This is certainly one possibility. Another, of course, is the fact that the inflammation may be different or that the magnitude of the changes in the airway have reached a point where steroids can no longer interfere with them. All of these are important issues to address.

DR. BUSSE: The histology of severe asthma reveals very severe compromise in the airways with exudation of proteinaceous material in the lumen, injury to epithelium, and infiltration of inflammatory cells into the submucosa. Is it possible that the use of corticosteroids in this situation prevents further injury to the airway and thus allows for a recovery of this lesion? Furthermore, the recovery of this process is slow and the potential benefit from steroids is to prevent continued progression of the disease.

DR. McFADDEN: I accept your point. It would be critical to perform the appropriate investigations to determine whether steroids make a difference in the recurrence rate of such individuals once they leave the emergency room or hospital. We are in the process of performing that study. As yet, we do not have any data to share with you.

DR. O'BYRNE: The studies which have modeled airway structure and functions in asthma suggest that airway smooth muscle thickness is the most important structural change responsible for airway hyperresponsiveness. It is presently unknown how important the subbasement membrane collagen deposition is in relation to the smooth muscle in changing airway function.

DR. DURHAM: There is one study that showed a dose-response effect of oral prednisolone (0.2, 0.4, and 0.6 mg/kg for 10 days) in patients developing asthma exacerbations in an outpatient setting. (Webb JR Dose response of patients to oral corticosteroid treatment during exacerbations of asthma. Br Med J 1986; 292:1045-1047.) I suspect the reason for the discrepancy in the effects of steroids on acute asthma (and changes in airway responsiveness) relate to the asthma severity and the dose and duration of steroid used in different studies.

DR. McFADDEN: I agree with your comment. There are no data of which I am aware that relate the effects of steroids to asthma severity in acute situations. In chronic asthma, as you know, the more severe patients do less well on inhaled and perhaps oral steroids. This is another area that requires investigation before we can resolve these important clinical issues.

DR. HARGREAVE: Failure to respond to glucocorticoids may be due to differences in types of inflammation. For example, Fahy reported severe exacerbations with sputum neutrophilia (which might not respond to steroid therapy). (Fahy JV, Kim KW, Liu J, Boushey HA. Prominent neutrophilic inflammation in sputum from subjects with asthma exacerbation. J Allergy Clin Immunol 1995; 95:843-852).

DR. McFADDEN: As I indicated earlier, I agree that the degree and/or type of inflammation may not be the same in patients at different points in their disease process. All that I am attempting to show is that there is a group of patients who present to an emergency room at various periods in their illness who are very resistant to therapy for relatively short periods of time. At other times in their natural history, they respond quite well to bronchodilators.

DR. GLEICH: Several comments. First, we have conducted several analyses of the pathology of asthma. In studies of asthma deaths using autopsy tissues in Rochester, Minnesota, we found the classic pathological markers of the disease. More recently, in analyses of fatal asthma in conjunction with Dr. Bruce Hyme, the Dade County Medical Examiners officer, Dr. S. Su in our laboratory found a difference in the relative frequencies of eosinophils and neutrophils depending on the time between the onset of the attack and death; neutrophils were more frequent in tissues from patients dying up to 2 hr and eosinophils were more frequent in tissues after 2 hr. One could query whether glucocorticoids alter these pathological patterns. One can also query why the predominant neutrophil infiltrate occurs. Is it due to an acute allergenic insult? Is it due to inhalation of endotoxin-laden particles? Clearly this is an area where we need further information. Third, I have been impressed at the pathological findings in patients who died of asthma after repeated visits to the emergency room. For example, one patient I reviewed had been turned away from the emergency room, because she was believed to be neurotic. At autopsy, her bronchial tree showed classic and quite marked changes of asthma. I mention this point because I suspect that many believe that the pathology of asthma is particularly marked in patients who die. I submit the comparable degrees of abnormality are present in patients with flares of chronic asthma.

Dr. McFadden: At present, we have a relatively small data base to compare the pathology of asthma at various stages of activity. Deaths still remain relatively uncommon, and although many people are doing biopsies, they tend to do them in individuals with mild disease. Therefore, rigorous comparisons of pathology can not be undertaken. We absolutely need data on these points if we are going to make any sense out of how inflammation ties into clinical disease.

Dr. Howarth: I enjoyed your talk, it is a very elegant data base you have established. From this is it possible to answer whether the speed of recovery is related to duration of deterioration? (That is, Do those who respond to β-agonists only have a short history where those patients with a progressive slow decline over weeks before presenting take longer to recover, consistent with Bill Russe's point that these patients have established structural changes that take time to respond?)

Dr. McFadden: I cannot answer your question specifically. Work that we have done in the past shows that there are no relationships between the duration of an asthma attack and the presenting signs and symptoms or response to therapy. Because of this, we have not critically looked at those variables in the current sample. However, it would be important to reexamine the data. Thank you for your suggestion.

Dr. Liu: Were there differences in the type or amount of medications used prior to the emergency room visit between patient who were admitted to the hospital and those sent home?

DR. MCFADDEN: There are no discernible differences in the type or amount of medication used prior to the emergency room visit in those who were admitted or sent home.

DR. THOMPSON: What objective means will you use to evaluate compliance in your studies on the value of steroids taken at home to prevent or reduce repeated asthma attacks?

DR. MCFADDEN: We hope to overcome the issue of compliance by following the patients closely. One of my associates, Dr. Ileen Gilbert, has recently begun to work with physicians in the inner city to set up an asthma program that has direct contact with the patients leaving our emergency room. We also hope to make home visits to assess patient status. Our plans are to follow the people who leave the hospital and the emergency department at regular intervals and measure their lung function. We also hope to be able to have them fill our quality of life and symptom questionnaires.

References

1. Weiss KB, Gergen PJ, Hodgson TA. An economic evaluation of asthma in the United States. N Engl J Med 1992; 326:862–866.
2. Overview of approaches to asthma therapy. In: Guidelines for the Diagnosis and Management of Asthma: National Asthma Education Program expert panel report. Bethesda, MD, Department of Health and Human Services, 1991:89–115 (NIH publication no. 91-3042).
3. Britton MG, Collins JV, Brown D, et al. High-dose corticosteroids in severe acute asthma. Br Med J 1976; 2:73–74.
4. Sue MA, Kwong FK, Klaustermeyer WB. A comparison of intravenous hydrocortisone, methylprednisolone, and dexamethasone in acute bronchial asthma. Ann Allergy 1986; 56:406–409.
5. Pierson WE, Bierman CW, Kelley VC. A double-blind trial of corticosteroid therapy in status asthmatics. Pediatrics 1974; 54:282–288.
6. Baigelman W, Chodosh S, Pizzuto D, Cupples LA. Sputum and blood eosinophils during corticosteroid treatment of acute exacerbations of asthma. Am J Med 1983; 75:929–936.
7. Flowers RJ. Lipocortin and the mechanism of action of the glucocorticoids. Br J Pharmacol 1986; 94:987–1015.
8. Ellul-Micallef R, Fenech FF. Intravenous prednisolone in chronic bronchial asthma. Thorax 1975; 30:312–315.
9. McFadden ER Jr, Kiser R, DeGroot W, Holmes B, Kiker R, Visir G. A controlled study of the effect of single doses of hydrocortisone on the resolution of acute attacks of asthma. Am J Med 1976; 60:52–59.
10. Molema J, Lammers J-WJ, van Herwaarden CLA, Folgering H. Effects of inhaled

beclomethasone dipropionate on β_2-receptor function in the airways and adrenal responsiveness in bronchial asthma. Eur J Clin Pharmacol 1988; 34:577-583.

11. Ellul-Micallef R, Borthwick RC, McHardy GJR. The time-course of response to prednisolone in chronic bronchial asthma. Clin Sci Molec Med 1974; 47:105-117.

12. Klaustermeyer WB, Hale FC. The physiologic effect of an intravenous glucocorticoid in bronchial asthma. Ann Allergy 1976; 37:80-86.

13. Collins JV, Clark TJH, Brown D, Townsend J. The use of corticosteroids in the treatment of acute asthma. Q J Med 1975; 174:259-273.

14. Haskell RJ, Wong BM, Hansen JE. A double-blind, randomized clinical trial of methylprednisolone in status asthmaticus. Arch Intern Med 1983; 143:1324-1327.

15. Fanta CH, Rossing TH, McFadden ER Jr. Glucocorticoids in acute asthma, a critical controlled trial. Am J Med 1983; 74:845-851.

16. Ramsdell JW, Berry CC, Clausen JL. The immediate effects of cortisol on pulmonary function in normals and asthmatics. J Allergy Clin Immunol 1983; 71:69-74.

17. Kattan M, Gurwitz D, Levison H. Corticosteroids in status asthmaticus. J Pediatr 1980; 96:596-599.

18. Storr J, Barrell E, Barry W, et al. Effect of a single oral dose of prednisolone in acute childhood asthma. Lancet 1987; 2:879-882.

19. Harfi H, Hanissian AS, Crawford LV. Treatment of status asthmaticus in children with high doses and conventional doses of methylprednisolone. Pediatrics 1978; 61:829-831.

20. Younger RE, Gerber PS, Herrod HG, et al. Intravenous methylprednisolone efficacy in Status Asthmaticus of childhood. Pediatrics 1987; 80:225-230.

21. MRC subcommittee on clinical trials in asthma: Controlled trial of effects of cortisone acetate in status asthmaticus. Lancet 1956; 2:803-806.

22. Luksza AR. Acute severe asthma treated without steroids. Br J Dis Chest 1982; 76:15-19.

23. Tanaka RM, Santiago SM, Kuhn GJ, et al. Intravenous methylprednisolone in adults in status asthmaticus, comparison of two dosages. Chest 1982; 82:438-446.

24. Raimondi AC, Figueroa-Casa JC, Roncoroni AJ. Comparison between high and moderate doses of hydrocortisone in the treatment of Status Asthmaticus. Chest 1986; 89:832-835.

25. Ratto D, Alfaro C, Sipsey J, et al. Are intravenous corticosteroids required in status asthmaticus? JAMA 1988; 260:527-529.

26. Engel T, Dirksen A, Frolund L, et al. Methylprenisolone pulse therapy in acute severe asthma. A randomized, double-blind study. Allergy 1990; 45:224-430.

27. Bowler JD, Mitchell CA, Armstrong JG. Corticsterstoids in acute severe asthma: effectiveness of low doses. Thorax 1992; 47:584-587.

28. Morell F, Orriols R, de Gracia J, Curull V, Pujol A. Controlled trial of intravenous corticosteroids in severe acute asthma. Thorax 1992; 47:588-591.

29. Ling H, Landau LI, Le Souef, PN. Lack of efficacy of single-dose prednisolone in moderately severe asthma. Med J Australia 1994; 160:701-704.

30. Harrison BDW, Hart GJ, Ali NJ, et al. Need for intravenous hydrocortisone in addition to oral prednisolone in patients admitted to hospital with severe asthma without ventilatory failure. Lancet 1986; 1:181-184.

31. Littenberg B, Gluck EH. A controlled trial of methyprednisolone in the emergency treatment of acute asthma. N Engl J Med 1986; 314:150–152.
32. Scarfone RJ, Fucks SM, Nager AL, Shane SA. Controlled trial of oral prednisone in the emergency department treatment of children with acute asthma. Pediatrics 1993; 92:513–518.
33. Chapman KR, Verberk PR, White JG, Rebuck AS. Effect of a short course of prednisone in the prevention of early relapse after the emergency room treatment of acute asthma. N Engl J Med 1991; 324:788–794.
34. Stein LM, Cole RP. Early administration of corticosteroids in emergency room treatment of acute asthma. Ann Intern Med 1990; 112:822–827.
35. McFadden R Jr., Elsanadi N, Dixon L, Takacs M, Deal EC, Boyd KK, Idemoto BK, Broseman LA, Panuska JR, Hammons T, Smith B, Caruso F, McFadden CB, Shoemaker L, Warren EL, Hejal R, Strauss L, Gilbert IA. Protocol therapy for acute asthma: therapeutic benefits and cost savings. Am J Med 1995; 99:651–661.
36. Fiel SB, Swartz NA, Glanz K, Frances ME. Efficacy of short-term corticosteroid therapy in outpatient treatment of acute bronchial asthma. Am J Med 1983; 75:259–262.
37. McNamara RM, Rubin, JM. Intramuscular methylprednisolone acetate for the prevention of relapse in acute asthma. Ann Emerg Med 1993; 22:1829–1835.
38. Shapiro GG, Furukawa CT, Pierson WE, Gardinier R, Bierman CW. Double-blind evaluation of methylprednisolone versus placebo for acute asthma episodes. Pediatrics 1983; 71:510–514.
39. Harris JB, Weinberger MM, Nassif E, et al. Early intervention with short courses of prednisone to prevent progression of asthma in ambulatory patients incompletely responsive to bronchodilators. J Peds 1987; 110:627–633.

21

Corticosteroids in the Treatment of Allergic Rhinitis

PETER H. HOWARTH

University Medicine
Southampton General Hospital
Southampton, England

I. Introduction

Allergic rhinitis is an inflammatory condition of the nasal mucosa characterized by the symptoms of nasal itch, sneeze, rhinorrhea, and nasal stuffiness. There is also often an impairment of the sense of smell in more chronic disease. The symptoms arise in individuals on exposure to agents to which they are sensitized. These are commonly proteins present in aeroallergens such as pollens, mite fecal particles, or animal danders. Sensitization will also occur in individuals with occupational disease in whom there may be hypersensitivity to either proteins in the work environment related, for example, to laboratory animals or latex, or to chemicals such as low molecular weight compounds, including toluene diisocyanate.

In allergic disease, the generation of symptoms during continuous allergen exposure is associated with the development of nasal mucosal inflammation. In individuals with aeroallergen hypersensitivity, this relates to an interaction on the nasal mucosal surface between a foreign protein and cell surface–bound immunoglobulin E (IgE)(1). Nasal smear, nasal lavage, and nasal biopsy studies have helped elucidate the pathological processes underlying the clinical and physiological changes in rhinitis. These identify changes in relationship to mast cells, basophils, eosinophils, endothelial cells, Langerhan's cells, T lymphocytes, and epithelial cells (2). These cellular events are associated with the development of nasal hyperreactivity, such that patients also experience symptom exacerbation on exposure to nonspecific stimuli, such as strong odors, aerosol sprays, tobacco smoke, or change in temperature (3). These stimuli may be more apparent to the patient than the underlying allergic hypersensitivity, particularly with perennial disease. The timing of the disease will depend on the presence of the aeroallergen such that for pollens in the Northern Hemisphere (e.g., grass or ragweed), there is a classical seasonality, in patients with seasonal allergic rhinitis only experiencing symptoms for a short period of the year. This contrasts with perennial allergic rhinitis in which the sensitivity is commonly to the indoor allergens, such as house dust mites and animal danders, which are present all year round and cause symptoms throughout the year.

Glucocorticoid therapy is the most globally efficacious treatment for allergic rhinitis, when avoidance of the precipitating cause is not possible, as is usual with the exception of some forms of occupational disease. This is normally administered directly to the nasal mucosa as a topical therapy. To appreciate the influence of this therapeutic approach on the underlying pathological process as well as on the manifestations of the disease, this chapter initially details the mucosal inflammatory events in rhinitis, discusses this in relationship to the effect of topical corticosteroid therapy, and then details the clinical trial findings in the disease in relationship to placebo and other comparative agents before finally considering the adverse effect profile of this treatment in rhinitis.

II. Mucosal Inflammation and Rhinitis

Allergic rhinitis is characterized by the presence of basophilic cells and eosinophils in nasal smears, an epithelial accumulation of mast cells and eosinophils, epithelial cell activation, tissue eosinophilia, an increase in mucosal Langerhan's cells, T-lymphocyte accumulation and activation, and upregulation of the vascular endothelial expression of leukocyte adhesion molecules (2,4). Following immune activation and tissue cell recruitment, the symptoms can best be explained on the basis of mediator release from activated mast cells, basophils, and eosinophils (Table 1).

A. Mast Cells

Nasal biopsy studies have identified an increase in mast cells within the airway epithelium in both seasonal and perennial rhinitis compared with biopsy findings in nonatopic, nonrhinitic subjects (5-7). Although one study, employing

Table 1 Mediator Relevance to Rhinitic Symptoms

Symptom	Mediator	Mechanism	Receptor
Nasal itch	Histamine	Neural	H_1
Sneezing	Histamine	Neural	H_1
Rhinorrhoea	Histamine	Neural	H_1
	Histamine	Vascular	H_1 and H_2
	Leukotriene	Vascular	LT
	Kinins	Vascular	β_2
Blockage	Histamine	Vascular	H_1 and H_2
	Kinins	Vascular	β_2
	Leukotriene	Vascular	LT
	Prostaglandins	Vascular	DP
	Substance P	Neurovascular	SP

tinctorial staining of biopsies, also reported a seasonal increase in submucosal mast cells (8), this has not been substantiated by immunohistochemical studies using more specific mast cell markers (tryptase antibody) or by detailed transmission electronmicroscopic analysis (5-7,9).

The mast cell is in an activated state in symptomatic rhinitis, with both ultrastructural evidence of degranulation apparent on transmission electronmicroscopic examination of biopsies (9,10) and elevated levels of the mast cell mediators histamine and tryptase apparent in nasal lavage fluid (11,12). The mast cell mediators, in particular histamine, will contribute to the development of rhinitic symptoms. Nasal insufflation with histamine induces nasal itch, sneeze, rhinorrhea, and transient nasal blockage (13), whereas H_1-antihistamine pretreatment partially modifies the acute nasal response to allergen, although having little influence on nasal blockage (14,15). The development of nasal obstruction, which reflects the interaction of released mediators with vascular receptors within the nose, in contrast to the neural basis for the other symptoms (16), will also be influenced by the release of newly generated lipid mediators, such as leukotrienes, prostanoids, and platelet-activating factor (17) and the local generation of kinins (18). Following immunological activation, mast cells generate and release prostaglandin D_2 as their major prostanoid and the sulfidopeptide leukotriene (LT) C_4, which is metabolized to LTD_4 and LTE_4 (1). In addition, there is the generation of kinins in association with induced plasma protein leakage. Leukotrienes appear to be relatively more important than histamine in respect to nasal obstruction. Inhibitors of 5-lipoxygenase have been shown to inhibit allergen-induced nasal obstruction (19,20), and a LTD_4 receptor antagonist has been reported to confer clinical benefit in naturally occurring ragweed seasonal rhinitis (21).

In addition to the acute effects, mast activation can also be implicated in the tissue recruitment of eosinophils. The cytokines interleukin-4, interleukin-5, and interleukin-6 (IL-4, IL-5, IL-6) as well as tumor necrosis factor alpha (TNF-α) have been colocalized to nasal mast cells (6,22) and TNF-α demonstrated to be released during acute mast cell degranulation. There is also evidence of mast cell IL-4 release in both seasonal and perennial disease with increased mast cell immunostaining for secretory IL-4 in comparison with the normal nose. Both IL-4 and TNF-α will upregulate endothelial leukocyte adhesion molecule expression (4), and TNF-α and IL-5 can be implicated in tissue eosinophil recruitment (23).

B. Basophils

Basophilic cells are identifiable in nasal smear samples in naturally occuring rhinitis (24,25) as well as becoming apparent during the late-phase response to allergen challenge (26). Basophils will contribute to the histamine and leukotriene secretion within the nose. Like mast cells, basophils possess high-affinity high-density IgE receptors and interact with allergen. Basophils, also like mast cells, are derived from CD34 progenitor cells within the bone marrow (27), and there is evidence of their enhanced production in rhinitis, with increased circulating numbers of basophils observed in this disease (28). A number of cytokines have been reported to prime basophils in vitro for increased mediator release in response to subsequent stimulation. These stimuli include IL-1, IL-3, IL-5, and granulocyte-macrophage colony-stimulating factor (GM-CSF) (29,31). Subsequently, studies have also identified that IL-1β, IL-3, GM-CSF, and TNF-α are able to induce mediator release directly (32-35) although this has not been a consistent finding (36).

A number of other cytokines have more recently been identified that may be of greater relevance to basophil activation in rhinitis, as they are more potent and not solely restricted in their action to only a proportion of donors. These are "histamine-releasing factors" (HRFs), a terminology used to describe products released from activated mononuclear cells which are capable of inducing basophil histamine release (37,38). Histamine-releasing factors have been identified in nasal lavage (39). Several members of the chemokine family are now known to account for a proportion of this activity, including connective tissue–activating peptide III (CTAP III) and its derivative neutrophil-activating peptide-2 (NAP-2) (40,41) MCP-1 (42), RANTES (43), and MIP-1α and MIP-1β (44). The relevance of these observations to clinical rhinitis is as yet undetermined, but RANTES has been shown to be increased within the airway epithelium in rhinitis and to be released following nasal challenge. In addition, it is now also appreciated that human basophils themselves also generate cytokines, such as IL-4 and IL-8 (45,46). Their relevance to rhinitis in this respect is, however, undefined, as immunohistochemical staining for IL-4 colocalizes this cytokine to tryptase-positive cells (mast cells) and IL-8 is predominantly colocalized to epithelial cells (6,7).

C. Eosinophils

Immunohistochemical staining of nasal mucosal biopsies identifies that eosinophils are evident in nasal mucosal biopsies within the submucosa and epithelium in active rhinitis (5–7) and their recovery is increased in nasal smear specimens (47,48). Eosinophils are not a normal cellular constituent of the nose. Transmission electron microscopic examination of nasal biopsies from patients with rhinitis reveals evidence of ultrastructural granular changes of eosinophil activation (Fig. 1). The eosinophil granule contains basic proteins, such as major basic protein (49), eosinophil cationic protein (ECP), eosinophil-derived neurotoxin (EDN), and eosinophil peroxidase (EPX) as well as numerous enzymes such as ribonucleases, gelatinases, and histaminase (49,50). Eosinophils in nasal biopsies in rhinitis have also been demonstrated to contain in a preformed state the cytokines IL-4 and IL-5 (6). Eosinophil activation is associated both with the release of granule components and with the de novo generation of arachidonic acid products. The major lipoxygenase arachidonic acid cleavage product is LTC_4 and eosinophils, primed by chemotactic factors and

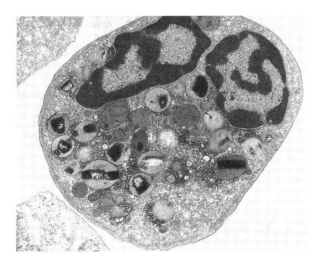

Figure 1 Transmission electon micrograph of tissue eosinophil in rhinitis (magnification ×16K), with some normal granules demonstrating electron-dense core and other granules with loss of electron-dense core.

cytokines such as IL-3, IL-5, and GM-CSF, have an enhanced state of activation and exhibit exaggerated LTC_4 generation and release (51–53). The generation of LTC_4 by eosinophils will contribute to nasal obstruction and to rhinorrhea.

An elevation in immunoreactive LTC_4 is evident in nasal lavage fluid in seasonal allergic rhinitis (54). In addition to an eosinophil source, LTC_4 may also be generated following either mast cell or basophil activation (55). A marker which is more specific for eosinophil activation is ECP, and a seasonal increase in nasal lavage ECP is evident in seasonal rhinitis (56), and elevated nasal lavage ECP levels can also be identified in perennial allergic rhinitis.

D. T Lymphocytes

The T lymphocyte represents a significant nonstructural cell within the nasal mucosa. An increase in certain T-cell populations has been described in nasal biopsy specimens both from patients with seasonal (57–59) and those with perennial (57) rhinitis, although this is not a consistent finding (60). These cells have been reported to be activated (61), although IL-2 receptor expression is low and usually no different from that identified in normal controls (59,60), and there is no seasonal change within grass pollen–sensitive subjects when symptomatic and nonsymptomatic periods are compared (57). Where there is a T-cell increase, this is largely related to an increase in the CD4 cell population which has the potential to generate proinflammatory cytokines such as IL-3, IL-4, IL-5, GM-CSF, and TNF-α (62). Following nasal allergen challenge, an increase in IL-4, IL-5, and GM-CSF mRNA-positive cells has been described in association with a mucosal eosinophilia (63), and T-cell clones derived from nasal mucosa challenged with allergen in vivo have a cytokine profile comparable with a TH2-like population (64). These findings are consistent with allergen-related T-lymphocyte activation and cytokine generation and with a contribution by this cell population to tissue leukocyte cell recruitment. At present, little information is available about T-cell cytokine synthesis in naturally occurring disease, but basal levels of T-cell mRNA expression appear to be low in nasal biopsies of patients with mild seasonal allergic rhinitis (63).

E. Langerhans' Cells

For T-cell activation, there has to be an interaction with antigen-presenting cells. Within the airways, the dendritic, or Langerhans', cell appears to be the capable antigen-presenting cell, as this function is poorly served by macrophages. These cells form a dendritic network within the mucosa, and a naturally occurring increase in mucosal Langerhans' cells has been described in seasonal rhinitis (65) which can be mimicked by repeated allergen challenge and is inhibited by the topical corticosteroid fluticasone propionate (66).

F. Endothelial Cells

In addition to the interaction between inflammatory mediators and the vascular endothelium, with respect to plasma protein exudation (67), there is also an interaction between mediators and cytokines with respect to inflammatory cell recruitment. The initial process of tissue leukocyte recruitment involves the adherence of circulating cells on the vascular endothelium prior to their diapedesis into the extravascular environment. This process involves the luminal expression on the vascular endothelium of leukocyte endothelial cell adhesion molecules (LECAMs) and their specific interaction with ligands expressed on the cell surface of leukocytes (4). Several LECAMs are considered to be involved in allergic inflammation: the selectins, P-selectin and E-selectin, and two members of the immunoglobulin supergene family, intracellular adhesion molecule-1 (ICAM-1) and vascular cell adhesion molecule-1 (VCAM-1).

Immunohistochemical staining of nasal biopsies for the LECAM's and quantifying their expression in relationship to the total vascular component within biopsies has identified a seasonal increase in VCAM-1 in naturally occuring seasonal allergic rhinitis (68). VCAM-1 has very low or absent basal expression out of season, and the modest increase in season is associated with tissue eosinophil recruitment. VCAM-1 recognizes the integrin $\alpha_4\beta_1$, present on eosinophils, basophils, and T lymphocytes but not neutrophils. In contrast to other LECAM-ligand interactions, VCAM-1–$\beta_1\alpha_4$ interactions confer some specificity with respect to tissue eosinophil accumulation (69). In perennial allergic disease, a condition that may be compounded by secondary infection and structural alterations, ICAM-1 has also been reported to have enhanced expression along with VCAM-1 when the results are compared to those from nonrhinitic subjects (70). There is thus ongoing cell recruitment in active rhinitis and consistent with this there is in perennial allergic disease, an increase in cells within the submucosa expressing lymphocyte function–associated antigen-1 $^+$ (LFA-1 $^+$), a cell surface ligand for ICAM-1.

G. Epithelial Cells

The airway epithelium is now increasingly being recognized as an active cell population involved in the inflammatory process. There is upregulation of the epithelial expression of ICAM-1 evident in both nasal smears (71) and nasal biopsies (72) in seasonal allergic rhinitis. Through its interaction with LFA-1, this would provide a mechanism for eosinophil retention at this site. The epithelium can also generate cytokines relevant to tissue cell recruitment.

Cultured human airway epithelial cells have been shown to synthesise GM-CSF, IL-6, and IL-8 (73,74). The presence of IL-8 immunoreactivity has been demonstrated with airway epithelium in nasal biopsies (6), although there does not appear to be an increased expression in rhinitis.

III. Inflammatory Model of Rhinitis

Following allergen-related activation of mast cells through cross linking of cell surface–bound IgE, there will be mediator generation and release with histamine, kinins, prostaglandins D_2 and LTC_4/LTD_4 contributing to the clinical presentation of nasal itch, sneeze, rhinorrhea, and blockage. The release of these mediators will be association also with the rolling margination of leukocytes on the vascular endothelium through induction of endothelial expression of P-selectin (75). The immediate release of preformed cytokines (TNF-α, IL-4, IL-5) will contribute to the cytokine induction of E-selectin, ICAM-1, and VCAM-1 on the vascular endothelium and the firmer adherence of leukocytes and their transendothelial migration. The accumulation of tissue basophils, eosinophils, and T lymphocytes will elaborate the cytokine network within the nasal mucosa and perpetuate the inflammatory response, with additional histamine and leukotreine release from activated basophils and eosinophils.

With chronic allergen exposure, the local generation of cytokines such as TNF-α and IL-1β, the latter possibly derived from activated epithelial cells and macrophages, will enhance the production of Langerhan's cells (76) and their epithelial accumulation. Langerhans cells have been shown to process high-affinity IgE receptors (77), and through their direct interaction with allergen will stimulate T-lymphocyte activation. The local generation of cytokines of the TH2 gene such as IL-3, IL-5, and GM-CSF will perpetuate the mucosal eosinophilia in rhinitis, as these cytokines stimulate progenitor cell development and maturation, exert weak chemotactic activity, prime eosinophils for enhanced activation and chemotaxis to other stimuli, and inhibit apoptosis, thereby prolonging tissue survival (78–95). Activated eosinophils have themselves been shown to generate IL-3, IL-5, and GM-CSF (96–100); these cytokines then serve an autocrine function, as well as exhibit increased LTC_4 generation (78,90,91). The local generation of RANTES and GM-CSF by epithelial cells can account for the accumulation of eosinophils at this location in rhinitis, and the release of IL-8 from its encrypted storage sites, by mast cell tryptase, provides an explanation for the epithelial accumulation of metachromatic cells (101).

The change in epithelial cell populations in allergic rhinitis, with eosinophil, mast cell, and basophil accumulation at this site, can explain the clinical phenomenon of "priming." Nasal priming describes the situation in which patients experience greater symptoms on exposure to equivalent or lower pollen counts after a period of sustained exposure to allergen (102,103), as in seasonal rhinitis.

It is thus apparent from the understanding of the inflammatory processes which underly rhinitis that prevention of airway inflammation with prophylactic therapy is the optimal approach to control disease expression and that, while having efficacy, inhibition of individual mediator release or end organ receptor antagonism will not give complete disease control.

IV. Influence of Corticosteroid Therapy on Nasal Inflammation

Corticosteroids act intracellularly to modify gene transcription and in so doing downregulate mucosal inflammation either by the induction of factors having anti-inflammatory effects or by inhibition of the generation of proinflammatory cytokines. This latter process is likely to be the predominant action of corticosteroids in allergic rhinitis. By modifying the local cytokine milieu, corticosteroids wil influence several processes involved in tissue leukocyte recruitment, including progenitor cell maturation, endothelial leukocyte cell adhesion molecule expression, cell activation, and cell priming as well as influencing the availability of chemotactic stimuli and reducing tissue eosinophil survival by promoting apoptosis (Table 2). Thus, through these multiple effects, corticosteroids are associated with a reduction in both mucosal inflammation and mucosal cell activation. These effects have been identified both in acute rhinitis, as induced by laboratory nasal allergen challenge, and in naturally occuring rhinitis.

Nasal allergen challenge is associated with mast cell degranulation (104–113), which accounts for the immediate response, and is then followed by a late response associated with tissue accumulation of neutrophils, eosinophils, and T lymphocytes (63,114). These cells are in an activated state, and in situ hybridization studies identify an increase in cells mRNA positive for IL-4, IL-5, and GM-CSF during the late response (63) compatible with activation

Table 2 Influence of Corticosteroids on Mucosal Inflammation in Rhinitis

Cell population	Effect
Mast cells	Decrease epithelial accumulation
	Prevent seasonal increase in secretory IL-4
Basophils	Decrease presence in nasal smears
Eosinophils	Decrease presence in smears, epithelium, and submucosa
	Enhance apoptosis
Endothelium	Inhibit VCAM-1 expression
Langerhans' cells	Decrease seasonal epithelial accumulation
T lymphocytes	Decrease epithelial accumulation
	Prevent allergen-induced increase in IL-4 mRNA
B lymphocytes	Prevent seasonal increase in serum IgE

of a TH2-like population of T lymphocytes. Pretreatment with corticosteroids (inhaled or oral) has been shown to reduce the upregulation in IL-4 mRNA, to reduce the basophil and eosinophil tissue recruitment, and with prolonged therapy to inhibit the immediate release of mast cell mediators and the associated immediate clinical response (26,63,112,115–117).

In naturally occurring disease, inhaled corticosteroids have been demonstrated when used prophylactically to prevent the seasonal increase in mucosal eosinophils and to downregulate the expression of secretory IL-4 by mast cells (118). A reduction in nasal eosinophils with intranasal steroids is well recognized (118), and recent evidence from studies in seasonal allergic rhinitis has indicated that this could relate to inhibition of the endothelial expression of VCAM-1 (68). VCAM-1 has the potential to interact with eosinophils through binding to the cell surface expressed integrin $\alpha_4\beta_1$ (VLA-4), and these results indicate that this interaction has relevance in vivo in allergic nasal inflammation.

Corticosteroid therapy has also been found to reduce the presence of metachromatic cells (mast cells and basophils) on the epithelial surface and in nasal secretions (117–120). Treatment has, however, a lesser effect on submucosal mast cell numbers, with several studies demonstrating no effect (118,121,122). One study has, however, reported a diminution in a subpopulation of submucosal mast cells with nasal steroid therapy; formalin-sensitive mast cells but not formalin-resistant mast cells (119). The formalin-sensitive mast cells may represent the tryptase-only mast cells (MC_T) in contrast to the tryptase- and chymase-positive mast cells (MC_{TC}) which are more prominent within the submucosa. The MC_T population is more pronounced within the epithelium, is T-cell dependent, and generates proportionally greater IL-5, IL-6, and TNF-α than the MC_{TC} (123).

Similar to the findings with mast cells, no reduction in submucosal T-lymphocyte numbers is apparent with topical nasal steroid therapy in rhinitis even in studies up to 1 year in duration (66,124). This is irrespective as to whether analysis is related to $CD3^+$ cells, to the $CD4^+$ and $CD8^+$ subpopulations, or to cells expressing the activation marker CD25. There is, however, a reduction in epithelial $CD3^+$, $CD4^+$, and $CD8^+$ cells with 1 year of topical corticosteroid therapy. This change is, however, slow, as no epithelial reduction is apparent by 3 months. These findings thus indicate that modification of T-cell activation is likely to be a more critical effect of corticosteroid therapy than modulation of tissue residency. In this respect, the effect of topical corticosteroid therapy on mucosal antigen-presenting cells has relevance to T-lymphocyte activation. A long-term placebo-controlled study of fluticasone propionate in perennial allergic rhinitis identified within 3 months of treatment a steroid-related reduction in CD1-positive and HLA-DR–positive cells within both the epithelium and lamina propria (66). This effect was maintained through the year of therapy. By reducing the presence of the CD1-positive population of dendritic cells (Langerhan's cells), the ability to present antigen to T cells and induce T-cell activation will be impaired.

In addition to these effects on antigen presentation, it is also apparent that topical corticosteroid therapy modifies the B-lymphocyte response to allergen, as several studies have identified that regular nasal steroid therapy modifies the seasonal increase in serum IgE (125,126). Whether this is a direct effect on B-cell IgE synthesis or a secondary effect due to inhibition of IL-4 and possibly IL-13 synthesis is not known, although the second consideration is most probable. It is thus apparent that regular nasal steroid therapy can modify many aspects of nasal mucosal inflammation and, although a clear-cut relationship is not defined, a reduction in mucosal inflammatory events is the most likely explanation for the reduction in nasal hyperreactivity with regular nasal steroid therapy.

V. Clinical Effect of Corticosteroids in Rhinitis

Clinically, corticosteroids improve rhinitic symptoms, reducing nasal itch, sneeze, rhinorrhea, and nasal blockage in both seasonal and perennial disease. When used prophylactically in seasonal disease, regular topical nasal steroid therapy prevents the pollen-related exacerbation in nasal symptoms. In addition, nasal corticosteroids have been shown to improve impaired sense of smell. Thus, corticosteroid therapy is effective in relieving all nasal symptoms of rhinitis.

These nasal effects of corticosteroids are related to their local rather than any systemic effects. When an equivalent dose to that administered topically to the nose is taken orally, the oral dose is no different in effect to placebo, whereas the topical therapy has significant clinical benefit (127,128). With topical nasal steroid therapy, there is evidence to indicate a dose-response relationship (Fig. 2). This has been more evident in perennial rather than seasonal disease. A comparative study of placebo with two doses of budesonide (50 µg per nostril b.i.d. and 100 µg per nostril b.i.d.) identified that both doses of active medication were better than placebo in reducing nasal blockage, nasal discharge, and sneezing bouts and that 400 µg of budesonide per day had significantly greater effect than 200 µg of budesonide per day in reducing nasal blockage and nasal discharge over a 2-week treatment period, but that this difference was not significant for sneezing (129). Over a 12-month period, the topical nasal administration of beclomethasone dipropionate 200 µg b.i.d., was also found to be more effective than 100 µg b.i.d. in the treatment of perennial rhinitis (130). Increasing the intranasal dose of 800 µg/day of beclomethasone dipropionate does not appear to confer additional clinical benefit, sug-

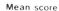

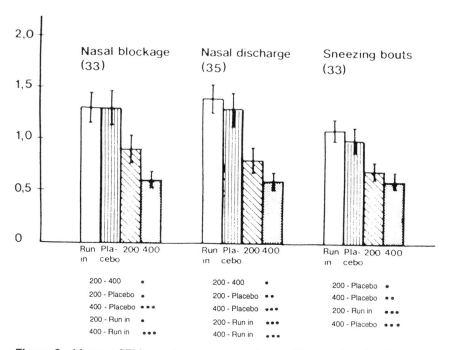

Figure 2   Means ±SEM symptom scores in patients with perennial allergic rhinitis during run-in period, placebo treatment, and treatment with budesonide 200 µg/day and 400/µg/day. Significant differences: *p < 0.05; **p < 0.01; ***p < 0.001). (From Ref. 129.)

gesting that a maximum therapeutic benefit is achieved at the 400-µg dose with this particular medication (130,131). In seasonal disease no difference has been reported between 200 and 400 µg per day of budesonide (132). This study, however, involved only small patient numbers, and when individuals responding to a lower dose were excluded in a separate study of fluticasone propionate in seasonal allergic rhinitis (65%), then a benefit of increasing the topical steroid dose (400 µg per day from 200 µg per day) was evident on nasal blockage symptoms (133). For topical nasal steroids to be most effective, they need to be taken on a regular rather than an as required basis (134) (Fig. 3).

A.   Seasonal Allergic Rhinitis

Regular topical nasal steroid therapy modifies season-related sneezing, rhinorrhea, and nasal blockage of allergic rhinitis in comparison with placebo (132). Comparative studies with H$_1$-antihistamines (135) and sodium cromoglycate

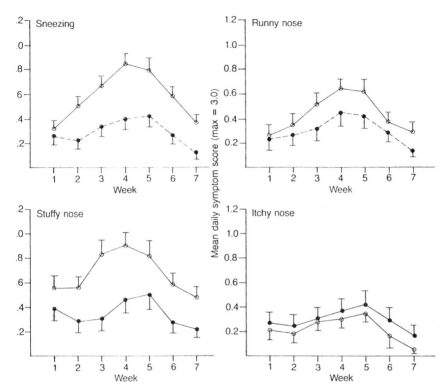

Figure 3 Mean ±SEM nasal symptoms during the ragweed season in patients receiving topical nasal beclomethasone as regular therapy, 200 μg b.d., *n* = 30, or as p.r.n. therapy, 100 μg, *n* = 30 (0). Significant differences in favor of regular therapy for sneezing, *p* = 0.0002; stuffy nose, *p* = 0.0015; runny nose, *p* = 0.025, with no difference in nasal itching, p = 0.37. (From Ref. 134.)

(136) identify the superiority of topical nasal steroid therapy in alleviating the spectrum of nasal symptoms (Fig. 4). This mode of therapy has greatest efficacy when used prophylactically and takes longer to exert its maximal effects if treatment initiation is delayed until symptoms are moderately troublesome. One comparative trial of prophylactic nasal budesonide therapy and immunotherapy identified greater benefit from the topical nasal steroid therapy (137), but the immunotherapy regimen was suboptimal and further comparative analysis is warranted.

B. Perennial Allergic Rhinitis

As for seasonal disease, topical nasal steroid therapy improves sneezing, nasal discharge, and nasal blockage in comparison to placebo. This has been

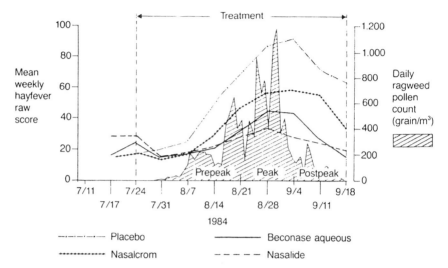

Figure 4 Mean weekly hay fever symptom scores for hay fever from 120 subjects randomly allocated to placebo, sodium cromoglycate, flunisolide, and beclomethasone dipropionate. (From Ref. 136.)

shown for all the topical steroid preparations, including beclomethasone (138), dexamethasone (139), beclomethasone dipropionate (140), flunisolide (141), budesonide (128), triamcinolone (142), and fluticasone propionate (143). Comparative studies with oral H_1-antihistamines (144–145) and topical sodium cromoglycate (146–147) have found topical corticosteroid therapy to be more efficacious in the treatment of perennial allergic disease. As disease is present when therapy is initiated in perennial allergic rhinitis, the maximum effect of treatment may not be seen until after 3–4 weeks of continuous therapy. When used at recommended doses, the nasal corticosteroid preparations generally have similar effects.

Brief reports exist of trials comparing intranasal budesonide with beclomethasone dipropionate and fluticasone propionate in the treatment of perennial allergic rhinitis (148,149). A parallel group comparison of fluticasone propionate, 200 μg, administered from a metered-dose inhaler (MDI), found no difference in the efficacy of this medication in improving symptoms than either 140 or 280 μg of budesonide administered from a Turbohaler (200 and 400 μg doses with 30% retained in nasal adaptor). Substantial or total control of symptoms was reported in the 6-week treatment period in 42, 43, and 57% of the three treatment groups, respectively (149). These improvements were all significantly greater than that identified with placebo (18%). Comparisons between beclomethasone dipropionate (BDP) and flunisolide report comparable effects when given at standard clinical doses (150,151), whereas budesonide, 400 µg, has been reported to be more efficacious than BDP at the same dose, although this is only with respect to nasal blockage (148).

VI. Adverse Effects

The local effects of the topical administration of nasal steroids include sneezing on application or a transient sensation of burning irritation. This occurs in about 10% of patients with MDI administration (152) and is less with aqueous or powder preparations (153). The use of propellants in MDIs, as well as the force of impact on the nasal mucosa with this mode of administration, is considered to be responsible for these side effects as well as for the nasal mucosal bleeding and crusting with MDI administration. These later adverse effects occur in about 2% of users and do not occur with alternative modes to topical steroid application and so cannot be related to the drug per se. Nasal mucosal biopsies obtained from perennial rhinitic subjects who had received continuous prophylactic therapy with beclomethasone dipropionate over a 5-year period identified no evidence for mucosal damage or mucosal atrophy (154,155), and similar evidence is available with flunisolide (156) and budesonide (157). Indeed, treatment over a 1-year period has been shown to normalize the nasal mucosa (157), and there does not appear to be any increase in nasal candidiasis with regular topical nasal steroid therapy (158).

Owing to the topical application and low-dose administered systemic effects are not a feature of intranasal steroid therapy. At standard clinical doses, topical nasal steroid therapy has no effect on plasma cortisol levels (159,160), has no significant effect on lower limb growth in children (161), and is not associated with the development of posterior subcapsular cataracts in the absence of oral steroid therapy (161,162).

VII. Conclusion

Intranasal steroids are thus efficacious and safe in the treatment of both seasonal and perennial allergic rhinitis. Their effects can be related to modification of the underlying airway inflammation in these disorders and nasal lavage and biopsy studies have identified an influence on many different aspects of allergic inflammation. This protean effect on airway inflammation accounts for their clinical superiority to alternative nasal therapies such as oral H_1-antihistamines, topical sodium cromoglycate, and nasal decongestants. For maximum efficacy, topical nasal steroids need to be taken regularly, and in seasonal disease are best initiated prophylactically prior to the seasonal appearance of pollen and then used continuously throughout the pollen season. Other than in patients with intermittent symptoms or very mild disease, topical nasal corticosteroid therapy represents the first-time treatment in patients with allergic rhinitis on account of their profile of action and safety.

Discussion

DR. A. LAITINEN: Have you looked at seasonal rhinitis patients out of season? How normal are the morphological findings, inflammatory cells, their activation, adhesion molecules, etc.? Are there any more permanent changes such as increased collagen deposition?

DR. HOWARTH: In pure grass pollen–sensitive seasonal rhinitis, nasal biopsies out of season when these patients are asymptomatic contain no mast cells or eosinophils within the epithelium, very few eosinophils within the submucosa, and normal expression of endothelial/leukocyte cell adhesion molecules. The collagen changes are of interest. The thickness of the collagen in the upper airways is similar to that found in asthmatics within the lower airways and thicker and denser than in the normal lower airways. These changes in the upper airways are also evident, however, in the apparent normal nose, and these changes may reflect the intermittent inflammation that occurs in the nose to nonallergic environmental stimuli. Consistent with this, ultrastructural studies of nasal biopsies reveal some evidence of mast cell degranulation in normal nonatopic patients.

DR. PERRETTI: (1) Do you find that steroids suppress cell adhesion molecule expression or not? If yes, is it an action specific for VCAM-1 or are they also active on other endothelial CAMs? (2) Similarly, do you observe that glucocorticoid treatment reduces IL-4 levels in mast cells? (3) Since you showed evidence that glucocorticoids reduce the number of mast cells found in your biopsies, if you normalized your IL-4 values to the cell number, do you still have a reduction in IL-4 by the steroids? That is, do steroids interfere directly with IL-4 synthesis in mast cells or do they reduce IL-4 levels via a reduction of the cell number?

DR. HOWARTH: In seasonal rhinitis, we find that regular therapy with topical corticosteroids prevents the seasonal increase in VCAM-1 expression in endothelial cells within the nasal mucosa. We have not, as yet, assessed glucocorticoid downregulation of adhesion molecule expression in perennial rhinitis. Similarly, although prophylactic glucocorticoid therapy prevents the seasonal increase in IL-4 immunoreactivity, we have not yet addressed the decrease in IL-4 expression in tissue biopsy specimens in perennial rhinitis. Optimally, it is necessary to have mRNA as well as protein immunohistochemical studies to investigate if the IL-4 regulation occurs at the gene level or whether the decrease relates to a decrease in cells containing IL-4. Indirectly, I can relate that mast cell numbers do not decrease, whereas IL-4 decreases, suggesting that it is at the gene level.

DR. LEUNG: Have you seen rhinitis patients with glucocorticoid resistance and have you studied them? (2) Did you look at the cytokine profile in glucocorticoid-resistant rhinitic patients?

DR. DURHAM: (1) Topical corticosteroids have more marked effects on inflammatory cells in the epithelium than the submucosa. (Rak S, Jacobson MR, Sudderick RM, et al. Influence of prolonged treatment with topical corticosteroid [fluticasone propionate] on early and late phase nasal responses and cellular infiltration in the nasal mucosa after allergen challenge. Clin Exp Allergy 1994; 24:930–939). (2) With regard to prolonged topical steroid treatment, Dr. Masuyama in our group has shown different effects on nasal allergen challenge compared with natural seasonal exposure. In both circumstances, T cells and eosinophil numbers are reduced, but with regard to cytokine mRNA expression, IL-4 is reduced more after challenge and IL-5 more during seasonal exposure. (Masuyama K, Jacobson MR, Rak S, et al. Topical glucocorticosteroid [fluticasone propionate] inhibits cells expressing cytokine mRNA for interleukin-4 in the nasal mucosa in allergen-induced rhinitis. Immunology 1994; 82:192–199; Masuyama K, Jacobson MR, Juliusson S. Topical corticosteroid [fluticasone propionate] inhibits seasonal rhinitis increases in IL-5 mRNA+ cells in the nasal mucosa (abstr). J Allergy Clin Immunol 1995; 95:300).

DR. GLEICH: Your observation of a reduction of IgE in the patients with allergic rhinitis treated with topical glucocorticoids is intriguing. Was the seasonal rise totally abolished? Presently, to my knowledge, only allergen immunotherapy abolished seasonal rises of IgE antibody.

DR. HOWARTH: The studies on topical corticosteroid therapy and inhibition of increments in plasma IgE in seasonal rhinitis were not undertaken in Southampton. The regular use of topical corticosteroid therapy prevents the seasonal increment in plasma IgE but does not appear to affect baseline IgE levels.

DR. SCHLEIMER: You have shown that the majority of the cytokine protein-positive cells are mast cells. Steve Durham and his colleagues have shown that T cells are the predominant mRNA-positive cells. Although I appreciate that some of these differences may relate to measuring RNA versus protein or challenge/disease status, I am frustrated by our apparent inability to nail down the relative importance of cellular sources. Regarding IgE, in vitro studies have actually shown an enhancement of immunoglobulin production by glucocorticoids.

Although the in vivo effect seen by Naclerio that you refer to may be due to local suppression of IL-4/IL-13 production, etc., Dr. Naclerio also suggested that it may relate to a diminution of antigen access to lymphoid cells as a result of steroid effects on permeability.

DR. HOWARTH: I do not think there is discrepancy between Dr. Durham's and our findings. There are several cell sources for cytokines; mast cells, T lymphocytes, epithelial cells, eosinophils, and matrix cells and the net effect at any one time will depend on the interactions between the cytokine pool. The model I have is that the mast cell is storing preformed cytokines is the acute responder and initiates the upregulation of cell adhesion molecules and eosinophil influx. The later activation and cytokine generation by T lymphocytes contributes to the chronicity of the disease along with continued cytokine production by mast cells in the presence of antigen. It awaits to be seen if there is a differential sensitivity to activation by antigen but at present corticosteroids will decrease cytokine synthesis by all cells and differentiation into proportional cell contribution will not help. Should other cell-specific therapies become available that modify cytokine synthesis/release, then this information would be of value. It is possible that IgE regulation is an indirect effect. Dr. Fokkens has demonstrated a decrease in Langerhan's cells with nasal steroid therapy, and this is considered to be the primary antigen-presenting cell. Regulation of IL-4 and IL-13 would also decrease IgE isotype switching by B cells, but it is interesting to note that the studies which suggest corticosteroid regulation of IgE production demonstrate an inhibition of the seasonal increase but no effect on the baseline level. It is thus possible that once B cells are committed, regulation of IL-4 and IL-13 does not inhibit established IgE synthesis.

DR. GLEICH: First, in our laboratory in spite of Dr. Hirohito Kita's efforts to torture eosinophils with virtually all known stimuli, we have not, as yet, been able to cause IL-5 production. Second, evidently you did not find TNF-α localization in eosinophils even though several reports have shown eosinophil localization of TNF-α. Do you have any explanation for this apparent discrepancy?

DR. HOWARTH: TNF-α is predominantly localized to mast cells in rhinitis. We have found TNF-α in eosinophils in nasal polyps and in postmortem specimens from asthma mortality, and the potential to upregulate cytokine gene expression is likely to depend on the strength of the local environmental stimuli and the state of cell priming. This will change within individuals and time depending on the status of their disease and the concomitant therapy.

DR. BOCHNER: I was wondering whether you could clarify the reasons for the different mast cell staining patterns seen with your two IL-4 antibodies. Is the ring staining due to cell surface IL-4? Also, does the staining pattern of mast cells change acutely after allergen challenge?

DR. HOWARTH: (1) We have found two patterns of immunoreactivity with two different IL-4 antibodies (4D9 and 3H4) which recognize different epitopes on the IL-4 protein. Monoclonal antibody 4D9 stains cytoplasmic IL-4 which is evident in both normal and rhinitic nasal mucosa and can be co-localized to tissue mast cells. Monoclonal antibody 3H4 gives a peripheral ring pattern of immunoreactivity which is evident in rhinitis but not very evident within the normal nose. Increases are seen in both seasonal and perennial rhinitis and a decrease occurs with corticosteroid therapy. The exact interpretation, whether this represents secretory or cell surface IL-4, awaits further clarification. It does appear to be related to disease activity and is also evident within the lower airways in asthma. (2) We find very few mast cells in lavage, so that flow cytometry is difficult to undertake. If sufficient cells could be obtained, then flow cytometry to monitor cell surface expression of IL-4 would be very reasonable.

DR. BUSSE: Can you comment on the specificity of staining for IL-5 protein product in the eosinophil? That is, do you have information on whether there is nonspecific attachment of IL-5 to the eosinophil or that the eosinophil IL-5 receptor has been activated by IL-5 and the detected IL-5 does not necessarily represent production of IL-5 but rather contact with the cytokine?

DR. HOWARTH: In both the upper and lower airways, we find IL-5 immunoreactivity co-localizing to airway eosinophils. Immunogold electron microscopy demonstrates that the IL-5 is located within eosinophil granules. The difference between these findings in vivo and efforts to demonstrate cytokine upregulation in eosinophils in vitro may relate to priming/activation processes occurring during tissue eosinophil recruitment which are not reproduced in vitro.

References

1. Howarth PH, Holgate ST. Basic aspects of allergic reactions. In: Naspitz C, Tinkelman DG, eds. Childhood Rhinitis and Sinusitis: Pathophysiology and Treatment. New York: Marcel Dekker, 1990:1-35.
2. Howarth PH. The cellular basis for allergic rhinitis. Allergy 1995:50(supll 23):6-10.
3. Mygind N. Essential Allergy. Oxford, UK: Blackwell Scientific, 1986:279-350.
4. Montefort S, Holgate ST, Howarth PH. Leucocyte-endothelial adhesion molecules and their role in bronchial asthma and allergic rhinitis. Eur Respir J 1993; 6:1044-1054.
5. Bentley AM, Jacobson MR, Cumberworth B, Barkans JR, Moqbel R, Schwartz

LB, Irani AA, Kay AB, Durham SR. Immunohistology of the nasal mucosa in seasonal allergic rhinitis: increases in activated eosinophils and epithelial mast cells. J Allergy Clin Immunol 1992; 89:821-829.

6. Bradding P, Feather IH, Wilson S, Bardin P, Holgate ST, Howarth PH. Immunolocalisation of cytokines in the nasal mucosa of normal and perennial rhinitis subjects: The mast cell as a source of IL-4, IL-5 and IL-6 in human allergic inflammation. 1993; 151:3853-3865.

7. Bradding P, Feather IH, Wilson S, Holgate ST, Howarth PH. The effects of seasonal exposure to allergic nasal cytokine immunoreactivity and its modulation by fluticasone propionate. Thorax 1993; 48:1059.

8. Viegas M, Gomez E, Brooks J, Davies RJ. The effect of the pollen season on nasal mast cell numbers. Br Med J 1987; 294:414.

9. Enerback L, Pipkorn U, Olafsson A. Intraepithelial migration of nasal mucosal mast cells in hay fever. Ultrastructural Observations. Int Arch Allergy Appl Immunol 1986; 88:289-297.

10. Trotter CM, Orr TSC. A fine structure of some cellular components in allergic reaction. 1. Degranulation of human mast cells in allergic asthma and perennial rhinitis. Clin allergy 1973; 3:411-425.

11. Rasp G, Hochstrasser K. Tryptase in nasal fluid is a unique marker of allergic rhinitis. Allergy 1993; 48:71-74.

12. Wilson SJ, Lau LCK, Howarth PH. Mediator and cellular events in naturally occurring seasonal allergic rhinitis. Clin Exp Allergy 1994; 24:977A.

13. Mygind N, Secter C, Kirkegaard J. Role of histamine and antihistamines in the nose. Eur J Respir Dis 1993; 64 (suppl 128):16-20.

14. Holmberg K, Pipkorn U, Bake P, Blychert L-D. Effects of topical treatment with H_1 and H_2 antagonists on clinical symptoms and nasal vascular reactions in patients with allergic rhinitis. Allergy 1989; 44:281-287.

15. Howarth PH, Harrison K, Smith S. The influence of Terfenadine and pseudoephedrine alone and in combination on allergen-induced rhinitis. Int Arch Allergy Immunol 1993; 107:318-321.

16. Rajakulasingam K, Howarth PH. Relation of disordered airway function to the treatment of rhinitis. In Busse WW, Holgate ST, eds. Asthma and Rhinitis. Cambridge, UK: Blackwell Scientific, 1995:1247-1254.

17. Howarth PH. Lipid mediators and allergic rhinitis. In: Robinson C, ed. Lipid Mediators in Allergic Diseases of the Respiratory Tract. Boca Raton, FL: CRC Press, 1993:109-119.

18. Rajakulasingam K, Polosa R, Church MK, Holgate ST, Howarth PH. Kinins and rhinitis. Clin Exp Allergy 1992; 22:734-740.

19. Knapp HR. Reduced allergen-induced nasal congestion and leukotriene synthesis with an orally active 5-lipoxygenase inhibitor. N Engl J Med 1990; 327:1745-1748.

20. Howarth PH, Harrison K, Lau LCK, Dube L, Cohn J. The influence of the 5-lipoxygenase inhibitor A-78773 on the nasal response to allergen in rhinitis. J Allergy Clin Immunol 1993; 93:297A.

21. Donnelly A, Glass M, Muller B, Smart S, Hutson J, Minkwitz MC, Casale R.

Leukotriene D_4 (LTD_4) antagonist ICI 204, 219 relives ragweed allergic rhinitis symptoms. J Allergy Clin Immunol 1993; 91:259.

22. Bradding P, Mediwake R, Feather IH, Madden J, Church MK, Holgate ST, Howarth PH. TNFα is localised to nasal mucosal mast cells and is released in acute allergic rhinitis. Clin Exp Allergy 1995; 25:406–415.

23. Howarth PH, Bradding P, Quint D, Redington AE and Holgate ST. Cytokines and airway inflammation. Ann NY Acad Sci 1994; 725:69–82.

24. Otsuka H, Denburg JA, Dolovitvh J, Hitch D, Lapp D, Rajan RS, Bienenstock J, Befus AD. Heterogeneity of instachromatic cells in human nose: significance of mucosal mast cells. J Allergy Clin Immunol 1985; 76:695.

25. Okuda M, Otsuka H, Kawabori S. Studies on nasal surface basophilic cells. Ann Allergy 1985; 54:69.

26. Bascom R, Wachs M, Naclerio RM, Pipkorn U, Galli SJ, Lichtenstein LM. Basophil influx occurs after nasal allergen challenge: Effects of topical corticosteroid pretreatment. J Allergy Clin Immunol 1988; 81:580–589.

27. Kirchenbaum AS, Kessler SW, Gott JP, Metcalfe DD. Demonstration of the origin of human mast cells from CD34+ bone marrow progenitor cells. J Immunol 1991; 146:1410–1415.

28. Charance M, Herbeth B, Kauffman F. Seasonal patterns of circulating basophils. Int arch Allergy Appl Immunol 1988; 86:462–464.

29. Massey WA, Randall J, Kagey-Sobotka A, Warner JA, MacDonald SM, Gillis S, Lichtenstein LM. Recombinant human IL-1α and IL-1β potentiate IgE dependent basophil histamine release. J Immunol 1989; 143:1875–1880.

30. Bischoff SC, De Weck AL, Dahinden CA. Interleukin-3 and granulocyte/macrophage-colony-stimulating factor render human basophils responsive to low concentrations of complement component C3a. Proc Natl Acad Sci USA 1990; 87:6813–6817.

31. Bischoff SC, Brunner T, De Weck AL, Dahinden CA. Interleukin 5 modifies histamine release and leukotriene generation by human basophils in response to diverse agonists. J Exp Med 1990; 172:1577–1582.

32. Heak-Frendscho M, Arai N, Arai K, Baeza ML, Finn A, Kaplan AP. Human recombinant granulocyte-macrophage colony-stimulating factor and interleukin 3 cause basophil histamine release. J Clin Invest 1988; 82:17–20.

33. MacDonald SM, Schleimer RP, Dagey-Sobotka A, Gillis S, Lichtenstein LM. Recombinant IL-3 induces histamine release from human basophils. J Immunol 1989; 142:3527–3532.

34. Haak-Frendscho M, Dinarell C, Kaplan AP. Recombinant human interleukin-1 beta causes histamine release from human basophils. J Allergy Clin Immunol 1988; 82:218–223.

35. Subramanian N, Bray MA. Interleukin 1 releases histamine from human basophils and mast cells in vitro. J Immunol 1987; 138:271–275.

36. Alam R, Wetter JB, Forsythe PA, Lett-Brown MA, Grant JA. Comparative effects of recombinant IL-1, -2, -3, -4 and -6, IFN-α, granulocyte-macrophage colony stimulating factor, tumour necrosis factor-γ and histamine releasing factors on the secretion of histamine from basophils. J Immunol 1989; 142:3431–3435.

37. Thueson DO, Speck LS, Lett-Brown MA, Grant JA, Histamine-releasing activity (HRA). 1. Production of a histamine releasing lymphokine by mitogen or antigen stimulated human mononuclear cells. J Immunol 1979; 123:623–632.
38. Thueson DO, Speck LS, Lett-Brown MA, Grant JA. Histamine-releasing activity (HRA). II. Interaction with basophils and physicochemical characterisation. J Immunol 1997; 123:633–639.
39. Sim TC, Hilsmeier KA, Alam R, Allan RK, Lett-Brown MA, Grant JA. Effect of topical corticosteroids on the recovery of histamine releasing factors in nasal washings of patients with allergic rhinitis. Am Rev Respir Dis 1992; 145:1316–1320.
40. Baeza ML, Riddigari SR, Kornfield D, Ramani N, Smith E, Hossler PA, Fischer T, Castor CW, Gorevic PG, Kaplan AP. Relationship of one form of human histamine-releasing factor to connective tissue activating peptide-III. J Clin Invest 1990; 85:1516–1521.
41. Reddigari SR, Kuna P, Miraliotta GF, Kornfield D, Baeza ML, Castor CW, Kaplan AP. Connective tissue-activating peptide-III and its derivative, neutrophil-activating peptide-2, release histamine from human basophils. J Allergy Clin Immunol 1992; 89:666–672.
42. Kuna P, Reddigari SR, Racinski D, Oppenheim JJ, Kaplan AP. Monocyte chemotactic and activating factor is a potent histamine-releasing factor for human basophils. J Exp Med 1992; 175:489–493.
43. Kuna P, Reddigari SR, Schall TJ, Rucinski D, Viksman MY, Kaplan AP. RANTES, a monocyte and T-lymphocyte chemotactic cytokine, releases histamine from human basophils. J Immunol 1992; 149:636–642.
44. Kuna P, Reddigari SR, Schall TJ, Rucinski D, Sadick M, Kaplan AP. Characterization of the human basophil response to cytokines, growth factors, and histamine releasing factors of the intercrine/chemokine family. J Immunol 1993; 150:1932–1943.
45. Brunner T, Heusser CH, Dahindem CA. Human peripheral blood basophils primed by interleukin-3 (IL-3) produce IL-4 in response to immunoglobulin E receptor stimulation. J Exp Med 1993; 177:605–611.
46. Elmedal B, Bjerke T. Rendiger N, Markvardsen P, Nielsen S, Schiotz PO. IL-8 is produced and prestored in human blood basophils. Allergy 1993; 16:2861.
47. Vaheri E. Nasal allergy with special reference to eosinophilia and histopathology. Acta Allergol 1956; 10:203–211.
48. Mullarkey MF, Hill JS, Webb DR. Allergic and non-allergic rhinitis: Their characterisation with attention to the meaning of nasal eosinophilia. J Allergy Clin Immunol 1980; 65:122–126.
49. Peters MS, Rodriguez M, Gleich GJ. Localisation of human eosinophil granules major basic protein, eosinophil cationic protein and eosinophils derived neurotoxin by immunoelectron microscopy. Lab Invest 1986; 54:656–662.
50. Bainton DF, Farquhar MG. Segregation and packaging of granule enzymes in eosinophilic leucocytes. J Cell Biol 1970; 45:54–73.
51. Owen Jr WF, Rothenberg ME, Silberstein DS, Gasson JG, Stevens RL, Austen KF, Soberman RJ. Regulation of human eosinophil viability, density and function

by granulocyte/macrophage colony-stimulating factor in the presence of 3T3 fibroblasts. J Exp Med 1987; 186:129–141.

52. Rothenberg ME, Owen Jr WF, Silberstein DS, Woods J, Soberman RJ, Austen KF, Stevens RL. Human eosinophils have prolonged survival, enhanced functional properties and become hypodense when exposed to interleukin-3. J Clin Invest 1988; 81:1986–1992.

53. Lopez AF, Sanderson CJ, Gamble JF, Campbell HD, Young IS, Vadas MA. Recombinant human interleukin 5 is a selective activator of human eosinophil function. J Exp Med 1988; 167:219–224.

54. Volovitz B, Osur SL, Berstein JM, Ogra PL. Leukotriene C_4 release in upper respiratory mucosa during natural exposure to ragweed in ragweed-sensitive children. J Allergy Clin Immunol 1988; 82:414–418.

55. Howarth PH. Allergic rhinitis: a rational choice of treatment. Respir Med 1989; 83:179–188.

56. Svensson C, Andersson M, Persson CG, Venge P, Alkrer U, Pipkorn U. Albumin, bradykinin and eosinophil cationic protein on the nasal mucosal surface in patients with hay fever during natural allergen exposure. J Allergy Clin Immunol 1990; 85:828–833.

57. Calderon MA, Lozewicz S, Prior A, Jordan S, Trigg CJ, Davies RJ. Lymphocyte infiltration and thickness of the nasal mucus membrane in perennial and seasonal allergic rhinitis. J Allergy Clin Immunol 1994; 93:635–643.

58. Saito H, Asakura K, Kataura A. Studies on the properties of infiltrating T-lymphocytes and ICAM-1 expression in allergic nasal mucosa. Acta Otolaryngol (Stockhm) 1994; 114:315–323.

59. Karlsson MG, Davidsson A, Hellquist HB. Increase in CD4+ and CD45Ro+ memory T-cells in the nasal mucosal of allergic patients. APMIS 1994; 102:753–758.

60. Fokkens WJ, Holm AF, Rijntjes E, Mulder PG, Vroom TM. Characterisation and quantification of cellular infiltrates in nasal mucosa of patients with grass pollen allergy, non-allergic patients and controls. Int Arch Allergy Appl Immunol 1990; 93:66–72.

61. Okuda M, Pawankar R. Flow cytometric analysis of intraepithelial lymphocytes in the human nasal mucosa. Allergy 1992; 47:255–259.

62. Mossman TR, Coffman RL. TH_1 and TH_2 cells: Different patterns of lymphokine secretion lead to different functional properties. Ann Rev Immunol 1989; 7:145–164.

63. Durham SR, Ying S, Varney VA, Jacobson MR, Sudderick RM, Mackay IS, Kay AB, Hamid QA. Cytokine messanger RNA expression of IL-3, IL-4, IL-5 and granulocyte/macrophage colony-stimulating factor in the nasal mucosa after local allergen provocation: Relationship to tissue eosinophilia. J Immunol 1992; 148:2390–2394.

64. Del-Prete GF, De Cari M, D'Elios MM, Maestrelli P, Ricci M, Fabbri L, Romagnani S. Allergen exposure induces the activation of allergen-specific Th2 cells in the airway mucosa of patients with allergic respiratory disorders. Eur J Immunol 1993; 23:1445–1449.

65. Fokkens WJ, Vroom T, Rinjtes E, Mulder P. Fluctuation of the number of CD1a(T6)-positive dendritic cells; presumably Langerhan's cells, in the nasal mucosa of patients with isolated grass pollen allergy before, during and after the grass pollen season. J Allergy Clin Immunol 1989; 84:39–43.

66. Holm AF, Fokkens WJ, Godthelp T, Mulder PG, Vroom TM, Rijntjes E. Effect of 3 months steroid therapy on nasal T cells and langerhans cells in patients suffering from allergic rhinitis. Allergy 1995; 50:204–209.

67. Persson CGA. Plasma exudation in the airways: Mechanisms and function. Eur Respir J 1991; 4:1268–1274.

68. Feather IH, Montefort S, Wilson SJ, Haskard DO, Howarth PH. Endothelial leucocyte adhesion molecule expression in seasonal allergic rhinitis: Relevance to disease expression and regulation by topical corticosteroid therapy. Am J Respir Cell Mol Biol (Submitted).

69. Bochner B, Luscinkas F, Gimbrone M, Newman W, Sterbinsky SA, Derse-Anthony CP, Klunk D, Schleimer RP. Adhesion of human basophils, eosinophils and neutrophils to IL-1 activated human vascular endothelial cells: contribution of endothelial cell adhesion molecule. J Exp Med 1991; 173:1553–1556.

70. Montefort S, Feather IH, Wilson SJ, Haskard DO, Lee TH, Holgate ST, Howarth PH. The expression of leucocyte-endothelial molecules in increases in perennial allergic rhinitis. Am J Respir Cell Mol Biol 1992; 7:393–398.

71. Ciprandi G, Pronzato C, Ricca V, Bagnasco M, Canonica GW. Evidence of intercellular adhesion molecule-1 expression on nasal epithelial cells in acute rhinoconjunctivitis raised by pollen exposure. J Allergy Clin Immunol 1994; 94:738–746.

72. Devalia JL, Calderon M, Sapsford RJ, McAulay AE, d'Ardenne AJ, Davies RJ. Cell adhesion molecules expressed by human nasal epithelial cells. Clin Exp Allergy 1991; 22:120.

73. Marini M, Soloperto M, Mazzetti M, Fasoli A, Matolli S. Interleukin-1 binds to specific receptors on human bronchial epithelial cells and upregulates granulocyte/macrophage colony stimulating factor synthesis and release. Am J Respir Cell Mol Biol 1991: 4:519–524.

74. Cromwell O, Hamid Q, Corrigan CJ, Barkans T, Meng Q, Collins PD, Kay AB. Expression and generation of interluekin-8, IL-6 and granulocyte-macrophage colony-stimulating factor by bronchial epithelial cells and enhancement by IL-1β and tumor necrosis factor-α. Immunology 1992; 77:330–337.

75. Hattorio R, Hamilton RK, Frigates RD, McEver RP, Sims PJ. Stimulated secretion of endothelial von Willebrand factor is accompanied by rapid redistribution to the cell surface of intracellular granule membrane protein GMP-140. J Biol Chem 1989; 264:7768–7771.

76. Schuler G, Steinman RM. Murine epidermal Langerhans' cells mature into potent immunostimulatory dendritic cells in vivo. J Exp Med 1985; 161:526–546.

77. Grabbe J, Haas N, Kolde G, Hakimi J, Czarnetzki BM. Demonstration of high affinity IgE receptor on human Langerhans cells in normal and diseased skin. Br J Dermatol 1993; 129:120–123.

78. Lopez AF, Williamson DW, Gamble JR, Begley CG, Harlan JM, Klebanoff SJ,

Waltersdorph A, Wong G, Clark SC, Vadas MA. Recombinant human granulocyte-macrophage colony-stimulating factor stimulates in vitro mature human neutrophil and eosinophil function, surface receptor expression, and survival. J Clin Invest 1986; 78:1220.

79. Campbell HD, Tucker WQJ, Hort Y, Martinson ME, Mayo G, Clutterbuck EJ, Sanderson CJ, Young IG. Molecular cloning, nucleotide sequence, and expression of the gene encoding human eosinophil differentiation factor (interleukin 5). Proc Natl Acad Sci USA 1987; 84:6629.

80. Clutterbuck EJ, Shields JG, Gordon J. Recombinant human interleukin 5 is an eosinophil differentiation factor but has no activity in standard human B cell growth factor assays. Eur J Immunol 1987; 17:1743.

81. Clutterbuck E, Hirst EMA, Sanderson CJ. Human interleukin-5 (IL-5) regulates the production of eosinophils in human bone marrow cultures: comparison and interaction with IL-1, IL-3, IL-6 and GM-CSF. Blood 1989; 73:1504.

82. Saito H, Hatake K, Dvorak AM, Lieferman KM, Donnenberg AD, Arai N, Ishizaka K, Ishizaka T. Selective differentiation and proliferation of haemopoietic cells induced by recombinant interleukins. Proc Natl Acad Sci USA 1988; 85:2288.

83. Clutterbuck EJ, Sanderson CJ. Regulation of human eosinophil precursor production by cytokines: a comparison of recombinant human interleukin-1 (rhIL-1), rhIL-3, rhIL-5, rhIL-6 and rh granulocyte-macrophage colony-stimulating factor. Blood 1990; 75:1774.

84. Wang JM, Rimaldi A, Biondi A, Chen ZG, Sanderson CJ, Mantovani A. Recombinant human interleukin 5 is a selective eosinophil chemoattractant. Eur J Immunol 1989; 19:701.

85. Warringa RAJ, Koenderman L, Kok PTM, Kreukniet J, Bruijnzeel PLB. Modulation and induction of eosinophil chemotaxis by granulocyte-macrophage colony-stimulating factor and interleukin-3. Blood 1991; 77:2694.

86. Sehmi R, Wardlaw AJ, Cromwell O, Kurihara K, Waltmann P, Kay AB. Interleukin-5 selectively enhances the chemotactic response of eosinophils obtained from normal but not eosinophilic subjects. Blood 1992; 79:2952.

87. Warringa RAJ, Mengelers HJJ, Kuijper PHM, Raaijmakers JAM, Bruijnzeel PLB, Koenderman L. In vivo priming of platelet-activating factor-induced eosinophil chemotaxis in allergic asthmatic individuals. Blood 1992; 79:1836.

88. Warringa RAJ, Schweizer RC, Maikoe T, Kuijper PHM, Bruijnzeel PLB, Koenderman L. Modulation of eosinophil chemotaxis by interleukin-5. Am J Respir Cell Mol Biol 1992; 7:631.

89. Schweizer R-C, Welmers BAC, Raaijmakers JAM, Zanen P, Lammers J-W, Koenderman L. RANTES- and interleukin-8–induced responses in normal human eosinophils: effect of priming with interleukin-5. Blood 1994; 83:3697.

90. Owen Jr WF, Rothenberg ME, Silberstein DS, Gasson JC, Stevens RL, Austen KF, Soberman RJ. Regulation of human eosinophil viability, density and function by granulocyte/macrophage colony-stimulating factor in the presence of 3T3 fibroblasts. J Exp Med 1987; 166:129.

91. Rotheberg ME, Owen Jr WF, Silberstein DS, Woods J, Soberman RJ, Austen

KF, Stevens RL. Human eosinophils have prolonged survival, enhanced functional properties, and become hypodense when exposed to human interleukin 3. J Clin Invest 1988; 81:1986.

92. Tai P-C, Sun L, Spry CJF. Effects of IL-5, granulocyte/macrophage colony-stimulating factor (GM-CSF) and IL-3 on the survival of human blood eosinophils in vitro. Clin Exp Immunol 1991; 85:312.

93. Valerius T, Repp R, Kalden JR, Platzer E. Effects of IFN on human eosinophils in comparison with other cytokines: A novel class of eosinophil activators with delayed onsent of action. J Immunol 1990; 145:2950.

94. Yamaguchi Y, Suda T, Ohna T, Tominaga K, Miura Y, Kasahara T. Analysis of the survival of mature human eosinophils: Interleukin 5 prevent apoptosis in mature human eosinophils. Blood 1991; 78:2542.

95. Stern M, Meagher L, Savill J, Haslett C. Apoptosis in human eosinophils: Programmed cell death in the eosinophil leads to phagocytosis by macrophages and is modulated by IL-5. J Immunol 1992; 148:3543.

96. Kita H, Ohnishi R, Okubo Y, Weiler D, Abrams JS, Gleich GJ. Granulocyte/macrophage colony-stimulating factor and interleukin 3 release from human peripheral blood eosinophils and neutrophils. J Exp Med 1991; 174:745–758.

97. Desreumanx P, Janin A, Colombel JF, Prin L, Phimas J, Emilie D, Torpier G, Capron A, Capron M. Interleukin-5 messenger RNA expression by eosinophils in the interstitial mucosa of patients with coeliac disease. J Exp Med 1992; 175:293–296.

98. Hamid Q, Barkaus J, Meng Q, Ying S, Abrams JS, Kay AB, Moqbel R. Human eosinophils synthesise and secrete interleukin-6 *in vitro*. Blood 1992; 80:1496–1501.

99. Braun RK, Hansel TT, de Vries IJM, Rits S, Blaser K, Evard F, Walker C. Human peripheral blood eosinophils have the capacity to produce IL-8. Eur J Immunol 1993; 23:956–960.

100. Moqbel R, Hamid Q, Ying S, Barkans J, Hartnell A, Tsicopoulos A, Wardlaw AJ, Kay AB. Expression of mRNA and immunoreactivity for the granulocyte/macrophage colony-stimulating factory in activated human eosinophils. J Exp Med 1991; 174:749–752.

101. Cairns JA, Walls AF. Mast cell tryptase is a mitogen for epithelial cells: Stimulation of IL-8 production and intracellular adhesion molecule-1 expression. J Immunol 1996; 156 (In press).

102. Connell JT. Quantitative intranasal pollen challenge: II. Effect of daily pollen challenge, environmental pollen exposure and placebo challenge on the nasal membrane. J Allergy 1968; 41:123–139.

103. Connell JT. Quantitative intranasal pollen challenge: III. The priming effect in allergic rhinitis. J Allergy 1969; 43:33–44.

104. Naclerio RM, Meier HL, Kagey-Sobotka A, et al. Mediator release after nasal airway challenge with allergen. Am Rev Respir Dis 1983; 128:597–602.

105. Raphael GD, Igrashi Y, White MV, Kaliner MA. The pathophysiology of rhinitis V. Sources of protein in allergen-induced nasal secretions. J Allergy Clin Immunol 1991; 88:33–42.

106. Nacleiro RM, Proud D, Togias AG, et al. Inflammatory mediators in late antigen-induced rhinitis. N Engl J Med 1985; 313:65–70.

107. Castells M, Schwartz LB. Tryptase levels in nasal-lavage fluid as an indicator of the immediate allergic response. J Allergy Clin Immunol 1988; 82:348–355.

108. Proud D, Bailey GS, Naclerio RN, et al. Tryptase and histamine as markers to evaluate mast cell activation during the responses to nasal challenge with allergen, cold, dry air, and hyperosmolar solutions. J Allergy Clin Immunol 1992; 89:1098–1110.

109. Proud D, Togias A, Naclerio RN, Crush SA, Norman PS, Lichtenstein LM. Kinins are generated *in vivo* following nasal airway challenge of allergic individuals with allergen. J Clin Invest 1983; 72:1678–1685.

110. Creticos PS, Peters SP, Adkinson Jr NF, et al. Peptide leukotriene release after antigen challenge in patients sensitive to ragweed. N Engl J Med 1984; 310:1626–1630.

111. Shaw RJ, Fitzharris P, Cromwell O, Wardlaw AJ, Kay AB. Allergen-induced release of sulphidopeptide leukotrienes (SRS-A) and LTB_4 in allergic rhinitis. Allergy 1985; 40:1–6.

112. Freeland HS, Pipkorn U, Schleimer RP, et al. Leukotriene B_4 as a mediator of early and late reactions of antigen in humans. The effect of systemic glucocorticoid treatments *in vivo*. J Allergy Immunol 1989; 83:634–642.

113. Kawabori S, Unno T. Degranulation of nasal epithelial mast cells after challenge of allergen. J Submicrosc Cytol Pathol 1983; 15:823–832.

114. Feather IH, Montefort S, Hibbert J, Wilson S, Howarth PH. The influence of allergen challenge on cell accumulation and leucocyte endothelial cell adhesion molecule (CAM) expression within the nasal mucosa in rhinitis. Eur Resp J 1994; 7(suppl 18):1605.

115. Pipkorn U, Proud D, Lichtenstein LM, Kagey-Sabotka A, Norman PS, Naclerio RM. Inhibition of mediator release in allergic rhinitis by pretreatment with topical glucocorticoids. N Engl J Med 1987; 316:1506–1510.

116. Andersson M, Andersson P, Venge P, Popkorn U. Eosinophils and eosinophil cationic protein in nasal lavages in allergen-induced hyperresponsiveness: Effects of topical glucocorticoid treatment. Allergy 1989; 44:342–348.

117. Bascom R, Wachs N, Naclerio R, Pipkorn U, Galli S, Lichtenstein L. Basophil influx occurs after nasal antigen challenge: effects of topical corticosteroid pretreatment. J Allergy Clin Immunol 1988; 81:580–589.

118. Bradding P, Feather IH, Wilson S, Holgate ST, Howarth PH. Cytokine immunoreactivity in seasonal rhinitis: Regulation by a topical corticosteroid. Am J Respir Crit Care Med 1995; 151:1900–1906.

119. Otsuka H, Denburg J, Befus A, et al. Effect of beclomethasone dipropionate on nasal metachromatic cell subpopulations. Clin Allergy 1986; 16:589–595.

120. Okuda M, Sakugachi KOH. Intranasal beclomethasone mode of action in nasal allergy. Ann Allergy 1983; 50:116–120.

121. Juliusson S, Holmberg K, Karlsson G, Enerback L, Pipkorn U. Mast cells and mediators in the nasal mucosa after allergen challenge. Effects of four weeks treatment with topical glucocorticoid. Clin Exp Allergy 1993; 23:591–599.

122. Lozewicz S, Wang J, Duddle J, Thomas K, Chalstrey S, Reilly G, Devalia JL, Davies J. Topical glucocorticoids inhibit activation by allergen in the upper respiratory tract. J Allergy Clin Immunol 1992; 89:951-957.

123. Bradding P, Okayama Y, Howarth PH, Church MK, Holgate ST. Heterogeneity of human mast cells based on cytokine content. J Immunol 1995; 155:297-307.

124. Peroni D, Feather I, Wilson S, Harrison K, Brewster H, Howarth PH. Fluticasone propionate aqueous nasal spray alleviates the symptoms of perennial allergic rhinitis without changing the mucosal inflammatory cell profile. J Allergy Clin Immunol 1993; 91:299.

125. Lichtenstein LM, Ishizaka K, Norman PS, Sabotka AK, Hill BM. IgE antibody measurements in Ragweed Hay Fever. J Clin Invest 1973; 52:472-482.

126. Naclerio RM, Adkinson NF, Creticos PS, Baroody FM, Hamilton RG, Norman PS. Intranasal steroids inhibit seasonal increases in ragweed-specific immunoglobulin E antibodies. J Allergy Clin Immunol 1993; 92:717-721.

127. Norman PS, Winkenwerder WL, Murgatroyd GW, Parsons JW. Evidence for the local action of intranasal dexamethasone aerosols in the suppression of hay fever symptoms. J Allergy 1986; 38:93-99.

128. Lindqvist N, Anderson M, Bende M, Loth S, Pipkorn U. The clinical efficacy of budesonide in hay fever treatment is dependent on topical nasal application. Clin Exp Allergy 1989; 19:71-76.

129. Balle VH, Pedersen U, Engby B. The treatment of perennial rhinitis with a new, non-halogenerated, topical, aerosol packed, steroid budesonide. Acta Otolaryngol 1982; 94:169-173.

130. Malm L, Wihl JA. Intranasal beclomethasone diproprionate in vasomolar rhinitis. Acta Allergol 1976; 31:227-238.

131. Siegel GC, Katz R, Rachelefsky GS, et al. Multicentre study of beclomethasone diproprionate nasal aerosol in adults with seasonal allergic rhinitis. J Allergy Clin Immunol 1982; 69:345-353.

132. Steensen H, Lindquist N. Treatment of grass-pollen induced hay fever with intranasal budesonide. Allergy 1991; 36:245-249.

133. Pedersen B, Dahl R, Richards DH, Jacques LA, Larsen BB, Pichler W, Nykanen KN. Once daily fluticasone propionate aqueous nasal spray controls symptoms in most patients with seasonal allergic rhinitis. Allergy 1995; 50:794-799.

134. Juniper EF, Guyatt GH, O'Byrne PM, Viveiros M. Aqueous beclomethasone dipropionate nasal spray: Regular versus "as required" use in the treatment of seasonal allergic rhinitis. J Allergy Clin Immunol 1990; 86:380-386.

135. Juniper EF, Kline PA, Hargreave FE, Dolovich J. Comparison of beclomethasone dipropionate aqueous nasal spray, astemizole, and the combination in the prophylactic treatment of ragweed pollen-induced rhinoconjunctivitis. J Allergy Clin Immunol 1989; 83:627-633.

136. Welsh PW, Stricker WE, Chu-Piu et al. Efficacy of beclomethasone nasal solution, flunisolide and cromolyn in relieving symptoms of ragweed allergy. Mayo Clinic Proc 1987; 62:125-134.

137. Juniper EF, Kline PA, Ramsdale EH, Hargreave FE. Comparison of efficacy and side effects of aqueous steroid nasal spray (budesonide) and allergen infection

therapy (Pollinex R) in the treatment of seasonal allergic rhinoconjunctivitis. J Allergy Clin Immunol 1990; 85:606–611.

138. Czarny D, Brostoff J. Effects of intranasal betamethasone-17-valerate on perennial rhinitis and adrenal function. Lancet 1968; 2:188.

139. McAllen MK, Langman MJS. A controlled trial of dexamethasone snuff in chronic perennial rhinitis. Lancet 1969; 1:968–971.

140. Brompton Hospital/Medical Research Council Collaborative Trial. Double-blind trial comparing two dosage schedules of beclomethasone dipropionate aerosol with a placebo in the treatment of perennial rhinitis for twelve months. Clin Allergy 1980; 10:239–251.

141. Incando G, Schatz M, Yamamoto F, Mellon M, Crepea S, Johnson JD. Intranasal flunisolide in the treatment of perennial rhinitis: correlation with immunologic parameters. J Allergy Clin Immunol 1980; 65:41–49.

142. Spector S, Bronsky E, Chervinsky P et al. Multi-centre double-blind, placebo-controlled trial of triamcinolone acetonide nasal aerosol in the treatment of perennial allergic rhinitis. Ann Allergy 1990; 64:300–305.

143. Van As A, Bronsky E, Dockhorn RJ et al. Once daily fluticasone proprinate is as effective for perennial allergic rhinitis as twice daily beclomethasone dipropionate. J Allergy Clin Immunol 1993; 91:1146–1154.

144. Robinson AC, Cherry JR, Daly S. Double-blind, cross-over trial comparing beclomethasone dipropionate and terfenadine in perennial rhinitis. Clin Exp Allergy 1989; 19:569–573.

145. Harding SM, Heath S. Intranasal steroid aerosol in perennial rhinitis: Comparison with an antihistamine compound. Clin Allergy 1976; 6:369–372.

146. Tandon MK, Strahan EG. Double-blind cross-over trial comparing beclomethasone dipropionate and sodium cromoglycate in perennial allergic rhinitis. Clin Allergy 1980; 10:459–462.

147. Hillas J, Booth RJ, Somerfield S, Morton R, Avery J, Wilson JD. A comparative trial of intranasal beclomethasone dipropionate and sodium cromoglycate in patients with chronic perennial rhinitis. Clin Allergy 1980; 10:253–258.

148. Brogden RN, McTavish D. Budesonide: An updated review of its pharmacological properties and therapeutic efficacy in asthma and rhinitis. Drugs 1992; 44:375–407.

149. Andersson M, Berglund R, Hammarlund A, Malcus 1, Olsson P, Sjolin I-L, Synnerstad B, Hedbys L. Fluticasone proprinate versus budesonide in patients with perennial allergic rhinitis. Thorax 1993; 48:459.

150. McAllen MK, Portillo PR, Parr EJ, Seaton A, Engler C. Intranasal flunisolide, placebo and beclomethasone dipropionate in perennial rhinitis. Br J Dis Chest 1980; 74:32–36.

151. Sahay JN, Chatterjee SS, Engler C. A comparative trial of flunisolide and beclomethasone dipropionate in the treatment of perennial allergic rhinitis. Clin Allergy 1980; 10:65–70.

152. Mygind N, Clark TJH (eds). Topical Steroid Treatment for Asthma and Rhinitis. London: Bailliere Tindall, 1980.

153. Orgel HA, Meltzer EO, Kemp JP, Welch MJ. Clinical rhinomanometric and cy-

tological evaluation of seasonal allergic rhinitis treated with beclomethasone diproprionate an aqueous nasal spray or pressurised nasal spray. J Allergy Clin Immunol 1986; 77:858–864.

154. Mygind N, Sorensen H, Pedersen CB. The nasal mucosa during long-term treatment with beclamethasone diproprionate aerosol. A light and scanning electron microscope study of nasal polyps. Acta Otolaryngol 1978; 85:437–443.

155. Holoperinen E, Malmberg H, Binder E. Treatment with intranasal beclomethasone dipropionate spray with long observation time; a clinical and histological study. Acta Otolaryngol. 1982; 386:270–273.

156. Sahery JN, Ibrahim NBN, Chatterjee SS, Nassar WY, Lodge KV, Jones CW. Long-term study of flunisolide treatment in perennial rhinitis with special reference to nasal mucosal histology and morphology. Ann Allergy 1980; 10:451–457.

157. Pipkorn U, Pukander J, Suonpan J, Makinen J, Lindqvist N. Long term safety of budesonide nasal aerosol: A 5.5 year follow-up study. Clin Allergy 1988; 18:253–259.

158. Sorensen H, Mygind N, Pedersen CB, Pugtz S. Long term treatment of nasal polyps with beclomethasone dipropionate aerosol III morphological studies and conclusions. Acta Otolaryngol 1976; 182:260-364.

159. Norman PS, Winkenwerder WL, Agbayani BF, Migeon CJ. Adrenal function during the use of dexamethasone aerosols in the treatment of ragweed hay fever. J Allergy 1967; 40:57-61.

160. Van As A, Bronsky EA, Grossman J, Meltzer EO, Ratner PH, Reed C. Dose tolerance study of fluticasone propionate aqueous nasal spray in patients with seasonal allergic rhinitis. Ann Allergy 1991; 67:156–162.

161. Wolthers OD, Pedersen S. Knemometric assessment of systemic activity of once daily intranasal dry-powder budesonide in children. Allergy 1994; 49:96–99.

162. Fraunfelder FT, Myer SM. Posterior subcapsular cataracts associated with nasal or inhalational corticosteroids. Am J Ophthamol 1990; 109:489–490.

163. X Toogood JH, Markov AE, Baskerville J, Dyson C. Association of occular cataracts with inhaled and oral steroid therapy during long term treatment of asthma. J of Allergy Clin Immunol 1993; 91:571–570.

22

Efficacy and Safety of Inhaled Corticosteroids in Children

SØREN E. PEDERSEN

Kolding Hospital
University of Odense
Kolding, Denmark

I. Introduction

Inhaled corticosteroids have been used for more than 25 years in the treatment of asthma in children. Initially, this therapy was reserved for children with very severe symptoms as an alternative to oral steroids. However, over the years, increasing knowledge and clinical experience have been accumulated about the beneficial and systemic effects of this treatment. As a result, the use of inhaled corticosteroids has expanded during the last decade, so that in 1996, these drugs are being introduced much earlier in the treatment of children with moderate asthma by many pediatricians, and the guidelines of some countries even recommend that these drugs be used as first-line therapy in all children with persistent, chronic symptoms. The appropriateness of such widespread use has been heavily debated. The debate has often been based on misconceptions and fears rather than scientific evidence. Therefore, the most important literature about clinical and systemic effects of inhaled steroids will be reviewed.

II. Pharmacodynamics

The dose-response relationships of the various inhaled steroids have only been sparsely studied in children. It seems that the clinical effect of a given dose of an inhaled corticosteroid depends on several factors, including:

The outcome measure studied
The duration of the administration of steroid
The severity of the disease
Perhaps also on the age of the patient and the duration of the asthma disease.

Furthermore, the various inhaled steroids differ in topical potency and the different inhalers vary in drug delivery to the intrapulmonary airways. This makes it very difficult in general terms to define an optimal daily dose of inhaled steroids in children. This dose probably varies with each inhaler-drug combination available on the market. Still it is worthwhile to make some general considerations about dose-response relationships of inhaled corticosteroids. This knowledge is important both when assessing the risk of systemic side effects and when comparisons of different drugs and inhalers or considerations about the place in the management strategy are made.

Normally quite marked and rapid clinical improvements and changes in lung functions are seen at already very low daily doses (around 100 µg) even in children with moderate and severe asthma (1) (Fig. 1). These improvements in lung function and symptoms precede and reach a plateau before the reduction in responsiveness (2). The additional improvement in these parameters with increasing doses is rather small, and often it takes an additional fourfold increase in dose to produce an additional significant effect on symptoms or peak flow measurements. Thus, after a marked initial steepness, the dose response curve becomes very shallow.

Low doses also have a significant effect on airway hyperresponsiveness or lower airways functions. However, the dose-response curve for these parameters is less steep, so that it is possible to demonstrate a significant log linear dose-response relationship over a much wider dose range on these parameters in children with moderate and severe asthma (1). A daily dose of 400 µg budesonide from a spacer produces about 80% of the maximum achievable protection against exercise-induced asthma. This indicates that the vast majority of school children can achieve optimal symptom control on quite low daily doses of inhaled steroids equivalent to 100–200 µg budesonide from a spacer (1,3), whereas somewhat higher doses and longer treatment is required to control hyperreactivity as assessed by protection against exercise-induced asthma (1,2,4–6). In agreement with this, a recent study reported that low doses of

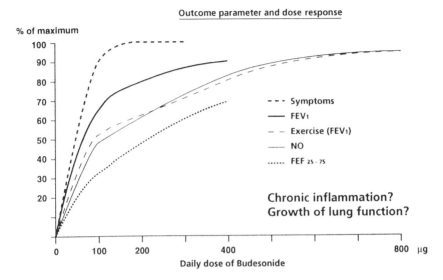

Figure 1 Steroid response relationships for various outcome parameters. The data on symptoms, lung function, and protection against exercise are taken from Ref. 1. The shape of the dose-response curves for normalization of the chronic inflammatory changes in the airways or maintaining normal growth of lung functions are not known.

inhaled steroid produced a marked effect on symptoms and lung functions, whereas somewhat higher doses were required to normalize nitric oxide (NO) concentration in exhaled air (7). The NO concentration in exhaled air is thought to parallel the inflammatory changes in the airways.

The effectiveness of low doses on symptoms and peak expiratory flow rates and the initial rapid increase followed by flatness of the dose-response curve on these parameters has also been confirmed in clinical trials in adults in which high doses (1500 µg/day) were no better than low doses (300 µg/day) in maintenance treatment of severe steroid-dependent patients when symptoms and peak expiratory flow rate were used as outcome parameter (8). In somewhat milder disease, Boe et al. did not find any statistically significant differences between the effect of daily doses of 400–800 µg budesonide or between 400 and 1000 µg beclomethasone on peak expiratory flow (PEF) and diary recordings (9). The lower dose of both drugs produced a marked and statistically significant effect. The same was the case in the study of Dahl et al. (10), which assessed the effect of 100–800 µg fluticasone propionate per day in 672 patients. Although a statistically significant dose-response relationship was found, the mean difference in morning PEF between the lowest and the highest dose was only around 14 L/min, and no statistically significant differences between individual dose steps were found (10).

These findings emphasize the importance of defining the aims of the treatment when the therapy is decided. Peak expiratory flow rate or symptoms may not be the best outcome measures to assess when inhaled steroids are used. Further studies are needed to clarify this.

No formal dose-response studies have been performed in preschool children, so the optimal dose in these age groups is not known. Daily doses of 200–800 µg from a spacer and 1000–2000 µg from a nebulizer have been found to be effective (11–15) in double-blind placebo-controlled trials.

III. Effect on Inflammation and Hyperreactivity

Steroids seem to have direct inhibitory actions on most of the inflammatory cells implicated in asthma (16) and on airway microvascular leak induced by inflammatory mediators. Furthermore, inhaled steroids inhibit the increased expression of granulocyte-macrophage colony-stimulating factor (GM-CSF) in airway epithelial cells of asthmatic patients (17) and the increased mucous secretion in the airways. As a result of these actions, steroids are very effective in controlling the chronic inflammation in asthmatic airways. This has been confirmed in several biopsy studies in adults, which have demonstrated normalization of the numbers of eosinophils, macrophages, mast cells, and lymphocytes; restoration of the disrupted epithelium; and normalization of the ciliated to goblet cell ratio after inhaled steroid treatment. There is also some evidence for a reduction in the thickness of the basement membrane (18–21), although in asthmatic patients receiving inhaled steroids for more than 10 years, some thickening of the basement membrane still seems to be present (22).

Inhaled steroids reduce airway responsiveness to both direct and indirect stimuli (23). Single doses reduce the late and continuous treatment reduces early and late responses to allergen and the subsequent increase in airway responsiveness (24–30). In accordance with this, chronic treatment reduces airway responsiveness to inhaled histamine and methacholine (24,25,29–39), the bronchoconstriction elicited by metabisulfite and bradykinin (which may be acting via neural mechanisms), and hyperosmolar, hyperventilation, and exercise challenges (which may act via mast cells) (5,6,37,40–45). These effects are probably a result of the reduction in the underlying inflammation, but the component of increased airway responsiveness caused by structural changes in the airway may be irreversible by steroids. Unlike all other drugs, steroids not only shift the dose-response curve to spasmogens to the right, but they also limit the maximum narrowing in response to the spasmogen (46) (Fig. 2).

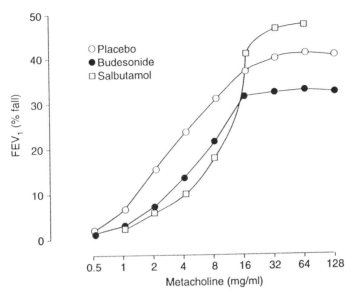

Figure 2 Dose-response curves to inhaled methacholine after treatment with placebo, inhaled steroids, and a β₂-agonist.

IV. Clinical Trials

A. School Children

Many controlled trials have established that inhaled steroids are effective in all patients irrespective of asthma severity. Continuous treatment controls asthma symptoms, reduces the frequency of acute exacerbations and the number of hospital admissions, and improves lung functions and bronchial hyperreactivity (3,36,47–50) both in patients treated at hospital clinics and in patients from general practice. Symptom control and improvements in peak expiratory flow rate occur rapidly (1–2 weeks) at low doses equivalent to 100 μg per day in children with moderate and severe asthma (1), whereas longer treatment (months) with somewhat higher doses (around 4–600 μg/day) is required to achieve maximum effect on bronchial hyperreactivity as assessed by exercise or histamine challenge tests (2,4–6,36,51). The protective effect against exercise-induced asthma is clinically important, as other drugs have to be taken just prior to exercise to confer a protective effect, and the duration of protection is too short for prolonged exercise (with the exception of long-acting inhaled β₂-agonist). A maximum effect against exercise-induced asthma is seen within

2 months after treatment is initiated (2,4–6), whereas a plateau in protection against histamine provocation seems to occur much later (around 20 months after the start of treatment) (4,36). The use of higher steroid doses in the beginning of treatment may reduce these time periods.

When the steroid treatment is discontinued, there is usually a deterioration of the asthma control and bronchial hyperreactivity to pretreatment levels within weeks to months, although in some patients, the effect is maintained much longer (51). So, for the majority of children, it seems that treatment with inhaled steroids suppresses the underlying mechanisms of asthma and causes remission of the condition but does not "cure" the disease (4,36). However, steroid discontinuation has only been evaluated after less than 2 years of continuous treatment and never in a group of children in whom the treatment has been initiated shortly after the start of the disease.

As for other asthma drugs, most clinical studies with inhaled corticosteroids have been of rather short duration. However, recently, two long-term studies have provided interesting information on the beneficial clinical effects and risk of side effects associated with long-term continuous use (36,50). One study on 116 children aged 7–16 years compared inhaled budesonide in a daily dose of 600 µg from a metered-dose inhaled (MDI) with treatment with an inhaled β_2-agonist during 22 months of treatment. Mean FEV_1 (forced expiratory volume in 1 sec) at entry was 80% of the predicted value. Marked improvements were seen in lung functions, peak flow variability, symptoms, and bronchial hyperresponsiveness in the budesonide group. The PD_{20} histamine rose progressively in the budesonide group throughout the whole study period but was unchanged in the β_2-agonist group. The differences between the two groups were maintained throughout the 22-month period (36). Furthermore, a high frequency (45%) of dropouts from the study because of symptoms and a worsening of lung functions was seen in the children not receiving budesonide. Similar differences were observed between budesonide treatment and treatment with combinations of other asthma drugs (β_2-agonist, theophylline, and disodiumcromoglycate) in another study which followed 278 children for 3 to 6 years on continuous budesonide treatment (50). In both studies, budesonide significantly increased the growth rate of lung function with age in comparison with the children not receiving inhaled steroids. Furthermore, in the study of Agertoft and Pedersen, the effect of budesonide on lung function was significantly greater when budesonide was started early (within 2 years) after asthma was diagnosed, so that children who started early had a more rapid response and obtained significantly better lung functions than the children in whom budesonide was not started until some years after the onset of asthma symptoms (50) (Fig. 3). In addition, in the children who started early, the accumulated dose of budesonide taken after 4.5 years of continuous treatment was significantly lower than the dose taken by the group of children in whom

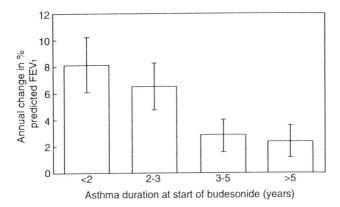

Figure 3 Influence of asthma duration at the start of inhaled steroid (budesonide) on the mean annual increase in FEV$_1$ measured after budesonide treatment (mean and 95% confidence intervals). Children who started early had a more rapid response and obtained significantly better lung functions than the children who did not receive the treatment until some years after the onset of asthma symptoms.

budesonide treatment was not initiated until after more than 5 years of continuous symptoms. FEV$_1$ in the control group not receiving inhaled steroids showed an annual decline of 1.3% against the predicted value. This together with the findings of higher lung functions at the use of lower doses of budesonide in children who started budesonide early provide evidence that early treatment with inhaled steroids may prevent the development of irreversible persistent structural changes, which have been reported to take place in the airways of children with chronic asthmatic symptoms (52–64). Recently, similar findings have been reported in adult studies, that is, early introduction of inhaled steroids produces a better clinical effect as compared with late introduction (65,66).

Finally, the hospitalization rate for acute severe asthma in the control group in the study by Agertoft was unchanged around 3% per year throughout the study. This figure was not different from the 2.8% which was seen in the budesonide group during the last 2 years before budesonide was initiated. During budesonide treatment, the hospitalization rate was reduced significantly to 0.14% per year. Similar effects on hospitalization rates have been reported by other investigators (67). No systemic side effects were seen in any of the two long-term studies (more details are given later).

Generally, the beneficial effects of inhaled steroids in children are more pronounced than for any other asthma drug as shown in several studies (3,36,37,47,48,50,68). In one study, children with mild and moderate asthma from general practice achieved markedly better symptom control and significantly higher morning and evening peak expiratory flow rates and lung functions during treatment with 50 μg fluticasone propionate twice a day as compared with children treated with disodium chromoglycate (DSCG), 20 mg four times a day (3). Similar results were reported by Østergaard and Pedersen comparing budesonide, 400 μg/day, with DSCG in children with mild and moderate asthma (37). In the two recent studies, 200 and 400 μg beclomethasone propionate per day was significantly more effective than continuous theophylline treatment in optimal doses and inhaled bronchodilators (47,48).

During recent years, cost-benefit evaluations have become an important factor when decisions about therapy are made. Such assessments have been made in both long-term studies (36,50). The results were quite similar. Inhaled steroids were a cost-effective treatment option that resulted net health care savings. In the Danish study, both direct medical costs and costs of necessary additional intervention, including hospitalizations, were reduced. In the Dutch study, direct medical costs were not reduced, because the steroid treatment was only compared with placebo and sabutamol treatment.

B. Preschool Children and Infants

Although the number of controlled studies in preschool children and infants is not so high as in school children, an increasing number of placebo-controlled clinical trials demonstrate the marked clinical effects of inhaled steroids, including improvement in lung functions, reduction of bronchial hyperresponsiveness, reduction in oral steroid requirement, and in the use of rescue bronchodilators (14,15,69,70). The results from these studies indicate that the same benefits are achieved in preschool children as in older children. A few trials have failed to demonstrate a significant beneficial effect (71–73). However, this seems to have been due to insufficient drug delivery from an inefficient nebulizer and/or a poor study design rather than a lack of effect of the drugs (74,75). Virus-induced wheeze, which is common in these age groups, is also modified (76), and two controlled trials have found that nebulized beclomethasone reduced the frequency (but not the severity) of respiratory symptoms and improved lung function in infants with postbronchiolitis wheezing (77,78). In one of these, 3 months of treatment after the virus-induced wheeze even reduced the occurrence of wheeze throughout the following year (78). Finally, three uncontrolled studies have observed clinical improvement in severe asthma in infancy, which had not responded to other treatment (79–81). The problem in young children and infants is—in addition to difficulties with effective drug delivery to the intrapulmonary airways—that in the daily clinical situation it is not possible to identify the children with recurrent wheeze who are asthmatics from nonasthmatic children who suffer from recurrent viral induced wheeze. The optimal use of inhaled steroids may differ between these two groups.

Like in older children, treatment with inhaled steroids has also been shown to be cost effective in children aged 1–3 years (82).

No formal comparisons with other treatments have been performed in young children. However, the children recruited for the controlled trials had all tried or were still on other asthma medication, including theophylline, inhaled and oral bronchodilators, DSCG, and alternate-day oral steroids, without achieving sufficient control. Still, inhaled steroids improved the condition indicating that this treatment is also more effective than any other asthma treatment in young children. Further studies are needed to assess this.

So, in summary, inhaled steroids are effective in all age groups of children with asthma. Low doses are as effective as or more effective than any other treatment in controlling symptoms and improving lung function. Early introduction of inhaled steroids after the debut of chronic symptoms seems to be preferable to late introduction. Further studies are needed to assess which measurement is the best outcome parameter when deciding the optimal dose of inhaled steroid. It seems that somewhat higher doses are required to produce a maximum effect on nitric oxide production or bronchial responsiveness than to achieve symptom control and maximum increase in peak expiratory flow rate. Finally, the doses required to ensure optimal growth of lung function or prevent the development of irreversible airway obstruction need further study.

V. Pharmacokinetics

Since the majority of drug deposited in the intrapulmonary airways is absorbed systemically, the pharmacokinetics of inhaled steroids are important in determining the systemic effects of the drug. A rapid biotransformation to inactive metabolites is important as is a high first-pass metabolism that reduces the amount of drug which becomes systemically bioavailable from the gastrointestinal tract. At present, only the pharmacokinetics of budesonide has been studied in children. It was found that school children metabolize budesonide about 40% faster than adults, the systemic bioavailability after oral dosing was approximately 15%, which is similar to that observed in adults, and finally the systemic availability of drug after inhalation from a spacer, Turbuhaler, or a nebulizer was around 25, 40, and 15% of the nominal dose, respectively (83,84). These studies were in school children. The pharmacokinetics in preschool children have not been studied.

VI. Delivery Systems

The systemic effect of an inhaled corticosteroid depends on the amount of drug which is systemically absorbed. When a corticosteroid is inhaled, the drug leaving the inhaler is deposited in the oropharynx and in the intrapulmonary airways (85–93). The part deposited in the oropharynx is swallowed and subsequently absorbed with a systemic bioavailability of less than 1% to about 50%, depending on the corticosteroid used (83,84,94,95). The systemic availability of the drug deposited in the intrapulmonary airways is not known. It is probably high, that is, close to 80% (95,96). Thus, the total systemic effect of a corticosteroid depends on the amount of drug deposited in the intrapulmonary airways and the amount absorbed and systemically available from the gastrointestinal tract. So a clinically very effective inhaler with a high intrabronchial deposition will also be expected to have a higher systemic effect than a clinically less effective inhaler. In contrast, the contribution of the orally deposited drug to the systemic effect is higher for an inhaler with a low intrapulmonary drug deposition, especially if the drug has a high gastrointestinal availability (Fig. 4).

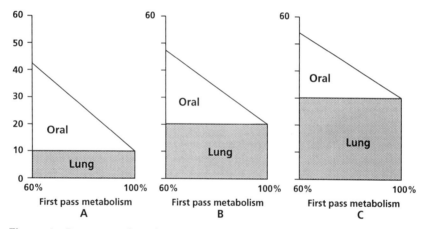

Figure 4 Percentage of nominal dose becoming systemically bioavailable from three different inhalers. The amount of systemically bioavailable drug depends on lung deposition (inhaler A = 10%, B = 20%, and C = 30% of nominal dose) and on the amount absorbed from the gastrointestinal tract; the latter being inversely related to the first-pass metabolism of the drug. If 400 µg corticosteroid from inhaler B reduces urinary cortisol excretion by 40% and 400 µg from inhaler A only reduces it by 20%, it may be concluded that inhaler A is preferable to inhaler B. If however, inhaler B is twice as effective as inhaler A clinically (as is the case in the figure), then there is no difference between the two inhalers, since the dose in inhaler B can be reduced by 50% and still be as effective as A. So for the same clinical effect the two inhalers have similar systemic effects. In fact, inhaler B may even be preferable to A if the steroid used has a low first-pass metabolism! Similar results on cortisol excretion could also be seen if the corticosteroid used had a high systemic bioavailability of drug deposited in the oropharynx and inhaler C was three times more effective than inhaler A but delivered a substantially lower dose to the oropharynx than inhaler A.

During recent years, a large variety of inhalers has been developed to make inhalation therapy easier for patients with asthma. These inhalers show a substantial variation in dose delivered to the patient and deposition pattern of the drug particles (85–92). Furthermore, both these parameters vary markedly with the inhalation technique used. For these reasons, it is important both to evaluate the effect and side effect profile of an inhaler so that an effect/side effect ratio (therapeutic ratio) can be defined for each inhaler-drug combination. If this is not done, false conclusions may be drawn from inhaler or drug comparisons, that is, if 400 μg corticosteroid from inhaler B reduced urinary cortisol excretion by 40% and 400 μg from inhaler A only reduces it by 20%, it may be concluded that inhaler A is preferable to inhaler B. If, however, inhaler B is twice as effective as inhaler A clinically, then there is no difference between the two inhalers, since the dose in inhaler B can be reduced by 50% and still be as effective as inhaler A. So, for the same clinical effect the two inhalers have similar systemic effects. In fact, inhaler B may even be preferable to inhaler A if the steroid used has a low first-pass metabolism! Similar results on cortisol excretion could also be seen if the corticosteroid used had a high systemic bioavailability of drug deposited in the oropharynx and inhaler C was three times more effective than inhaler A but delivered a substantially lower dose to the oropharynx than inhaler A (see Fig. 4)! Finally, conclusions from studies in adults may not be valid in children, who have a different inhalation technique and a different anatomy of the upper airways. At present, few pediatric studies have considered the importance of these aspects when evaluating inhaled steroids and their delivery systems.

Based on the findings in deposition studies in adults, spacers reduce oropharyngeal deposition of drug (85–92), and therefore these devices are theoretically preferable to other inhalers for delivering inhaled corticosteroids to patients, particularly when high doses of corticosteroids with a high gastrointestinal bioavailability are used. Most studies evaluating this issue in children have compared the systemic effect of the same dose of a corticosteroid delivered from two different inhalers without considering the question of clinically equieffective doses of the two inhalers. In such studies, it has been confirmed that microgram for microgram beclomethasone delivered via a spacer (Volumatic) has less systemic activity than the same dose delivered from a MDI (97–99) or a dry-powder inhaler (Diskhaler) (100). Since the Volumatic spacer seems to be at least as effective as these inhalers, the clinical effect/systemic effect ratio for the Volumatic spacer is probably better than the ratio for these inhalers.

Budesonide from a Nebuhaler has less systemic effect than budesonide from a Turbuhaler (83,84,101,102). Mouthwashing after Turbuhaler treatment seems to reduce this difference (101). This would also be expected from a recent pharmacokinetic study which shows that orally deposited drug contributes with about 15% of the total systemic effect of budesonide from a Turbuhaler in children (83). However, the Turbuhaler is more effective than these inhalers (102–104). So the higher systemic effect of the Turbuhaler is mainly due to a higher intrabronchial deposition, and hence the therapeutic ratio is almost the same for this inhaler and the Nebuhaler, since the budesonide dose can be reduced when a Turbuhaler is used.

In contrast with other studies, Toogood compared both the clinical effect and the systemic effect of a MDI alone and a MDI with a Nebuhaler in adults (105). He found an enhanced clinical effect of the Nebuhaler but also a somewhat higher systemic effect from this inhaler. The data also indicated that the effect/systemic effect ratio was better for the Nebuhaler. This is in agreement with the findings in a recent pharmacokinetic study in children (106).

The importance of inhalation device for the clinical and systemic effect of other steroids than budesonide has not been studied in children. For fluticasone propionate, the therapeutic ratio is probably very similar for all devices, because of the low gastrointestinal bioavailability of this drug. However, important differences in clinical effect and in systemic effect may exist between the various devices, if they deliver a different amount of drug to the intrapulmonary airways.

We have no knowledge about the clinical therapeutic ratio for the various nebulizer systems, although a recent study suggested that important differences may exist (107). Nose breathing, which is common in young children, would be expected to filter off the large particles, which for some drugs, are likely to be absorbed and cause systemic effects without adding to the clinical effect. Jet nebulizers with spacer-like reservoirs, which filter off the large particles, are likely to improve the therapeutic ratio.

Most studies assessed the adverse effects of the various inhalers on the hypothalamic-pituitary-adrenocortical (HPA) axis. The importance of inhaler on other systemic effects such as calcium metabolism needs further study, since it is possible that the swallowed drug may have a local gastrointestinal effect on calcium absorption (108,109).

A. Conclusion

Further studies are needed to define which the inhaler system is preferable for the delivery of inhaled corticosteroids in children. Generally, spacer systems seem to be advantageous to other inhalers for delivery of steroids which have a high gastrointestinal bioavailability. Recent findings with the dry-powder inhaler Turbuhaler indicate that the clinical effect/systemic effect ratio of this inhaler is quite similar to that of a spacer. Furthermore, the low gastrointestinal bioavailability of fluticasone also reduces the importance of a spacer for this drug. The difference in effect/systemic effect ratio between the various inhalers is clinically most important when high doses of inhaled corticosteroids are used.

VII. Systemic Effects

Although the benefits of inhaled steroids in asthma are clear, there are still concerns about systemic effects of these drugs, particularly as they are likely to be administered over very long periods. The safety and risk of systemic side effects have been extensively studied throughout the past 25 years without these terms being clearly defined. Often a measurable systemic effect is considered to be equivalent to a clinically relevant systemic side effect, but this is not necessarily the case. Whether a systemic effect is measurable or not entirely depends on the sensitivity of the method used for the measurement, so when more sensitive methods are being developed more systemic effects will become measurable. Therefore, it is important to realize that for a given drug or inhaler, there will always be a dose below which no systemic effects can be detected no matter which method is used. Then there will be a dose range within which systemic effects are measurable in one or more systems (this dose varies from system to system). However, these measurable effects merely reflect small changes within the normal range of the normal biological feedback system and they do not have any clinical relevance (Fig. 5). Finally, there will be a dose level which will also be associated with clinically important systemic side effects in one or more systems. Little information is available about the dose level at which the systemic effects become clinically relevant, and our knowledge about this issue is mainly confined to case reports on idiosyncratic reactions (110,111). In contrast, our knowledge about the dose level at which

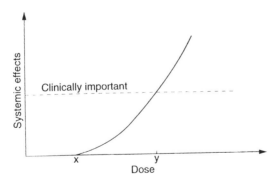

Figure 5 Dose-response curves for the systemic effects of an inhaled steroid. At low doses no detectable effects are seen. This is followed by a dose range (from dose x) in which measurable systemic effects can be detected with sensitive methods. These effects are without clinical importance. At dose y the measurable effects are so marked that they become clinically important, because the reduction in endogenous cortisol production cannot longer compensate the effects of the systemically bioavailable exogenous steroid.

measurable systemic effects are seen is quite good. This information is important, since it can normally assumed that doses which are not associated with any measurable systemic effects in sensitive laboratory test systems will be clinically safe. With this in mind, the present knowledge about various measurable systemic effects of oral and inhaled steroids will be briefly summarized with special emphasis on the lowest dose at which *measurable systemic effects* are seen.

The vast majority of all studies evaluating the risk of systemic effects have been on children older than 5 years, and if specific comments are not made, the findings presented are from studies on these age groups.

As mentioned previously, the systemic effect of an inhaled steroid depends on several factors, including the dose delivered to the patient, the pharmacokinetic fate of the particular inhaled steroid (extent of first-pass hepatic metabolism), the site of deposition of the drug (gastrointestinal tract and lung), and individual differences in steroid response between different patients. Many of these parameters are influenced by the choice of inhaler. Therefore, a summary of the literature will always be an oversimplification of a complex issue.

A. HPA Axis

Treatment with corticosteroids may cause hypothalamic-pituitary-adrenal suppression by reducing corticotropin (ACTH) production, which in turn leads to a reduced cortisol secretion by the adrenal gland. If this sequence of events continues, atrophy of the adrenal gland may follow. The degree of HPA suppression is dependent on the dose, duration, frequency, time of day, and route of administration of the steroid (112–114). The higher the plasma corticosteroid levels, the greater the HPA suppression until a certain critical levels is reached when maximum suppression occurs. The duration of treatment is important. A single dose will cause transient suppression of ACTH production, but recovery is rapid; however, when repeated doses are given, recovery of ACTH production is less rapid and with prolonged therapy, recovery in some individuals may take months.

Various tests are used to measure HPA axis function. Some assess *basal adrenal activity* (a single morning plasma cortisol level, 24-hr urinary free cortisol excretion, overnight urinary cortisol excretion, 24-hr integrated plasma cortisol, nocturnal integrated plasma cortisol). A single plasma cortisol level is the least sensitive, whereas repeated plasma cortisol determinations are very sensitive in detecting small changes in basal cortisol secretion rate. This method detects the small reductions in the frequent peaks in plasma cortisol concentrations that normally occur in patients at rest (115–118). It seems that these small peaks are the first to disappear in the sensitive feedback system of the HPA axis. However, the clinical relevance of the findings in such studies conducted under laboratory conditions, which are quite different from a normal day-to-day living, is not known, since these tests may detect changes at steroid doses which have been used for years without any clinical side effects or any measurable adverse effect on other HPA function tests.

Other test measures, the *HPA response* following stimulation (short tetracosactrin test, 6 AM metyrapone test) or stress (insulin-induced hypoglycaemia). The metyrapone and insulin hypoglycaemia tests measure the integrity and function of the entire HPA system. However, they are time consuming, may make the patient feel unwell, and, in the case of the insulin stress test, are potentially dangerous. Although the "gold standard" is claimed to be the insulin stress test (119), there is no general consensus as to the most sensitive, specific, and clinically relevant test to use (120–123). The short tetracosactrin test probably remains the one most frequently employed to provide information on the adrenal reserve (124), but the single-dose metyrapone test is often recommended to assess HPA function (122,124). As for the basal adrenal activity tests, the clinical importance of small, but statistically significant, reductions in response is not known, since the reduced response is often within the normal range of the test.

A large number of studies have assessed HPA axis function following inhaled glucocorticosteroids. The results are sometimes conflicting, mainly because the investigations have often been uncontrolled, patients have frequently previously been on oral glucocorticoid therapy, the duration of treatment has varied, different inhalers have been used, and different tests applied to monitor changes in HPA function.

Improvements in HPA axis function have been repeatedly shown in glucocorticoid-dependent patients when their oral steroid dose is reduced following the introduction of inhaled corticosteroids (125–131). This improvement has been shown both in tests assessing basal adrenal activity and in tests measuring HPA response after stimulation. However, the effect of chronic administration of oral steroids may continue for a long time after reduction of the oral dose.

No significant effects on *basal endogenous adrenal cortisol secretion rate* have been reported with doses of up to 400 µg budesonide per day from a spacer (12,132–140). Furthermore, urinary cortisol excretion are not suppressed at budesonide doses of up to 800 µg per day in many studies (132,135, 140,141), although some report significant effects on basal cortisol excretion by these doses (142). In contrast, 400 µg budesonide per day from a Turbuhaler seems to reduce urinary cortisol excretion (102,143). Finally, preschool children treated with daily budesonide doses of 200–300 µg for 3–5 years had normal adrenal function as assessed by very sensitive methods (81) such as frequent plasma cortisol measurements over 24 hr.

In studies in which plasma cortisol was measured at frequent intervals during nighttime or over a 24-hr period, 400–1000 μg beclomethasone dipropionate per day from a metered-dose inhaler (MDI) was associated with a significant reduction in the normal physiological secretion of cortisol (115–118,144). Similar findings have been reported for budesonide from a MDI with a spacer (144). In one study, the effect seemed to be dose dependent (115), whereas the other study found no correlation between dose and cortisol suppression (117,118). At variance with these results, the majority of studies have not observed any significant changes in urinary cortisol excretion in children treated with beclomethasone dipropionate up to 400 μg per day (112,145–151) although some studies do find significant changes in children receiving 400 μg per day from a Diskhaler or a MDI (152–154). However, the cortisol excretion was still within the normal range on this dose. This was also the case for the majority of children receiving long-term treatment with substantially higher doses—up to 2000 μg per day (141)—although the proportion of studies reporting significant effects on basal adrenal activity tests increases with increasing dose. Finally, the influence of a daily dose of 200 μg fluticasone propionate and 800 μg budesonide on plasma cortisol profile over a 24-hr period and an increase in plasma cortisol after ACTH stimulation has been evaluated (155). No significant effects were found on these parameters by any of the two drugs. Both had significantly less effect than 2.5–7.5 mg prednisolone per day.

The reports on other inhaled steroids are sparse. Nebulized flunisolide in doses up to 1.6 mg per day or MDI treatment with 1 mg/day did not seem to affect basal adrenal activity even if significant clinical improvements were seen at these doses (156,157). Furthermore, fluticasone propionate in daily doses of 200 and 400 μg has been shown to reduce cortisol excretion in the urine (143).

At present, one study has reported a somewhat reduced *HPA response* in asthmatic children only treated with inhaled corticosteroids (and no oral steroids) in high doses (142). Otherwise, no studies have found a reduced HPA response in asthmatic children only treated with inhaled corticosteroids (134,141,148, 150). Doses up to 800 μg per day have been the most extensively studied. One study found an abnormal insulin tolerance test in a group of 16 children, 9 of whom had also received oral steroids in the past, as compared with a group of normal nonasthmatic children (158). The dose of beclomethasone used was 300–500 μg daily. The results of that study were challenged (159) with regard to the timing of the tests and the fact that the control group was nonasthmatics.

As for adults, no cases of clinical adrenal insufficiency have been reported in patients only treated with inhaled corticosteroids.

The effect of different inhaled corticosteroids on the HPA axis has only been directly compared in a few studies in children. The effect of beclomethasone on urinary cortisol excretion was found to be more marked than that of budesonide in some studies, especially at high daily doses (≥800 μg)

(132,160,161). Other studies have not found any differences between the two drugs (144,162–165). Hoffmann-Streb found no significant difference in the effect of a daily dose of 200 μg fluticasone propionate and 800 μg budesonide on plasma cortisol profile over a 24-hr period or increase in cortisol after ACTH stimulation (155). Both drugs had significantly less effect on these parameters than 2.5–7.5 mg prednisolone per day. Finally, a recent dose-response study in our own clinic found that microgram for microgram fluticasone Diskhaler and budesonide Turbuhaler had the same effect on cortisol excretion in the urine (143).

B. Conclusion

The effects of the HPA axis seem to differ between the various inhaled corticosteroids and inhaler systems. Significant effects on basal adrenal cortisol secretion rate can be detected with some delivery systems in some studies at daily doses of some inhaled corticosteroids of around 400 μg. However, at present, no clinically relevant side effects on the HPA axis have been reported in children receiving such therapy for many years. There seems to be little point in performing routine monitoring of adrenal function in children treated with inhaled corticosteroids in standard pediatric doses.

VIII. Bone Turnover

In adults, up to 10% of bone is replaced each year, but the rate differs in cortical bone (about 5%), in trabecular bone (up to 20%), and at different individual sites. If bone mass is to remain constant, resorption and formation must be in balance. Systemic steroids can induce osteoporosis by increasing bone resorption and decreasing bone formation (166,167). Although no controlled prospective longitudinal studies have been performed, cross-sectional studies in children and adults suggest that steroid-induced osteoporosis is clinically important, since a large proportion of patients receiving long-term oral steroids experience rib or vertebral fractures (168–170).

The effect of exogenous steroids on bone can be evaluated by measurement of biochemical markers of bone metabolism (bone formation and degradation), bone mineral density (BMD), or frequency of fractures.

A. Markers of Bone Formation

Alkaline Phosphatase

Alkaline phosphatase exists as several isoenzymes, and it is synthesized by the liver, bone, kidney, intestines, and placenta. Therefore, it is important to measure *bone-specific serum alkaline phosphatase*. This enzyme is found in the membrane of preosteoblasts and active osteoblasts. Serum levels are higher during bone synthesis; that is, at times of high osteoblast activity. It shows no diurnal variation in plasma concentration and is a rather insensitive measure of *acute* changes in bone formation.

Procollagen Type I Carboxyterminal Propeptide (PICP) and Procollagen Type I N-Terminal Propeptide (PINP)

These markers of bone formation are released from the carboxyterminal end and the N-terminal end of procollagen, respectively, during synthesis of collagen. Serum levels of both correlate with collagen 1 synthesis. Collagen 1 is found in both bone and soft tissue. The disadvantage of these markers is that the contribution from soft tissue is not known. Furthermore, the concentration in serum is genetically determined in each individual, so it is of little use as a reference value. A small diurnal variation is seen, with maximum levels measured at night when the bone turnover is increased.

Osteocalcin

Osteocalcin is a calcium-binding, vitamin K–dependent gamma-carboxyglutamic acid–containing noncollagenous protein (also called bone Gla protein, or BGP) synthesized by the osteoblasts. It comprises 1–2% of bone protein. Osteoblastic synthesis of osteocalcin is increased by $1,25\text{-}(OH)_2$ and D_3, and the circulating levels reflect osteoblast activity. Osteocalcin levels show a small diurnal variation, with maximum levels during the night owing to increased bone turnover. Approximately 20–30% of the osteocalcin escapes into the circulation. *Intact osteocalcin* reflects bone formation and osteoblast activity, whereas *osteocalcin fragments* reflect osteoclast activity and degradation of bone. Therefore, it is important to have specific immunoassays that detect as much as possible of the intact osteocalcin molecule and no or little of the fragments. Correct handling of the serum samples is also important, because proteolytic enzymes in the serum will degrade the osteocalcin molecule into fragments. There are a number of different immunoassays for measuring osteocalcin, some using polyclonal antibodies and others monoclonal antibodies.

Markers of Bone Resorption and Degradation

Hydroxyproline

Urinary Hydroxyproline Excretion After a 12-hr Fast. Hydroxyproline is the specific amino acid of collagen which is released during collagen degradation. It is a nonspecific bone marker present in all collagens and in some other proteins. Approximately 10% is released into the urine, but only 50% of what is found in the urine originates from bone. Urinary levels are increased after ingestion of gelatin; however, a 12-hr fast eliminates this problem.

Glycosylated Hydroxylysine

This marker exists in two forms, GH and GHH. It is released from all types of collagens. GH is found in higher concentration than GHH in bone and in lower concentration than GHH in skin.

Tartrate-Resistant Acid Phosphatase (TRAP)

TRAP exists in several isoenzymes and is synthesized from blood cells, prostate, and bone. *Bone-specific TRAP* is abundant in osteoclasts and the levels of TRAP are thought to reflect osteoclast activity.

Pyridinoline/Desoxypyridinoline

Pyridinoline/desoxypyridinoline are used much more frequently than the two previous markers. They are collagen cross links released by the osteoclast during bone resorption. Pyridinoline is present both in bone and cartilage, whereas desoxypyridinoline is more bone specific. There is a diurnal, age, gender, and day-to-day variation which has to be kept in mind when using these markers.

Cross-Linked Carboxyterminal Telopeptide of Type I Collagen

ICTP is released into the circulation as fragments during collagen degradation. These fragments are intact and resist further degradation. ICTP increases during bone resorption and the serum level correlates with the bone resorption rate. There is a small diurnal variation, with increased levels during the night owing to increased bone turnover.

Urinary Calcium Excretion in Relation to Creatinine

After a 12-hr fast, urinary calcium excretion is a measure of the calcium coming mainly from bone. It is thought to reflect the difference between the rates of mineralization and resorption.

Bone Mineral Density (BMD)

At present, dual x-ray absorptiometry (DEXA) is the most commonly used and best-validated technique for measuring BMD. Although a low BMD in adults is associated with an increased risk of fracture as compared with patients with a high BMD, the association is statistical rather than clinically very useful. Considerable overlap exists in BMD levels between subjects, who have a fracture and those who do not. Generally, BMD is thought to predict fracture with the same relation as blood pressure predicts a stroke.

Recently, ultrasound of the calcaneus has been used to measure osteoporosis (quality of trabecular bone). Preliminary data look interesting, but further validation is needed to assess its value in detecting steroid induced osteoporosis.

In children, the rate of bone modeling/turnover is much higher than in adults. Furthermore, in adults, the skeletal mass is decreasing, whereas in children, it is increasing throughout childhood and adolescence until peak bone mass/density is reached in early adulthood. The increase in bone mass is not a constant process but varies with age and season of the year. The skeletal modeling/turnover rate and calcium retention being highest during spring and summer and during infancy and adolescence. Normally, most of the skeletal mass will be accumulated by late adolescence. As final height in relation to predicted adult height is the most important outcome when growth is studied in children so is *maximal peak bone mass density probably the most clinically relevant outcome measure to assess when the influence of steroids on bones in children is studied.* In addition to nutrition (including calcium intake), heredity (both parents), endocrine factors (sexual development), and physical activity appear to have profound effects on peak bone mass formation. Therefore, these confounding factors should be considered when the effects of steroids on bone metabolism are assessed.

Bone Markers and Steroids

The data on markers of bone metabolism are relative sparse in children. Reduced osteocalcin levels have been reported in children with asthma independent of whether the child received steroids or not (171). Serum levels of calcium, phosphate, magnesium, total and bone specific alkaline phosphatase, osteocalcin, parathyroid hormone, 1,25-dihydroxyvitamin D, or urinary hydroxyproline excretion have been found to be unaffected by daily doses of budesonide and beclometasone dipropionate up to 800 μg and fluticasone propionate up to 400 μg per day (138,154,171,172).

TRAP was significantly reduced in children treated with beclomethasone dipropionate, 300–800 μg/day (171), indicating a reduced degradation. Finally, serum levels of PICP and ICTP and hydroxyproline excretion in the urine were not affected by treatment with budesonide, 400 μg/day (173–175), but at 800 μg, a significant reduction in PICP and ICTP has been reported (173–175), suggesting a reduction in both formation and degradation of collagen 1 at this dose. Low doses (2.5–5.0 mg) of prednisolone cause significant reductions in serum levels of osteocalcin, PICP, and ICTP and in hydroxyproline excretion in the urine of children (172,176).

So no adverse effects on markers of bone formation and degradation have been reported at standard paediatric doses of inhaled steroids. High doses cause significant changes, which suggest a reduced bone turnover rate (reduced formation and reduced degradation). The importance of these significant changes during steroid treatment (which is often short term) has yet to be elucidated. It is probably most clinically relevant to consider the net effect of bone formation and bone resorption. If, for instance, formation and resorption decrease to the same extent, the changes may not be important, since the net effect may be zero. In contrast, a treatment is normally considered to be more of a problem if formation markers decrease more than resorption markers or if resorption markers increase together with a decrease in formation markers. The appropriateness of this assumption needs further study, since it has still not been shown that such changes in short-term studies have any clinical relevance (177). Fracture is the only important endpoint when the effect of steroids on bones is assessed. Markers of bone turnover and bone mineral density are surrogates, although the latter seems to relate to some extent to the risk of fractures.

Bone Density and Steroids

It appears that asthmatic children and adolescents never treated with exogenous corticosteroids may have decreased bone density and reduced osteocalcin levels in the blood when compared with normal nonasthmatic children (171). The reason for this is not known. When the clinical condition of a child improves as a result of therapy, the physical activity and dietary habits of the patient may change. These factors have been shown to affect bone density (178,179). Thus, in adult patients with rheumatoid arthritis, prednisolone treatment may actually increase bone density (180). This might also be the case for children with asthma. Therefore, conclusions from studies on the effects of inhaled corticosteroids in healthy children or children not requiring the therapy may not be relevant for asthmatic children requiring the treatment (81).

At present, bone densitometry has only been sparsely applied to assess the bone mineral density in children receiving inhaled corticosteroids. In a cross-sectional study, 4.5 years' treatment with inhaled budesonide at a mean dose of 691 µg per day was not associated with lower bone density in children as compared with children who had never received exogenous steroids. Furthermore, bone density did not correlate with years of budesonide treatment or current or accumulated dose of budesonide (181) (Fig. 6). Similar findings were reported in 26 children treated with beclomethasone dipropionate, 300–800 µg/day for 2 years (171) and in a similar number of children aged 5–18 years receiving inhaled steroids for at least 1 year (182). In accordance with these cross-sectional studies, increases in vertebral bone density over a period of 6 months in a group of 14 children treated with beclomethasone propionate were found to be similar to the increases seen in a comparable group of 16 children treated with sodium cromoglycate (183). So at present there are no indications that long-term treatment with inhaled corticosteroids is associated with an increased risk of osteoporosis or fracture in children. However, further prospective long-term studies are needed.

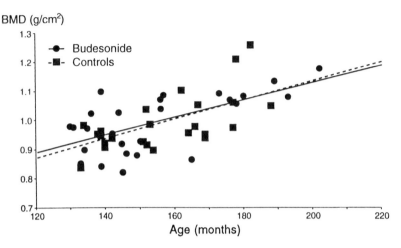

Figure 6   Bone mineral density as a function of age in two groups of children with asthma. Group A had never been treated with exogenous steroids. Group B had been treated with inhaled budesonide at a mean daily dose of 691 μg for an average of 4.5 years. No significant differences were seen between the two groups.

No controlled studies have evaluated the effect of long-term steroid treatment on the clinically most important parameter; that is *peak* bone mass/density. Most studies have been of short-term (< 6 months) or intermediate-term (> 6 months to several years) duration. It is not known how the findings in such studies relate to peak bone mass/density (184). It may be similar to growth studies (see later) where findings in short-term studies do not relate at all to long-term growth, that is, height velocity computed over a period of 3 years in childhood explains only about one-third of the variation in final height (185).

Conclusion

Inhaled corticosteroids have now been used extensively for more than 20 years, and so far there are no indications that long-term treatment with these drugs is associated with an increased risk of osteoporosis or fracture in children. Standard pediatric doses are not associated with any changes in biochemical markers of bone formation or degradation, whereas low doses of prednisolone (2.5–5.0 mg/day) adversely affect these parameters. Further controlled prospective studies are needed to assess the effect of long-term treatment on peak bone mass/density.

IX. Growth

When the effects of steroids on growth in children are assessed, it is important to appreciate that growth may be divided into three distinct age-related components (186):

1. The rapid, but rapidly decelerating, growth of the first 2–3 years of life. This phase is probably controlled by the same factors which are important for fetal growth; the main one being nutrition.
2. Childhood growth which occurs from age 3 to 10–11 years. This phase mainly represents the contribution of the endocrine system, particularly growth hormone.
3. Pubertal growth, which largely depends on a combination of growth hormone and sex corticosteroids.

Since the importance of the various factors which affect growth seems to differ between these three phases, studies should preferably be performed in all three age groups and conclusions from results obtained in one age group not transferred to the other age groups.

A. Influence of Disease

Most chronic diseases of childhood have been shown to affect adversely the normal growth pattern of a child. However, little is known about the mechanisms through which the growth is affected. The most commonly observed influence of the asthmatic condition on growth is a reduction in growth rate, which is most often seen toward the end of the first decade of life (187–194) (Fig. 7). This reduced growth rate continues into the mid-teens and is associated with a delay in the onset of puberty. This prepubertal deceleration of growth velocity resembles growth retardation. However, the delay in pubertal maturation is also associated with a delay in skeletal maturation, so that the bone age of the child corresponds to the height and that ultimately there is no reduction in final height, which is reached at a later than normal age (187–194). This difference in growth patterns seems to be unrelated to the use of inhaled corticosteroids, but it seems to be more pronounced in children with the most severe asthma. Abnormalities of adrenal androgen release have been suggested as a cause of this growth reduction and delayed puberty. However, to date, there has been no formal testing of this hypothesis in children with asthma.

Recent studies suggest that poorly controlled asthma may in itself affect growth in populations of children who have never received inhaled corticosteroids. Thus, the height standard deviation scores have been found to correlate significantly with the pulmonary functions (50) and the degree of asthma con-

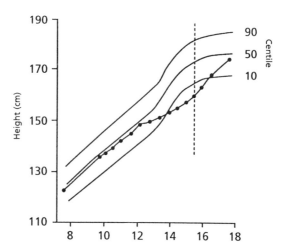

Figure 7 The most commonly observed influence of the asthmatic condition on growth is a reduction in growth rate which is most often seen toward the end of the first decade of life. The reduced growth rate continues into the mid-teens and is associated with a delay in the onset of puberty. This prepubertal deceleration of growth velocity resembles growth retardation. However, the delay in pubertal maturation is also associated with a delay in skeletal maturation so that the bone age of the child corresponds to the height, and that, ultimately, there is no reduction in final height, which is reached at a later than normal age. This difference in growth patterns seems to be unrelated to the use of inhaled corticosteroids, but it seems to be more pronounced in the children with most severe asthma.

trol (195,196). Exactly which mechanisms operate in poorly controlled asthma is unclear. However, acute hypoxia has been shown to reduce circulating levels of testosterone and dehydroepiandrosterone sulfate levels in the blood (197), and it is tempting to hypothesize that poorly treated airways disease could lead to a similar situation.

The deviant growth pattern seen in many children with asthma complicates the interpretation of results from cross-sectional studies comparing the heights of asthmatic children treated with inhaled corticosteroids with the heights of normal children or children with asthma who are not treated with inhaled corticosteroids. The results of Littlewood (198) illustrate this problem. Littlewood found that a group of asthmatic children (mean age = 10.9 years) treated with inhaled beclomethasone had lower height standard deviations scores than a group of children never treated with inhaled corticosteroids (mean age = 6.6 years). Based on the results of other studies (187–194), this difference was probably due to differences in age rather than differences in treatment between the two groups.

B. Effects of Exogenous Steroids

When the effect of exogenous corticosteroids on growth is evaluated, it is convenient to divide the studies into:

Short-term studies, which assess growth during periods of 6 months or less

Intermediate-term studies, which evaluate growth during periods longer than 6 months but which do not assess final adult height

Long-term studies, which assess growth for many years and also include final adult height in relation to predicted adult height

Growth marker studies, which measure steroid induced changes in various serum markers which are thought to reflect bone formation/degradation or growth

When the results from growth studies are evaluated, it is important to realize that an effect on growth found in short- or intermediate-term studies is not necessarily equivalent to an effect on final adult height. Therefore, long-term studies are by far the most clinically relevant.

Over the years, growth of asthmatic children with inhaled corticosteroids has been studied extensively. Although there have been flaws in the designs of most studies, some conclusions can be made.

C. Oral Steroids

Short-term knemometric studies and long-term studies have found that treatment with oral steroids retards growth and induces changes in blood levels of biochemical markers of growth (113,176,194,199–205) even at doses as low as 2.5 and 5.0 mg prednisolone per day (113,176,199,203). The suppressive effect seems to depend on the duration of treatment, dose, and frequency (201,202), and when treatment is stopped, catch-up growth may occur (204,205). However, growth retardation caused by daily and alternate-day administration of large doses of systemic corticosteroids for extended periods of time may be permanent (194,199).

Short-Term Studies

Recently, knemometry has made it possible to measure changes in short-term linear growth of the lower leg within weeks. This may be a valuable adjunct/alternative to traditional growth studies, since knemometry allows very controlled designs. However, the clinical implication of knemometry findings still needs further study. Thus, it was found that daily treatment with 2.5 mg prednisolone totally stopped lower leg growth (206). This indicates that knemometry is too sensitive and probably amplifies or exaggerates the growth-stunting effects of exogenous steroids. On the other hand, it also means that *if an exogenous steroid has no adverse effect on lower leg growth in a knemometric study, it is most unlikely that such treatment will be associated with any growth suppression during long-term treatment.*

Several knemometric studies have evaluated the influence of inhaled budesonide delivered from a Nebuhaler on short-term growth in school children (207–210). In these studies, daily doses ≤400 μg were found not to affect growth adversely. Later, the data from these two studies were pooled with the data from two other knemometric studies. Analysis of these results from 61 children also failed to show any growth suppression of doses ≤400 μg per day (209). In contrast, 800 μg budesonide per day from a Nebuhaler or 400 μg/day from the dry-powder Turbuhaler significantly reduced lower leg growth rate in the three studies evaluating these inhaler-dose combinations (207–209,211). This effect, however, was less than the effect observed during treatment with 2.5 mg prednisolone per day (206). All children participating in these studies were mild asthmatics not requiring inhaled corticosteroids.

In preschool children, 200 μg budesonide per day from a Nebuhaler did not affect short-term lower leg linear growth in children aged 13–36 months (212), whereas 800 μg per day was associated with a significant reduction. In agreement with this finding, preschool children treated with 200–300 μg budesonide per day grew normally during 3–5 years of continuous treatment (81).

Beclomethasone delivered from a Diskhaler has been assessed in two knemometric studies with different designs (213,214). In both studies, treatment with a daily dose of 400 μg was associated with a significant growth suppression of lower leg growth. In the study of Wolthers and Pedersen (213), the growth suppressive effect of beclomethasone was significantly higher than that observed during treatment with 200 μg fluticasone propionate per day in the same children and of the same magnitude as the effect of 2.5 mg prednisolone in another study of similar design (206).

Budesonide from a Turbuhaler and fluticasone from a Diskhaler have been compared in a recent dose-response study (211). It was found that microgram for microgram the two drug-delivery combinations had similar effects. The dose of 200 μg/day did not adversely affect the lower leg growth rate, whereas treatment with 400 μg/day was associated with a slight reduction in lower leg growth, which was significant for budesonide. This indicates that 400 μg budesonide per day from a Turbuhaler has a higher systemic effect than 400 μg budesonide per day from a Nebuhaler. This is in good agreement with the findings on cortisol excretion in the urine and the observation that the Turbuhaler is clinically more effective than the Nebuhaler in children (102–104). No other inhaled corticosteroids have been compared with placebo in knemometric studies.

Intermediate-Term Studies

Many intermediate-term longitudinal growth studies have been conducted over the years (47,50,81,118,134,149,187,188,195,215–236). Until 1993, none included a control group. Some studies have been historical follow-up studies, whereas others have been prospective more or less controlled studies. A MDI or a Diskhaler were used for the administration of beclomethasone and a Nebuhaler for budesonide administration. None of these studies, which comprised more than 2000 children treated for a mean period 1–13 years, found any adverse effect of the inhaled corticosteroid on growth. To give an idea of the design of the studies, a few representative ones are summarized briefly.

An early study (234), which looked at 40 children who had previously been treated with oral corticosteroids, showed that the rate of growth in these children improved when inhaled beclomethasone was substituted for systemic corticosteroids.

Ferguson and Murray (190) reviewed the growth of 183 children with asthma. They found that the mean height was significantly less than the predicted mean, but the use of inhaled corticosteroids did not appear to have a significant effect on growth. This was also found in another study (149), which observed the growth of 26 children receiving various doses of beclomethasone for 13–20 months. The investigators concluded that the subjects continued to grow along their predicted percentile. More than 40% of the children were below the 25th percentile for height on entry to the study, and 18 of the subjects had been receiving systemic corticosteroids. Four years later, Godfrey et al. (221) reviewed 19 of these original 26 children together with 22 new subjects. The children were followed for 3–5 years, and the investigators concluded that their height increased along the predicted percentile.

A study by Graf-Lonnevig and Kraepelien (224) involved 31 children, all of whom were prepubertal on entry into the study. The subjects received inhaled beclomethasone for 16–40 months at doses that started at 400 μg/day but which were reduced to the minimum at which each child's symptoms were controlled. Before the start of the study, the height standard deviation score for these children was less than that for healthy children, and bone age was also somewhat retarded. The treatment with inhaled beclomethasone had neither a positive nor negative influence on these parameters.

Nassif et al. (223) studied growth for an average of 2 years in 32 children treated with inhaled beclomethasone and 24 children receiving prednisolone on alternate days. The groups were not truly comparable, in that those taking prednisolone were significantly younger and had an earlier onset of asthma than those taking beclomethasone. Children in both groups were shorter than expected before starting corticosteroids. There was no evidence of any growth deceleration in either group, and the mean height remained on the 35th percentile throughout the 2-year observation period.

Ninan et al. (195) measured height velocity in 58 prepubertal children with chronic asthma before they were treated with inhaled corticosteroids and for a mean of 4.9 years after such treatment was started. The height velocity standard deviation score was maximal when the asthma was well controlled both before and after starting inhaled corticosteroids. The effectiveness of asthma control correlated significantly with the height SD score both before and after the inhaled corticosteroids were started. Inhaled corticosteroids did not adversely affect growth.

McKenzie followed 43 children on continuous treatment with 200 µg fluticasone propionate per day for 1 year and found that growth was unaffected by the treatment when compared with the expected growth in children of that age (237).

Few studies have examined growth in asthmatic children taking doses of inhaled corticosteroids in excess of 800 µg/day. One group (220) reported their observations in 50 children with a mean age of 11 years, who were receiving 750–1.500 µg beclomethasone, for an average of 19 months. Six showed a decrease in height percentile. In four of these, the growth deceleration might be explained by physiological delay in the onset of puberty.

There is little information about the long-term effects of inhaled corticosteroids on growth in preschool children. However, recent studies with budesonide allow some analysis of this age group (81,134,218,220). No adverse effect on height velocity or bone age was found with inhaled budesonide in a dose of 200 µg/day (134), or of doses ranging between 200 and 1100 $µg/m^{-2}$/day for a year (218,220), or of 2–300 µg budesonide per day delivered from a Nebuhaler for 2–5 years (81).

At present, only four controlled, prospective studies including controls have been published: two using budesonide (50,235) and two (47,236) beclomethasone.

In a controlled, prospective study, Agertoft and Pedersen (50) measured growth and pulmonary function in children with asthma during long-term treatment with inhaled budesonide and compared these findings with those obtained from children not treated with corticosteroids. The 216 children were followed at 6 monthly intervals for 1–2 years without inhaled budesonide and then for 3–6 years on inhaled budesonide. Also followed were 62 asthmatic children treated with theophylline, β_2-agonists, and disodiumcromoglycate but not with inhaled steroids for 3–7 years (controls). During the period of budesonide therapy, the mean daily dose decreased from 710 to 430 µg ($p < .01$).

A positive correlation between height SDS and percentage predicted FEV_1 in the controls and in the children on budesonide was found during the run-in period indicating that asthma severity influenced growth. No statistically significant differences were seen between the two groups in measured height or height SDS at study entry or at the end of the run-in period when mean measured height in the two groups was 124 cm (controls) and 125 cm (budesonide). Compared with run-in and with the control group treatment, inhaled budesonide did not cause any statistically significant changes in growth rate during the 3–6 years of treatment. Over the whole period, the annual increase in height was 5.62 cm (controls) and 5.48 cm (budesonide). Furthermore, the mean annual change in height SDS was similar in the two groups and not significantly affected by the budesonide treatment: –0.004 (budesonide run-in), –0.012 (budesonide treatment), and –0.002 (control group). Because the dose of budesonide varied in each individual child during the treatment period, the influence of budesonide dose on growth could not be accurately assessed. However, when high doses were used (>700 µg/day), both growth rate and lung functions were lower than during run-in and during treatment with 400 µg/day, indicating that either high doses or poor asthma control (or both) may adversely affect growth.

The prospective investigation of Merkus et al. (235) corroborated these findings. These investigators studied 40 asthmatic children who were randomized to treatment with 600 µg budesonide per day or placebo for 2 years. In addition, growth in these two groups was compared with the growth of 80 matched healthy control subjects. The mean difference in growth rates between patients treated with placebo and their controls was –0.70 cm/year; that between children treated with budesonide and their controls was –0.44 cm/year. The observed mean (SEM) case-control difference between treatment groups was +0.27 (0.58) in favor of budesonide treatment. The investigators concluded that asthmatic children (especially the boys) have a prepubertal growth delay and that budesonide in a daily dose of 600 µg does not adversely affect growth over a 2-year period.

Tinkelman et al. (47) compared 100 µg beclomethasone four times per day from a MDI dose inhaler with sustained-release theophylline twice daily in a controlled, randomized, prospective study on 195 asthmatic children between the ages of 6 and 16 years. The duration of the study was 2 years and the observed mean growth rate for all children, who had their first and last measurement greater than 100 days apart (linear regression on height measurements), was 4.2 cm/year for the children taking beclomethasone and 5.5 cm/year for those taking theophylline ($p < .005$). The growth-retarding effect was mainly observed in boys, and there was no significant difference between the two groups when the girls were studied separately.

Doull et al. (236) assessed the effect of daily doses of 400 beclomethasone µg from a Diskhaler on virus-induced wheezing episodes of 7- to 9-year-old children, who, between these episodes (around five per year), had no asthma symptoms requiring continuous inhaled corticosteroid treatment. Out of 4800 children, 200 were eligible, and of these, 104 entered a randomized double-blind group parallel comparison between beclomethasone and placebo. Ninety-four children completed the study, the duration of which was 31 weeks. Statural height was measured at least once a month. After the double-blind period, there was a 17-week washout period during which the children were seen twice. Growth rate during beclomethasone treatment was significantly lower than during placebo treatment, so that the children on placebo grew on average 1 cm more during the 31 weeks of study. No catch-up growth was seen during the washout period.

Long-Term Studies

At present, no long-term studies have been conducted. However, Balfour-Lynn (187,188) followed 66 children for an average of 13.1 years. He found no difference in overall growth rate between children who received beclomethasone dipropionate and those who did not. Final heights were reported to be within the expected range in the children treated with beclomethasone dipropionate. No data on predicted height estimated from parental height were given (187,188). Other investigators have reported similar results, and recently, a metanalysis performed on 21 studies representing 810 patients compared attained height with expected height of children with asthma treated with inhaled or oral steroids (238). The analysis found a significant weak growth impairment in children receiving oral steroids, whereas children treated with inhaled steroids attained normal height. Furthermore, there was no statistical evidence for inhaled steroid therapy to be associated with growth impairment at higher doses or longer therapy durations. So, although no firm conclusions can be made about the effect of inhaled corticosteroids on final height, the studies addressing that question indicate that children with asthma treated with inhaled steroids usually attain a normal final height.

The effect of other inhaled corticosteroids on growth has not been thoroughly assessed, although a retrospective study did not find any adverse effect on growth by 1 year's treatment with triamcinolone (228).

D. Growth Factors

During recent years, the blood levels of various biochemical markers, such as growth hormone, somatomedin-1 (IgF-1), IGF-binding protein 3 (IgFBP-3), carboxyterminal propeptide type 1 procollagen (PICP), and the aminoterminal propeptide of type 3 procollagen (PIIINP), have been found to correlate to some extent with growth rate. However, the predictive value of drug-induced changes in the levels of these markers is not known. The effect of inhaled steroids on some of these markers has been discussed earlier (see discussion of bone markers in Section VIII.A). In our own studies, we have found that treatment with even low doses of prednisolone (2.5–5.0 mg/day) are associated with significant reductions in the levels of some of these markers, whereas daily doses of beclomethasone or budesonide, $\leq$400 µg, and fluticasone propionate, 200 µg, do not affect any of the markers, giving further support to the view that such doses of steroid are safe (154,172–174,176). Furthermore, daily doses of beclomethasone and budesonide around 400 µg (range 200–1200 µg) do not adversely affect the output of urinary growth hormone (144,239).

E. Problems in Growth Assessment—Individual Sensitivity to Steroids?

In spite of the many studies not finding an adverse effect of inhaled steroids on growth, the interindividual variation in sensitivity to the growth-inhibiting effects of steroids is often discussed. Case reports sometimes suggest that growth inhibition in individual children may be seen (240). When such reports are evaluated, it must be remembered that growth is a very complex process which may be affected by a host of factors, including disease severity, psychological factors, growth factors, receptor affinity, nutrition, body composition, age, puberty, genetic factors, and treatment. Children show spontaneous fluctuations in growth velocity often with seasonal variations—most children growing faster in the summer when compared with the winter (241). More recently, it has also become clear that in some children fluctuations are not purely seasonal, but cycles of growth may span 2 or more years (242) (Fig. 8). This leads to a very poor correlation between the growth velocity in 1 year and that in the next year (243). These variations in combination with a standard error of the height measurement, which for trained observers is around 0.2–0.3 cm, and the abnormal growth pattern seen in many asthmatic children unrelated to the use of inhaled steroids, mean that case reports of apparently reduced growth in association with an asthma treatment should be interpreted with caution and not lead to too firm conclusions about cause-effect relationships (Fig. 9).

Because growth is such a complex and volatile process, many studies have demonstrated poor correlations between short-term height velocity and annual height velocity (185,244) or between steroid-induced changes in short-term lower leg growth rate and statural growth during the subsequent year. One-month lower leg length velocity explains virtually nothing of the variation in annual statural height velocity (185,244). In addition, the correlation between two consecutive annual height velocity values for normal prepubertal children is also very poor; a low gain in 1 year is not necessarily followed by a low gain the next year and vice versa (185). The correlation between 1-, 2-, 3-, and 4-year values are only partially correlated with one another (185), and height velocity computed over a period of 3 or 4 years in childhood only explains 34 and 38% of the variation in final height, respectively. *Therefore, the only clinically important outcome measure of human growth is the final height in rela-*

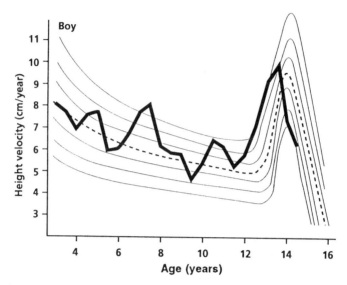

Figure 8 Individual growth velocity curve in a normal child. Marked variations in annual growth rate are seen. If a steroid treatment had been started at age 7 and stopped at age 9.5, it would have been concluded that the treatment caused growth stunting.

tion to expected final height allowing for gender and midparental height differences.

F. Summary and Conclusions of Growth Data

In general, the literature on the effects of inhaled corticosteroids on growth is reassuring, considering that the majority of children with mild and moderate asthma only require low doses of inhaled corticosteroids to be optimally con-

---

Figure 9 Individual growth curve in an asthmatic normal girl (curve A). At age 8, inhaled steroid was started in a daily dose of 400 µg. This treatment was continued throughout the observation period with minor dose adjustments. During the first years, it could easily have been concluded that the treatment caused growth stunting. However, growth gradually caught up, so that height returns to the original percentile even if the treatment was not changed. A similar growth pattern is seen in the asthmatic boy (curve B). In this patient, treatment was initiated at age 8.5 and changed at 11.5. If the treatment given at age 8.5 had been an inhaled steroid and this treatment was stopped at age 11.5, it would probably have been concluded that the inhaled steroid caused growth stunting. However, the treatment given at age 8.5 was sodium cromoglycate, which at age 11.5 was changed to inhaled budesonide.

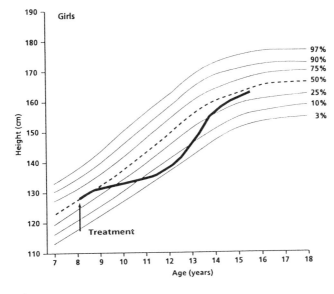

(A)

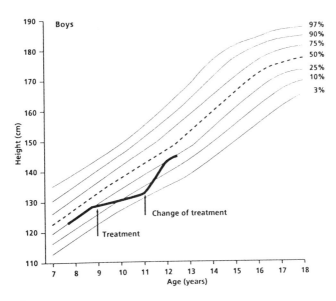

(B)

trolled. The conclusions for the various products and inhalers are as follows: Low doses of oral steroids equivalent to 2.5–5.0 mg prednisolone per day significantly stunts short- and intermediate-term growth and long-term oral steroid treatment can reduce final predicted height.

Treatment with inhaled budesonide in daily doses up to 400 µg from a Nebuhaler does not adversely affect growth in children with asthma. Treatment with 800 µg budesonide per day from a Nebuhaler or 400 µg/day from a Turbuhaler reduces short-term lower leg linear growth in children with mild asthma. The clinical relevance of this needs further study, since prospective long-term studies with continuous use of these doses in children with severe asthma have not been performed.

Treatment with 400 µg beclomethasone per day from a MDI or a Diskhaler reduces short-term lower leg linear growth and recent studies also indicate that this treatment may reduce intermediate-term statural growth in children with mild asthma, although a large number of intermediate-term studies have not been able to confirm this effect. These studies seem to have been on more severe asthmatics and did not include a control group not receiving beclomethasone.

Fluticasone propionate in doses up to 400 µg/day from a Diskhaler does not adversely affect short-term lower leg growth, and 200 µg/day for 1 year does not seem to affect intermediate-term statural growth.

No firm conclusions can be made about the effect of inhaled steroids on final height, although the studies addressing this question strongly suggest that children with asthma treated with inhaled steroids usually attain a normal final height.

The question about the possibility of individually increased sensitivity to a growth-retarding effect of inhaled steroids needs further study. Some data suggest that it exists; however, the normal fluctuation in growth rate and deviant growth pattern in asthmatic patients not receiving inhaled steroids complicates the interpretation of individual growth data.

Finally, although results from short-term studies reflect systemic effects, they do not predict intermediate or long-term growth. Similarly, results from intermediate-term studies are poor predictors of final statural height.

X. Cataracts

Cataract formation as a complication of continuous treatment with oral steroids is limited to the posterior subcapsular type (PSC) (245,246). When the risk of cataract as a complication to inhaled therapy with corticosteroid is assessed, it is important to include carefully matched control groups of patients never treated with oral or inhaled steroids, since atopic patients, particularly patients with atopic eczema, may have a higher occurrence of cataracts than nonatopic patients (247).

Several studies have evaluated the risk of PSC in children receiving long-term treatment with inhaled corticosteroids. The conclusions were the same; that is, continuous treatment with inhaled corticosteroids is not associated with an increase occurrence of cataract development in children (181,223,248–250).

At present, only one study has been performed (181), so our information on this issue is based on case reports in selected groups of patients.

PSC has been reported in a few adults or children treated for asthma or rhinitis with beclomethasone dipropionate or dexamethasone aerosol (223,251–254). The risk is generally assumed to be much lower with inhaled corticosteroids than with systemic steroids, although no systematically collected data are available to quantify the supposed advantage. However, in a few patients, preexisting PSC has been reported to resolve after converting from regular prednisone to inhaled corticosteroid therapy (255), and the prevalence rates are normally markedly higher in patients who have received oral steroids (15–20%) than in patients who have only been treated with inhaled steroids (1–3%) (181,246,248–250). Nassif reported a single case of PSC among 32 children treated for less than 3 years with low-dose beclomethasone, a prevalence rate no different from that found in 24 children receiving alternate-day prednisolone (223) or in 25 children who had never received any oral or inhaled steroids (181). In the latter study, no PSC was observed in the 27 children who had been treated with inhaled budesonide at a mean daily dose of 691 μg per day for 3–7 years (mean 4.5 years) (181). No other publication allows an estimate of the incidence or prevalence rates, because the size of the population at risk is not stated. Furthermore, in many cases, past or current oral steroid therapy confounds the interpretation of the causative role attributed to the inhaled steroid (223,251,254).

A. Conclusion

At present, there are no indications that inhaled corticosteroids increase the risk of cataract in children.

XI. Metabolic Effects

A. Glucose Metabolism

Systemic corticosteroids have an effect on glucose metabolism, decreasing cellular uptake and utilization and enhancing the formation of glucose from other metabolic precursors. Therefore, a number of studies have evaluated glucose metabolism in patients treated with inhaled corticosteroids. In children, beclomethasone dipropionate, 250–800 μg/day, for at least 3 months and flunisolide,

1600 µg/day, for 2 months had no effect on fasting glucose and hemoglobin A_{1c} (150,256). Turpeinen also did not find an effect on fasting glucose and insulin levels or glucose tolerance test by treatment with budesonide, 800 µg/day (257). However, in that study, an increased serum insulin/glucose ratio was seen after the glucose tolerance test.

So inhaled corticosteroids do not affect fasting glucose and hemoglobin A_{1c}. But, as expected, high-dose therapy may be associated with an increase in the fasting insulin, peak glucose, and insulin/glucose ratio after glucose tolerance tests.

B. Lipic Metabolism

Turpinen found no significant changes in the mean cholesterol level in children treated with budesonide, 800 µg/day. High-density lipoprotein cholesterol increased by 22% in children on 800 µg/day of budesonide, but there were no changes in children receiving 400 µg/day (257). Triglycerides were unchanged. In another study, Giorgi (256) found no effect on triglycerides, cholesterol, or phospholipids in children receiving flunisolide, 1600 µg/day.

XII. Central Nervous System Effects

The use of systemic corticosteroids for different illnesses has been associated with the appearance of psychoses in 2.4% and acute psychological changes in 3% of cases (258). These changes seem to be dose related and usually occur within the first 6 days of therapy. Previous personality does not seem to be predictive (259), and the manifistations are nonspecific: emotional lability, anxiety, euphoria, depression, and insomnia.

For inhaled corticosteroids, the evidence is limited to isolated case reports in a total of eight patients (two adults and six children) (260–263). The manifestations have been hyperactive behavior, aggressiveness, insomnia, uninhibited behavior, and impaired concentration. One case involved a nasal spray of beclomethasone (260) and the rest were associated inhaled budesonide, 200–1200 µg/day. In most cases, the changes occurred within the first 2 days, and sometimes the causality was proved by improvement on discontinuation and recurrence on reintroducing the same drug. A few patients tolerated lower doses of the same drug or switching from budesonide to beclomethasone. All returned to normal after discontinuation of the inhaled corticosteroid.

XIII. Oral Candidiasis

Clinical thrush is seldom a problem in children treated with inhaled or systemic steroids. The occurrence seems to be related to dose, dose frequency, and inhaler—spacers seem to reduce the incidence (264–268). Mouthrinsing has not been reported to be beneficial. The condition is easily treated and rarely necessitates withdrawal of the treatment.

XIV. Dysphonia

Hoarseness of the voice is a much more common problem than candidiasis, and it occurs in 20–30% of patients receiving inhaled steroids (264–268). This symptom may be due to a local steroid myopathy of laryngeal muscles, which is reversible after withdrawal of treatment, but unlike thrush, it tends to recur when the treatment is reintroduced. Spacers to not appear to protect against dysphonia.

XV. Other Local Side Effects

There is no evidence of an increase in infections, including tuberculosis, of the lower respiratory tract after chronic use of inhaled steroids. Although thinning of the skin around the mouth may occur in young children treated with nebulized corticosteroids through a face mask, there is no evidence for a similar process in the airways.

XVI. Summary

Inhaled corticosteroids have now been used for the treatment of childhood asthma for more than 25 years. During that time, a substantial number of studies have been set up to evaluate the safety and efficacy of this therapy. Generally, the results have been reassuring. No clinically important side effects have been associated with the treatment. However, so far, the majority of studies have evaluated doses up to 400 μg per day, and the long-term experience with high-dose therapy is still rather limited. Since the occurrence of measurable systemic effects increases with dose, the lowest dose which controls the symptoms should always be used. Furthermore, inhaler-steroid combinations with a high clinical effect/systemic effect ratio should be preferred. When these precautions are taken, inhaled corticosteroids can be used as an effective, safe treatment of childhood asthma (50). Indeed, recent findings suggest that early introduced long-term treatment with inhaled steroids improves long-term outcome of pulmonary functions, reduces the risk of development of irreversible airways obstruction, and reduces the dose of steroid required to control the disease (50). This has not been shown for any other drug. So in the future, more complex evaluations, including the child's risk of developing irreversible airway obstruction and the risk of a reduced quality of life with an increased number of exacerbations, should be made when the safety issues of the various asthma drugs are being discussed.

Discussion

DR. BUSSE: Your data would suggest that the improvement in lung growth occurs early in the course of corticosteroid treatment. Does this suggest that early intervention suppresses the activity of asthma disease and its adverse effect in lung disease and the timing of treatment intervention is key?

DR. PEDERSEN: We saw an initial quite marked and rapid improvement which had become close to maximal within the first 6 months. After this period, the lung functions stayed on the percentile reached, and during the coming years the lung function grew along their percentile. I think that the initial marked improvement is due to reduction in inflammation and clinical improvement. Once the maximum effect has been achieved, the continued steroid treatment ensures that the lung functions will continue to grow along their percentile. If inhaled steroids are not given, lung functions will not continue to grow along this percentile but tend to deviate progressively from it, so that they lose an average 1.3% per year from this percentile. So, inhaled steroids can ensure normal growth of lung functions. However, they can not totally normalize lung functions if the asthma has not been treated for some years. This indicates that some irreversible damage can develop from poorly treated disease, but this is not seen to the same extent when steroids are used.

DR. MCFADDEN: The data on declining lung function in children with asthma not treated by steroids are not supported by observations in adults. If such a phenomenon persisted, adults with asthma whose disease began in childhood would have severely compromised lung function at an early age with all that this entails regarding morbidity and mortality. Further, one would expect an ever-increasing number of such individuals to be in the population, thus the number of severe asthmatics would increase. This does not seem to be the case. Do you think that it is possible that the event that you are describing may be a transient one that stops at some later point in time.

DR. PEDERSEN: We do not know if the number of severe asthmatics is increasing or not, or if it would increase to a greater extent if steroids were not used. We do not know whether the event is transient, we only know that it seems to be constant over a 4-year period. A recent study from Copenhagen found a significant irreversible reduction in FEV_1 of around 11% in young adults who had had asthma for an average of 9 years during childhood but who had not grown out of their disease. It is interesting that their finding of a 1.2% loss in FEV_1 per year is similar to our finding of a 1.3%. We still do not know how severe the disease should be before such a loss is seen or whether it would continue for a longer period than 9 years. If this were the case, one would expect a 50-year-old person who has had persistent asthma continuously for 40 years to have a FEV_1 around 50% of predicted normal. I do not know how frequently this is seen, but it strikes me that in the literature the lung function of adult asthmatics does not seem to normalize to nearly the same extent as we see in children started early on inhaled steroids.

DR. LEUNG: (1) In children who are losing lung function due to chronic asthma, is there an effect on lung growth? (2) Is the loss of lung function irreversible? (3) What is the basis for the loss of lung function?

DR. PEDERSEN: (1) We do not know whether there is an effect on lung growth. The parameters studied by us and others are FEV_1, $FEV_{25-75\%}$, and FEV_1/VC ratio. These parameters all seem to grow less than predicted. (2) It seems that the reduction is irreversible, since treatment with steroids or β_1-agonists does not normalize the measurement. (3) We do not know the basis for the loss of lung function.

DR. MCFADDEN: There are few data that show that adult asthmatics have persistent irreversible obstruction. Again, I can not help but wonder if the changes that you are describing in your children are not transient. They appear to be of equal or of similar magnitude to those seen in patients with cystic fibrosis and exceed the losses that develop in adults with chronic bronchitis. If such a progression was not halted, it would limit the life expectancy of adult asthmatics.

DR. PEDERSEN: The annual decline (loss) from normal lung growth in children not receiving inhaled steroids was 1.3%. This figure is lower than the decline seen in cystic fibrosis and somewhat higher than the decline seen in normal children exposed to passive smoking. An annual reduction of 1.3% would, if it continues throughout life, mean that you would see lung functions around 50% of the predicted normal in adults who have had continuous moderate/severe asthma for 40 years without receiving continuous treatment with inhaled steroids. When I see results from studies in 50-year-old patients, it is my impression that you often see such patients with FEV_1 in that range, but of course they have not been followed continuously for 40 years. Such proof would be very difficult to obtain. Furthermore, when you evaluate our results, you should remember that FEV_1 before they received inhaled steroids had been around 70% of predicted for at least 1 year. So our patients were not as mild as we anticipated in 1986 when the study was started.

DR. GLEICH: I am impressed by the accuracy of your measurements. Can you truly measure leg length to 1 mm? Are these measurements (of the leg) related to total growth?

DR. PEDERSEN: The method is very standardized, because we use the same nurse and very vigorous measuring conditions which are described in details in our publications. The technical error in our studies has been brought down to 0.1 mm. An average weekly growth of the lower leg would be 0.5 mm/week.

DR. LEMANSKE: I would like to emphasize that one needs to keep in mind that the effects of corticosteroids on growth, as well as the process of growth itself, are very complex. Therefore, although analysis of group mean trends of inhaled corticosteroids on growth can provide us with some useful guidelines, one must keep in mind that individual patient responses may vary significantly from the mean and side effects at certain safe doses may still occur.

DR. PEDERSEN: In all of our knemometric studies, 800 μg budesonide/day reduces lower leg growth rate. Treatment with 200 or 400 μg budesonide doses do not. It is important when you interpret these data to realize that (1) a negative finding (i.e., no effect is very good at predicting that there will be no effect during long-term treatment); (2) a significant suppression in a knemometric study is not a good predictor for a reduced growth rate in a long-term study; and (3) lower leg length increases in lulls and spurts. Because of these cycles, knemometry cannot be used to predict anything about individual sensitivity—there will always be a marked interindividual variation. A child with low growth during one period may have increased growth during another period even if the treatment has not been changed.

DR. LEUNG: Was the 1.3% decrease in lung function a gaussian distribution or were there a few "outliers?" Do glucocorticoids have an effect on lung growth? Is there any data that if you do not get glucocorticoids as a child you get decreasing function—besides yours? Do adult asthmatics have decreased lung function?

DR. PEDERSEN: (1) No, outliers did not cause the result. (2) Yes, budesonide treatment ensured a normal lung growth along a parallel to the predicted percentile. It did not reduce growth or accelerate growth after the initial marked change in lung function, which I believe was due to the antiasthmatic effects of the drug. There are other data suggesting that asthma can cause irreversible damage to the airways. These differences are given in my paper.

DR. MCFADDEN: Were the criteria for entry well defined? What about prior therapy?

DR. PEDERSEN: We did have fixed criteria for being included into the study, and the study population was very accurately characterized, because we had been following them for 1–2 years at entry. Furthermore, the treatment required was very clear and written down in the protocol. So this is a very controlled study, but it is not randomized.

DR. ROCKLIN: Are you following markers of bone metabolism in these children and, if so, what are the results? Also, do any abnormalities found (if any) correlate with long-term growth results?

DR. PEDERSEN: There have been studies showing that there is a significant correlation between some of the growth markers and long-term growth. We are analyzing our data at present. It seems as if PICP may show the best correlation. However, the predictive value of changes in the markers is not known.

References

1. Pedersen S, Hansen OR. Budesonide treatment of moderate and severe asthma in children. A dose response study. J All Clin Immunol 1995; 1:29–33.
2. Shapiro GG. Childhood asthma: update. Pediatr Res 1992; 13:403–412.
3. Price JF. Comparative data in childhood asthma. Eur Respir J 1992; 5(suppl 15):3265.
4. Waalkens JH, van Essen Zandvliet EE, Gerritsen J, Duiverman EJ, Kerrebijn KF, Knol K. The effect of an inhaled corticosteroid (budesonide) on exercise-induced asthma in children. Dutch CNSLD Study Group. Eur Respir J 1993; 6:652–656.
5. Henriksen JM, Dahl R. Effects of inhaled budesonide alone and in combination with low-dose terbutaline in children with exercise-induced asthma. Am Rev Respir Dis 1983; 128:993–997.
6. Henriksen JM. Effect of inhalation of corticosteroids on exercise-induced asthma: randomised double blin cross-over study of budesonide in asthmatic children. Br Med J 1985; 291:248–249.
7. Alving KH, Lundberg JON, Nordvall SL. Dose-dependent reduction of exhaled nitric oxide in asthmatic children by inhaled steroids. Am J Respir Crit Care Med 1995; 151:129.
8. Hummel S, Lehtonen L. Comparison of oral-steroid sparing by high-dose and low-dose inhaled steroid in maintenance treatment of severe asthma. Lancet 1992; 340:1483–1487.
9. Boe J, Rosenhall L, Alton M, et al. Comparison of dose response effects of inhaled beclomethasone dipropionate and budesonide in the management of asthma. Allergy 1989; 44:349–455.
10. Dahl R, Lundback B, Malo J, et al. A dose ranging study of fluticasone propionate in adult patients with moderate asthma. Chest 1993; 5:1352–1258.
11. Greenough A, Pool J, Gleeson JG, Price JF. Effect of budesonide on pulmonary hyperinflation in young asthmatic children. Thorax 1988; 43:937–938.
12. Gleeson JG, Price JF. Controlled trial of budesonide given by the nebuhaler in preschool children with asthma. Br Med J 1988; 297:163–166.
13. Bisgaard H, Schiötz PO. Treatment of asthmatic bronchitis in young children with steroid inhalation. Ugeskr Laeger 1993; 155:181–182.
14. Bisgaard H, Munck SL, Nielsen JP, Petersen W, Ohlsson SV. Inhaled budesonide for treatment of recurrent wheezing in early childhood. Lancet 1990; 336:649–651.

15. Connett GJ, Warde C, Wooler E, Lenney W. Use of budesonide in severe asthmatics aged 1–3 years. Arch Dis Child 1993; 69:351–355.

16. Schleimer RP. Effects of glucocorticoids on inflammatory cells relevant to their therapeutic application in asthma. Am Rev Respir Dis 1990; 141:59–69.

17. Sousa AR, Poston RN, Lane SJ, Narhosteen JA, Lee TH. Detection of GM-CSF in asthmatic bronchial epithelium and decrease by inhaled corticosteroids. Am Rev Respir Dis 1993; 147:1557–1561.

18. Laitinen LA, Laitinen A, Haahtela T. A comparative study of the effects of an inhaled corticosteroid, budesonide, and of a beta-2-agonist, terbutaline, on airway inflammation in newly diagnosed asthma. J Allergy Clin Immunol 1992; 90:32–42.

19. Djukanovic R, Wilson JW, Britten YM, et al. Effect of an inhaled corticosteroid on airway inflammation and symptoms of asthma. Am Rev Respir Dis 1992; 145:699–674.

20. Jeffery PK, Godfrey RW, Ädelroth E, Nelson F, Rogers A, Johansson S. Effect of treatment on airway inflammation and thickening of basement membrane reticular collagen in asthma. Am Rev Respir Dis 1992; 145:890–899.

21. Burke C, Power CK, Norris A, Condez A, Schmekel B, Poulter LW. Lung function and immunopathological changes after inhaled corticosteroid therapy in asthma. Eur Respir J 1992; 5:73–79.

22. Lungren R, Söderberg M, Horstedt P, Stenling R. Morphological studies on bronchial mucosal biopsies from asthmatics before and after ten years treatment with inhaled steroids. Eur Respir J 1988; 1:883–889.

23. Barnes PJ. Effect of corticosteroids on airway hyperresponsiveness. Am Rev Respir Dis 1990; 141:70–76.

24. Benoist MR, Brouard JJ, Rufin P, et al. Dissociation of symptom scores and bronchial hyperreactivity: study in asthmatic children on long-term treatment with inhaled beclomethasone dipropionate. Pediatr Pulmonol 1992; 13:71–77.

25. Boner AL, Piacentini GL, Bonizzato C, Dattoli V, Sette L. Effect of inhaled beclomethasone dipropionate on bronchial hyperreactivity in asthmatic children during maximal allergen exposure. Pediatr Pulmonol 1991; 10:2–5.

26. Cockroft DW, Murdoch KY. Comparative effects of inhaled salbutamol, sodium cromoglycate and BDP on allergen-induced early asthmatic responses, late asthmatic responses and increased bronchial responsiveness to histamine. J Allergy Clin Immunol 1987; 79:734–740.

27. Burge PS. The effects of corticosteroids on the immediate asthmatic reaction. Eur J Respir Dis 1982; 63(suppl 122):163–166.

28. Dahl R, Johansson S. Importance of duration of treatment with inhaled budesonide on the immediate and late bronchial reaction. Eur J Respir Dis 1982; 62(suppl 122):5167–5175.

29. deBaets FM, Goetyn M, Kerrebijn KF. The effect of two months of treatment with inhaled budesonide on bronchial responsiveness to histamine and house-dust mite antigen in asthmatic children. Am Rev Respir Dis 1990; 142:581–586.

30. De Baets FM, Goeteyn M, Kerrebijn KF. The effect of two months of treatment with inhaled budesonide on bronchial responsiveness to histamine and house-dust mite antigen in asthmatic children. Am Rev Respir Dis 1990; 142:581–586.

31. Molema J, van Herwaarden CLA, Folgering HTM. Effect of long-term treatment with inhaled cromoglycate and budesonide on bronchial hyperresponsiveness in patients with allergic asthma. Eur Respir J 1989; 2:308–316.

32. Kraan J, Koeter GH, Van der Mark TW, Sluiter HJ, De Vries K. Changes in bronchial hyperreactivity induced by 4 weeks of treatment with antiasthmatic drugs in patients with allergic asthma: a comparison between budesonide and terbutaline. J Allergy Clin Immunol 1985; 76:628–336.

33. Kerrebijn KF, van Essen-Zandvliet EEM, Neijens HL. Effect of long-term treatment with inhaled corticosteroids and beta-agonists on bronchial responsiveness in asthmatic children. J Allergy Clin Immunol 1987; 79:653–659.

34. Dutoit JI, Salome CM, Woolcock AJ. Inhaled corticosteroids reduce the severity of bronchial hyperresponsiveness in asthma, but oral theophylline does not. Am Rev Respir Dis 1987; 136:1174–1178.

35. Bel EH, Timmers MC, Hermans JO, Dijkman JH, Sterk PJ. The longer term effects of nedocromil sodium and beclomethasone dipropionate on bronchial responsiveness to methacholine in non-atopic asthmatic subjects. Am Rev Respir Dis 1990; 141:21–28.

36. Van Essen-Zandvliet EE, Hughes MD, Waalkens HJ, Duiverman EJ, Pocock SJ, Kerrebijn KF. Effects of 22 months of treatment with inhaled corticosteroids and/or beta-2-agonists on lung function, airway responsiveness and symptoms in children with asthma. Am Rev Respir Dis 1992; 146:547–554.

37. Østergaard P, Pedersen S. The effect of inhaled disodium cromoglycate and budesonide on bronchial responsiveness to histamine and exercise in asthmatic children: a clinical comparison. In: Godfrey S, ed. Glucocorticosteroids in Childhood Asthma. 1987:55–65.

38. Bennati D, Piacentini GL, Peroni DG, Sette L, Testi R, Boner AL. Changes in bronchial reactivity in asthmatic children after treatment with beclomethasone alone or in association with salbutamol. J Asthma 1989; 26:359–364.

39. Kraemer R, Sennhauser F, Reinhardt M. Effects of regular inhalation of beclomethasone dipropionate and sodium cromoglycate on bronchial hyperreactivity in asthmatic children. Acta Paediatr Scand 1987; 76:119–123.

40. Groot CAR, Lammers JJ, Molema J, Festen J, van Herwaarden CLA. Effect of inhaled beclomethasone and nedocromil sodium on bronchial hyperresponsiveness to histamine and distilled water. Eur Respir J 1992; 5:1075–1082.

41. O'Connor BJ, Rigde SM, Barnes PJ, Fuller RW. Greater effect of inhaled budesonide on adenosine 5-monophosphate-induced than on metabisulfite-induced bronchoconstriction in asthma. Am Rev Respir Dis 1992; 146:560–564.

42. Vanthenen AS, Knox AJ, Wisnierski A, Tattersfield AE. Effect of inhaled budesonide on bronchial reactivity to histamine exercise and eucapnic dry air hyperventilation in patients with asthma. Thorax 1991; 46:811–816.

43. Fuller RW, Choudry NB, Eriksson G. Actions of budesonide on asthmatic airway hyperresponsiveness. Effects on directly and indirectly acting bronchodilators. Chest 1991; 100:670–674.

44. Rodwell LT, Anderson SD, Seale JP. Inhaled steroids modify bronchial responses to hyperosmolar saline. Eur Respir J 1992; 5:953–962.

45. Østergaard P, Pedersen S. Bronchial hyperreactivity in children with perennial extrinsic asthma. In: Oseid S, Edwards AM, eds. The Asthmatic Child in Play and Sport. London: Pitman, 1982:326–331.

46. Bel EH, Timers MC, Zwinderman AH, Dijkman JH, Sterk PJ. The effect of inhaled corticosteroids on the maximal degree of airway narrowing to methacholine. Am Rev Respir Dis 1991; 143:109–113.

47. Tinkelman DG, Reed CE, Nelson HS, Offord KP. Aerosol beclomethasone dipropionate compared with theophylline as primary treatment of chronic, mild to moderately severe asthma in children (see comments). Pediatrics 1993; 92:64–77.

48. Meltzer EO, Orgel HA, Ellis EF, Eigen HN, Hamstreet MPB. Long-term comparison of three combinations of albuterol, theophylline, and beclomethasone in children with chronic asthma. J Allergy Clin Immunol 1992; 90:2–11.

49. Pedersen S, Agertoft L. Effect of long-term budesonide treatment on growth, weight and lung function in children with asthma. Am Rev Respir Dis 1993; 147:A265.

50. Agertoft L, Pedersen S. Effects of long term treatment with an inhaled corticosteroid on growth and pulmonary function in asthmatic children. Respir Med 1994; 88:373–381.

51. Waalkens HJ, Van Essen-Zandvliet EE, Hughes MD, et al. Cessation of long-term treatment with inhaled corticosteroid (budesonide) in children with asthma results in deterioration. Am Rev Respir Dis 1993; 148:1252–1257.

52. Mosfeldt Laursen E, Kaae Hansen K, Backer V, Bach-Mortensen N, Prahl P, Koch C. Pulmonary function in adolescents with childhood asthma. Allergy 1993; 48:267–272.

53. Silverman M, Tausig LM, Martinez F, et al. Early childhood asthma: what are the questions? Am J Respir Crit Care Med 1995; 151:S1–42.

54. Kraemer R, Meister B, Schaad UB, Rossi E. Reversibility of lung function abnormalities in children with perennial asthma. J Pediatr 1983; 102:347–350.

55. Brown PJ, Greville HW, Finucane KE. Asthma and irreversible airflow obstruction. Thorax 1984; 39:131–136.

56. Sherrill D, Sears MR, Lebowitz MD, et al. The effects of airway hyperresponsiveness, wheezing, and atopy on longitudinal pulmonary function in children: a 6-year follow-up study. Pediatr Pulmonol 1992; 13:78–85.

57. Sherrill DL, Martinez FD, Lebowitz MD, et al. Longitudinal effects of passive smoking on pulmonary function in New Zealand children. Am Rev Respir Dis 1992; 145:1136–1141.

58. Martin AJ, McLennan LA, Landau LI, Phelan PD. The natural history of childhood asthma to adult life. Br Med J 1980; 280:1397–400.

59. Yaacob I, Mohammad M. Pulmonary function in symptom-free asthmatics. Singapore Med J 1993; 34:522–523.

60. Martinez FD, Wright AL, Taussig LM, Holberg CJ, Halonen M, Morgan WJ. Asthma and wheezing in the first six years of life. N Engl J Med 1995; 332:133–138.

61. Cade JF, Pain MC. Pulmonary function during clinical remission of asthma how reversible is asthma. Aus NZ J Med 1973; 3:545.

62. Kelly WJ, Hudson I, Raven J, Phelan PD, Pain MC, Olinsky A. Childhood asthma and adult lung function. Am Rev Respir Dis 1988; 138:26–30.
63. Martin AJ, Landau LI, Phelan PD. Lung function in young adults who had asthma in childhood. Am Rev Respir Dis 1980; 122:609–617.
64. Kokkonen J, Linna O. The state of childhood asthma in young adulthood. Eur Respir J 1993; 6:657–661.
65. Haahtela T, Järvinen M, Kava T, et al. Effects of reducing or discontinuing inhaled budesonide in patients with mild asthma. N Engl J Med 1994; 331:700–705.
66. Selroos O, Backman R, Forsen KO, et al. The effect of inhaled corticosteroids in asthma is related to the duration of pretreatment symptoms. Am J Respir Crit Care Med 1994; 149:A211.
67. Resnick A, Greenberger PA. A corticosteroid program for prevention of hospitalization for status asthmaticus in children. NER Allergy Proc 1987; 8:104–107.
68. Edmunds AT, Goldberg RS, Duper B, Devichand P, Follows RM. A comparison of budesonide 800 micrograms and 400 micrograms via Turbohaler with disodium cromoglycate via Spinhaler for asthma prophylaxis in children. Br J Clin Res 1994; 5:11–23.
69. Noble V, Ruggins NR, Everad ML, Milner AD. Inhaled budesonide via a modified Nebuhaler for chronic wheezing in infants. Arch Dis Child 1992; 67:285–288.
70. Greenough A, Pool J, Gleeson JG, Price JF. Effect of budesonide on pulmonary hyperinflation in young asthmatic children. Thorax 1988; 43:937–938.
71. Van Bever JP, Schuddinck L, Wojciechowski M, Stevens WJ. Aerosolised budesonide in asthmatic infants. Pediatr Pulmonol 1990; 9:177–180.
72. Storr J, Lenney CA, Lenney W. Nebulised beclomethasone dipropionate in preschool asthma. Arch Dis Child 1986; 61:270–273.
73. Webb MSC, Milner AD, Hiller EJ, Henry RI. Nebulised beclomethasone dipropionate suspension. Arch Dis Child 1986; 61:1108–1110.
74. O'Callaghan C. Particle size of beclomethasone dipropionate produced by 2 nebulisers and spacers. Thorax 1990; 45:109–111.
75. Lodrup Carlsen KC, Nikander K, Carlsen K-H. How much nebulised budesonide reaches infants and toddlers? Arch Dis Child 1992; 67:1077–1079.
76. Connett G, Lenney W. Prevention of viral induced asthma attacks using inhaled budesonide. Arch Dis Child 1993; 68:85–87.
77. Maayan C, Itzhaki T, Bar-Yishay E, Gross S, Tal A, Godfrey S. The functional response of infants with persistent wheezing to nebulized beclomethasone dipropionate. Pediatr Pulmonol 1986; 2:9–14.
78. Carlsen KH, Leegard J, Larsen S, Orstravik I. Nebulised beclomethasone dipropionate in recurrent obstructive episodes after acute bronchiolitis. Arch Dis Child 1988; 63:1428–1433.
79. Godfrey S, Avital A, Rosler A, Mandelberg A, Uwyyed K. Nebulised budesonide in severe infantile asthma. Lancet 1987; 2:851–852.
80. de Jongste JC, Duiverman EJ. Nebulised budesonide in severe childhood asthma. Lancet 1989; 1:1388.
81. Volovitz B, Amir J, Malik H, Kauschansky A, Varsano I. Growth and pituitary-

adrenal function in children with severe asthma treated with inhaled budesonide. N Engl J Med 1993; 329:1703–1733.

82. Connett GJ, Lenney W, McConchie SM. The cost effectiveness of budesonide in severe asthmatics aged one to three years. Br J Med Econ 1993; 6:127–134.

83. Pedersen S, Steffensen G, Ohlsson SV. The influence of orally-deposited budesonide on the systemic availability of budesonide after inhalation from a Turbuhaler. Eur J Clin Pharmacol 1993; 36:211–214.

84. Pedersen S, Steffensen G, Ekman I, Tönneson M, Borgå O. Pharmacokinetics of budesonide in children after oral deposition and inhalation from two different inhalers. Eur J Clin Pharmacol 1987; 31:579–582.

85. Dolovich M, Ruffino RE, Roberts R, Newhouse MT. Optimal delivery of aerosols from metered dose inhalers. Chest 1981; 80(suppl 65):911–915.

86. Dolovich M, Ruffino R, Corr D, Newhouse MT. Clinical evaluation of a simple demand-inhalation MDI aerosol delivery device. Chest 1983; 84:36–41.

87. Morén F. Drug deposition of pressurized inhalation aerosols. I. Influence of actuator tube design. Int J Pharmacol 1978; 1:205–212.

88. Newman SP, Pavia D, Morén F, Sheahan NF, Clarke SW. Deposition of pressurized aerosols in the human respiratory tract. Thorax 1981; 36:52–55.

89. Newman SP, Morén F, Pavia D, Little F, Clarke SW. Deposition of pressurized suspension aerosols inhaled through extension devices. Am Rev Respir Dis 1981; 124:317–320.

90. Newman SP, Pavia D, Clarke SW. Improving the bronchial deposition of pressurized aerosols. Chest 1981; 80(suppl 65):909–911.

91. Newman SP, Pavia D, Garland N, Clarke SW. Effects of various inhalation modes on the deposition of radioactive pressurized aerosols. Eur J Respir Dis 1982; 63(suppl 119):57–65.

92. Newman SP. Deposition and Effects of Inhalation Aerosols. Rahms Tryckeri, Lund, Ph.D. dissertation, 1983.

93. Short MD, Singh CA, Few JDE. The labelling and monitoring of lung deposition of an inhaled synthetic anticholinergic bronchodilating agent. Chest 1981; 80:918–921.

94. Martin LE, Tanner RJN, Clarke THJE. Absorption and metabolism of orally-administered beclomethasone dipropionate. Clin Pharmacol Ther 1974; 15:267–275.

95. Ryrfeldt Å, Edsbäcker S, Tönneson ME. Pharmacokinetics and metabolism of budesonide, a selective glucocorticoid. Eur J Respir Dis 1981; 63:86–95.

96. Johanson SÅ, Anderson KE, Brattsand RE. Topical and systemic glucocorticoid potencies of budesonide and beclomethasone dipropionate in man. Eur J Clin Pharmacol 1982; 22:523–539.

97. Prahl P, Jensen T. Decreased adrenocortical suppression utilizing the Nebuhaler for inhalation of steroid aerosols. Clin Allergy 1987; 17:393–398.

98. Farrer M, Francis AJ, Pearce SJ. Morning serum cortisol concentrations after 2 mg inhaled beclomethasone dipropionate in normal subjects: effect of a 750 ml spacing device. Thorax 1990; 46:891–894.

99. Brown PH, Blundell G, Greening AP, Crompton GK. Do large volume spacer devices reduce the systemic effects of high dose inhaled corticosteroids? Thorax 1990; 45:736–739.

100. Pedersen S. Safety aspects of corticosteroids in children. Eur Respir Rev 1994; 4:33–43.
101. Selroos O, Halme M. Effect of a volumatic spacer and mouth-rinsing on systemic absorption of inhaled corticosteroids from a metered dose inhaler and a dry powder inhaler. Thorax 1991; 46:891–894.
102. Pedersen S, Hansen OR. Treatment of asthmatic children with budesonide from a Turbuhaler and a MDI with a Nebuhaler. 35th Nordic Congress of Pneumonology, 1990:35.
103. Borgström L. Methodological studies on lung deposition. Evaluation of inhalation devices and absorption mechanisms. Acta Univ Ups 1993:1–51.
104. Engel T, Heinig JH, Malling HJ, Scharling B, Nikander K, Madsen F. Clinical comparison of inhaled budesonide delivered either via pressurized metered dose inhaler of Turbuhaler. Allergy 1989; 44:220–225.
105. Toogood JH, Jennings B, Baskerville J, Johansson SÅ. Use of spacers to facilitate inhaled corticosteroid treatment of asthma. Am Rev Respir Dis 1984; 129:723–729.
106. Pedersen S, Steffensen G, Borgaa O. Pharmacokinetics of budesonide after two different modes of inhalation and oral deposition in children with asthma. Eur J Clin Pharmacol 1995;
107. Dahlström K, Larsson P. Lung deposition and systemic availability of budesonide inhaled as nebulised suspension from different nebulisers. J Aer Med 1995;
108. Klein RG, Arnaud SB, Gallagher JC, DeLuca HF, Riggs BL. Intestinal calcium absorption in exogenous hypercortisonism. J Clin Invest 1977; 60:253–259.
109. Hahn TJ, Halstead LR, Teitelbaum SL, Hahn BH. Altered mineral metabolism in glucocorticoid-induced osteopenia: effects of 25-hydroxy vitamin D administration. J Clin Invest 1979; 64:655–665.
110. Hollmann GA, Allen DB. Overt glucocorticoid excess due to inhaled corticosteroid therapy. Pediatrics 1988; 81:452–455.
111. Priftis K, Everard ML, Milner AD. Unexpected side-effects of inhaled steroids: a case report. Eur J Pediatr 1991; 150:448–449.
112. Meltzer EO, Kemp JP, Welch MJ, Orgel HA. Effect of dosing schdule on efficacy of beclometasone dipropionate aerosol in chronic asthma. Am Rev Respir Dis 1985; 131:732–736.
113. Byron MA, Jackson J, Ansell BM. Effect of different corticosteroid regimens on hypothalamic–pituitaryadrenal axis and growth in juvenile chronic arthritis. J R Soc Med 1983; 76:452–457.
114. Sherman B, Weinberger M, Chen-Waldren H, et al. Further studies of the effects of inhaled glucocorticoids on pituitary-adrenal function in healthy adults. J Allergy Clin Immunol 1982; 69:208–212.
115. Law CM, Honour JW, Merchant JLE. Nocturnal adrenal suppression in asthmatic children taking inhaled beclomethasone dipropionate. Lancet 1986; 1:942–944.
116. Law CM, Preece MA, Warner JO. Nocturnal adrenal suppression in children inhaling beclomethasone dipropionate. Lancet 1986; 1:321–323.
117. Tabacknik E, Zadik Z. Diurnal cortisol secretion during therapy with inhaled beclomethasone dipropionate in children with asthma. J Pediatr 1991; 118:294–297.
118. Philip M, Aviram M, Leiberman Ee. Integrated plasma cortisol concentration in

children with asthma receiving long-term inhaled corticosteroids. Pediatr Pulmonol 1992; 12:84–89.

119. Stewart PM, Seckl JR, Corrie J, Edwards CR, Padfield PL. A rational approach for assessing the hypothalamo-pituitary-adrenal axis. Lancet 1988; 28:1208–1210.

120. Brown PH, Blundell G, Greening AP, Crompton GK. Screening for hypothalamo-pituitary-adrenal axis suppression in asthmatics taking high dose inhaled corticosteroids. Respir Med 1991; 85:511–516.

121. Hartzband PI, Van Herle AJ, Sorger L, Cope D. Assessment of hypothalamic-pituitary-adrenal (HPA) axis dysfunction: comparison of ACTH stimulation, insulin-hypoglycemia and metyrapone. J Endocrinol Invest 1988; 11:769–776.

122. Holt PR, Lowndes DW, Smithies E, Dixon GT. The effect of an inhaled steroid on the hypothalamic-pituitary-adrenal axis—which tests should be used? Clin Exp Allergy 1990; 20:145–149.

123. Jasani MK, et al. Studies of the rise in plasma 11-hydroxy-corticosteroids in corticosteroid treated patients with rheumatoid arthritis during surgery: correlations with the functioning integrity of the hypothalamic-pituitary-adrenal axis. Q J Med 1968; 37:407–421.

124. Linder BL, Esteban NV, Yergey AL, Winterer JC, Loriaux DL, Cassoria F. Cortisol production rate in childhood and adolescence. J Pediatr 1990; 117:892–896.

125. Ädelroth E, Rosenhall L, Glennow C. High dose inhaled budesonide in the treatment of severe steroid-dependent asthmatics—a 2-year study. Allergy 1985; 40:58–64.

126. Stiksa G, Nemcek K, Glennow C. Adrenal function in asthmatics treated with high-dose budesonide. Respiration 1985; 48:91–93.

127. Laursen J, Wynn V, James V. The adrenocortical response to insulin-induced hypoglycaemia. J Clin Endocrinol Metab 1963; 27:183–189.

128. Tarlo SM, Broder I, Davies GM, Leznoff A, Mintz S, Corey PN. Six-month double-blind, controlled trial of high dose, concentrated beclomethasone dipropionate in the treatment of severe chronic asthma. Chest 1988; 93:998–1002.

129. Glazer I, Geni M, Racz I, Molcho M, Weissenberg R, Lunenfeld B. Bechlometasone dipropionate aerosol in the treatment of steroid-dependent chronic bronchial asthma in adults. Monogr Allergy 1977; 12:249–252.

130. Bulow KB, Kalen N. Local and systemic effects of bechlometasone inhalation in steroid-dependent asthmatic patients. Curr Ther Res 1974; 16:1110–1118.

131. Maberly DJ, Gibson GJ, Butler AG. Recovery of adrenal function after substitution of bechlometasone dipropionate for oral corticosteroids. Br Med J 1973; 1:778–782.

132. Bisgaard H, Damkjaer Nielsen M, Andersen B, et al. Adrenal function in children with bronchial asthma treated with beclomethasone dipropionate or budesonide. J Allergy Clin Immunol 1988; 81:1088–1095.

133. Clissold SP, Heel RC. Budesonide: a preliminary review of its pharmacodynamic properties and therapeutic efficacy in asthma and rhinitis. Drugs 1984; 28:485–518.

134. Varsano I, Volovitz B, Malik H, Amir Y. Safety of 1 year of treatment with budesonide in young children with asthma. J Allergy Clin Immunol 1990; 85:914–920.

135. Bisgaard H, Pedersen S, Damkjaer Nielsen M, Osterballe O. Adrenal function in asthmatic children treated with inhaled budesonide. Acta Paediatr Scand 1991; 80:213–217.

136. Field HV, Jenkinson PMA, Frame MH, Warner JO. Asthma treatment with a new corticosteroid aerosol budesonide administered twice daily by spacer inhaler. Arch Dis Child 1982; 57:864–866.

137. Field HV, Jenkinson PMA, Frame MH, Warner JO. Budesonide in childhood asthma. Eur J Respir Dis 1982; 63(suppl 122):273–274.

138. Pedersen S. Safety of inhaled glucocorticosteroids. Excerpta Med 1989;40–51.

139. Bisgaard H, Damkjaer Nielsen M, Andersen B, et al. Adrenal function in children with bronchial asthma treated with beclomethasone dipropionate or budesonide. J Allergy Clin Immunol 1988; 81:1088–1095.

140. Wolthers OD, Pedersen S. Measures of systemic activity of inhaled glucocorticosteroids in children: a comparison of urine cortisol excretion and knemometry. Respir Med 1995;

141. Prahl P, Jensen T, Bjerregaard-Andersen H. Adrenocortical function in children on high-dose steroid aerosol therapy. Results of serum cortisol, ACTH stimulation test and 24 hour urinary free cortisol excretion. Allergy 1987; 42:541–544.

142. Nina TK, Reid IW, Carter PE, Smail PJ, Russell G. Effects of high doses of inhaled corticosteroids on adrenal function in children with severe persistent asthma. Thorax 1993; 48:599–602.

143. Agertoft L, Pedersen S. Short term lower leg growth and urinary cortisol excretion in children treated with fluticasone propionate and budesonide dry powder inhalers. Arch Dis Child 1995;

144. Nicolaizik WH, Marchant JL, Preece MA, Warner JO. Endocrine and lung function in asthmatic children on inhaled corticosteroids. Am J Respir Crit Care Med 1994; 150:624–628.

145. Feigang B, Asthford DR. Adrenal corticol function after long-term beclometasone aerosol therapy in early childhood. Ann Allergy 1990; 64:342–346.

146. Godfrey S, König P. Beclomethasone aerosol in childhood asthma. Arch Dis Child 1973; 48:665–670.

147. Dickson W, Hall CE, Ellis M, Horrocks RH. Beclomethasone dipropionate aerosol in childhood asthma. Arch Dis Child 1973; 48:671–675.

148. Klein R, Waldman R, Kershnar H, et al. Treatment of chronic childhood asthma: I. A double-blind cross-over trial in nonsteroid dependent patients. Pediatrics 1977; 60:7–13.

149. Godfrey S, König P. Treatment of childhood asthma for 13 months and longer with beclomethasone dipropionate aerosol. Arch Dis Child 1974; 49:591–595.

150. Goldstein DE, König P. Effect of inhaled bechlometasone dipropionate on hypothalamic-pituitary-adrenal axis function in children with asthma. Pediatrics 1983; 72:60–64.

151. Katz RM, Rachelefsky GS, Siegel SC, Spector SL, Rohr AS. Twice-daily beclomethasone dipropionate in the treatment of childhood asthma. J Asthma 1986; 23:1–7.

152. Chang CC, Tam AY. Suppression of adrenal function in children on inhaled steroids. J Paediatr Child Health 1991; 27:232-234.
153. Wyatt R, Waschek J, Weinberger M, Sherman B. Effects of inhaled beclomethasone dipropionate and alternate-day prednisone on pituitary-adrenal function in children with chronic asthma. N Engl J Med 1978; 299:1387-1391.
154. Wolthers O, Kaspersen Nielsen H, Pedersen S. Bone turnover in asthmatic children treated with dry powder inhaled fluticasone propionate and beclomethasone dipropionate. Eur Paediatr Respir Soc 1993; 86.
155. Hoffmann-Streb A, L'Allemand D, Niggemann B, Buttner P, Wahn U. Adrenocortical function in children with bronchial asthma under fluticasone treatment. Monatsschr Kinderheilkd 1993; 141:508-512.
156. Piacentini GL, Sette L, Peroni DG, Bonizzato C, Bonetti S, Boner AL. Double-blind evaluation of effectiveness and safety of flunisolide aerosol for treatment of bronchial asthma in children. Allergy 1990; 45:612-616.
157. Sly RM, Imseis M, Frazer M, Joseph F. Treatment of asthma in children with triamcinolone acetonide aerosol. J Allergy Clin Immunol 1978; 62:76-82.
158. Vaz R, Senior B, Morris M, Binkiewicz A. Adrenal effects of beclomethasone inhalation therapy in asthmatic children. J Pediatr 1982; 100:660-662.
159. König P, Goldstein DE. Adrenal function after beclometasone inhalation therapy. J Pediatr 1982; 101:646-647.
160. Brown PH, Matusiewicz, Shearing C, Tibi L, Greening AP, Crompton GK. Systemic effects of high dose inhaled steroids: a comparison of beclomethasone dipropionate (BDP) and budesonide (BUD). Thorax 1992; 48:845.
161. Johansson SA, Andersson K, Brattsand R, et al. Topical and systemic glucocorticoid potencies of budesonide and beclometasone dipropionate in man. Eur J Clin Pharmacol 1982; 22:523-529.
162. Ebden P, Jenkins A, Houston G, Davies BH. Comparison of two high dose corticosteroid aerosol treatments, beclomethasone dipropionate (1500 g/day) and budesonide (1600 g/day) for chronic asthma. Thorax 1986; 41:869-874.
163. Svendsen UG, Frelund L, Heinig JH, Madsen F, Nielsen NH, Weeke B. High-dose inhaled steroids in the management of asthma: a comparison of the effects of budesonide and beclomethasone dipropionate on pulmonary function, symptoms, bronchial responsiveness and the adrenal function. Allergy 1992; 47:174-186.
164. Springer C, Avital A, Maayan CH, Rosler A, Godfrey S. Comparison of budesonide and beclomethasone dipropionate for treatment of asthma. Arch Dis Child 1987; 62:815-819.
165. Baran D. A comparison of inhaled budesonide and beclomethasone dipropionate in childhood asthma. Br J Dis Chest 1987; 81:170-175.
166. Reid IR. Pathogenesis and treatment of steroid osteoporosis. Clin Endocrinol 1989; 30:83-103.
167. Smith R. Corticosteroids and osteoporosis. Thorax 1990; 45:573-575.
168. Greenberger PA, Hendrix RW, Patterson R, Chmiel JS. Bone studies in patients on prolonged systemic corticosteroid therapy for asthma. Clin Allergy 1982; 12:363-368.
169. Adinoff AD, Hollister JR. Steroid-induced fracture and bone loss in patients with asthma. N Engl J Med 1983; 309:265-268.

170. Dykman TR, Gluck OS, Murphy WA, Hahn TJ, Hahn BH. Evaluation of factors associated with glucocorticoid-induced osteopenia in patients with rheumatoid diseases. Arthritis Rheum 1985; 28:361–368.

171. König P, Hillman G, Cervantes CE. Bone metabolism in children with asthma treated with inhaled beclomethasone dipropionate. J Pediatr 1993; 122:219–226.

172. Wolthers OD, Juel Riis B, Pedersen S. Bone turnover in asthmatic children treated with oral prednisolone or inhaled budesonide. Pediatr Pulmonol 1993; 16:341–346.

173. Wolthers O, Juul A, Hansen M, Müller J, Pedersen S. The insulin-like growth factor axis and collagen turnover in asthmatic children treated with inhaled budesonide. Acta Paediatr 1995; 84:393–397.

174. Wolthers O, Juul A, Hansen M, Müller J, Pedersen S. Growth factors and collagen markers in asthmatic children treated with inhaled budesonide. Eur Respir J 1993; 6(suppl 17):261

175. Sorva R, Turpeinen M, Juntunen-Backman K, Karonen SL, Sorva A. Effects of inhaled budesonide on serum markers of bone metabolism in children with asthma. J Allergy Clin Immunol 1992; 90:808–815.

176. Wolthers O, Juul A, Hansen M, Müller J, Pedersen S. The insulin-like growth factor axis and collagen turnover during prednisolone treatment. Arch Dis Child 1994; 71:409–413.

177. Reid IR, Veale AG, France JT. Glucocorticoid osteoporosis. J Asthma 1994; 31:7–18.

178. Prince RL, Smith M, Dick IME. Prevention of postmenopausal osteoporosis. N Engl J Med 1991; 325:1189–1195.

179. Johnston CC, Miller JZ, Slemenda CWE. Calcium supplementation and increases in bone mineral density in children. N Engl J Med 1992; 327:82–87.

180. Reid DM, Kennedy NSJ, Smith MAE. Bone loss in rheumatoid arthritis and primary generalised osteoarthrosis: effects of corticosteroids, suppressive anti-rheumatic rugs and calcium supplements. Br J Rheum 1986; 138:57–61.

181. Agertoft L, Pedersen S. Bone density in children during long-term treatment with budesonide. Eur Respir J 1993; 6:261S.

182. Kinberg KA, Hopp RJ, Biven RE, Gallagher JC. Bone mineral density in normal and asthmatic children. J Allergy Clin Immunol 1994; 94:490–497.

183. Baraldi E, Bollini MC, De Marchi A, Zacchello F. Effect of beclomethasone dipropionate on bone mineral content assessed by X-ray densitometry in asthmatic children: a longitudinal evaluation. Eur Respir J 1994; 7:710–714.

184. Matkovic V. Calcium and peak bone mass. J Intern Med 1992; 231:151–160.

185. Karlberg J, Gelander L, Albertsson-Wikland K. Distinctions between short- and long-term human growth studies. Acta Paediatr 1993; 82:631–634.

186. Karlberg J, Engstrom I, Karlberg P, Fryer JG. Analysis of linear growth using a mathematical model. 1. From birth to three years. Acta Paediatr Scand 1987; 76:478–488.

187. Balfour Lynn L. Effect of asthma on growth and puberty. Pediatrician 1987; 14:237–241.

188. Balfour-Lynn L. Growth and childhood asthma. Arch Dis Child 1986; 61:1049–1055.

189. Armenio L, Baldini G, Bardare M, et al. Double blind, placebo controlled study of nedocromil sodium in asthma. Arch Dis Child 1993; 68:193–197.
190. Fergusson AC, Murray AB, Tze WJ. Short stature and delayed skeletal maturation in children with allergic disease. J Allergy Clin Immunol 1982; 69:461–465.
191. Sprock A. Growth pattern in 200 children with asthma. Ann Allergy 1965; 23:608–611.
192. Hauspie R, Susanne C, Alexander F. A mixed longitudinal study of the growth in height and weight in asthmatic children. Human Biol 1976; 48:271–276.
193. Hauspie R, Susanne C, Alexander F. Maturational delay and temporal growth retardation in asthmatic boys. J Allergy Clin Immunol 1977; 59:200–206.
194. Martin AJ, Landau LI, Phelan PD. The effect on growth of childhood asthma. Acta Pediatr Scand 1981; 70:683–688.
195. Ninan TK, Russell G. Asthma, inhaled corticosteroid treatment, and growth. Arch Dis Child 1992; 67:703–705.
196. Russel G, Ninan T, Carter P, et al. Effects of inhaled corticosteroids on HPA function and growth in children. Res Clin Forums 11 1989; 3:77–86.
197. Semple PA, Watson WS, Beastall GH, Hume R. Endocrine and metabolic studies in unstable cor pulmonale. Thorax 1983; 38:45–49.
198. Littlewood JM, Johnson AW, Edwards PA, Littlewood AE. Growth retardation in asthmatic children treated with inhaled beclomethasone dipropionate (letter). Lancet 1988; 1:115–116.
199. Oberger E, Engström I, Karlberg J. Long-term treatment with glucocorticoids/ACTH in asthmatic children. Acta Paediatr Scand 1990; 79:77–83.
200. Falliers CJ, Tan LS, Szentivanyi J, Jorgensen JR, Bukrantz SC. Childhood asthma and steroid therapy as influences on growth. Am J Dis Child 1963; 105:127–137.
201. Morris HG. Growth and skeletal maturation in asthmatic children: effect of corticosteroid treatment. Pediatr Res 1975; 9:579–583.
202. Chang KC, Miklich DR, Barwise G, Chai H, Miles-Lawrence R. Linear growth of chronic asthmatic children: the effect of the disease and various forms of steroid therapy. Clin Allergy 1982; 12:369–378.
203. Kerrebijn KF, De Kroon PM. Effect on height of corticosteroid therapy in asthmatic children. Arch Dis Child 1968; 43:556–661.
204. Blodgett FM, Burgin L, Iezzoni D, Gribetz D, Talbot NB. Effects of prolonged cortisone therapy on the statural growth, skeletal maturation and metabolic status of children. N Engl J Med 1956; 254:636–641.
205. Van Metre TE, Pinkerton HL. Growth suppression in asthmatic children receiving prolonged therapy with prednisone and methylprednisolone. J Allergy 1959; 30:103–113.
206. Wolthers OD, Pedersen S. Short term linear growth in asthmatic children during treatment with prednisolone. Br Med J 1990; 301:145–148.
207. Wolthers OD, Pedersen S. Growth of asthmatic children during treatment with budesonide: a double blind trial (see comments). Br Med J 1991; 303:163–165.
208. Wolthers OD, Pedersen S. Controlled study of linear growth in asthmatic children during treatment with inhaled glucocorticosteroids. Pediatrics 1992; 89:839–842.
209. Wolthers O, Pederson S. Growth in asthmatic children during treatment with budesonide. Pediatrics 1992; 91:517–518.

210. Wolthers O, Pedersen S. Inappropriate statistics. Pediatrics 1993; 91:517–518.
211. Agertoft L, Pedersen S. Short term lower leg growth in children during treatment with fluticasone propionate and budesonide. A dose response study. Am J Respir Crit Care Med 1995; 151:150.
212. Bisgaard H. Systemic activity from inhaled topical steroid in toddlers studied by knemometry. Acta Paediatr Scand 1993; 82:1066–1071.
213. Wolthers OD, Pedersen S. Short-term growth during treatment with inhaled fluticasone propionate and beclomethasone dipropionate. Arch Dis Child 1993; 68:673–676.
214. McKenzie CA, Wales JKH. Growth in asthmatic children. Br Med J 1991; 303:416.
215. Ribeiro LB. Budesonide: safety and efficacy aspects of its long-term use in children. Pediatr Allergy Immunol 1993; 4:73–78.
216. Kerrebijn KF. Beclomethasone dipropionate in long-term treatment of asthma in children. J Pediatr 1976; 89:821–826.
217. Varsano I, Volovitz B, Malik He. Safety of 1 year of treatment with budesonide in young children with asthma. J Allergy Clin Immunol 1990; 85:914–920.
218. Ruiz RG, Price JF. Growth and adrenal responsiveness with budesonidein young asthmatics. Respir Med 1994; 88:17–20.
219. Ruin RGG, Price JF. Growth and adrenal responsiveness in young asthmatic children on inhaled corticosteroids. Am Rev Respir Dis 1990; 141:A625.
220. Delacourt C, Chomienne F, DeBile J. Preservation of growth velocity in asthmatic children treated with high doses of beclomethasone dipropionate. Eur Respir J 1991; 4(suppl 14):593s.
221. Godfrey S, Balfour-Lynn L, Tooley M. A three to five year follow-up of the use of aerosol steroid, beclomethasone dipropionate, in childhood asthma. J Allergy Clin Immunol 1978; 62:335–339.
222. Nassif E, Weinberger M, Sherman e. Extrapulmonary effects of maintenance corticosteroid therapy with alternate-day prednisone and inhaled beclomethasone in children with chronic asthma. J Allergy Clin Immunol 1987; 80:518–529.
223. Nassif E, Weinberger M, Sherman B, Brown K. Extrapulmonary effects of maintenance corticosteroids therapy with alternate-day prednisone and inhaled beclomethasone in children with chronic asthma. J Allergy Clin Immunol 1987; 80:518–529.
224. Graff-Lonnevig V, Kraepelien S. Long term treatment with beclomethasone dipropionate aerosol in asthmatic children, with special reference to growth. Allergy 1979; 34:57–61.
225. Lee-Hong E, Collins-Williams C. The long term use of beclomethasone dipropionate for the control of asthma in children. Ann Allergy 1977; 38:242–244.
226. Francis RS. Long-term beclomethasone dipropionate aerosol therapy in juvenile asthma. Thorax 1976; 31:309–314.
227. Gilliam GL, McNicol KN, Williams HE. Chest deformity, residual airways obstruction and hyperinflammation, and growth in children with asthma. Arch Dis Child 1970; 45:789–799.
228. Brown DCP, Savacool AM, Letizia CM. A retrospective review of the effects of

one year of triamcinolone acetonide aerosol treatment of the growth patterns of asthmatic children. Ann Allergy 1989; 63:47–51.

229. Ribeiro LB. A 12 month tolerance study with budesonide in asthmatic children. Excerpta Med 1987; 95–108.

230. Hiller EJ, Groggins RC, Lenney W, Stokes M, Milner AD. Bechlomethasone dipropionate powder inhalation treatment in chronic childhood asthma. Prog Respir Res 1981; 17:285–289.

231. Clay MM, Pavia D, Newman SP, Lennard-Jones T, Clarke SW. Assessment of jet nebulisers for lung aerosol therapy. Lancet 1983; 2:592–594.

232. Brown HB, Bhowmik M, Jackson FA, Thantrey N. Bechlometasone dipropionate aerosols in the treatment of asthma in childhood. Practitioner 1980; 224:847–851.

233. Verini M, Verotti A, D'Arcangelo A, Misticoni G, Chiarelli F, Morgese G. Long-term therapy in childhood asthma: clinical and auxological aspects. Eur Rev Med Pharmacol Sci 1990; 12:169–173.

234. Morrow Brown H, Storey G. Bechlometasone dipropionte steriod aerosol in treatment of perennial allergic asthma in children. Br Med J 1973; 3:161–164.

235. Merkus PJ, van Essen Zandvliet EE, Duiverman EJ, van Houwelingen HC, Kerrebijn KF, Quanjer PH. Long-term effect of inhaled corticosteroids on growth rate in adolescents with asthma. Pediatics 1993; 91:1121–1126.

236. Doull IJ, Freezer NJ, Holgate ST. Growth of asthmatic children on inhaled corticosteroids. Am Rev Respir Dis 1993; 147:A265.

237. MacKenzie CA, Wales JKH. Clinical experience with inhaled fluticasone proprionate—childhood growth. Eur Respir J 1993; 6(suppl 17):262s.

238. Allen DB, Mullen ML, Mullen B. A meta-analysis of the effect of oral and inhaled corticosteroids on growth. J Allergy Clin Immunol 1994; 93:967–976.

239. Zeitlin S, Wood P, Evans A, Radford M. Overnight urine growth hormone, cortisol and adenosine 3'5' cyclic monophosphate excretion in children with chronic asthma treated with inhaled beclomethasone dipropionate. Respir Med 1993; 87:445–448.

240. Thomas BC, Stanhope R, Grant DB. Impaired growth in children with asthma during treatment with conventional doses of inhaled corticosteroids. Acta Paediatr 1994; 83:196–199.

241. Marshall W. Evaluation of growth rate in height over periods of less than one year. Arch Dis Child 1971; 46:414–420.

242. Butler GE, McKie M, Ratcliffe SG. The cyclical nature of prepubertal growth. Ann Hum Bio 1990; 17:177–198.

243. Voss LD, Wilkin TJ, Balley BJR, Betts PR. The reliability of height and weight velocity in the assessment of growth (the Wessex Growth Study). Arch Dis Child 1991; 66:833–837.

244. Karlberg J, Low L, Yeung CY. On the dynamics of the growth process. Acta Paediatr 1994; 83:777–778.

245. Spaeth GP, Von Smallman L. Corticosteroids and cataracts. Int Ophthalmol Clin 1966; 6:915–929.

246. Bhagat RG, Chai H. Development of posterior subcapsular cataracts in asthmatic children. Pediatrics 1984; 73:626–630.

247. Massarano AA, Hollis S, Devlin J, David TJ. Growth in atopic eczema. Arch Dis Child 1993; 68:677–679.
248. Simons FER, Persaud MP, Gillespie CA, Cheang M, Shuckett EP. Abscens of posterior subcapsular cataracts in young patients treated with inhaled glucocorticoids. Lancet 1993; 342:776–778.
249. Sevel D, Weinberg EG, van Niekerk CH. Lenticular complications of long-term steroid therapy in children with asthma and eczema. J Allergy 1977; 60:215–217.
250. Toogood JH, Markov AE, Baskerville J, Dyson C. Association of ocular cataracts with inhaled and oral steroid therapy during long-term treatment of asthma. J Allergy Clin Immunol 1993; 91:571–579.
251. Kewley GD. Possible association between beclomethasone dipropionate aerosol and cataracts. Aust Paediatr J 1980; 16:117–118.
252. Karim AKA, Thompson GM, Jacob TJC. Steroid aerosols and cataract formation. Br Med J 1987; 299:918.
253. Fraunfelder FT, Meyer SM. Posterior subcapsular cataracts associated with nasal or inhalation corticosteroids. Am J Ophthalmol 1990; 109:489–490.
254. Allen MB, Ray SG, Leitch AG, Dhillon B, Cullen B. Steroid aerosols and cataract formation. Br Med J 1989; 299:432–433.
255. Rooklin AR, Lampert SI, Jaeger EA, McGeady SJ, Mansmann HC, JR. Posterior subcapsular cataracts in steroid-requiring asthmatic children. J Allergy Clin Immunol 1979; 63:383–386.
256. Giorgi PL, Oggiano N, Biraghi M, Kantar A. Effect of high doses of inhaled flunisolide on hypothalamic-pituitary-adrenal axis function in children with asthma. Curr Ther Res 1991; 49:778–783.
257. Turpeinen M, Sorva R, Juntunen-Backman K. Changes in carbohydrate and lipid metabolism in children with asthma inhaling budesonide. J Allergy Clin Immunol 1991; 88:384–389.
258. Mitchell DM, Collins JV. Do corticosteroids really alter mood? Postgrad Med J 1984; 60:467–470.
259. Hall RCW, Popkin MK, Stickney SK, Garnder ER. Presentation of the steroid psychosis. J Nerv Ment Dis 1979; 167:229–236.
260. Phelan MC. Beclomethasone mania. Br J Psychiatr 1989; 155:871–872.
261. Meyboom RHB. Budesonide and psychic side-effects. Ann Intern Med 1988; 109:683.
262. Connett G, Lenney W. Inhaled budesonide and behavioural disturbances. Lancet 1991; 338:634.
263. Lewis LD, Cochrane GM. Psychosis in a child inhaling budesonide. Lancet 1983; 2:634.
264. Selroos O, Backman R, Forsen KO, et al. Local side-effects during 4-year treatment with inhaled corticosteroids—a comparison between pressurized metered-dose inhalers and Turbuhaler. Allergy 1994; 49:888–890.
265. Müns G, Bergmann KC. Local and systemic side effects of inhalatory corticosteroids—what has been confirmed? Pneumologie 1993; 47:201–208.
266. Williams J, Cooper S, Wahedna I, Wong CS, MacFarlane JT. Inhaled steroids and

their effects on voice and throat—a questionnaire survey. Am Rev Respir Dis 1992; 145:A741.

267. Matusiewicz S, Williamson I, Brown P, Greening AP, Crompton GK. A survey of voice problems and cough in patients taking inhaled aerosol corticosteroids. Eur Respir J 1991; 4:484s.

268. Settipane GA, Kalliel JN, Klein DE. Rechallenge of patients who developed oral candidiasis or hoarseness with beclomethasone dipropionate. N Engl Reg Allergy Proc 1987; 8:95-97.

23

Effects of Inhaled Steroid Therapy for Asthma on Skeletal Metabolism

JOHN H. TOOGOOD

University of Western Ontario
London, Ontario, Canada

I. Introduction

Skeletal complications are a frequent cause of major morbidity in asthmatic patients dependent on long-term oral or parenteral glucocorticoid therapy (1). It is surprising therefore that, until recently, few data existed to document the effects of inhaled steroid therapy on skeletal metabolism and the risk of fracture. The need for such data is becoming increasingly urgent in view of current trends toward the use of larger daily doses of these drugs in clinical practice and a worldwide shift toward their earlier introduction in the course of the disease.

II. Pathogenesis of Glucocorticoid-Induced Osteoporosis

Administered systemically or orally, glucocorticoids act directly—probably mainly in the jejunum—to inhibit the transmucosal transport and systemic absorption of dietary calcium. They also act directly on the renal tubule to inhibit the resorption of calcium from the glomerular filtrate. The combined effects of these processes may trigger secondary hyperparathyroidism, which then acts to increase bone resorption. In addition, glucocorticoids also act directly on bone by inhibiting osteoblast activity. These interactions between the extraskeletal and skeletal effects of the drug result in a decrease of bone formation and an increase in bone resorption.

Host factors interact with these drug-related factors to determine the degree of risk of glucocorticoid-induced osteoporosis in a particular individual. These host factors may reflect inherent or acquired intersubject differences in glucocorticoid metabolism (2) and/or mineral metabolism and/or other inherited familial and ethnic factors known to determine the attainment of peak bone mass during youth (3–5).

III. Metabolic Indices

The serum levels of 1,25-dihydroxyvitamin D_3 and serum parathormone normally rise homeostatically in response to any incipient drop in serum calcium concentration. Thus, changes in these indices provide an indirect measure of any inhibitory effect that a glucocorticoid drug may exert on calcium absorption from the gut. Alternatively, this effect may be assessed directly by measuring the absorption of orally administered radiolabeled calcium or strontium.

The 24-hr urinary calcium output provides a measure of the direct effect of glucocorticoids on the kidney, and also any increase in the absorption of calcium from bone that may occur as a consequence of secondary hyperparathyroidism.

The effects of these drugs on bone formation are measurable by changes in the serum level of several products of osteoblast activity: the carboxypropeptide of type I procollagen (PICP), osteocalcin (Gla protein), and alkaline phosphatase. Procollagen production relates to the formation of the osteoid matrix; the others relate to mineralization of the matrix.

Bone resorption is measurable indirectly in terms of the urinary output of several breakdown products of the osteoid matrix: hydroxyproline, pyridinoline, or deoxypyridinoline (collagen phosphatase, cross links) or variations in the serum level of tartrate-resistant acid phosphatase (TRAP). In addition, the serum levels of calcitonin, androstenodione, and dihydroepiandrosterone reflect bone resorption indirectly, since these normally modulate bone resorption.

IV. Data Available for Inhaled Steroid

The effects on skeletal metabolism of the formulations of inhaled steroid that are currently marketed in the United States, that is, triamcinolone acetonide and flunisolide, have not been adequately studied to date. Therefore, this chapter is focused mainly on data derived from studies of beclomethasone dipropionate and budesonide—mainly the latter, since, to date, the bulk of the available data pertain to this drug.

V. Effects of Budesonide on Mineral Metabolism

Studies spanning a dose range from 0.6 to 3.2 mg of budesonide per day (nominal dose)* have consistently shown an increase in serum phosphate levels (6,7). On the other hand, no decrease in serum calcium has been observed when the drug is administered in doses as high or higher than 2.4 mg/day (6,8). Nor has budesonide manifested any effect on the serum levels of parathormone or 1,25-dihydroxyvitamin D_3, when given in doses up to 2.4 mg per day (6). Thus, there is no evidence to suggest that inhaled budesonide inhibits the absorption of calcium from the gut.

However, in all these studies, the drug was administered from a pressurized aerosol via a spacer. Whether dry-powder inhalation devices or a metered-dose inhaler (MDI) without a spacer, are similarly free of effect is not known. When the latter devices are used instead of a pressurized aerosol with spacer, a much larger fraction of each nominal dose is deposited in the oropharynx, whence it may be swallowed. Because of its high topical potency, the swallowed portion might act directly on the gut mucosa to inhibit calcium absorption—and this in fact has been demonstrated to occur in healthy subjects to whom beclomethasone was administered orally (9). As yet, no similar data are available for any of the other inhaled steroids used to treat asthma.

The effects of budesonide on the resorption of calcium from the glomerular filtrate are variable. Daily doses of 1.2 (10), 2.4 (6), or 3.2 mg (8) did not increase the 24-hr urinary calcium output. However, in one of these studies, the data indicate that each of the four divided doses given during the day triggered a transient hypercalciuria, which was offset subsequently by a compensatory nocturnal hypocalcuria; thus, the urinary output of calcium per 24 hr remained unchanged (6). In contrast, in a different study that utilized the same daily dose of budesonide (i.e., 2.4 mg) but administered it morning and evening in two rather than four divided doses, the 24-hr urinary calcium output increased significantly (10). Whether these conflicting findings reflect the chronopharmacological effects of different dosing schedules, or the action of uncontrolled extraneous factors such as differences in the dietary intake of

---

*"Nominal" dosage signifies the amount of drug emitted from the valve of the MDI with each activation of the pressurized aerosol. It is not adjusted for losses that may occur within the delivery device or add-on spacer if attached.

calcium by different groups of test subjects, or interactions between such factors, is unclear. Nevertheless, the data are sufficient to establish that high doses of budesonide, and possibly other inhaled steroids, can evoke significant hypercalciuria under some circumstances. Conceivably, this might prove clinically significant in persons who conserve calcium poorly as a result of inherent or acquired metabolic inefficiencies in their intestinal absorption and/or renal resorption of calcium.

Hypercalciuria has been observed clinically in preschool children treated for acute asthma with steroid aerosols administered via a face mask with spacer (11). The risk of urinary lithiasis is a concern. Since the drug and dosing regimen used were not reported, it is not possible to estimate to what extent this hypercalciuria may relate to the particular drug used, or the dose or dosing schedule, and/or the mode of drug delivery.

VI. Effects of Budesonide on Bone Turnover

A. Bone Formation

If budesonide is administered in doses up to 3.2 mg/day, it does not adversely affect serum alkaline phosphatase levels (7,8,12,13). On the other hand, a significant, dose-dependent suppression of the production of osteocalcin by osteoblasts has been demonstrated with budesonide in doses of 1.2 mg/day or higher, although not with lower doses (7,8,13). This inhibitory effect on the normal, diurnally cyclic production of osteocalcin is probably not ameliorated by scheduling the entire daily dose of budesonide to be given in the forenoon instead of diurnally (10). Budesonide treatment partially inhibits the normal responsiveness of osteoblasts to vitamin D_3 stimulation, as illustrated in Figure 1. These direct effects of the drug on osteocalcin production need to be distinguished from the preexisting reduction in osteocalcin levels that may be demonstrated, independent of inhaled steroid therapy, in some asthmatic children (14).

Budesonide treatment may also inhibit the production of procollagen. This effect appears to be slower in onset and more sustained than the accompanying inhibition of osteocalcin production (7,8,12,15). These dynamic disparities may reflect differences between the two indices with respect to their specificity as markers of osteoblast activity (16). The inhibition of procollagen production appears more readily discernible in males than in females (12). This might be relevant to the sex-related differences that have been observed in some other studies with regard to patient susceptibility to growth inhibition during inhaled steroid treatment (17).

B. Bone Resorption

No increase in the urinary output of hydroxyproline or deoxypyridinoline has been observed with budesonide doses up to 3.2 mg/day (7,8,13). Indeed, several observers have noted a paradoxical reduction in hydroxyproline output in response to doses of 1.6 mg/day budesonide per day or higher (7,10). This implies a downregulation of osteoclast activity in response the steroid-induced inhibition of osteoblast activity and, in consequence, a reduction rather than an increase in bone resorption. Lower doses of budesonide do not affect hydroxyproline excretion.

Large doses of budesonide do not affect the serum level of calcitonin (18). A dose-dependent suppression of the production of androgen by the adrenal cortex occurs with budesonide treatment (6,7). We have observed that the androgen production of some postmenopausal women may approximate zero after 1 week of high-dose budesonide treatment (6). This change could be clinically important. Estrogen deficiency is a major risk determinant of osteoporosis and fracture in postmenopausal women, who are entirely dependent for their residual supply of estrogen on biotransformation of these androgens of adrenocortical origin; thus, the glucocorticoid-induced reduction in androgen output may augment the risk of bone complications in some older women treated for asthma with high-dose inhaled steroid or a combined inhaled/oral steroid regimen in the absence of an estrogen supplement. An analogous high-risk situation was observed after 2 years of high-dose beclomethasone treatment in a young man who had asthma and an unrelated problem, primary testicular failure not treated with an adequate testosterone supplement (19).

VII. Comparisons of Budesonide Versus Prednisone

The presence or absence of a particular adverse effect of budesonide on bone metabolism appears less important clinically than its magnitude relative to the therapeutic alternative. In patients with moderate or severe asthma, the alternative is usually oral prednisone.

None of the budesonide doses yet tested (up to 3.2 mg/day) affect bone turnover as much as therapeutically equivalent doses of prednisone (8,13,15,20). Either budesonide or prednisone can inhibit the responsiveness of osteoblasts to vitamin D_3, as illustrated in Figure 1. The estimated ED_{50} for this effect is about 3.6 mg budesonide per day or 20 mg prednisolone per day, and the potency ratio is $\sim 1.0{:}5.5$ (budesonide:prednisolone).

Comparisons of the effects of graded doses of prednisone versus inhaled steroid on selected indices of systemic glucocorticoid activity provide a basis for estimating a "safe dose" cutoff for budesonide or any other inhaled steroid (20). A clinically meaningful cutoff may be defined empirically as that dose of inhaled steroid which displays systemic activity equivalent to that of 15 mg prednisone per day administered to a 70-kg adult. The basis for choosing such a cutoff criterion is the accumulated clinical experience that has shown adult doses of prednisone higher than 15 mg/day to be associated with a relatively

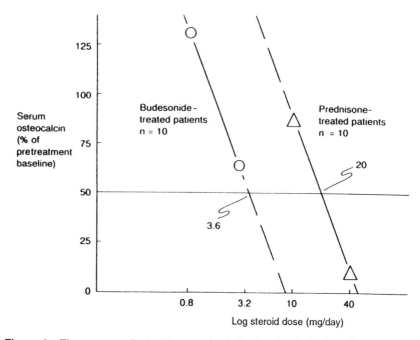

Figure 1 The response of osteoblasts to stimulation by vitamin D_3 in patients pretreated with high or low doses of budesonide (O) or prednisone (Δ). Group means are shown for the AM serum osteocalcin level after 7 days of treatment with vitamin D_3 2.0 µg/day PO. The ED_{50} for suppression of the vitamin D_3 response is 3.6 mg budesonide or 20 mg prednisone. (Adapted from Ref. 8.)

high incidence of serious bone complications and doses less than 15 mg/day to be associated with a lower and more clinically acceptable level of risk (20).

Based on this empiric convention, some estimates of a "safe" dose cutoff for budesonide were derived from measurements of its effect upon four different response indices (7,8,20,21). These are shown in Table 1. The estimates vary from about 2 to 6 mg/day. The prudent choice would be the lowest estimate: 2 mg/day.

VIII. Comparisons of Budesonide Versus Beclomethasone*

In respect to bone formation, either budesonide or beclomethasone may inhibit osteocalcin production (8,10,21,22,23). The effect is discernible within a week

---

*The basis for categorizing the daily dosage of inhaled steroid as "low," "intermediate," or "high" is illustrated in Table 2.

Table 1 Estimates of a "Safe-Dose" Cutoff (Milligrams of Budesonide per Day)[a]

Serum osteocalcin: vitamin D_3 Stimulated		Dehydro Epiandrosterone	Androstenedione	Serum Cortisol 8 A.M.
no	yes			
2.0 (8)	2.7 (8)			1.8 (20)
5.2 (7)		6.0 (7)	2.9 (7)	3.0 (7)

[a]Based on systemic bioequivalence of the inhaled steroid to effects of 15 mg of prednisone per day.

of commencing the treatment (8,22), and beclomethasone appears more potent in this regard than budesonide (24,25). With beclomethasone, the normal diurnally cyclic pattern of osteocalcin production is conserved despite sharply depressed serum levels (22). Presumably the same would apply with any other inhaled steroid, but no similar data are available as yet.

High-dose budesonide (see Table 2) does not inhibit alkaline phosphatase production (24,25), whereas beclomethasone may do so when given in doses equal to or higher than 2 mg/day (26). Some studies have not substantiated this effect of beclomethasone on alkaline phosphatase (23,24).

Low-dose budesonide (see Table 2) may inhibit procollagen production in asthmatic patients (12). Shorter periods of treatment of nonasthmatic test subjects have not demonstrated such an effect when high doses were used (15). Whether beclomethasone similarly inhibits procollagen production has not yet

Table 2 Basis for Categorizing Daily Dosage of Inhaled Steroid as Low, Intermediate, or High

Dose category[a]	Nominal daily dose		% of inhaled steroid users[b] (n = 296)
	mg/70 kg adult	µg/kg	
Low	<1.0	<14	55
Intermediate	1.0–2.0	14–29	40
High	>2.0	>29	5

[a]The designations of dose category applied throughout this chapter are empirically derived and based on considerations of potential risk. Doses designated as "low" are generally accepted as free from clinically important adverse effects. Those designated as "high" show a level of systemic activity equivalent to that of 15 mg of prednisone per day as judged by a bioequivalence comparison of budesonide versus prednisone in adults with moderate to severe asthma (20).
[b]Data from a 1989–1990 audit of the entire adult population receiving ambulatory care for asthma from three specialist physicians in a tertiary health care facility (50).

ben determined. The only study reported to date found no effect after 3 weeks' treatment with 2 mg/day (23).

With respect to bone resorption, 2 mg of beclomethasone per day may increase the urinary hydroxyproline output (24,26), but budesonide has not done so when given at the same time or higher dosage (7,8,24). At low dosage, neither of these drugs increases the hydroxyproline output (8,24,27). Either drug may paradoxically reduce hydroxyproline output, which implies a reduction in bone resorption (10,23,24,26). Similarly, children treated with intermediate (see Table 2) doses of beclomethasone showed some evidence of reduced bone resorption as measured by the serum level of tartrate-resistant acid phosphatase (14). Either drug may inhibit androgen production from the adrenal cortex, and they appear to have similar systemic potencies in this respect (6,24).

IX. Clinical Outcomes

To determine whether any of the effects that inhaled steroid drugs have on laboratory indices of skeletal metabolism signal a clinically important increase in the risk of fracture, it is necessary to determine the impact of the treatment on bone density. The lifetime risk of an osteoporotic fracture has been estimated to increase about 1.5- to 3-fold for each standard deviation decrease in bone density from the normalized values of persons of the same age and sex (28,29,30).

X. Effects of Inhaled Steroid Therapy on Bone Density

Among 11 studies available for review at the present time, 9 are cross-sectional surveys and 2 are controlled prospective studies. In one of the latter, Luengo et al. compared the effect of low-dose beclomethasone supplemented by intermittent prednisone versus daily low-dose prednisone alone in two matched groups of adult patients followed for 2 years (31). In the group treated with daily prednisone alone, bone density declined at a rate about eight times faster than normal. However, in the patients treated with low-dose beclomethasone supplemented by infrequent short courses of prednisone, bone loss proceeded at a normal rate (31).

In the other prospective study (32), the mean bone density of asthmatic children who had received 0.3–0.4 mg of beclomethasone per day for at least 6 months did not differ from that of age- and sex-matched asthmatic controls not treated with inhaled steroid. However, the expected increase in bone mass during a further 6-month treatment period was about 40% less in the beclomethasone-treated patients than in the controls not treated with beclomethasone. The clinical implications of this observation remain to be determined by longer follow-up. Of concern is the possibility that failure to attain maximal bone density in youth is known to be a major determinant of the risk of osteoporotic fracture in later life (33).

Among the nine cross-sectional surveys published to date in full or abstract form, seven studied adults. Reid et al. found that inhaled steroid treatment at a nominal dose averaging less than 1 mg/day was associated with significantly reduced levels of total body calcium in comparison with normal subjects (34). However, a confounding effect from past oral or parenteral steroid therapy could not be excluded in these patients (35). In contrast, Wolfe et al. found no reduction in the mean bone density of a small group of asthmatic adults treated for 1.6–4.0 years with low doses of various inhaled steroids (36). Nevertheless, one patient among the study group had exceptionally low bone density, and the possibility that this might be partly or wholly attributable to his inhaled steroid treatment could not be excluded. Stead et al. found low bone densities in asthmatic patients treated with an intermediate dose of inhaled steroid (37), but the causal role of the inhaled steroid remains ambiguous, because the patients were postmenopausal and had also taken unverifiable amounts of prednisone. Packe et al. found a substantial reduction in bone density in asthmatic patients treated with intermediate doses of inhaled steroid (1–2 mg/day). However, the possible confounding effect of past or recent oral steroid usage could not be excluded (38). Boulet et al. found a slight reduction of bone density in asthmatic patients treated with low or intermediate doses of inhaled steroid, but there was no discernible relationship between bone density and the daily dosage used (39). Similarly, Ip et al., surveying asthmatic adults who had received long-term, low-dose beclomethasone treatment, found bone density values that were marginally lower than those of healthy controls (40). However, in the absence of a comparison group of untreated patient controls, it is uncertain whether the observed reduction in bone density relates to the inhaled steroid treatment per se or to some other correlate of chronic asthma such as reduced physical activity.

One of the two pediatric cross-sectional surveys published to date found no reduction in bone density in children treated with an intermediate dose of inhaled steroid for an average of 2–3 years (14). These patients were compared with asthmatic children not receiving inhaled steroid therapy and also with healthy control subjects. The other pediatric study (41) found that the bone density of 30 children treated with beclomethasone at a dose averaging about 0.6 mg/day did not differ significantly from that of normal controls. Furthermore, no significant correlations were found between the bone density of these individuals and their daily dose or lifetime cumulative dose of inhaled steroid. These findings do not exclude the possibility that higher doses and/or longer treatment might adversely affect bone density.

To try to resolve the uncertainties engendered by these conflicting findings, we measured bone density in 69 adult patients attending our asthma clinic (42). The survey was specifically designed to facilitate differentiation between any effect of the inhaled steroid that might be observed and that due to past or current oral steroid usage or to nonsteroidal factors such as age, physical activity, or the postmenopausal state. The key observations are as follows:

1. In these adults, inhaled steroid treatment was associated with a dose-dependent and statistically significant reduction in bone density. Density dropped by an average of 0.5 standard deviations for each increment of inhaled steroid dosage by 1 mg/day (nominal dose).

2. This bone-depleting effect was offset to a clinically valuable degree by an opposing effect that related to the cumulative lifetime dose of inhaled steroid. This resulted in an increase in bone density and a reduction in the risk of fracture (Fig. 2). We hypothesize that this reflects bone reconstitution consequent to withdrawal of the patients from their previously used prednisone after they switched to inhaled steroid. This repair process was not prevented by the use of beclomethasone or budesonide in doses averaging 1.2 mg/day.

3. The postmenopausal women in this group who had received prolonged inhaled steroid therapy, as evidenced by their lifetime dose of more than 3 g, had normal bone density on average. Furthermore, this applied regardless of how much prednisone they had used in the past and despite their current use of budesonide or beclomethasone at a high dose, averaging 1.6 mg/day. All these women had received an estrogen supplement as well, and their bone density correlated positively with the duration of their estrogen therapy.

4. About 55% of the variability in bone density that was observed in our survey group could not be explained by their past or current glucocorticoid treatment. This presumably relates mainly to genetic factors, since the latter are known to be the major determinants of the variability in bone density that can be seen in any randomly selected population (43–47). This suggests that some patients treated with inhaled steroid may be at significantly greater risk than others if the adverse effect of these drugs on bone is added to that of pre-existing, non–drug-related factors.

In summary, the data from this survey indicated that the daily dose, but not the duration, of inhaled steroid therapy may adversely affect bone density, and that estrogen therapy may offset this bone-depleting effect in postmenopausal women. Further studies are needed to test the hypotheses generated from this study; that is, (1) the existence of two opposing effects of inhaled steroid

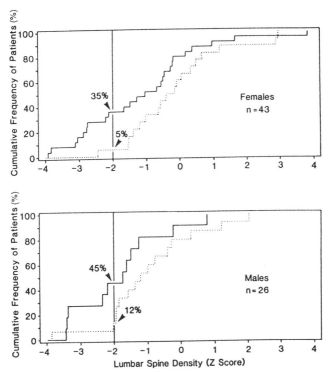

Figure 2 Influence of the cumulative dose of inhaled steroid on the frequency distribution of Z-scores for lumbar spine density among women (above) and men (below), subdivided at the median cumulative dose of inhaled steroid: ≤3 g (–) and >3 g (- - -). The Z-score quantifies the number of standard deviations that the measured bone density differs from the density of healthy persons of the same age and sex. The lifetime risk of fracture increases 1.5- to 3-fold for each standard deviation decrease in bone density. A larger lifetime exposure to inhaled steroid was associated with more normal lumbar spine density values (*P* = .02) and a reduction in the number of patients at risk of fracture (42). These advantages were more prominent in women than in men.

therapy on bone density—one a direct effect of the daily dose and the other an indirect effect of prolonged use of the drug with an accompanying abstention from oral or parenteral steroid use; and (2) the apparent capacity of supplemental estrogen therapy to prevent and/or correct glucocorticoid-induced osteoporosis in women in addition to its expected effect on involutional osteoporosis.

Furthermore, it remains to be determined whether the maximum bone density achieved by young adults may be adversely affected if they receive substantial amounts of inhaled steroid prior to 30 years of age. This is an important question, because failure to achieve maximum bone density during youth may lead to an increase in the incidence of osteoporotic fracture when those individuals reach the sixth decade of life and older.

XI. Effects on Occurrence of Fractures

The effects of inhaled and oral steroid treatment on the prevalence of vertebral fracture have been compared in two cross-sectional radiographic surveys (31,48).

Fractures were found in 56% of a nonrandomly selected group of 25 adults receiving low-dose daily prednisone. However, in a matched group treated with low-dose beclomethasone supplemented by infrequent short courses of prednisone, significantly fewer fractures were found: 8% ($P = .02$) (31).

In another survey of 63 adults, regression analysis of the relationships between the cumulative lifetime dose of inhaled steroid and the duration of oral steroid therapy versus the prevalence of vertebral fracture showed that (1) the longer these patients had used prednisone, the lower their bone density ($P = .10$), and (2) the higher their cumulative lifetime dose of inhaled steroid, the higher their bone density ($P = .02$) and the fewer the number of vertebral fractures ($P = .02$) (48). This confirms that the positive association between the lifetime inhaled steroid dosage and higher bone densities that was observed in these patients (49) is, in fact, clinically beneficial.

XII. Summary

There is no evidence that inhaled budesonide or beclomethasone inhibits the absorption of calcium from the intestine when these drugs are administered in conventional dosage via a pressurized aerosol with a spacer. Whether larger doses administered without a spacer, or in a different formulation such as a dry powder or nebulizer solution, are equally free of any discernible effect on calcium absorption, and how this may relate to the particular drug or dosage used has yet to be determined.

The effect of inhaled steroid treatment on the normal urinary conservation of calcium may be influenced by interactions between the dosing regimen, the drug and/or delivery system used, and also by patient-related factors such as age and variations in dietary calcium content or physical activity. There is as yet no systematically collected body of data that would allow these relationships or their possible clinical importance to be evaluated.

Inhaled steroid drugs can partially inhibit osteoblast function in a dose-dependent fashion, as evidenced by their effects on the production of osteocalcin and procollagen. Budesonide or beclomethasone may increase, decrease, or exhibit no effect on osteoclast activity and bone resorption depending on the dose and drug given. Beclomethasone appears to be more potent than budesonide in this respect.

Notwithstanding the adverse effects that inhaled steroids have been shown to exert on bone turnover, the magnitude of these effects is less than that of prednisone when the inhaled and oral drugs are compared at therapeutically equivalent dosages. The latter observation derives from a comparative study of budesonide versus prednisone (8), but the principle probably applies to all inhaled steroids as a class.

Furthermore, although prednisone therapy is known to increase the risk of vertebral fracture substantially, preliminary data derived from patients who commenced using regular glucocorticoid treatment after attaining adulthood suggest that long-term budesonide or beclomethasone treatment may materially reduce this risk—presumably by facilitating a reduction in prednisone usage and an increase in physical activity, with consequent restitution of the bone previously depleted by systemic glucocorticoid treatment. Further investigations are needed to substantiate these findings.

XIII. Caveats

The conclusions summarized above are largely inferential and based on a small and fragmentary body of data. Therefore, they must be viewed as tentative at best. Furthermore, they relate almost exclusively to budesonide and beclomethasone. There is an urgent need for similar data for triamcinolone acetonide and flunisolide and for investigational new drugs such as fluticasone. The latter appears to be the most promising of the antiasthmatic inhaled steroids undergoing development at this time.

Most importantly, the impact of inhaled steroid treatment on bone density and the risk of fracture requires further study. Particular attention needs to be paid to subsets of patients who may be at greater than average risk. This would include postmenopausal women and children, adolescents, and young adults who have not attained peak bone density prior to commencing regular inhaled steroid therapy.

The interactions between drug-related risk factors and inherent or acquired physiological inefficiencies in calcium conservation and/or bone mass development also merit systematic study.

Discussion

DR. THOMPSON: What factors contribute to variable patient responses vis-à-vis the bone effects of glucocorticoids.

Dr. Toogood: It is well known that people vary in their susceptibility to the systemic effects of glucocorticoid drugs, and this has been thought to relate, at least in part, to inherent or acquired differences in glucocorticoid metabolism. The McMaster group has identified a proportion of asthmatic children treated with inhaled steroid who seem unusually susceptible to growth inhibition, and this susceptibility appears to apply selectively to growth and not to other organ systems normally targeted by glucocorticoid activity. I do not know whether this increase in risk applies to bone density as well as to growth.

Dr. Hargreave: (1) How was the budesonide given? (2) Should we assume that the equivalent of 2 mg/day by MDI is 1 mg/day by Turbuhaler?

Dr. Toogood: (1) All the patients who participated in our study of bone density were treated with a MDI, and almost all of these inhaled the drug via a large volume (750 ml) spacer (Nebuhaler). No one received treatment with a dry-powder formulation. (2) In my opinion, this would not be a safe assumption, because conflicting results have been observed in comparative studies of these two delivery devices. For example, we found in a controlled prospective study that there was considerable variation between subjects but, on average, the two devices were essentially equivalent in terms of intrapulmonary drug delivery and potential systemic toxicity. Others have noted a twofold difference. I suspect these discrepancies reflect interstudy differences with respect to the inhalation technique employed by the patients when using one or other of the test devices.

Dr. Pedersen: What about the increase in bone mass during adolescence?

Dr. Toogood: Because peak bone mass is not attained until about 30 years of age, and because the peak value attained is a major determinant of the risk of fracture in patients who reach 60 years of age or older, it is important that the effects of inhaled steroid therapy on the attainment of peak bone mass be systematically studied through adolescence and the third decade of life. To the best of my knowledge, there are as yet no data that address this issue. Potentially confounding factors are very important in adults as well as children. Extraneous, nonsteroidal factors such as calcium intake and absorption may act as important codeterminants of the degree of risk of osteoporosis incurred by individual patients receiving inhaled steroid treatment. This was illustrated in our bone density survey by the substantial amount of unexplained variation in bone density that we observed (R^2 0.45) after controlling for the effects of the daily dose of inhaled steroid and the additional risk factors analyzed. This indicates a strong influence from some unexplained factor or factors, possibly genetic, acting alone or possibly in conjunction with the daily dose of inhaled steroid as determinants of bone density.

DR. LANE: (1) How soon do you see a steroid effect on biochemical markers in the serum (e.g., osteocalcin)? (2) What are the most sensitive markers of bone resorbtion/formation? (3) Can you change bone turnover with high-dose oral steroids and use the suppression as a predictor of subsequent risk of osteoporosis?

DR. TOOGOOD: The dose per day is the most important determinant of whether a significant effect on osteocalcin production is discernible with either oral or inhaled steroid therapy. If a sufficient dose of inhaled steroid is given, a significant drop in the serum osteocalcin level may be seen within 1 week. Other markers of bone formation such as procollagen may respond more slowly. Densitometry provides the most useful measure of bone mass, since it provides a basis for estimating the risk of fracture. The clinical use of biochemical markers of bone turnover was reviewed by Delmas (Delmas TD. Biochemical markers of bone turnover methodology and clinical use in osteoporosis. Am J Med 1991; 91:59S–63S). It is my opinion, there is no convincing evidence that any single index of skeletal metabolism is more reliable than another for the purpose of identifying glucocorticoid treated patients at risk from osteoporosis. With respect to osteocalcin in particular, in the patients who participated in our cross-sectional survey of bone density, their serum osteocalcin levels were low on the average and did not correlate significantly with their bone density either by regression or multiple regression analysis. The need for diagnostic densitometry ought to be based on clinical considerations rather than any particular metabolic index such as the osteocalcin level. With respect to drug safety studies, we found in a post hoc comparison of various laboratory markers of bone turnover marked variability between the seven indices measured when they were rank ordered according to their statistical power for detecting between-drug or between-dose differences. Our conclusion was that, in order to minimize the likelihood of type II error (which is a primary requisite for "safety studies"), it is desirable to measure a combination of indices. The specificity of procollagen assays as a measure of bone turnover may be compromised by co-existing inflammatory disease such as asthma or arthritis (O.D.Wolthers, personal communications).

DR. SCHLEIMER: You mentioned that BDP and budesonide both decrease bone formation but only BDP increases bone resorption. Unless this is only a matter of dose, I cannot envision a good explanation for it. How do you explain it?

DR. TOOGOOD: The disparity presumably does not reflect a qualitative difference between beclomethasone and budesonide in regard to their respective effects on bone but rather a difference in relative toxicity. One may reasonably assume that any inhaled steroid drug will increase bone resorption provided one administers a high enough dose. Using graded-dose comparisons, it should be quite feasible to determine an ED_{50} for this particular effect for each of the different inhaled steroids currently used.

DR. BRATTSAND: The expression of one important bone protein, bone sialo-protein, is in fact upregulated by glucocorticoids. (Oldberg A, Jirskog-Hed B, Axelsson S, et al. Regulation of bone sialoprotein mRNA by steroid hormones. J Cell Biol 1989; 109:3183–3186.)

DR. TOOGOOD: If I understand correctly, this questions asks whether low-dose glucocorticoid treatment might conserve bone mineral density by inhibiting bone resorption. I imagine the genesis of the question lies in the serendipitous observation by several investigators of a reduction in urinary hydroxyproline output (which implies reduced bone resorption) in response to treatment with budesonide doses of 1.6 mg/day or higher. This is the reverse of what would have been expected based on past experience with oral or systemic glucocorticoid therapy. These relationships have not been systematically investigated as yet. However, a priori, it seems likely that the reduced hydroxyproline output in response to budesonide treatment reflects a homeostatic downregulation of osteoclasts secondary to a primary inhibiting effect of the inhaled steroid on osteoblast function. (These two cell populations are functionally linked.) The net effect would be to help conserve bone density in the face of a slight reduction in bone formation caused by the inhaled steroid treatment.

DR. DURHAM: You showed that estrogen replacement in postmenopausal women protects against corticosteroid-induced osteoporosis. Might there be a similar role for testosterone in older males who develop severe glucocorticoid-induced osteoporosis?

DR. TOOGOOD: The role of androgen therapy in the treatment of osteoporosis remains ambiguous. Virilizing side effects may limit their use, and long-term follow-up of their effects on lipids as well as bone mass is required. Although oral steroids may suppress endogenous testosterone production up to 50%, it would appear that inhaled steroid therapy even at doses ≥ 1 mg/day does not significantly reduce testosterone levels in young or elderly males with normal gonads. Thus, there is no indication for testosterone replacement in males with normal gonads who require inhaled steroid treatment for asthma. However, if high-dose inhaled steroid is administered to a man with primary hypogonadism who is not taking an adequate testosterone supplement, this may materially increase the risk of osteoporotic fracture, because it inhibits production of androgens from his only source of a residual supply—the adrenal cortex. Postmenopausal women not receiving supplemental estrogen may also incur some risk owing to androgen insufficiency as a complication of the use of inhaled steroids.

We observed in some postmenopausal women that the androgen production from their adrenal cortex approximated zero after 1 week of high-dose budesonide treatment. Because estrogen deficiency is known to be a major risk determinant of osteoporosis and fracture in postmenopausal women, and because they are entirely dependent for their residual supply of estrogen on biotransformation of these androgens of adrenocortical origin, the glucocorticoid-induced reduction in androgen output may augment the risk of bone complications in some older women if they are treated for asthma with high-dose inhaled steroid or a combined inhaled/oral steroid regimen in the absence of an estrogen supplement.

DR. O'BYRNE: Why do the daily doses of glucocorticoids relate to reduced bone density and why does total lifetime dose appear to protect?

DR. TOOGOOD: We hypothesize the existence of two separate effects of the inhaled steroid: (1) a direct bone-depleting effect of the current daily dose that relates to the action of the drug on bone turnover and (2) an indirect effect that probably reflects the restitution of previously osteoporotic bone consequent to the withdrawal of prednisone after the commencement of inhaled steroid treatment. The design of our study (in particular, the criteria for patient selection and the use of ANCOVA to control for the effects of confounding variables) made it possible to distinguish these opposing effects from one another in a patient population that had been exposed to both oral and inhaled steroids.

References

1. Lukert BP, Raisz LG. Glucocorticoid-induced osteoporosis: Pathogenesis and management. Ann Intern Med 1990; 112:352–364.
2. Gambertoglio JG et al. Prednisolone disposition in cushingoid and noncushingoid kidney transplant patients. J Clin Endocrinol Metab 1980; 51:561.
3. Pocock NA, Eisman JA, Hooper JL, Yeates MG et al. Genetic determinants of bone mass in adults: a twin study. J Clin Invest 1987; 80:706–710.
4. Seeman E, Hooper JL, Bach LA, et al. Reduced bone mass in daughters of women with osteoporosis. N Engl J Med 1989; 320:554–558.
5. Morrison NA, et al. Prediction of bone density from Vitamin D receptor alleles. Nature 1994; 367:284–287.
6. Toogood JH, Crilly RG, Jones G, Nadeau J, Wells GA. Effect of high dose inhaled budesonide on calcium and phosphate metabolism and the risk of osteoporosis. Am Rev Respir Dis 1988; 138:57–61.
7. Jennings BH, Anderson K-E, Johansson S-A. Assessment of systemic effects of inhaled glucocorticoids: comparison of the effects of inhaled budesonide and oral prednisoloone on adrenal function and markers of bone turnover. Eur J Clin Pharmacol 1991; 40:77–82.

8. Hodsman AB, Toogood JH, Jennings B, Fraher LJ, Baskerville JC. Differential effects of inhaled budesonide and oral prednisolone on serum osteocalcin. J Clin Endocrinol Metab 1991; 72:530-540.
9. Smith BJ, Phillips PJ, Pannall PR, Cain HJ, Leckie WJH. Effect of orally administered beclomethasone dipropionate on calcium absorption from the gut in normal subjects. Thorax 1993; 48:890-893.
10. Toogood JH, Jennings B, Hodsman AB, Baskerville J, Fraher LJ. Effects of dose and dosing schedule of inhaled budesonide on bone turnover. J Allergy Clin Immunol 1991; 88:572-580.
11. Bentur L, Bibi H, Rubin AE, Bentur Y. Inhaled corticosteroids in young children: associated with hypercalciuria. Am Rev Respir Dis 1993; 147:A265.
12. Sorva R, Turpeinen M, Juntunen-Backman K, Karonen SL, Sorva A. Effects of inhaled budesonide on serum markers of bone metabolism in children with asthma. J Allergy Clin Immunol 1992; 90:808-815.
13. Wolthers OD, Riis BJ, Pedersen S. Bone turnover in asthmatic children treated with oral prednisolone or inhaled budesonide. Pediatr Pulmon 1993; 16:341-346.
14. Konig P, Hillman L, Cervantes C, Levine C, Maloney C, Douglass B, Johnson L, Allen S. Bone metabolism in children with asthma treated with inhaled beclomethasone dipropionate. J Pediatr 1993; 122:219-226.
15. Markov AE, Toogood JH, Hodsman AB, Steer B, Fraher LJ. Differential effects of inhaled budesonide and oral prednisone on biochemical markers of skeletal and adrenal functions. J Bone Min Res 1992; 7:S97.
16. Wolthers OD. University Hospital, Aarhus, Denmark 1994. Personal communication, February 1994.
17. Tinkelman DG, Reed CE, Nelson HS, Offord KP. Aerosol beclomethasone dipropionate compared with theophylline as primary treatment of chronic, mild to moderately severe asthma in children. Pediatrics 1993; 92:64-77.
18. Jennings BH. The effects of inhaled budesonide vs oral prednisolone on calcium metabolism. In: The Assessment of Systemic Effects of Inhaled Glucocorticoids. Ph.D. dissertation. University of Lund, Sweden, 1990; IV:1-IV:11.
19. Chalkley SM, Chisholm DJ. Cushing's syndrome from an inhaled glucocorticoid. Med J Aust 1994; 160:611-615.
20. Toogood JH, Baskerville J, Jennings B, Lefcoe NM, Johansson S-A. Bioequivalent doses of budesonide and prednisone in moderate and severe asthma. J Allergy Clin Immunol 1989; 84:688-700.
21. Toogood JH, Jennings B, Hodsman A, Fraher L, Baskerville J. Effect of inhaled budesonide (BUD) on osteoblast function. J Allergy Clin Immunol 1990; 85:144.
22. Pouw EM, Prummel MF, Oosting H, Roos CM, Endert E. Beclomethasone inhalation decreases serum osteocalcin concentrations. Br Med J 1991; 302:627-628.
23. Puolijoki H, Lippo K, Herrala J, Salmi J, Tala E. Inhaled beclomethasone decreases serum osteocalcin in postmenopausal asthmatic women. Bone 1992; 13:285-288.
24. Jennings BH. A comparison of budesonide and beclomethasone dipropionate in healthy volunteers. In: The Assessment of Systemic Effects of Inhaled Glucocorticoids. Ph.D. dissertation. University of Lund, Sweden, 1990; VII:1-VII:14.

25. Leech JA, Hodder RV, Ooi DS, Gay J. Effects of short-term inhaled budesonide and beclomethasone dipropionate on serum osteocalcin in premenopausal women. Am Rev Respir Dis 1993; 148:113–115.
26. Ali NJ, Capewell S, Ward MJ. Bone turnover during high dose inhaled corticosteroid treatment. Thorax 1991; 46:160–164.
27. Peretz A, Bourdoux PP. Inhaled corticosteroids, bone formation, and osteocalcin. Lancet 1991; 338:1340.
28. Wasnich RD, Ross PD, Davis JW, Vogel JM. A comparison of single and multisite BMC measurements for assessment of spine fracture probability. J Nucl Med 1989; 30:1166–1171.
29. Kanis JA. What constitutes evidence for drug efficacy in osteoporosis? Drugs and Aging 1993; 3:391–399.
30. Cummings SR, Black DM, Nevitt M, Browner W, Cauley J, Ensrud K, Genant HK, Palermo L, Scott J. Bone density at various sites for prediction of hip fractures. Lancet 1993; 341:72–75.
31. Luengo M, Del Rio L, Guanabens N, Picado C. Long-term effect of oral and inhaled glucocorticoids on bone mass in chronic asthma. A two year follow-up study. Eur Respir J 1991; 4:342s.
32. Baraldi E, Bollini MC, De Marchi A, Zacchello F. Effect of beclomethasone dipropionate on bone mineral content assessed by X-ray densitometry in asthmatic children: a longitudinal evaluation. Eur Respir J 1994; 7:710–714.
33. Kreipe RE. Bones of today, bones of tomorrow. Am J Dis Child 1992; 146:22–25.
34. Reid DM, Nicoll JJ, Smith MA, Higgins B, Tothill P, Nuki G. Corticosteroids and bone mass in asthma: comparisons with rheumatoid arthritis and polymyalgia rheumatica. Br Med J 1986; 293:1463–1466.
35. Crompton GK. Corticosteroids and bone mass in asthma. Br Med J 1987; 294:123.
36. Wolff AH, Adelsberg B, Aloia J, Zitt M. Effect of inhaled corticosteroid on bone density in asthmatic patients: a pilot study. Ann Allergy 1991; 67:117–121.
37. Stead RJ, Horsman A, Cooke NJ, Belchetz P. Bone mineral density in women taking inhaled corticosteroids. Thorax 1990; 45:792.
38. Packe GE, Douglas JG, McDonald AF, Robbins SP, Reid DM. Bone density in asthmatic patients taking high dose inhaled beclomethasone dipropionate and intermittent systemic corticosteroids. Thorax 1992; 47:415–417.
39. Boulet LP, Giguere MC, Milot J, Brown J. Long-term effects of high dose inhaled steroids on bone turnover and density. Am Rev Respir Dis 1993; 147:A293.
40. Ip M, Lam K, Yam L, Kung A, Ng M. Decreased bone mineral density in premenopausal asthma patients receiving long term inhaled steroids. Chest 1994; 105:1722–1727.
41 Kinberg KA, Hopp RJ, Biven RE, Gallagher JC. Bone mineral density in normal and asthmatic children. J Allergy Clin Immunol 1994; 94:490–497.
42. Toogood JH, Baskerville JC, Markov AE, et al. Bone mineral density and the risk of fracture in patients receiving long-term inhaled steroid therapy for asthma. J Allergy Clin Immunol 1995; 96:157–166.
43. Pocock NA, Eisman JA, Hopper JL, Yeates MG, Sambrook PN, Eberl S. Genetic determinants of bone mass in adults: a twin study. J Clin Invest 1987; 80:706–710.

44. Dequeker J, Nijs J, Verstaeten A, Geusens P, Gevers G. Genetic determinants of bone mineral content at the spine and the radius: a twin study. Bone 1987; 8:207–209.

45. Moller M, Horman A, Harvarld B, Hauge M, Henningsen K, Nordin BEC. Metacarpal morphometry in monozygotic and dizygotic elderly twins. Calcif Tissue Res 1978; 25:197–201.

46. Smith DA, Nance WE, Wong Kang K, Christian JC, Johnston CC Jr. Genetic factors in determining bone mass. J Clin Invest 1973; 52:2800–2808.

47. Seeman E, Hopper JL, Bach LA, et al. Reduced bone mass in daughters of women with osteoporosis. N Engl J Med 1989; 320:554–558.

48. Hodsman A, Haddad R, Markov A, Baskerville J, Toogood JH. Association of long-term inhaled (I-S) or oral steroid (O-S) therapy with vertebral fracture in asthmatic adults. Clin Invest Med 1993; 6:B6.

49. Toogood JH, Markov A, Hodsman A, Fraher L, Baskerville J. Bone mineral density (BMD) in asthmatic adults receiving long-term inhaled steroid (I-S) or prednisone (PRED) therapy. Clin Invest Med 1993; 6:B6.

50. Laity A, Toogood JH, Mazza J, Moote DW. Profile of ambulatory care for chronic asthma in a tertiary referral clinic. Clin Invest Med 1991; 14:A6.

24

Steroid-Resistant Asthma

DONALD Y. M. LEUNG

National Jewish Center for Immunology and Respiratory Medicine
and University of Colorado Health Sciences Center
Denver, Colorado

I. Introduction

Various studies have now demonstrated that airway inflammation and immune activation play an important role in the pathogenesis of chronic airway obstruction and bronchial hyperreactivity in chronic asthma (1,2). Recent trends in the treatment of asthma have, therefore, focused on the use of anti-inflammatory therapy, particularly inhaled glucocorticoids (3). Asthmatics, however, vary in their responses to glucocorticoid therapy (4,5). Although the majority of patients respond to regular inhaled glucocorticoid therapy, a subset of patients have poorly controlled asthma even when treated with high doses of oral prednisolone or its equivalent. These patients represent a challenging problem for clinicians.

In the evaluation of patients with a history of "steroid-resistant" (SR) asthma, it is important to be aware that most patients who present with a poor response to steroids have other confounding factors which contribute to difficulty in their management. These include poor compliance with use of prescribed medications, inadequate medication technique, for example, with metered-dose inhalers, incorrect diagnosis, ongoing exposure to environmental allergens, psychosocial disturbances, or abnormal glucocorticoid pharmaco-kinetics. This chapter examines the role of immune mechanisms and altered glucocorticoid receptors (GRs) in the pathogenesis of persistent airway inflammation in the subset of patients who appear to be resistant to the immuno-suppressive effects of glucocorticoids. Since these patients likely evolve over time, understanding mechanisms involved in steroid resistance could lead to earlier identification of this challenging group of asthmatics and provide important insights into the pathogenesis of chronic asthma.

II. Control of Airway Inflammation by Glucocorticoids

A number of controlled clinical studies have demonstrated that treatment of most asthmatics with inhaled and/or systemic glucocorticoids is accompanied by a decrease in bronchoalveolar lavage (BAL) fluid concentrations of eosinophil cationic protein, as well as a reduction in the numbers of BAL eosinophils and activated T cells in asthmatic airways (6,7). In atopic patients, glucocorticoid treatment blocks the appearance of the late-phase asthmatic response following experimental allergen challenge in the lungs (8). A detailed examination of glucocorticoid action is reviewed in the literature (9) and elsewhere in this book. Nevertheless, for the purposes of this chapter, before considering mechanisms of steroid resistance, it is useful to summarize briefly some of the effects of glucocorticoid treatment on individual cell types involved in airway inflammation.

In vitro studies have demonstrated that glucocorticoids inhibit T-lympho-cyte proliferation and cytokine production. These effects result, in part, from the reduction of interleukin-2 (IL-2) synthesis and inhibition of IL-2 receptor (CD25) expression on T cells (10). Glucocorticoids also inhibit IL-1 produc-tion by macrophages, an event that is important for IL-2 secretion. An addi-tional aspect of glucocorticoid action likely occurs from modulating the pattern of cytokine secretion by T cells. In this regard, recent studies indicate that ste-roid-sensitive (SS) asthmatics respond to oral prednisolone therapy with a de-crease in activated T cells expressing IL-4 and IL-5 mRNA transcripts but a concomitant increase in γ-interferon (IFN-γ) mRNA expression (11).

Glucocorticoid treatment also reduces the production of cytokines (e.g., IL-5 and granulocyte-macrophage colony-stimulating factor [GM-CSF]), and mediators (e.g., RANTES) that affect eosinophils. These cytokines are produced by T lymphocytes, eosinophils, mast cells, airway epithelial cells, endothelial cells, eosinophils (autocrine stimulation), and macrophages. The capacity of glucocorticoids to inhibit the release of these cytokines is thought to play a critical role in the inhibition of eosinophil differentiation and effector function.

Macrophages in BAL bear IgE receptors (CD23 and possibly FcεRI) and participate in IgE-dependent activation with formation of leukotrienes, PAF, IL-1, and tumor necrosis factor (TNF-α). IL-1 and TNF-α are known to activate vascular endothelium and initiate leukocyte recruitment via the induction of endothelial leukocyte adhesion molecules. Administration of glucocorticoids markedly diminishes the number of circulating monocytes and inhibits the release of arachidonic acid metabolites as well as the release of PAF, IL-1, TNF-α, and GM-CSF. By inhibiting the release of these mediator and cytokines, glucocorticoids indirectly block the expression of leukocyte adhesion molecules on vascular endothelial cells, eosinophil activation, and macrophage support of lymphocyte-mediated responses.

In summary, glucocorticoids influence airway inflammation by changing the spectrum of locally released mediators and cytokines involved in the recruitment, proliferation, and activation of inflammatory effector cells (e.g., eosinophils, and T lymphocytes). Other proposed mechanisms of steroid action in asthma include upregulation of the β-adrenergic receptor which mediates smooth muscle relaxation (12). Corticosteroids also enhance the formation of lipocortin, a cellular protein that inhibits the action of phospholipase A_2 (13). This could then inhibit formation of lipid mediators such as prostaglandin (PG) D_2, leukotrienes, and PAF. Nevertheless, current data strongly suggest the primary beneficial effect of glucocorticoids lies in their potent anti-inflammatory and immunosuppressive properties.

III. Definition of Steroid-Resistant Asthma

In 1968, Schwartz and colleagues (14) first introduced the term *steroid-resistant* (SR) asthma to describe a group of six asthmatics who had poor clinical responses to high-dose systemic glucocorticoid therapy. Of note, following the intravenous infusion of 40 mg of hydrocortisone into these SR asthmatics, a blunted eosinopenic response was observed in these patients as compared with SS asthmatics. Additional studies by these investigators suggested that accelerated plasma cortisol clearance could account, at least in part, for the subsequent steroid resistance.

Subsequently, in 1981, Carmichael and colleagues reported on a group of 58 patients with chronic poorly controlled asthma (15). These patients had a baseline FEV_1 (forced expiratory volume in 1 sec) of less than 60% predicted and a 30% or greater increase in FEV_1 after administration of a bronchodilator. However, they failed to increase their FEV_1's by greater than 15% after a course of prednisolone, 20 mg daily for 7 days, and were therefore called steroid resistant. In contrast, SS asthmatics, were found to have an increase in FEV_1 by >30% with this treatment. Furthermore, compared with SS asthma, several other factors also appeared to distinguish patients with SR asthma. These included a longer duration of symptoms, relatively lower morning peak expiratory flow rates, and increased bronchial hyperresponsiveness. It should be noted these factors may be more related to an increased severity of clinical disease than specifically to steroid resistance.

In 1984, Löfdahl and colleagues highlighted drug interactions as a possible mechanism for apparent steroid resistance (16). For example, if glucocorticoid clearance from the body is enhanced by another medication, the actual tissue concentrations of glucocorticoids are reduced, and would thus result in a diminished therapeutic response. In subsequent studies of SR asthma by Corrigan and colleagues (17) as well as Alvarez and colleagues (18), pharmacokinetic abnormalities were considered and ruled out as a confounding factor prior to a diagnosis of SR asthma. Thus, it appears that a subset of asthmatics resistant to glucocorticoid therapy does indeed exist.

It should be noted that at the present time, there is no universally accepted definition of SR asthma. For example, in a report by Corrigan et al. (17), SR asthma was defined as the failure to demonstrate an increase in baseline FEV_1 by greater than 15% after a course of 20 mg daily of oral prednisolone for 1 week followed by 40 mg daily for a second week. The difficulty in defining SR asthma stems in part from the lack of a definition of an adequate trial of systemic glucocorticoid therapy. To address this issue, Kamada and colleagues studied asthmatic children whose morning prebronchodilator FEV_1 was <70% predicted and requiring a burst of prednisone therapy (19). Over 60% of patients who responded demonstrated a >15% improvement of the morning prebronchodilator FEV_1 within 3 days, and 93% showed a significant improvement within 10 days of initiating glucocorticoid therapy. Prolongation of the course of therapy beyond 10 days did not cause significantly greater improvement of FEV_1. From this it was concluded that 10–14 days of high-dose systemic glucocorticoid therapy ($\geq$20 mg twice daily) was an adequate trial to assess steroid responsiveness.

IV. Cellular Responses to Glucocorticoids

A number of abnormalities in immune cell-mediated responses have been reported in patients with SR asthma (Table 1). In 1981, Kay et al. (21) reported that peripheral blood monocytes from SR asthmatics, as compared with SS patients, failed to demonstrate a reduction in complement receptor expression following glucocorticoid treatment. Subsequently, in 1984, Poznansky and colleagues reported on the surface markers and functional response of mononuclear cells from SR asthmatics incubated with phytohemagglutinin (PHA) (22). In SS and SR asthmatics, there was no difference at baseline in the phe-

Table 1 Cellular Features of Steroid-Resistant Asthma

Failure to inhibit PHA-Induced T-cell proliferation
Increased levels of T-cell activation
Failure to decrease cytokine production in vivo and in vitro
Increased IL-2 and IL-4 gene expression in the airways
Persistent eosinophil activation

notype of freshly isolated peripheral blood mononuclear cells (PBMCs); that is, the proportion of T cells, CD4$^+$ T cells, OKM1$^+$ monocytes, CD8$^+$ T cells, or HLA-DR$^+$ cells. When mononuclear cells were coincubated with methylprednisolone, at doses as low as 10^{-8} M, T-lymphocyte proliferation in the SS asthma group was inhibited by greater than 60%. In contrast, cells from the SR asthmatics did not demonstrate a significant decrease in proliferation at the same methylprednisolone concentration. This study, therefore, suggested a functional abnormality in mononuclear cell responsiveness to glucocorticoids but no difference in the phenotype of cells from SR asthmatics.

In 1989, Wilkinson and colleagues first examined the possibility that cytokines or mediators involved in the modulation of inflammation may not be inhibited by glucocorticoid treatment of cells from SR asthmatics (23). They identified a 3-kDa monocyte-derived neutrophil-activating factor. PBMCs from SS asthmatics were cultured in the absence and presence of hydrocortisone. When the supernatants of these cultures were added to calcium-ionophore–activated neutrophils, leukotriene B$_4$ production was suppressed by supernatants from the cells coincubated with hydrocortisone. In contrast, with supernatants from hydrocortisone-treated cells derived from SR asthmatics, no suppression of leukotriene B$_4$ production was observed. These data suggested that a monocyte-derived factor in SR asthmatics enhances the proinflammatory potential of infiltrating neutrophils and its production is not inhibited by glucocorticoid treatment.

Further evidence that mononuclear cells from patients with SR asthma are poorly responsive to glucocorticoids was reported by Vecchiarelli et al. (24). They studied lipopolysaccharide (LPS)–induced production of IL-1 and TNF-α by PBMCs from 14 acute asthmatics before and after 1 week of prednisolone (25 mg/day) treatment. At baseline, levels of LPS-induced IL-1 and TNF-α production were similar in both groups of asthmatics. However, following glucocorticoid treatment, TNF-α production by PBMCs from SS, but not SR, patients was significantly reduced. Furthermore, in SS patients, the degree of TNF-α inhibition correlated with the clinical response to steroids. Steroid therapy did not change IL-1 production in either asthma group.

Since T lymphocytes play a critical role in the pathogenesis of asthma, there have been an increasing number of studies examining the role of T cells in SR asthma. In 1991, Corrigan and colleagues demonstrated that persistent activation of T cells in vitro may play a role in the pathogenesis of SR asthmatics. They found that PHA-induced proliferation of peripheral blood T cells was inhibited by dexamethasone in SS asthmatics but not in SR asthmatics (17). In a second report, these investigators reported an increased expression of CD25 (IL-2 receptor) and HLA-DR activation antigens on peripheral blood T cells of SR asthmatics (25). They also demonstrated that dexamethasone inhibited PHA-induced T-lymphocyte proliferation as well as IL-2 and IFN-γ production in cells from SS asthmatics but not in cells from SR asthmatics. Interestingly, cyclosporin A inhibited proliferation and cytokine production in lymphocytes from both SS and SR asthmatics.

Alvarez and colleagues (18) have also shown that PBMCs from SR asthmatics have a reduced inhibition of PHA-induced lymphocyte proliferation when incubated with methylprednisolone. Indeed, at lower methylprednisolone concentrations (10^{-9} to 10^{-10} M), PHA-induced proliferation was actually increased in PBMCs from patients with SR asthma as compared with patients with SS asthma. Of note, when coincubated with troleandomycin (TAO), a macrolide antibiotic that inhibits methylprednisolone but not prednisolone metabolism, proliferation was reduced in a dose-dependent fashion in lymphocytes from both SS and SR asthmatics. This suggests that clinically steroid resistance is a reversible phenomenon. Of potentially greater clinical importance is that although SR asthma is associated with refractoriness to glucocorticoids, these patients can be sensitive to other drugs potentially useful in the treatment of asthma, including β-agonists, cyclosporin, and TAO.

Lee and Lane recently used the tuberculin delayed-type hypersensitivity skin reaction to investigate the in vivo responsiveness of mononuclear cells to oral prednisolone in SS and SR asthmatics in a double-blind, crossed-over, placebo-controlled study (26). In the SS, but not in the SR group, prednisolone suppressed the cutaneous tuberculin response and infiltration of macrophages, eosinophils, and T cells. These data provided further evidence of an in vivo defect in the responsiveness of the macrophage–T cell interaction to the suppressive effects of glucocorticoids in SR asthma and suggested that resistance to glucocorticoids is not organ specific.

The above studies demonstrate that peripheral blood and skin-infiltrating mononuclear cells from patients with SR, but not SS, asthma are functionally resistant to the immunosuppressive effects of glucocorticoids. Recently, Leung and colleagues (27) extended such studies to examine *bronchoalveolar lavage* BAL cells from SS and SR asthmatics prior to and after a 1-week course of daily high-dose (40 mg daily) prednisone. At baseline, they found no significant difference between BAL total white cell counts, total eosinophils, or numbers of activated T cells in the SR versus SS asthma group. However, after prednisone therapy, there was a significant decrease in BAL eosinophil counts as well as number of BAL-activated T cells in the SS asthma group. In contrast, in the SR asthma group, prednisone therapy was not accompanied by any significant changes in BAL eosinophil counts or number of BAL-activated T cells.

Since cytokine expression plays a critical role in the pathogenesis of airway inflammation, studies were extended to determine the expression of cytokine messenger RNA (mRNA) in BAL cells. At baseline, BAL cells from patients with SR asthma, as compared with cells from SS asthma, had a significantly higher number of cells expressing mRNA for IL-2 and IL-4 (Fig. 1). However, no significant differences between these two patient populations were observed in the expression of IL-5 mRNA and IFN-γ mRNA at baseline. After prednisone therapy, BAL cells from SS, but not SR, asthmatics demonstrated a significant decrease in the number of cells expressing IL-4 mRNA and IL-5 mRNA. Furthermore, although small reductions in the numbers of BAL cells per 1000 positive for IL-2 mRNA accompanied prednisone therapy in each patient group, these differences were not significant.

Treatment of SS asthmatics with prednisone resulted in a significant rise in the number of BAL cells expressing IFN-γ mRNA for (27). In contrast, when

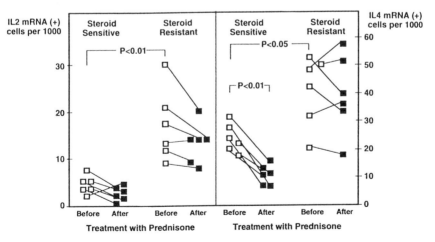

Figure 1 Number of cells with positive hybridization signals for IL-2 and IL-4 mRNA in BAL fluid from six patients with SS asthma and six patients with SR asthma obtained before and after treatment for 1 week of 40 mg daily prednisone. Before prednisone therapy, there were significantly more cells expressing IL-2 ($P < .01$) and IL-4 ($P < .05$) mRNA in the BAL fluid of patients with SR asthma as compared with SS asthma. Values were compared by the Mann-Whitney U-test. (From Ref. 27.)

SR asthmatics were treated with prednisone, their BAL cells demonstrated a decrease in the numbers of IFN-γ mRNA (+) cells. These divergent responses resulted in a highly significant difference in IFN-γ gene expression following prednisone treatment between the SR versus SS asthmatic groups. Taken together, these data demonstrate that the airway cells from patients with SR, as compared with SS, asthma have a distinct pattern of cytokine gene expression and response to glucocorticoid therapy.

V. Mechanisms of Glucocorticoid Resistance

A. Glucocorticoid Resistance in Nonasthmatic Conditions

Familial Glucocorticoid Resistance

A syndrome of familial end-organ glucocorticoid resistance is well described (28,29). These patients usually have elevated total plasma cortisol concentrations but do not develop Cushingoid features. The molecular basis for end-organ glucocorticoid resistance in the various reported kindreds are heterogeneous and includes either reduced GR numbers, decreased binding affinity for glucocorticoids, or poor DNA binding of the GR to glucocorticoid-responsive elements (GRE). PBMCs and cultured fibroblasts from these patients have reduced GR numbers or decreased binding affinity for glucocorticoid. Epstein-Barr virus (EBV)–transformed cells from two such patients have been shown to have a decreased level of GR mRNA, and the genomic DNA of both individuals showed an altered restriction enzyme pattern. These genomic differences could be detected with a probe specific for the putative steroid binding domain of the human GR gene (30).

Malignancies

Glucocorticoids are an important modality for the treatment of lymphomas and leukemias. Bloomfield et al. (31) found that malignant lymphoma cells from patients who respond to dexamethasone treatment had more GR sites per cells and greater in vitro sensitivity to glucocorticoid-induced inhibition of proliferation than did tumor cells from nonresponders. Molecular studies have also been carried out on mutant murine lymphoma cell lines selected for glucocorticoid resistance. S49 lymphoma cell lines lyse in the presence of dexamethasone. Yamamoto reported the isolation of four classes of SR S49 cells after selection for growth in 10^{-6} M dexamethasone (32). These mutant lines expressed the following GR abnormalities: (1) GR defective in dexamethasone binding, (2) GR defective in DNA binding and nuclear localization, (3) a 40-kDa GR that bound steroid and DNA but did not contain the domain that modulates transcription, and (4) *deathless* mutants that apparently expressed a normal GR but were defective in some other step of the lysis pathway. These studies suggested that glucocorticoid action requires multiple events and that defects may occur at any step in this process translating into steroid resistance.

Autoimmune Disorders

Poor response to steroids have been observed in patients with systemic lupus erythematosus (SLE), rheumatoid arthritis (RA), sarcoidosis, chronic urticaria, bullous pemphigoid, Crohn's disease, and dermatomyositis (33–37). Of interest, patients with these SR conditions can be sensitive to other immunosuppressive drugs such as cyclosporin or methotrexate (34–38). The GR binding characteristics of these patients have not been studied. Antibodies to lipocortin, a 37-kDa protein that inhibits phospholipase A_2 and whose formation is induced by corticosteroids, have also been described in some patients with systemic lupus erythematosus and rheumatoid arthritis (38). They have also been found in a relatively high proportion of patients with asthma. However, their presence does not correlate with resistance to steroids or to treatment (39).

B. Role of Altered Glucocorticoid Receptors in Steroid-Resistant Asthma

Glucocorticoids bind to a specific intracellular receptor to inhibit T-cell activation by various stimuli (reviewed in Ref. 40). Since patients with familial glucocorticoid resistance and steroid-resistant malignancies have alterations in their GR, it is possible that the poor glucocorticoid response in SR asthma is due to an alteration in GR number or binding affinity. In this regard, Sher and colleagues have recently reported abnormalities in GR binding of PBMCs from patients with SR asthma (20). In their study, a [^{3}H]dexamethasone radioligand binding assay and Scatchard analysis was carried out in 17 patients with SR asthma (Fig. 2): 15 of the patients who had a significant increase in their GR K_d that is, a decrease in binding affinity for glucocorticoids,) in the nuclear fraction of their PBMCs when compared with normal subjects or SR asthma patients. This defect was designated as type I SR asthma. Two other patients with SR asthma had normal GR K_d values but a markedly decreased number of GR binding sites per cell; that is, < 3 SD below the normal range. This defect was designated as type II SR asthma.

Since SR asthma has been found to be associated with persistent T-cell activation even when patients are treated with glucocorticoids, it was of interest to determine whether the altered GR binding parameters were restricted to specific subsets of PBMCs (20). Therefore, GR binding parameters in their T-cell and non–T-cell subpopulations were analyzed (Fig. 3). A fourfold significant increase in T-cell nuclear GR K_d over non–T cells was observed in the PBMCs from type I SR asthma patients. The T cells from type I SR asthma patients also had a significantly higher GR K_d than T cells from normal con-

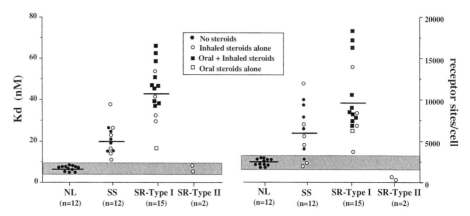

Figure 2   The GR binding parameters of 12 normal (NL) controls, 17-steroid resistant asthmatics, and 12 steroid-sensitive asthmatics. Normal ranges for both GR parameters are indicated by the shaded bar. The solid bar indicates the mean for each group. All groups were significantly different ($P = .0001$, ANOVA) from each other. (From Ref. 20.)

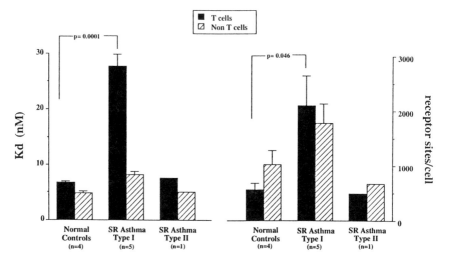

Figure 3   The GR number and binding affinity in fractionated T- and non–T-cell populations of patients with type I SR asthma. The increased dissociation constant (K_d) and receptor sites per cell of nuclear GR are limited to the T-cell population of type I SR asthmatics and are significantly different from normal controls ($P = .0001$ K_d; $P = .046$ GR sites/cell). No difference in nuclear GR binding parameters in the non–T-cell fraction was observed. Each bar represents the mean $\pm$ SEM. (From Ref. 20.)

trols. These results were consistent with an earlier observation by Lane and Lee (41) that peripheral blood monocytes from SR asthmatics had normal GR binding affinity and receptor numbers. In contrast, the abnormally low GR number observed in a type II SR asthma patient was not limited to T cells but was also present in non–T cells as well (20).

Since patients with SR asthma frequently have a history of prolonged glucocorticoid therapy, it is of some concern that the abnormalities in GR binding parameters observed in SR asthma might be induced by systemic glucocorticoid therapy. Several observations suggest that this is not operative: First, in a group of stable patients with SR asthma who were not receiving maintenance oral prednisone therapy, no significant change in GR binding parameters were observed following a 1-week course of high-dose "burst" prednisone (20). Second, in patients with interstitial lung disease receiving chronic high-dose prednisone therapy, the same degree of abnormality in GR K_d as the type I or GR number as the type II SR asthmatics was not observed (20). Third, a number of patients presenting with type I (abnormal GR binding affinity) SR asthma have not previously received oral prednisone (20; Y. M. Leung and S. J. Szefler, unpublished observations). Fourth, previous studies have reported that glucocorticoid treatment induces a modest downregulation of the number of GRs, which differs from the alterations seen in type I SR asthma (42). Finally, Spahn et al. (43) examined GR binding affinity in 10 patients with poorly controlled asthma prior to and after a course of high-dose prednisone therapy. These patients demonstrated significantly decreased GR binding affinity at baseline. However, after prednisone treatment, there was an associated reduction in airway inflammation accompanied by a significant decrease in GR K_d toward normal values.

Since there is only one human GR gene (44), the clinical observation that patients with type I SR asthma can develop severe side effects from chronic treatment with systemic steroids combined with the observation that their GR defect is restricted to T cells suggest that type I SR asthma is acquired, possibly as the result of a particular pathway of immune activation. In contrast, since type II SR asthma is not associated with the development of sterid-induced side effects and is not limited to T cells, it may be analogous to patients with primary cortisol resistance and would therefore be expected to be an irreversible GR defect (Table 2).

To determine whether the altered PBMC GR binding in patients with SR asthma is reversible, Sher et al. (20) measured GR binding in PBMCs prior to and following incubation for 48 hr in culture medium (Fig. 4). When PBMCs from patients with type I SR asthma were incubated in medium alone, they showed a significant change in GR binding with normalization of both GR K_d and GR number after 48 hr of incubation as compared with baseline values on freshly isolated cells. In contrast, incubation of PBMCs from normal donors

Table 2 Clinical and Laboratory Features of Steroid-Resistant Asthma

Features	Type I	Type II
AM Cortisol[a]	Suppressed	No
Cushingoid side effects[a]	Yes	No
GR binding affinity	Reduced	Normal
GR number	High	Low
Reversibility of GR defect	Yes	No

[a]Feature on high-dose systemic steroids.

under similar culture conditions did not result in any significant change in GR binding. These data suggest that the decreased GR binding affinity found in T cells from patients with type SR asthma is an acquired defect and is consistent with a recent study by Lane and Lee demonstrating in patients with SR asthma that there was no polymorphism within the functional domains of their GR cDNA (45).

As already noted, airway cells from patients with SR asthma express increased levels of IL-2 mRNA and IL-4 mRNA (27). Therefore, it was of interest to determine whether the combination of IL-2 and IL-4 could alter GR binding affinity in PBMCs from normal individuals. In this regard, Kam et al. (46) demonstrated that GR abnormalities similar to those observed in cells from SR asthmatics can be induced in PBMCs from normal donors by incubation of their cells with the combination of IL-2 and IL-4. In contrast, incubation of normal PBMCs with IL-1, IL-5, and IFN-γ for 48 hr, as compared with culture medium alone, did not induce a significant elevation in GR K_d.

These data support the notion that the GR binding alterations in type I SR asthma are acquired as a response to increased secretion of certain cytokines. As a proof of concept, we examined the effects of IL-2 and IL-4 on GR binding parameters in patients with type I SR asthma (20). In this regard, the reduced GR binding affinity in PBMCs from type I SR asthmatics was sustained in culture over the 48-hr period when their cells were incubated in the presence of combination IL-2 + IL-4.

The effect of in vitro 48-hr incubation with media alone and with combination IL-2 and IL-4 on the patients with type II SR asthma with low GR numbers have also been studied (20). In contrast to the type I SR asthma patients, PBMCs from patients with type II SR asthma did not demonstrate any changes in GR binding when incubated in culture medium alone. Furthermore, although the combination of IL-2 and IL-4 increased the number of GRs in normal PBMCs, these cytokines had no effect on GR binding parameters from these two type II SR asthma patients. Thus, it appears that the low GR numbers in type II SR asthma patients is an irreversible defect, whereas the reduced GR binding affinity in type I SR asthma patients is an acquired reversible defect.

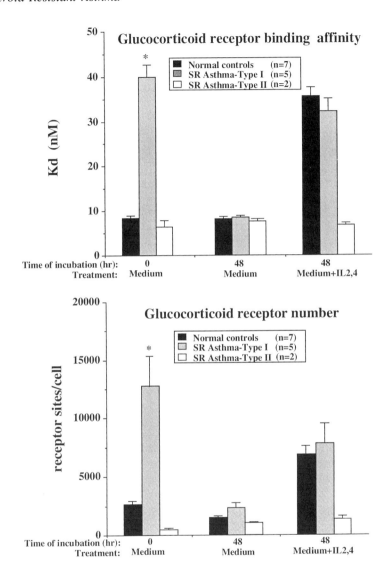

Figure 4 Time course of nuclear GR binding parameters in PBMCs from type I and type II SR asthma patients and normal donors. Freshly isolated PBMCs from five type I SR asthmatics (time 0 hr) have significantly elevated GR K_d (*P = .0001) as compared with normals and revert to normal GR binding when cultured in medium alone for 48 hr. Incubation of PBMCs from seven normal subjects and two Type II SR asthma patients show no change in GR binding parameters when cultured in medium alone for 48 hr. Combination IL-2 + IL-4 significantly increases GR K_d and GR number (P = .0001) of normal donors and alters GR binding parameters in PBMCs from type I SR asthmatics but not PBMCs from type II SR asthmatic patients. Each bar represents the mean ± SEM. (From Ref. 20.)

The precise mechanisms by which different patterns of cytokines or immune activation might result in decreased steroid responsiveness in asthma remain unclear. The observation that the GR binding defect in type I SR asthma is localized to the nuclear, but not cytosolic, GR may be an important clue (20,46). It is well known that the GR changes its structure and conformation when translocated between the cytosol and nucleus (reviewed in Ref. 40). The activated GR nuclear complex regulates transcription by binding to specific DNA GREs. The induction or repression of GR target genes ultimately results in the altered expression of glucocorticoid-regulated proteins (47). This latter action is mediated by direct binding of the modulatory domain of the GR with transcription factors, such as AP-1 or NFκB. However, overexpression of AP-1 or other transcription factors has been found to interfere with GR function (48). Since SR asthma appears to be associated with much higher levels of cytokine activation than SS asthma, the activation of particular transcription factors such as AP-1 (49) may provide an explanation for the nuclear localization of the GR binding defect in SR asthma and differences in patterns of steroid responsiveness in asthma.

Taken together, these studies raise the intriguing possibility that type I SR asthma, which represents the majority of patients who present with SR asthma, may be the end result of ongoing immune activation which no longer comes under the control of the immunoresuppressive effects of steroids. This is consistent with the observations that PHA-induced T-cell proliferation and cytokine production by PBMCs from patients with SR asthma are poorly inhibited by the addition of dexamethasone or methylprednisolone in vitro (17,18). Indeed, cyclosporin A, a new drug whose major action is inhibition of T-cell proliferation and cytokine secretion, improves the clinical symptoms of several patients with SR asthma (50). These observations are again consistent with the notion that ongoing asthma inflammation and cytokine secretion may contribute to the acquired GR defect found in SR asthma.

It is of interest that SS asthmatics also have reduced GR binding affinity as compared with normal donors but less than that observed in type I SR asthma (Fig. 2). This observation is of interest, because it suggests that chronic asthma may be associated with a spectrum of GR binding abnormalities with SR asthma being at the extreme end of this range. The degree of change in GR binding affinity may be related to the magnitude of airway inflammation and immune activation. This phenomenon along with the possibility of irreversible changes in the airway structure could explain refractoriness to conventional therapy. Although not as yet specifically addressed in any studies, it is possible that the significantly reduced GR binding affinity in SS asthma patients may have clinical relevance, since recent studies indicate that endogenous cortisol levels regulate IgE-dependent late-phase allergic reactions (51). Since endogenous cortisol levels are significantly lower than levels achieved following administration of therapeutic doses of steroids, even the moderate abnormalities in GR found in SS asthmatics may have an influence on the ability of endogenous glucocorticoids to suppress airway inflammation. Furthermore, even modest doses of inhaled glucocorticoids have the potential to reduce nocturnal plasma cortisol concentrations, further compromising the availability of endogenous cortisol during the critical nighttime period when pulmonary function is lowest in patients with severe asthma (52,53). Consequently, inhaled glucocorticoids may provide symptomatic relief, whereas incompletely resolving the inflammatory process. Thus, an understanding of the mechanisms which underlie SR asthma may have important implications for controlling inflammation in milder forms of asthma.

VI. Summary and Implications for Therapy

In summary, SR asthma is associated with persistent immune activation and airway inflammation which is resistant to the immunosuppressive and anti-inflammatory effects of inhaled and/or systemic glucocorticoids. There appears to be at least two mechanisms which contribute to SR asthma (see Table 2). Type I SR asthma is associated with an abnormally reduced GR binding affinity as compared with normal controls and SS asthmatics (20). This defect is localized to the T-cell population, a group of cells thought to have a central role in the pathogenesis of asthma. Conversely, SR asthma with the type II binding abnormality is associated with normal binding affinity but a markedly reduced number of GRs per cell. An important distinction between these two types of SR asthma is that the GR defect in type I SR asthma is reversible in culture but is sustained by incubation with combination IL-2 and IL-4 but not by either cytokine alone. In contrast, the GR binding defect in type II SR asthma is irreversible and does not respond to coincubation with combination IL-2 + IL-4. Aside from ligand-receptor binding abnormalities, further studies are needed to determine whether steroid resistance may arise from abnormal binding of the GR to the GRE in nuclear DNA. Furthermore, it will be of interest to ascertain whether patient factors, for example, allergen exposure, known to contribute to poorly controlled asthma have an effect on GR binding affinity (54).

These studies on SR asthma have several important clinical implications: First, with the increasing use of corticosteroids in the treatment of asthma, it is important to recognize that patients vary in their response to steroids. Second, the observation of a distinctive pattern of cytokine gene expression in SR asthma is consistent with the possibility that different patterns of cytokine expression and immune activation alter response to therapy. Although many of these patients may respond to an extremely high dose of glucocorticoids, such treatment carries the risk of serious side effects. In this regard, the newer generation of inhaled synthetic glucocorticoids may be useful in the treatment of poorly controlled asthma owing to their enhanced binding affinity for the GR (55).

Continued research will be needed to define the mechanisms of action for ongoing airway immune activation, correlation of response to particular treatment strategies, and identification of the most appropriate treatment regimen for a particular pathway of cellular activation. An understanding of the mechanisms by which glucocorticoids fail to resolve inflammation in asthma may provide important new insights into the mechanisms which perpetuate chronic airway inflammation. Although this chapter has focused primarily on patients with SR asthma, it is likely that patients who are steroid dependent, that is, patients who require systemic or inhaled glucocorticoid therapy to maintain control of their asthma, are part of the same spectrum of disease and bear similar mechanisms which result in severe asthma. New information on mechanisms for steroid resistance may therefore also have application to newer approaches for treatment of milder forms of asthma.

Acknowledgments

Supported in part by USPHS grants HL-36577, RR-00051, and AR-41256.

The author wishes to thank Maureen Plourd-Sandoval for assistance in preparing this manuscript.

Discussion

DR. MIESFELD: What is the link (mechanistic) between decreased ligand binding affinity and decreased GRE binding? Is there a DNA binding defect in normal individuals?

DR. LEUNG: All patients have the ligand binding abnormality. More than half of them also have the DNA binding defect. At this time, we do not understand the mechanism for decreased GRE, although we suspect cytokine-induced glucocorticoid receptor binding defects may occur following GR binding to transcription factors. Yes, normal PBMCs can develop the DNA binding defect, but only if their cells are preincubated with IL-2 and IL-4.

DR. LIU: (1) How do the dose-response effects of IL-2 and IL-4 interact? (2) Can IL-13 act alone to produce the binding defect or is it just a replacement for IL-4?

DR. LEUNG: (1) The higher the IL-2 and IL-4 concentrations, the greater the inducible GR defect. (2) Excess IL-2 or IL-4 would not allow induction of a

GR defect. They must be equimolar. IL-13 does not act on T cells. It induces abnormalities in the non–T-cell fraction.

DR. DENBURG: Your hypothesis would predict that only immune activation via a TH2-type mechanism (producing both IL-2 and IL-4) would lead to the reduced GR binding. In putatively TH1-mediated immune diseases, such as SLE or RA, have you had a chance to examine GR binding?

DR. LEUNG: We have not looked at glucocorticoid receptor binding in other diseases associated with immune activation. This is certainly worth doing.

DR. BARNES: It is important to recognize that there may be different types of glucocorticoid resistance in asthma and that different mechanisms may be involved. In the studies we have conducted in collaboration with Drs. Lane and Lee, we have identified a defect in GRE binding in peripheral blood mononuclear cells. It is unlikely that these cells have been exposed to significant levels of cytokines, and we believe that this is a primary defect, whereas the effects you describe in T lymphocytes appear to be secondary to cytokine exposure.

DR. LEUNG: Yes, I agree the steroid resistance is likely to be the final common pathway with multiple etiologies and mechanisms.

DR. LANE: (1) Is the defect in DNA binding you see in some patients secondary to the defect in ligand binding? (2) Can you speculate on how IL-2 and IL-4 are interacting with the ligand binding function of the GR?

DR. LEUNG: (1) The defect in DNA binding could certainly occur as the result of defective ligand binding. (2) IL-2 and IL-4 are known to signal increases in NF-κB and other transcription factors via different pathways of receptor activation. The activation via both pathways may cause excess NF-κB expression which binds to GRs via protein-protein interactions and prevent GR binding.

DR. JORDANA: Have you examined whether IL-10 inhibits or reverses the effects induced by IL-2 and IL-4 on glucocorticosteroid binding on lymphocytes?

DR. LEUNG: No.

DR. LIU: Could the requirement for both IL-2 and IL-4 be explained by effects of these cytokines on a heterogeneous population of lymphocytes in peripheral blood?

DR. LEUNG: Possibly. This could be addressed by examining cell lines or T-cell clones.

DR. HERSCHMAN: Can you investigate the IL-2/IL-4 effect in established human leukemic T-cell lines?

DR. LEUNG: We have tried various established cell lines; for example, Jurkat and EBV cell lines without success. However, these cell lines may not express high-affinity IL-2 and IL-4 receptors.

DR. HARGREAVE: (1) What is your clinical definition of glucocorticoid-resistant asthma (physiological changes and inflammatory indices)? (2) Have you done sputum studies on eosinophil infiltration?

DR. LEUNG: (1) Our current definition is physiological; that is, failure of pre-bronchodilator AM FEV_1 to improve by at least 15% after 1–2 weeks of 40 mg daily of prednisone. I agree, we should incorporate inflammatory markers into the definition. (2) Sputum studies may be a convenient way to monitor eosinophil infiltrations but have not been done.

DR. SCHLEIMER: Trying to connect the observations of Drs. Saatcioglu and Karin and your group, I wonder whether underexpression of IKB and failure to induce it may be a primary abnormality in your steroid-resistant subjects or in normals individuals after cytokine treatment?

DR. LEUNG: I agree, this is worth looking at.

DR. LANE: Do you think that IL-4 is a marker for corticosteroid-resistant asthma on the basis of your BAL data? If so, how do you explain the lack of atopic association with glucocorticoid-resistant asthma?

DR. LEUNG: No, the steroid resistance is mediated primarily by the combination of IL-2 and IL-4. Perhaps the response of cells to IL-2 and IL-4 will be a better marker for steroid resistance. Most of our patients with steriod-resistant asthma are atopic.

DR. O'BYRNE: In patients with just the abnormality in affinity for the GR, does increasing the dose of glucocorticoids provide a clinical effect?

DR. LEUNG: Yes, in patients with type I steroid-resistant asthma and reduced ligand binding affinity, we expect patients would respond to the introduction of glucocorticoids with high binding affinity.

DR. SZEFLER: There appear to be a spectrum of relative resistance. *Steroid resistance* is not a good term. It is a clinical and operational definition. Our suspicion is that in patients who are characterized by the clinical definition as steroid resistant, response can still be identified by several strategies; for example, using higher affinity steroid, increased dosing frequency, administration at critical times of the day (chronopharmacological approach). This may be more difficult to accomplish in the patients with a type 2 abnormality where the receptor number is markedly reduced. These patients would require alternative therapeutic strategies to bypass these observations to regulation of inflammation.

DR. GAULDIE: In glucocorticoid-resistant patients, how widespread is the resistance? What cells are resistant or are all cells resistant?

DR. LEUNG: Steroid resistance appears to be localized to immune effector cells, particularly T cells in patients with steroid-resistant asthma. Most patients with steroid-resistant asthma can develop severe side effects (e.g., hypertension, osteoporosis, cataracts, skin striae) from chronic high-dose steroid use. The latter observation suggests that outside of immune effector cells, most other cells are quite sensitive to the biological effects of steroids. The exact prevalence of steroid-resistant asthma is unknown and is probably underreported, since the syndrome is frequently unrecognized.

References

1. Kay AB. Asthma and inflammation. J Allergy Clin Immunol 1991; 87:893–910.
2. Bousquet J, Chanez P, Lacoste JY, Barneon G, Ghavanian N, Enander I, Venge P, Ahlstedt S, Simony-Lafontaine J, Godard P, Michel F-B. Eosinophilic inflammation in asthma. N Engl J Med 1990; 323:1033–1039.
3. U. S. Department of Health and Human Services, Public Health Service, International Concensus Report on Diagnosis and Management of Asthma, 1992, National Institutes of Health Publication no. 92-3091.
4. Dutoit JI, Salome CM, Woolock AJ. Inhaled corticosteroids reduce the severity of bronchial hyperresponsiveness in asthma but oral theophylline does not. Am Rev Respir Dis 1987; 136:1174–1178.
5. Kerrebijn KF, van Essen-Sandvliet EEM, Neijens HJ. Effect of long-term treatment with inhaled corticosteroids and beta-agonists on the bronchial responsiveness in children. J Allergy Clin Immunol 1987; 79:653–659.
6. Djukanovic R., Wilson, J.E.W., Britten, K.M., Wilson, S.J., Wallis, A. F., Roche, W. R., Howarth, P.H., and Holgate S.T. Effect of an inhaled corticosteroid on airway inflammation and symptoms in asthma. Am Rev Respir Dis 1992; 1145:669–674.
7. Adelroth E, Rosenhall L, Johansson S-A, Linden M, Venge P. Inflammatory cells and eosinophilic activity in asthmatics investigated by bronchoalveolar lavage: the effects of anti-asthmatic treatment with budesonide or terbutaline. Am Rev Respir Dis 1990; 142:91–99.
8. Cockcroft DW, Murdock KY. Comparative effects of inhaled salbutamol, sodium cromoglycate, and beclomethasone dipropionate on allergen-induced early asthmatic responses, late asthmatic responses, and increased bronchial responsiveness to histamine. J Allergy Clin Immunol 1987; 79:734–740.
9. Schleimer RP. Effects of glucocorticoids on inflammatory cells relevant to their therapeutic applications in asthma. Am Rev Respir Dis 1990; 141:S59–S69.
10. Reed JC, Abidi AH, Alpers JD, Hoover RG, Robb RJ, Nowell PC. Effect of cyclosporin A and dexamethasone on interleukin 2 receptor gene expression. J Immunol 1986; 137:150–154.

11. Robinson D, Hamid Q, Ying S, Bentley A, Assoufi B, Durham S, Kay AB. Prednisolone treatment in asthma is associated with modulation of bronchoalveolar lavage cell interleukin-4, interleukin-5, and interferon-γ cytokine gene expression. Am Rev Respir Dis 1993; 148:401–406.

12. Morris HG. Pharmacology of corticosteroids in asthma. In: Middleton E, Reed CE, Ellis EF, eds. Allergy Principles and Practice. St. Louis: Mosby, 1978:464–480.

13. Lundgren JF, Hirata F, Marom Z, Logun C, Steel L, Kaliner M, Shelhamer J. Dexamethasone inhibits respiratory glycoconjugate secretion from feline airways in vitro by the induction of lipocortin (lipomodulin) synthesis. Am Rev Respir Dis 1988; 137:353–357.

14. Schwartz HJ, Lowell FC, Melby JC. Steroid resistance in bronchial asthma. Ann Intern Med 1968; 69:493–499.

15. Carmichael J, Paterson IC, Diaz P, Crompton GE, Kay AB, Grant IWB. Corticosteroid resistance in chronic asthma. Br Med J 1981; 282:1419–1422.

16. Löfdahl C-G, Mellstrand T, Svedmyr N. Glucocorticoids and asthma. Studies of resistance and systemic effects of glucocorticoids. Eur J Respir Dis 1984; 65:69–77.

17. Corrigan CJ, Brown PH, Barnes NC, Szefler SJ, Tsai J-J, Frew AJ, Kay AB. Glucocorticoid resistance in chronic asthma: Glucocorticoid pharmacokinetics, glucocorticoid receptor characteristics, and inhibition of peripheral blood T cell proliferation by glucocorticoids in vitro. Am Rev Respir Dis 1991; 144:1016–1025.

18. Alvarez J, Surs W, Leung DYM, Iklé D, Gelfand EW, Szefler SJ. Steroid-resistant asthma: Immunologic and pharmacologic features. J Allergy Clin Immunol 1992; 89:714–721.

19. Kamada AK, Leung DYM, Gleason MC, Hill MR, Szefler SJ. High-dose systemic glucocorticoid therapy in the treatment of asthma: a case of resistance and patterns of response. J Allergy/Clin Immunol 1992; 90:685–687.

20. Sher ER, Leung DYM, Surs W, Kam JC, Zieg G, Kamada AK, Harbeck R, Szefler SJ. Steroid resistant asthma: cellular mechanisms contributing to inadequate response to glucocorticoid therapy. J Clin Invest 1994; 93:33–39.

21. Kay AB, Diaz P, Carmichael J, Grant IWB. Corticosteroid-resistant chronic asthma and monocyte complement receptors. Clin Exp Immunol 1981; 44:576–580.

22. Poznanzky MC, Gordon ACH, Douglas JG, Krajewski AS, Wyllie AH, Grant IWB. Resistance to methylprednisolone in cultures of blood mononuclear cells from glucocorticoid-resistant asthmatics patients. Clin Sci 1984; 67:639–645.

23. Wilkinson JR, Crea AEG, Clark TJH, Lee TH. Identification and characterization of a monocyte-derived neutrophil-activating factor in corticosteroid-resistant bronchial asthma. J Clin Invest 1989; 84:1930–1941.

24. Vecchiarelli A, Siracusa A, Cenci E, Puliti M, Abbriiti G. Effect of corticosteroid treatment on interleukin-1 and tumour necrosis factor secretion of monocytes from subjects with asthma. Clin Exp Allergy 1992; 22:365–370.

25. Corrigan CJ, Brown PH, Barnes NC, Tsai J-J, Frew AJ, Kay AB. Glucocorticoid resistance in chronic asthma. Am Rev Respir Dis 1991; 144:1026–1032.

26. Lane SJ, Sousa AR, Poston RN, Lee TH. In vitro cutaneous tuberculin response to prednisolone in corticosteroid resistant bronchial asthma. J Allergy Clin Immunol 1993; 91:222A.

27. Leung DYM, Martin RJ, Szefler SJ, Sher ER, Ying S, Ming Q, Kay AB, Hamid Q. The airways of steroid resistant vs steroid sensitive asthma are associated with different patterns of cytokine gene expression. J Exp Med 1995;

28. Chrousos GP, Vingerhoeds A, Brandon D, Eil C, Pugeat M, DeVroede M, Loriaux L, Lipsett MB. Primary cortisol resistance in man: A glucocorticoid receptor-mediated disease. J Clin Invest 1982; 69:1261-1269.

29. Hurley DM, Accilli D, Stratakis CA, Karl M, Vamvakopoulos N, Rorer E, Constantine K, Taylor SI, Chrousos GP. Point mutation causing a single amino acid substitution in the hormone binding domain of the glucocorticoid receptor in familial glucocorticoid resistance. J Clin Invest 1991; 87:680-686.

30. Linder MJ, Thompson EB. Abnormal glucocorticoid receptor gene and mRNA in primary cortisol resistance. J Steroid Biochem 1989; 32:243-249.

31. Bloomfield CD, Peterson BA, Zaleskas J, Frizzera G, Smith KA, Hildebrandt L, Gajl-Peczalska KJ, Munck A. In-vitro glucocorticoid studies for predicting response to glucocorticoid therapy in adults with malignant lymphoma. Lancet 1980; 1:952-956.

32. Yamamoto KR, Gehring U, Stampfer MR, Sibley C. Genetic approaches to steroid hormone action. Recent Prog Horm Res 1976; 32:3-11.

33. Frieri M, Madden J. Chronic steroid-resistant urticaria. Ann Allergy 1993; 70:13-20.

34. Hammond JM, Bateman ED. Successful treatment of life-threatening steroid-resistant pulmonary sarcoidosis with cyclosporin in a patient with systemic lupus erythematosus. Respir Med 1990; 84:77-79.

35. Curley AK, Holden CA. Steroid-resistant bullous pemphigoid treated with cyclosporin A. Clin Exp Dermatol 1991 ;16:68-69.

36. Dundar S, Ozdemir O, Ozcebe O. Cyclosporin in steroid-resistant auto-immune haemolytic anaemia. Acta Haematol 1991; 86:200-202.

37. Coman E, Reinus JF. Cyclosporine use in steroid-resistant Crohn's disease—grasping at new straws? Acta Haematol 1990; 86:758-759.

38. Flower RJ. Lipocortin and the mechanism of action of the glucocorticosteroids. Br J Pharmacol 1988; 94:987-1015.

39. Chung KF, Podgorski MR, Goulding NG, Flower RJ, Barnes PJ. Circulating autoantibodies to recombinant lipocortin-1 in asthma. Respir Med 1991; 85:121-124.

40. Munck A, Mendel DB, Smith LI, Orti E. Glucocorticoid receptors and actions. Am Rev Respir Dis 1990; 141:S2-S10.

41. Lane SJ, Lee TH. Glucocorticoid receptor characteristics in monocytes of patients with corticosteroid-resistant bronchial asthma. Am Rev Respir Dis 1991; 143:1020-1024.

42. Vedeckis WV, Ali M, Allen HR. Regulation of glucocorticoid receptor protein and mRNA levels. Cancer Res 1989; 49:2295s-2302s.

43. Spahn J, Leung DYM, Surs W, Nimmagadda SR, Szefler SJ. Effect of prednisone treatment on glucocorticoid receptor binding parameters in poorly controlled asthma. J Allergy Clin Immunol 1994; 93:384A.

44. Hollenberg SM, Weinberger C, Ong ES, Cerelli G, Oro A, Lebo R, Thompson EB, Rosenfeld MG, Evans RM. Primary structure and expression of a functional human glucocorticoid receptor cDNA. Nature 1985; 318:635-641.

45. Lane SJ, Arm JP, Staynov DZ, Lee TH. Chemical mutational analysis of the human glucocorticoid receptor cDNA in glucocorticoid-resistant bronchial asthma. Am J Respir Cell Mol Biol 1994; 11:42–48.
46. Kam J, Szefler SJ, Surs W, Sher E, Leung DYM. The combined effects of IL-2 and IL-4 after the binding affinity of the glucocorticoid receptor. J Immunol 1993; 151:3460–3466.
47. Diamond MI, Miner JM, Yoshinaga SK, Yamamoto KR. Transcription factor interactions: selectors of positive or negative regulation from a single DNA element. Science 1990; 249:1266–1272.
48. Jain J, McCaffrey PG, Valge-Archer VE, Rao A. Nuclear factor of activated T cells contains Fos and Jun. Nature 1992; 356:801–804.
49. Yang-Yen H-F, Chambard J-C, Sun Y-L, Smeal T, Schmidt TJ, Drouin J, Karin M. Transcriptional interference between c-Jun and the glucocorticoid receptor: Mutual inhibition of DNA binding due to direct protein-protein interaction. Cell 1990; 62:1205–1215.
50. Alexander AG, Barnes NC, Kay AB. Trial of cyclosporin A in corticosteroid-dependent chronic severe asthma. Lancet 1992; 339:324–328.
51. Herrscher RF, Kasper C, Sullivan TJ. Endogenous cortisol regulates immunoglobulin E–dependent late phase reaction. J Clin Invest 1992; 90:596–603.
52. Law CM, Honour JW, Marchant JL, Preece MA, Warner JO. Nocturnal adrenal suppression in asthmatic children taking inhaled beclomethasone dipropionate. Lancet 1986; 1:942–944.
53. Tabachnik E, Zadid Z. Diurnal cortisol secretion during therapy with inhaled beclomethasone dipropionate in children with asthma. J Pediatr 1991; 118:294–297.
54. Nimmigadda SR, Szefler SJ, Surs W, Spahn JD, Leung DYM. Effects of allergens on glucocorticoid receptor binding affinity in patients with asthma. J Allergy Clin Immunol 1994; 93:385A.
55. Landwehr LP, Spahn JD, Kamada AK, Surs W, Leung DYM, Szefler SJ. Effects of hydrocortisone vs synthetic glucocorticoids on lymphocyte activation in steroid resistant asthmatics. J Allergy Clin Immunol 1995;

Part Five

PROSPECTS

25

Inhaled Glucocorticoids in Asthma
Current Understanding and Future Directions

PETER J. BARNES

National Heart and Lung Institute
Imperial School of Medicine
London, England

I. Introduction

Glucocorticoids are by far the most effective therapy for asthma currently available, and inhaled glucocorticoids have now become the mainstay of treatment in patients with chronic asthmatic symptoms (1). The recognition that even patients with mild asthma and episodic symptoms have eosinophilic inflammation in their airway mucosa has provided a scientific rationale for the early use of inhaled glucocorticoids in adults and children (2,3), Yet, despite their efficacy and widespread use in asthma, the molecular mechanisms of topical glucocorticoids in asthma are not yet well understood. Asthma is a complex chronic inflammatory disease involving many cells, mediators, and inflammatory effects. Glucocorticoids are likely to act at on several steps in this complex inflammatory process, including recruitment and activation of inflammatory cells, production of inflammatory mediators, and the inflammatory response itself. Indeed, it is the widespread spectrum of actions of glucocorticoids that may account for their unrivaled efficacy in the control of asthma of all types and severity (4).

The purpose of this chapter is to discuss current concepts of the mechanism of action of inhaled glucocorticoids in asthma and how this knowledge might lead to new therapeutic approaches in the future. Although most patients with asthma respond well to glucocorticoid therapy, some patients have a less satisfactory response; understanding the determinants of glucocorticoid responsiveness may be important in the future.

II. Cellular Targets for Inhaled Glucocorticoids

A. Effects on Asthmatic Inflammation

Steroids are remarkably effective in controlling the inflammation in asthmatic airways, and it is likely that they have multiple cellular effects. Biopsy studies in patients with asthma have now confirmed that inhaled glucocorticoids reduce the number and activation of inflammatory cells in the airway (5–9). Similar results have been reported in bronchoalveolar lavage of asthmatic patients, with a reduction in both eosinophil number and eosinophil cationic protein concentrations, a marker of eosinophil degradation, after inhaled budesonide (10). These effects may be due to inhibition of cytokine synthesis in T lymphocytes and other inflammatory and structural cells. There was also restoration of the disrupted epithelium and a normalization of the ciliated to goblet cell ratio (5). There is also some evidence for a reduction in the thickness of the basement membrane (9), although in asthmatic patients taking inhaled glucocorticoids for over 10 years, the characteristic thickening of the basement membrane was still present (11). A surprising finding is an apparent increase in the number of fibroblasts in the airway after steroid treatment (5), possibly related to the fact that glucocorticoids increase the production of platelet-derived growth factor, a fibroblast mitogen, from alveolar macrophages (12).

B. Effect on Inflammatory and Airway Cells

Glucocorticoids may have indirect inhibitory actions on several inflammatory cells implicated in asthma (13). It is likely that inhaled glucocorticoids exert their anti-inflammatory effects topically on airway cells, although it is possible that some of the antiasthma effects of inhaled glucocorticoids may be due to the systemic actions of the inhaled drug on target cells outside the lung. In studies in dogs, inhaled budesonide in clinically relevant doses has an inhibitory effect on the bone marrow precursors of leukocytes, although it is not certain whether this effect is direct or indirect via inhibition of some airway-derived colony-stimulating factor(s) (14).

Macrophages

Glucocorticoids inhibit the release of inflammatory mediators and cytokines from alveolar macrophages in vitro (15), although their effect after inhalation in vivo is not impressive (16). Glucocorticoids may be more effective in inhibiting cytokine release from alveolar macrophages than in the inhibition of lipid mediators and reactive oxygen species (17,18). Oral prednisone inhibits the increased gene expression of interleukin-1β (IL-1β) in alveolar macrophages obtained by bronchoalveolar lavage from asthmatic patients (19).

Eosinophils

Glucocorticoids have a direct inhibitory effect on mediator release from eosinophils, although they are only weakly effective in inhibiting the secretion of reactive oxygen species and eosinophil basic proteins (20). Glucocorticoids appear to inhibit the permissive action of cytokines such as granulocyte-macrophage colony-stimulating factor (GM-CSF) and IL-5 on eosinophil survival (21,22), possibly by activation of an endonuclease that breaks up DNA and results to programmed cell death. One of the best-described actions of glucocorticoids in asthma is a reduction in circulating eosinophils, which may reflect an action on eosinophil production in the bone marrow (23). In asthmatic patients, there is an increase in the proportion of low-density eosinophils in the circulation, which may reflect an effect of cytokines (24). Inhaled glucocorticoids inhibit the increase in circulating eosinophil count at night in patients with nocturnal asthma and also reduce plasma concentrations of eosinophil cationic protein (25). After inhaled glucocorticoids (budesonide, 800 μg b.i.d.), there is a marked reduction in the number of low-density eosinophils, presumably reflecting the inhibition of cytokine production in the airways (26).

T Lymphocytes

An important target cell in asthma may be the T lymphocyte, since glucocorticoids are very effective in the inhibition of activation of these cells and in blocking the release of cytokines, which are likely to play an important role in the recruitment and survival of several inflammatory cells involved in asthmatic inflammation. In an experimental model of asthma which involves sensitization and repeated exposure to allergen in an IgE-producing strain of rat, there is an influx of eosinophils and lymphocytes into the lung with a concomitant increased airway responsiveness to inhaled methacholine (27). Pretreatment with glucocorticoids completely inhibits the increased eosinophil and lymphocyte numbers and the increase in airway responsiveness, whereas pretreatment with cyclosporin A, which similarly inhibits cellular influx, fails to block the increased airway responsiveness (28). This suggests that the effect of glucocorticoids on airway hyperresponsiveness may be through some cell other than the T lymphocyte.

Mast Cells

Although glucocorticoids do not appear to have a direct inhibitory effect on mediator release from lung mast cells (29,30), chronic steroid treatment is associated with a marked reduction in mucosal mast cell number (5,6). This may be linked to a reduction in stem cell factor (c-kit ligand) production, which appears to be necessary for mast cell expression in mucosal tissues. Mast cells also secrete various cytokines, but whether this is inhibited by glucocorticoids has not yet been reported.

Neutrophils

Neutrophils are not prominent in the biopsies of asthmatic patients, and they are not very sensitive to the effects of glucocorticoids. There is some evidence that neutrophils are prominent in sudden severe asthma, which may not be responsive to glucocorticoid therapy (31).

Endothelial Cells

Steroid receptor gene expression in the airways is most prominent in the endothelial cells of the bronchial circulation and airway epithelial cells (32). Glucocorticoids do not appear directly to inhibit the expression of endothelial adhesion molecules, although they may inhibit cell adhesion indirectly by suppression of cytokines involved in the regulation of adhesion molecule expression (13). Glucocorticoids may have an inhibitory action on airway microvascular leak induced by inflammatory mediators (33,34). This appears to be a direct effect on postcapillary venular endothelial cells. The mechanism for this antipermeability effect has not been fully elucidated, but there is evidence that synthesis of a 100-kDa protein distinct from lipocortin-1, termed vasocortin, may be involved (35). Although there have been no direct measurements of the effects of glucocorticoids on airway microvascular leakage in asthmatic airways, regular treatment with inhaled glucocorticoids decreases the elevated plasma proteins found in bronchoalveolar lavage fluid of patients with stable asthma (36).

Epithelial Cells

Epithelial cells may be one of the most important targets for inhaled glucocorticoids in asthma (Fig. 1). Glucocorticoids inhibit the increased transcription of the IL-8 gene induced by tumor necrosis factor (TNF-α) in cultured human airway epithelial cells in vitro (37,38) and the transcription of the RANTES gene in an epithelial cell line (39). Inhaled glucocorticoids inhibit the increased expression of GM-CSF and RANTES in the epithelium of asthmatic patients (9,40,41).

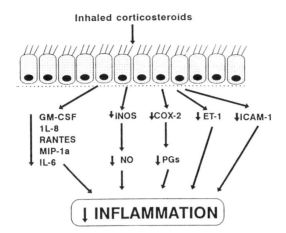

Figure 1 Effect of inhaled glucocorticoids on airway epithelial cells. Inhaled gluco-corticoids may reduce asthmatic inflammation by inhibiting synthesis of several inflammatory mediators, including cytokines (IL-8; GM-CSF; RANTES; released by normal T cells activated and secreted; macrophage inflammatory protein [MIP - 1α]), NO by inhibition of iNOS, prostaglandins (PG) by inhibition of inducible cyclo-oxygenase (COX-2), endothelin-1 (ET-1), and intercellular adhesion molecule-1 (ICAM-1).

There is expression of the inducible form of nitric oxide synthase (iNOS) in the airway epithelium of patients with asthma which is not observed in normal individuals (42). This may account for the increase in nitric oxide (NO) in the exhaled air of patients with asthma compared with normal subjects (43,44). Asthmatic patients who are taking regular inhaled steroid therapy, however, do not show such an increase in exhaled NO (43), suggesting that glucocorticoids have suppressed epithelial iNOS expression. Furthermore, double-blind randomized studies show that oral and inhaled glucocorticoids reduce the elevated exhaled NO in asthmatic patients to normal values (45,46).

Submucosal Glands

Glucocorticoids inhibit mucous secretion in airways, and this may be a direct action of glucocorticoids on submucosal gland cells (47). The inhibitory effect of glucocorticoids may involve lipocortin-1 synthesis (48). In addition, there are indirect inhibitory effects due to the reduction in inflammatory mediators that stimulate increased mucous secretion. Whether glucocorticoids have any effect on goblet cell secretion or goblet cell hyperplasia is not yet certain. Inhaled glucocorticoids appear to reverse the increased numbers of goblet cells in the airway epithelium of asthmatic patients (5).

III. Key Gene Targets of Inhaled Glucocorticoids

Glucocorticoids produce their effect on responsive cells by activating glucocorticoid receptors (GRs) to regulate directly or indirectly the transcription of target genes (49,50) (Fig. 2). The number of genes *directly* regulated by GRs in a given cell may be between 10 and 100 (51), although the number of genes regulated indirectly via effects is likely to be very much greater. Many genes that do not appear to have glucocorticoid response elements (GREs) in their promoter sequence are regulated by glucocorticoids, and this is likely to be via an effect of glucocorticoids of GRs on the activity of transcription factors that regulate expression of these genes. The number of GREs and their position relative to the transcriptional start site may be an important determinant of the magnitude of the transcriptional response to glucocorticoids. Thus, an increased number of GREs and proximity to the TATA box increases the steroid inducibility of a gene. Interaction with other transcription factors may also be important in determining differential steroid responsiveness in different cell types. Other transcription factors binding in the vicinity of GREs may have a pow-

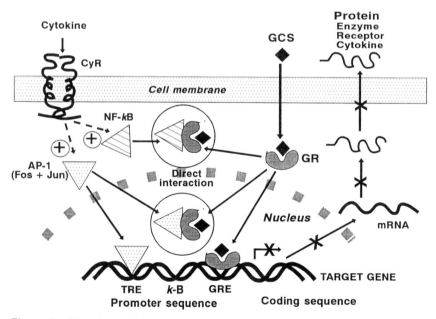

Figure 2   Direct interaction between the transcription factors AP-1 and NF-κB and the activated GR may result in mutual repression. In this way, glucocorticoids may counteract the chronic inflammatory effects of cytokines that activate these transcription factors. These interactions may occur in the nucleus or in the cytoplasm.

erful influence on steroid inducibility, and the relative abundance of different transcription factors may contribute to the steroid responsiveness of a particular cell type. GRs may interact with other transcription elements at *composite* response elements (at which two distinct transcription factors must be present for activation), which may be important in determining cell-specific responses to glucocorticoids (52). GR-DNA interaction changes DNase I sensitivity, indicating that there may be a change in the configuration of DNA or chromatin, which may expose previously masked areas, resulting in increased binding of other transcription factors and the formation of a more stable transcription initiation complex.

Inhaled glucocorticoids may have effects on several genes in the control of asthmatic inflammation (53) (Table 1).

A. Cytokines

Although it is not yet possible to be certain of the most critical aspects of steroid action in asthma, it is likely that their inhibitory effects on cytokine synthesis are of particular relevance. Multiple cytokines appear to play a critical role in orchestrating asthmatic inflammation (54,55). Glucocorticoids inhibit the transcription of several cytokines that are relevant in asthma, including IL-1, TNF-α, GM-CSF, IL-3, IL-4, IL-5, IL-6, IL-8, and RANTES (56). These effects may be mediated via interaction of GRs with a negative GRE (nGREs), resulting in a direct reduction in gene transcription. Cytokine genes may be particularly sensitive to the inhibitory effects of glucocorticoids; for example,

Table 1 Effect of Glucocorticoids on Transcription of Genes Relevant to Asthma

Increased transcription
    lipocortin-1
    β_2-adrenoceptor
    endonucleases
    secretory leukocyte inhibitory protein
Decreased transcription
    cytokines (IL-1, IL-2, IL-3, IL-4, IL-5, IL-6, IL-8, IL-11, IL-12,
        IL-13, TNF-α, GM-CSF, RANTES, MIP-1α, SCF)
    inducible nitric oxide synthase (iNOS)
    inducible cyclo-oxygenase (COX-2)
    inducible phospholipase A$_2$ (cPLA$_2$)
    endothelin-1
    NK$_1$-receptors
    Adhesion molecules (ICAM-1)

in the IL-6 gene, there are at least four nGREs close to the promoter site and a "blocking" GREs located very close to the start site of transcription (57).

There may not be such a nGRE consensus sequence in the promoter region of many cytokines, suggesting that glucocorticoids inhibit transcription via different molecular mechanisms. Thus, the 5'-promoter sequence of the human IL-2 gene has no GRE consensus sequences, yet glucocorticoids are potent inhibitors of IL-2 gene transcription in T lymphocytes. Transcription of the IL-2 gene is predominantly regulated by a cell-specific transcription factor, nuclear factor, of activated T cells (NF-AT), which is activated in the cytoplasm of T-cell receptor stimulation via calcineurin (58). A nuclear factor is also necessary for increased activation, and this factor appears to be similar to AP-1, which binds directly to NF-AT to form a transcriptional complex (59). Glucocorticoids inhibit IL-2 gene transcription indirectly by binding to the transcription factor activator protein-1 (AP-1), thus preventing increased transcription owing to NF-AT (60). Another example is provided by the inhibitory effect of glucocorticoids on IL-8 gene transcription, which is regulated predominantly via nuclear factor-kappa B (NF-κB) (61).

For some cytokines, such as IL-1, IL-3, and GM-CSF, increased breakdown of mRNA has also been demonstrated (62,63). Glucocorticoids may not only block the synthesis of cytokines but may also block their effects in several ways. First, glucocorticoids may inhibit the synthesis of certain cytokine receptors, such as the IL-2 receptor (64). Second, several cytokines produce their cellular effects by activating transcription factors, such as AP-1 and NF-κB, that activate or repress target genes that are regulated in an opposing manner by GRs. For example, TNF-α activates both AP-1 and NF-κB in human lung, and this is counteracted by glucocorticoids (65). T-lymphocyte activation is mediated partly by the activation of AP-1, which leads to the induction of a number of target genes such as IL-2, IL-2 receptor, and cell proliferation (66). This activation is potently inhibited by glucocorticoids. Furthermore, there is a direct interaction between AP-1 and the GR, so that glucocorticoids can directly counteract the cellular action of cytokines, as discussed below.

B. Nitric Oxide Synthase

Nitric oxide synthase NOS may be induced by various cytokines, resulting in increased nitric oxide production. NO may increase airway blood flow and plasma exudation and may amplify the proliferation of TH2 lymphocytes which orchestrate eosinophilic inflammation in the airways (67,68). The induction of the inducible form of NOS (iNOS) is potently inhibited by glucocorticoids (69,70). In cultured murine and human pulmonary epithelial cells, proinflammatory cytokines result in increased expression of iNOS and increased NO formation (71,72). This is due to increased transcription of the iNOS gene and is inhibited by glucocorticoids. There is no obvious nGRE in the promoter sequence of the murine or human iNOS gene (73,74), but NF-κB appears to be the most important transcription factor in regulating iNOS gene transcription (75). Since TNF-α and oxidants may activate NF-κB in airway epithelial cells, this may account for their activation of iNOS expression (76). Glucocorticoids may therefore prevent induction of iNOS by inactivating NF-κB; thereby inhibiting transcription.

C. Inflammatory Mediators

Glucocorticoids inhibit the synthesis of several inflammatory mediators implicated in asthma. Glucocorticoids also inhibit the induction of the gene coding for inducible cyclo-oxygenase (COX-2) in monocytes and epithelial cells (77,78), and this also appears to be via NF-κB activation (79). Glucocorticoids also inhibit the gene transcription of a form of PLA_2 induced by cytokines (80). Whether glucocorticoids also modulate expression of the 5-lipoxygenase has not yet been established.

Glucocorticoids increase the synthesis of lipocortin-1, a 37-kDa protein that has an inhibitory effect on phospholipase A_2, and therefore may inhibit the production of lipid mediators, such as leukotrienes (LTs), prostaglandins, and platelet-activating factor. Glucocorticoids induce the formation of lipocortin-1 in rat and human leukocytes (81,82). Recombinant lipocortin-1 has acute anti-inflammatory properties and inhibits the release of lipid mediators from lungs (83). Although this action of glucocorticoids was at one time believed to be their most important anti-inflammatory effect (84), it is now evident that lipocortin-1 has rather nonspecific effects (85), and there have been doubts about the ability of glucocorticoids to induce lipocortin-1 in some cells (86).

Glucocorticoids also inhibit the synthesis of endothelin-1 in lung (87) and airway epithelial cells (88), and this effect may also be via inhibition of transcription factors.

Glucocorticoids may also modulate the effects of inflammatory mediators. Thus LTB_4 and platelet-deriving factor induce the expression of c-*fos* and c-*jun* and activate AP-1 binding in inflammatory cells (89), and this may be inhibited by glucocorticoids.

D. Receptors

Glucocorticoids also decrease the transcription of genes coding for certain receptors. Thus, the NK_1-receptor, which mediates the inflammatory effects of substance P in the airways may show increased gene expression in asthma (90). This may be inhibited glucocorticoids though an interaction with AP-1 as the NK_1 receptor gene promoter region has no GREs but it has an AP-1 response element.

Glucocorticoids increase the expression of β_2-adrenoceptors by increasing the rate of transcription (91) and the human β_2-receptor gene has at least three potential GREs (92). Glucocorticoids increase β_2-receptor gene transcription in human lung in vitro (93). This may be relevant in asthma, as it may prevent downregulation in response to prolonged treatment with β_2-agonists. In rats, glucocorticoids prevent the downregulation and reduced transcription of β_2-receptors in response to chronic β-agonist exposure (94).

IL-1 acts on two types of surface receptor, designated IL-1RI and IL-1RII. The inflammatory effects of IL-1β are mediated exclusively via IL-1RI, whereas IL-1RII has no signaling activity but binds IL-1 and, therefore, acts as a molecular trap that interferes with the actions of IL-1. Glucocorticoids are potent inducers of this decoy IL-1 receptor and result in release of a soluble form of the receptor, thus reducing the functional activity of IL-1 (95,96).

E. Enzymes

There may be increased transcription of other relevant genes. Glucocorticoids increase the mRNA level and expression of neutral endopeptidase in cultured airway epithelial cells (97), and this may result in increased degradation of bronchoconstrictor peptides, such as bradykinin, tachykinins, and endothelin-1. This effect may explain the inhibitory effect of glucocorticoids on neurogenic plasma extravasation in airways which is due to the release of tachykinins from sensory nerves (98). However, other studies have reported no effect of glucocorticoids on airway epithelial neutral endopeptidase (NEP) expression (99), and the inhibitory effects of glucocorticoids on neurogenic inflammation may be via inhibition of NK$_1$-receptor expression. Angiotensin-converting enzyme is also involved in the degradation of bradykinin and is induced by glucocorticoids (100).

Glucocorticoids markedly reduce the survival of certain inflammatory cells, such as eosinophils. Eosinophil survival is dependent on the presence of certain cytokines, such as IL-5 and GM-CSF. Exposure to glucocorticoids blocks the effects these cytokines and leads to programmed cell death or apoptosis (22). This may involve the activation of specific endonucleases (101). Glucocorticoids may activate endonucleases, and this may be relevant to the action of glucocorticoids on eosinophil and mast cell survival in the airways of asthmatic patients.

F. Adhesion Molecules

Adhesion molecules play a key role in the trafficking of inflammatory cells to sites of inflammation. The expression of many adhesion molecules on endothelial cells is induced by cytokines and glucocorticoids may lead indirectly to a reduced expression via their inhibitory effects on cytokines, such as IL-1β and TNF-α. Glucocorticoids may also have a direct inhibitory effect on the expression adhesion molecules, such as intracellular adhesion molecule-1 (ICAM-1) and E-selectin at the level of gene transcription) (102). ICAM-1 expression in bronchial epithelial cell lines and monocytes is inhibited by glucocorticoids (103). ICAM-1 expression is dependent on NF-κB activation (104), and this may account for the inhibitory effects of glucocorticoids.

G. Other Effects

Glucocorticoids exert a number of other anti-inflammatory effects which are not yet understood at a molecular level. Glucocorticoids have a direct inhibitory effect on plasma exudation from postcapillary venules at inflammatory sites. The onset of effect is delayed, suggesting that gene transcription and protein synthesis are involved. The mechanism for this antipermeability effect has not been fully elucidated, but there is evidence that synthesis of a 100-kDa protein distinct from lipocortin-1, termed vasocortin, may be involved (35).

IV. Molecular Mechanisms of Anti-inflammatory Actions

Most attention has focused on the interaction of the GR with DNA as a mechanism of action of glucocorticoids in the control of inflammation. Although at one time, it was believed that the anti-inflammatory effect of glucocorticoids could be explained by increased transcription of lipocortin-1, this has not been supported by recent evidence. Most of the anti-inflammatory actions of glucocorticoids appear to be due to the reduced transcription of genes encoding inflammatory proteins and enzymes (53).

A. Direct Gene Repression

The mechanisms involved in gene repression are even less well understood. In some instances, this may be due to the fact that GR binding to nGRE results in steric hindrance to the binding of transcription factors that may induce the same gene. GRs may also form complexes with activating transcription factors in the nucleus to inhibit their effect, so that glucocorticoids may exert an inhibitory effect on the transcription of genes (such as IL-2, IL-8, and RANTES) which do not have a nGRE in their promoter sequence.

B. Messenger RNA Stability

GRs may also inhibit protein synthesis by reducing the stability of mRNA via enhanced transcription of specific ribonucleases that break down mRNA containing constitutive gold (AU)–rich sequences in the untranslated 3′-region, thus shortening the turnover time of mRNA (105). This is the case with certain cytokines, but little is known of the specificity of RNAse enzymes.

C. Interaction with Other Transcription Factors

GRs may interact directly with other transcription factors, which bind to each other via so-called leucine zipper interactions (106,107). This could be an important determinant of steroid responsiveness and is a key mechanism whereby glucocorticoids exert their anti-inflammatory actions (53). This interaction was first demonstrated for the collagenase gene which is induced by the transcription factor AP-1, which is a heterodimer of *Fos* and *Jun* oncoproteins, the products of the protooncogenes c-fos and c-jun. AP-1 binds to a specific DNA binding site (TRE or TPA response element, TGACTCA). Glucocorticoids are potent inhibitors of collagenase gene transcription induced by TNF-α and phorbol esters which activate AP-1. AP-1 forms a protein-protein complex with activated GRs, and this prevents GRs from interacting with DNA and thereby reduces steroid responsiveness (108–110). In cell-free systems, recombinant c-*jun* and c-*fos* inhibit GR binding to DNA (110). Conversely, glucocorticoids may inhibit the effects of those cytokines that produce their effects on gene transcription via activation of AP-1 (Fig. 2). The GR is likely to interact with the *Fos* component of AP-1 (111). In human lung and monocytes, TNF-α and phorbol esters increase AP-1 binding to DNA, and this is inhibited by glucocorticoids (65,112). GRs may interact with other transcription factors, including NF-κB in a similar manner (65,112,113). There is evidence that β-agonists via cyclic AMP formation and activation of protein kinase A result in the activation of the transcription factor (CREB) that binds to a cyclic AMP–responsive element (CRE) on genes (114). A direct interaction between CREB and GR has been demonstrated (115). β-Agonists increase CRE binding in human lung in vitro and at the same time reduce GRE binding, suggesting that there may be a protein-protein interaction between CREB and GR within the nucleus (116,117). These interactions between activated GRs and transcription factors occur within the nucleus, but recent observations suggest that these protein-protein interactions may also occur in the cytoplasm (118).

D. Posttranscriptional Modulation

The GRs may also influence protein synthesis by affecting the stability of mRNA via enhanced transcription of specific ribonucleases that break down mRNA containing constitutive AU-rich sequences in the untranslated 3′-region, thus shortening the turnover time of mRNA (105).

V. Glucocorticoid Responsiveness

Although most patients with asthma respond to relatively low doses of inhaled glucocorticoids, a proportion require much higher doses. Some patients may not be controlled even on high doses of inhaled glucocorticoids and require oral glucocorticoids (steroid-dependent asthma), whereas a few patients may show no response, even with high doses of oral glucocorticoids (steroid-resistant asthma) (Fig. 3). There may be several mechanisms that determine glucocorticoid responsiveness, but there is little understanding of the molecular mechanisms involved.

There is little evidence for pharmacokinetic differences in the handling of inhaled glucocorticoids between different patients (119), suggesting that differences in cellular responsiveness are more important. Large differences in the cellular response to glucocorticoids are seen in vitro. There may be different responses to glucocorticoids, depending on the response measured, as some genes may be more susceptible to suppression or induction than others. Similarly, inflammatory cells may show differential responsiveness to the inhibitory effects of glucocorticoids. For example, neutrophils and mast cells appear to be relatively resistant to the effects of glucocorticoids, whereas T lymphocytes, macrophages, and epithelial cells are very sensitive.

Another major problem in investigating responsiveness to inhaled glucocorticoids in asthma is the difficulty in measuring a response, since the effects of glucocorticoids on airway function may be slow to evolve. It has often proved difficult to demonstrate a dose response to inhaled steroids, although this

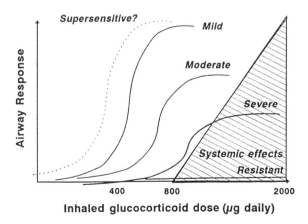

Figure 3 Differences in glucocorticoid responsiveness between patients.

may depend on the outcome measure used. For spirometric measurements, little response may be seen after inhaled glucocorticoids, although symptoms are markedly improved and there may be a dramatic reduction in the frequency of asthma exacerbations (4). Some studies have found no dose response even with widely separated doses (120). This may reflect the fact that, for some patients with milder asthma, small doses of inhaled glucocorticoids may have reached the maximum on the dose-response curve, whereas for other patients with more severe inflammation in their airways, there may be a dose response (see Fig. 3). More direct measurements of inflammation may give a more meaningful dose response. Although it is not feasible to repeatedly biopsy airways from asthmatic patients with different doses of inhaled glucocorticoids, it may be possible to use less invasive measurements, such as induced sputum (121) and exhaled NO (46,122), to monitor responses.

A. Regulation of the GR

GR expression may be regulated by several factors (123). Downregulation occurs after exposure to glucocorticoids (124), but it is not certain how important this is in chronic steroid therapy. A marked reduction in GR mRNA occurs in human lung after exposure to glucocorticoids in vitro for 24 hr (32), but it is not certain whether this persists after prolonged treatment. Studies with transgenic mice that express antisense GR mRNA, resulting in lower GR levels, have demonstrated that even a reduction in GR expression by twofold caused various abnormalities, including an increase in circulating cortisol and an increase in body fat (125). It seems unlikely that downregulation of the GR is an important factor in asthma therapy, as most evidence suggests that the dose of inhaled glucocorticoids needed to control asthma usually reduces with time as the asthmatic inflammation comes under control (126,127). This can be understood in terms of the functional antagonism between GRs and transcription factors, such as AP-1 and NF-κB.

B. Effect of Cytokines

Reduced glucocorticoid responsiveness may result from cytokine-mediated inflammation owing to the functional antagonism by activated transcription factors, such as AP-1 and NF-κB. Increased expression of c-*fos* and c-*jun*, components of AP-1, inhibits the effects of glucocorticoids on gene expression (110). This would account for the reduced responses to inhaled glucocorticoids in patients with severe asthma (Fig. 4). It may also explain why acute severe asthma responds poorly to intravenous glucocorticoids, when presumably there is intense inflammation of the airway wall (128). It is possible that there are individual differences in the degree of transcription factor activation induced by proinflammatory cytokines (possibly due to differences in the kinases and phos-

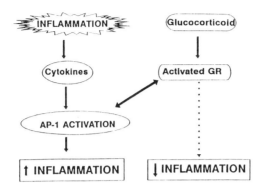

Figure 4 Cytokine-mediate reduction in airway responsiveness to glucocorticoids. By increasing AP-1 activation, GRs are complexed, and this leads to reduced glucocorticoid responsiveness.

phatases that regulate their expression and activation within cells), and that this accounts for differences in glucocorticoid responsiveness between patients. In patients with glucocorticoid-resistant asthma, there is a decrease in GR binding affinity which is confined to T lymphocytes and may be mimicked by exposing T lymphocytes in vitro to high concentration of of Il-2 and IL-4 simultaneously (129).

C. Effect of β-Adrenergic Agonists

High concentrations of β-agonists activate the transcription factor CREB in human lung and in cells such as monocytes (112,116). There appears to be a direct protein-protein interaction between CREB and ligand-activated GRs resulting in reduced GRE binding (Fig. 5). Thus, in rat lung, there is a concentration-dependent reduction in GRE binding as the concentration of albuterol increases, with a 50% reduction in binding at concentrations at 10^{-4} M (130). This effect of β-agonists is blocked by propranolol, indicating that β-adrenoceptors are involved, and is mimicked by forskolin, which increases cyclic AMP by directly activating adenylyl cyclase. This inhibitory effect of β-agonists on GRE binding also occurs in epithelial cells and T lymphocytes (117), where such interactions are likely to occur in patients treated with high doses of inhaled β-agonists. A recent clinical study demonstrated that the normal protection against allergen challenge provided by 3 weeks of treatment with an inhaled glucocorticoid was lost when the inhaled steroid was administered with a relatively high dose of inhaled β-agonist (131). This suggests that high concentrations of β-agonists may be deleterious is asthma by reducing the anti-inflammatory actions of glucocorticoids. This secondary glucocorticoid resis-

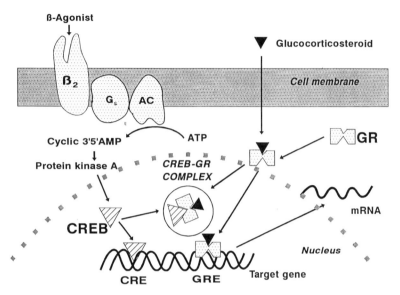

Figure 5 Effect of a β_2-agonist on GRs. High doses of β_2-agonists increase cyclic AMP and activate CREB. CREB may interact directly with GRs, resulting in reduced glucocorticoid responsiveness.

tance would be overcome by increasing the dose of inhaled glucocorticoids. This interaction may account for some of the association between high doses of inhaled β-agonists and an increase in asthma morbidity and mortality (132–134). If high doses of inhaled β-agonists reduce glucocorticoid responsiveness, it follows that a reduction in the total dose of β-agonists may be beneficial in such patients. In an open study, gradual reduction in the dose of nebulized β-agonists in patients with severe asthma resulted in improved control of asthma and a reduced requirement for oral glucocorticoids (135).

D. Glucocorticoid-Resistant Asthma

Glucocorticoid-resistant asthma, defined by < 15% increase in FEV_1 (forced expiratory volume in 1 sec) or peak expiratory flow after 2 weeks of oral prednisolone (20–40 mg) , is very rare (136). Resistance to the anti-inflammatory and immunomodulatory effects of glucocorticoids is described in several inflammatory and immune diseases, including rheumatoid arthritis and transplant rejection. This resistance differs from the extremely rare familial glucocorticoid resistance, as it is not associated with high circulating concentrations of cortisol or adrenocorticotropin (ACTH), and is not accompanied by hypertension, hypokalemia, or androgen excess (137,138). This suggests that any abnormality is unlikely to be due to the same abnormalities in the steroid binding domain of the GR that are described in familial glucocorticoid resistance (139). Indeed, recent chemical mutational analysis of the GR has failed to demonstrate any major abnormality in the predicted structure in glucocorticoid-resistant asthma compared with glucocorticoid-sensitive asthma (140). Glucocorticoid resistance may be primary (inherited or acquired of unknown cause) or secondary to some factor known to reduce glucocorticoid responsiveness (glucocorticoids themselves, cytokines, β-adrenergic agonists), as discussed above.

Glucocorticoid resistance has been documented in both T lymphocytes and monocytes of glucocorticoid-resistant patients, and the abnormality is widespread as the cutaneous blanching responses to topical steroids is also impaired (141). Since circulating cells and cells in the skin are unlikely to be exposed to inflammatory cytokines, this suggests that the abnormality is primary. There is no major abnormality in the binding affinity of glucocorticoids to GRs or in the density of cytoplasmic GRs (142–144). There is similarly no defect in nuclear localization of GRs after ligand binding. However, there appears to be a defect in the binding between GRs and GREs, with a markedly reduced number of GRs available for binding to DNA (145). This may be secondary to interaction with transcription factors, since there is also a defect in the glucocorticoid-induced inhibition of AP-1 binding and in PMA-induced activation of AP-1 (146). This suggests that there may be an abnormality in AP-1 itself, and there is an increased basal activation of AP-1 in peripheral blood mononuclear cells of glucocorticoid-resistant patients (147). There is no obvious abnormality in the sequence of c-*fos* or c-*jun*, which are the main components of AP-1 (I.M. Adcock, unpublished data), suggesting that the defect may be in the enzymes that control the activation of AP-1 (such as *Jun*-kinases). By contrast, the interaction between the GR and CREB or NF-κB is not impaired. This suggests that the defect is confined to the AP-1–inhibitory effects of glucocorticoids, and this may explain why the anti-inflammatory actions of glucocorticoids are impaired, whereas metabolic and homeostatic actions are not.

VI. Future Clinical Use of Inhaled Glucocorticoids

A. Early Use of Inhaled Glucocorticoids

Inhaled glucocorticoids are being increasingly used for the control of asthma. Although there is no question about their role in the management of moderate to severe asthma, their use in the treatment of mild asthma is still being debated, particularly in children. The major concern about the use of inhaled glucocorticoids early in the treatment of asthma is the possibility that long-term systemic effects may be deleterious. However, extensive studies using sensitive markers of systemic effects of glucocorticoids have been reassuring (1,4). When inhaled glucocorticoids are used early in the course of asthma, it is likely that only low doses are needed, with a low risk of systemic effects. Whether early use of inhaled glucocorticoids alters the natural history of asthma is uncertain, and careful long-term studies are needed to address this issue. A recent study has demonstrated that even when inhaled glucocorticoids are introduced, early asthma symptoms recur when steroids are withdrawn after 2 years of treatment (127). When glucocorticoids are used in the treatment of established asthma, they suppress the disease but need to be taken continuously. Cessation of treatment with inhaled glucocorticoids results in the recurrence of asthmatic symptoms in days to weeks, indicating that glucocorticoids do not have a curative effect (148,149).

Recent studies in adults and children suggest that the early introduction of inhaled steroids gives improved lung function compared with treatment with bronchodilators, and that the longer the delay in introduction of inhaled steroids, the less improvement in lung function occurs (126,127,150). These important studies suggest that inhaled steroids should be started at the time the diagnosis of asthma is made irrespective of asthma severity. Delay in the introduction of inhaled steroids may lead to irreversible changes in the airways. Further prospective controlled studies are now needed, particualrly in children.

B. Steroid-Sparing Therapies

In patients with more severe asthma, higher doses of inhaled glucocorticoids are needed, with increased risks of adverse effects. There are several medications used in the treatment of asthma which may reduce the requirement of oral or inhaled steroids, although there is some ambiguity about the term *steroid sparing*. For example, β-agonists, which control the symptoms of asthma, do not appear to suppress the chronic inflammatory response and yet may give improved control of asthma when added to inhaled steroids. Steroid sparing is normally taken to mean that the treatment has an effect on the underlying disease process. To date, steroids are the only asthma treatment that has been demonstrated to reduce the inflammation in asthmatic airways. Steroid-sparing therapies may be useful in reducing the dose of inhaled steroid required for asthma control when high doses of inhaled steroids are needed, and would have an advantage if local side effects such as dysphonia were a limiting factor in the dose of inhaled steroid that was needed. Several therapies for asthma have been considered as alternatives to steroid therapy.

Cromones

Both cromolyn sodium (CS) and nedocromil sodium (NS) have antiasthma effects which are believed to be mediated by control of the inflammatory process

(151,152). Both drugs are indicated in the control of mild asthma and need to be taken regularly. NS has been compared with inhaled steroids in studies of airway hyperesponsiveness and has been found to be less effective than a low dose (400 μg daily) of inhaled steroid (153,154). Inhaled NS and inhaled BDP both reduce histamine responsiveness, but only the inhaled steroid reduces responsiveness to fog, improves baseline lung function, and peak flow variability and reduces inhaled β_2-agonist usage (155). Some studies have demonstrated that NS controls asthma when either oral or inhaled glucocorticoids were withdrawn (156,157) or provides additional control when added to high-dose inhaled steroids (158), whereas others have not shown any steroid-sparing effect (159).

Immunosuppressive Therapy

Several immunosuppressive agents have been shown to have antiasthma effects, including methotrexate (160–162), oral gold (163,164), and cyclosporin A (165,166). These therapies all have side effects that may be more troublesome than those of oral steroids and are therefore only indicated as an additional therapy to reduce the requirement of oral glucocorticoids. Because of side effects, these treatments cannot be considered as a way to reduce the requirement for inhaled steroids. Several other therapies, including azathioprine, dapsone, and hydroxychloroquine, have not been found to be beneficial.

The molecular mechanism of action of cyclosporin A (CsA) and the related immunosuppressant tacrolimus (FK 506) is now established (58). Both drugs, after binding to a specific immunophilin, prevent the activation of calcineurin and thus interfere with the cytoplasmic component of NF-AT. Glucocorticoids block the nuclear component of NF-AT, which is now identified as AP-1 (60). This predicts that there might be a synergistic interaction between CsA and glucocorticoids in suppresion of transcription of IL-2, IL-4, and IL-5 genes (Fig. 6). This has recently been confirmed in human peripheral T cells in vitro (167). It may be possible to take advantage of this synergistic interaction to optimize immunosuppresion in asthmatic airways by giving low doses of CsA systemically to avoid nephrotoxicity and to localize synergy to the airways by high-dose inhaled steroids.

β-Agonists

Although bronchodilators act predominantly on airway smooth muscle, it is possible that they may have additional effects to regulate asthmatic inflammation. Whether β-agonists have anti-inflammatory effects in asthma is controversial, partly because of the definition of anti-inflammatory treatment (132). β-Agonists are potent inhibitors of mast cell mediator release in vitro (168) and probably after inhalation in vivo (169), but they do not appear to have an effect on the chronic inflammation of asthma (5). This also applies to long-act-

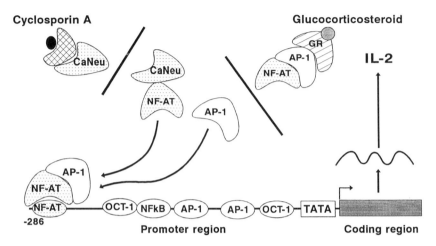

Figure 6 Interaction between cyclosporin A and glucocorticoids (GCs) on the activity of NF-AT on the IL-2 gene promoter. Cyclosporin A binds to an immunophilin that blocks calcineurin (CaNeu), thus preventing activation of the cytoplasmic component of NF-AT. GRs bind to AP-1, the nuclear component of NF-AT, thus resulting in a synergistic inhibition of IL-2 gene transcription.

ing inhaled β_2-agonists, such as salmeterol, which has no effect on the inflammation in asthmatic airways (170). In a large study in general practice, the addition of salmeterol gave a greater improvement in lung function in patients still symptomatic on taking BDP, 400 µg daily, than increasing the dose of inhaled glucocorticoids to 1200 µg (171). Furthermore, there was no difference in the number of exacerbations between the group of patients treated with salmeterol and the group treated with the increased dose of glucocorticoids.

Theophylline

Theophylline is normally classified as a bronchodilator, but the concentrations required to relax human airway smooth muscle in vitro suggest that this is unlikely to be very important in its antiasthma effects (172). Theophylline is able to block the late response to allergen at a time when it should not be having any bronchodilator action, and withdrawal of theophylline leads to reduced control of asthma (173,174), with an increase in activated CD4[+] T cells in the airways (174). There is some evidence that theophylline has a steroid-sparing effect (175) and may have similar effects in the control of asthma to low-dose inhaled glucocorticoids (176). It is not yet certain whether there is a synergistic interaction between the effects of theophylline and glucocorticoids on asthmatic inflammation.

VII. Future Developments

Because inhaled glucocorticoids are the most effective therapy currently available for asthma, perhaps the most useful advances in asthma therapy in the future may be the improvement of inhaled glucocorticoids so that systemic and local adverse effects are less likely. The use of new delivery devices has partly achieved the desired reduction in local and systemic effects, but novel types of glucocorticoids for inhalation or the development of nonsteroidal drugs that mimic the essential antiasthma effects of glucocorticoids are also a possibility. There is a single type of GR (177), and therefore it is not possible to develop novel steroids that have a greater selectivity. Improvements in inhaled glucocorticoids must, therefore, be based on pharmacokinetic differences. It is likely that inhaled glucocorticoids exert their antiasthmatic effects topically in the airways rather than via a systemic effect, although it is possible that there may be some systemic action on the bone marrow.

New inhaled steroids may be developed by increasing the inactivation of the systemic component of the inhaled steroid and/or by potentiating the topical anti-inflammatory action of steroids in the airways (178).

A. Increased Metabolism

The fraction of inhaled steroid deposited in the oropharynx and swallowed is available for absorption from the gastrointestinal tract. First-pass metabolism in the liver is, therefore, important in limiting the systemic effect of inhaled steroids. Budesonide and fluticasone propionate have very efficient first-pass metabolism. The swallowed fraction of inhaled steroids is also markedly reduced by the use of a large volume spacer device or by mouthwashing. However, the major component of inhaled steroid which reaches the systemic circulation is derived from the respiratory tract. The fraction of the inhaled dose that is absorbed via the lungs may be inactivated in the lung or in the circulation by esterases. Examples of such a steroids are fluocortinbutyl ester (hydrolyzed in tissue and blood) and tixocortol pivalate (inactivated by blood by S-methyltransferases) (178). However, the same properties reduce the topical potency of these steroids, resulting in local metabolism in the airways, and neither of these steroids has useful antiasthma effects. It is possible that steroids with a higher receptor affinity could be developed to exert a topical action before metabolism occurs.

B. Increased Binding

Currently, effective inhaled steroids derived from lipophilic substitution in the $17\alpha,17\beta$ positions of the glucocorticoid structure have a high affinity for the GR and also have a high mucosal uptake and retention in airways and lung

(178–180). However, increasing the local tissue retention time carries the risk of more troublesome local effect, in the oropharynx. More selective targeting of the inhaled steroid to the key target cells may be another approach in the future, although it is likely that several target cells are involved in asthma. One possibility is to target airway macrophages by the use of liposomes coated with surface receptors that trigger phagocytosis (178).

C. Genomic Selectivity

Steroids exert their anti-inflammatory and immunomodulatory effect by regulating gene transcription via several different mechanisms, as discussed above. By the use of the site-directed mutagenesis of the GR, it is possible to differentiate some of these mechanisms so that some receptor mutants may more selectively mediate a particular type of genomic mechanism. It is possible that different types of steroids might be developed in the future which may cause conformational changes in the receptor to lead to more selective genomic effects.

D. Transcription Factor Inhibitors

As discussed above, many of the key anti-inflammatory actions of glucocorticoids may be mediated via an inhibitory effect of the ligand-activated GR on activated transcription factors by a direct protein-protein interaction. In the future, it is possible that drugs may be developed that mimic this inhibitory action by blocking the synthesis or activation of transcription factors, such as NF-κB or AP-1. Some drugs have already been identified that have relatively specific inhibitory effects on these transcription factors, including dithiocarbamates for NF-κB (181) and curcumin for AP-1 (182). It is unlikely that with high-output screening assays, other such drugs will be discovered in the future, particularly as the critical enzymes that regulate the synthesis and activation of transcription factors are characterized. Such drugs may be useful in the management of chronic inflammatory diseases such as asthma.

E. Novel Anti-inflammatory Drugs

New anti-inflammatory drugs may be developed in the future that either replace glucocorticoids or may be used as steroid-sparing drugs (183). Leukotriene antagonists and 5-lipoxygenase inhibitors appear to have antiasthma effects in clinical trials (184,185), although it is unlikely that they will have significant anti-inflammatory effects. However, glucocorticoids are not very effective in inhibiting leukotriene production (186), and there may, therefore, be added benefit of combining a leukotriene antagonist with inhaled glucocorticoids. Phosphodiesterase (PDE4) inhibitors appear to have inhibitory effects against mast cells, eosinophils, T lymphocytes, and macrophages, and therefore have potential as anti-inflammatory drugs in asthma and may mimic the effect of glucocorticoids (187,188). Several selective PDE4 inhibitors are currently undergoing clinical trial in asthma, but the major limitation is nausea and vomiting. Other anti-inflammatory approaches include the development of IL-4 and IL-5 inhibitors or antagonists, although it may prove difficult to find nonpeptide drugs with these properties.

Discussion

Dr. PERRETTI: You have briefly mentioned sensory neurons and asthma. What is the role of neurogenic inflammation in contributing to the inflammatory response in asthma? And, if they have a role, do you think glucocorticoid treatment may alter their action; that is, the action and/or release of substance P and so on?

Dr. BARNES: Neurogenic inflammation may be important in some types of asthma. It is likely that glucocorticoids may reduce neurogenic inflammation in several ways. They may inhibit the induction of preprotachykinin genes, inhibit the expression of tachykinin NK_1 receptors, and inhibit the formation of mediators, such as bradykinin, that activate neurogenic inflammation.

Dr. BRATTSAND: The studies on steroid resistance suggest that too much steroid receptor is mopped up by transcription factors like AP-1. What are the most important GRE interactions, which are lost in that way?

Dr. BARNES: We propose that activated GR interacts with other transcription factors, such as NF-κB, CREB, and AP-1. This will reduce the number of GRs in a cell, and this will reduce interactions with DNA (i.e., GRE binding) but also interactions with other transcription factors (protein-protein interactions) resulting in inhibition of genomic and nongenomic actions of glucocorticoids. Perhaps of greater importance is the inhibition of cytokine gene expression via nongenomic effects.

Dr. HERSCHMAN: I want to sound a note of caution. We know that over a dozen stimuli that activate a number of different transcription factors can all induce PGS-2/COX-2. Moreover, although the same inducer activates the same second-messenger pathway and induces several distinct immediate-early genes (IEGs), glucocorticoids suppress one IEG but not another despite the use of four orders of magnitude higher drug. Although I hate to be a mystic, I think there is likely to be an as yet undiscovered mechanism at the gene structure/chromatin level that is shared by the fraction of immediate-early genes whose induction is suppressed by glucocorticoids.

Dr. Barnes: It is likely that glucocorticoids have several molecular effects—some of these will be short term, such as the interactions with transcription factors like NF-κB, AP-1, or CREB, as I described. Other interactions may be longer term and may inhibit different molecular mechanisms, which remain to be defined.

Dr. Persson: (1) The hypothesis of neurogenic inflammation is entirely built on data obtained in guinea pig and rat airways where typically capsaicin and nicotine evoke neurogenic exudation (inflammation). Now, these potent neural stimulants produce pain and secretion in human airways but not the slightest tendency of plasma exudation, not even when painful doses of capsaicin are applied on already inflamed and hyperreactive airways (Greiff et al. Thorax, in press). Hence, the neurogenic exudation/inflammation hypothesis is a phantom phenomenon in our current state of knowledge of human airway mechanisms. (2) I think NO in airway epithelium may not cause inflammation but may rather suppress the permeability of the subepithelial microcirculation. Thus, when we apply NO synthase inhibitors on the airway mucosa, we record a significant plasma exudation response in stark contrast to the effect recorded when NOs inhibitors are given intravenously.

Dr. Barnes: Neurogenic inflammation may not be important in the majority of patients with asthma, but it may be relevant in some patients with severe disease. NO may have beneficial and deleterious effects. In small amounts, as produced by constitutive enzymes, it may have anti-inflammatory actions, but when produced in large amounts from the inducible enzyme (iNOS) , it may amplify inflammation in the airways. One of the beneficial effects of glucocorticoids may be to inhibit NOS but to preserve constitutive NOS function.

Dr. Laitinen: Asthma is a syndrome, and therefore will be several genes involved. How much overlapping do these genes have with the genes controlling atopy or hyperreactivity?

Dr. Barnes: Glucocorticoids may be particularly effective at blocking the induction of inducible genes induced in inflammation (e.g., iNOS, COX-2, chemokines, and cytokines), but they do not have an inhibitory effect on noninducible genes such as IgE. This may explain why glucocorticoids do not cause severe immune depression.

Dr. Leung: (1) As a point of clarification, in the salbutamol-CREB/glucocorticoid receptor studies you mentioned, was this done in vivo or in vitro? (2) Is there any in vivo data on β-agonists upregulating CREB?

Dr. Barnes: We have demonstrated that β-agonists increase CREB binding in monocytes and T lymphocytes and that this reduces GRE binding in vitro. We have not studied this in vivo, as the concentrations of β-agonists may not be attained in plasma but are feasible in the airways after high doses of β-agonists.

References

1. Barnes PJ. Inhaled glucocorticoids for asthma. New Engl J Med 1995; 332:868–875.
2. Barnes PJ. A new approach to asthma therapy. N Engl J Med 1989; 321:1517–1527.
3. Barnes PJ. Antiinflammatory therapy in asthma. Ann Rev Med 1993; 44:229–249.
4. Barnes PJ, Pedersen S. Efficacy and safety of inhaled steroids in asthma. Am Rev Respir Dis 1993; 148:S1–S26.
5. Laitinen LA, Laitinen A, Haahtela T. A comparative study of the effects of an inhaled corticosteroid, budesonide, and of a β_2-agonist, terbutaline, on airway inflammation in newly diagnosed asthma. J Allergy Clin Immunol 1992; 90:32–42.
6. Djukanovic R, Wilson JW, Britten YM, et al. Effect of an inhaled corticosteroid on airway inflammation and symptoms of asthma. Am Rev Respir Dis 1992; 145:699–674.
7. Jeffery PK, Godfrey RW, Ädelroth E, et al. Effects of treatment on airway inflammation and thickening of basement membrane reticular collagen in asthma. Am Rev Respir Dis 1992; 145:890–899.
8. Burke C, Power CK, Norris A, et al. Lung function and immunopathological changes after inhaled corticosteroid therapy in asthma. Eur Respir J 1992; 5:73–79.
9. Trigg CJ, Manolistas ND, Wang J, et al. Placebo-controlled immunopathological study of four months inhaled corticosteroids in asthma. Am J Respir Crit Care Med 1994; 150:17–22.
10. Ädelroth E, Rosenhall L, Johansson S-A, et al Inflammatory cells and eosinophilic activity in asthmatics investigated by bronchoalveolar lavage. Am Rev Respir Dis 1990; 142:91–99.
11. Lungren R, Soderberg M, Horstedt P, et al. Morphological studies on bronchial mucosal biopsies from asthmatics before and after ten years of treatment with inhaled steroids. Eur Respir J 1988; 1:883–889.
12. Haynes AR, Shaw RJ. Dexamethasone-induced increase in platelet-derived growth factor (B) mRNA in human alveolar macrophages and myelomonocytic HL60 macrophage-like cells. Am J Respir Cell Mol Biol 1992; 7:198–206.
13. Schleimer RP. Effects of glucocorticoids on inflammatory cells relevant to their therapeutic application in asthma. Am Rev Respir Dis 1990; 141:S59–S69.
14. Woolley MJ, Denburg JA, Ellis R, et al. Allergen-induced changes in bone marrow progenitors and airway responsiveness in dogs and the effect of inhaled budesonide on these parameters. Am J Respir Cell Mol Biol 1994; 11:600–606.
15. Fuller RW, Kelsey CR, Cole PJ, et al. Dexamethasone inhibits the production of thromboxane B_2, and leukotriene B_4 by human alveolar and peritoneal macrophages in culture. Clin Sci 1984; 67:693–696.

16. Bergstrand H, Björnson A, Blaschke E, et al. Effects of an inhaled corticosteroid, budesonide, on alveolar macrophage function in smokers. Thorax 1990; 45:362-368.
17. Martinet N, Vaillant P, Charles T, et al. Dexamethasone modulation of tumour necrosis factor-α (cachectin) release by activated normal human alveolar macrophages. Eur Respir J 1992; 5:67-72.
18. Standiford TJ, Kunkel SL, Rolfe MW, et al. Regulation of human alveolar macrophage and blood monocytge-derived interleukin-8 by prostaglandin E_2 and dexmaethasone. Am J Respir Cell Mol Biol 1992; 6:75-81.
19. Borish L, Mascali JJ, Dichuck J, et al. Detection of alveolar macrophage-derived IL-1β in asthma. Inhibition with corticosteroids. J Immunol 1992; 149: 3078-3082.
20. Kita H, Abu-Ghazaleh R, Sanderson CJ, et al. Effect of steroids on immunoglobulin-induced eosinophil degranulation. J Allergy Clin Immunol 1991; 87:70-77.
21. Lamas AM, Leon OG, Schleimer RP. Glucocorticoids inhibit eosinophil responses to granulocyte-macrophage colony-stimulating factor. J Immunol 1991; 147:254-259.
22. Wallen N, Kita H, Weiller D, et al. Glucocorticoids inhibit cytokine-mediated eosinophil survival. J Immunol 1991; 147:3490-3495.
23. Baigelman W, Chodosh S, Pizzuto D, et al. Sputum and blood eosinophils during corticosteroid treatment of acute exacerbations of asthma. Am J Med 1983; 75:929-936.
24. Owen WF, Rothenberg ME, Silberstein DS, et al. Regulation of human eosinophil viability, density and function by granulocyte/macrophage colony-stimulating factor in the presence of 3T3 fibroblasts. J Exp Med 1987; 166:129-141.
25. Wempe JB, Tammeling EP, Köeter GH, et al. Blood eosinophil numbers and activity during 24 hours; effects of treatment with budesonide and bambuterol. J Allergy Clin Immunol 1992; 90:757-765.
26. Evans PM, O'Connor BJ, Fuller RW, et al. Effect of inhaled corticosteroids on peripheral eosinophil counts and density profiles in asthma. J Allergy Clin Immunol 1993; 91:643-649.
27. Elwood W, Lotvall JO, Barnes PJ, et al. Characterisation of allergen-induced bronchial hyperresponsiveness and airway inflammation in actively-sensitised Brown Norway rats. J Allergy Clin Immunol 1992; 88:951-960.
28. Elwood W, Lötvall JO, Barnes PJ, et al. Effect of dexamethasone and cyclosporin A on allergen-induced airway hyperresponsiveness and inflammatory cell responses in sensitized Brown Norway rats. Am Rev Respir Dis 1992; 145: 1289-1294.
29. Schleimer RP, Schulman ES, MacGlashan DW, et al. Effects of dexamethasone on mediator release from human lung fragments and purified human lung mast cells. J Clin Invest 1983; 71:1830-1835.
30. Cohan VL, Undem BJ, Fox CC, et al. Dexamethasone does not inhibit the release of mediators from human lung mast cells residing in airway, intestine or skin. Am Rev Respir Dis 1989; 140:951-954.
31. Sur S, Crotty TB, Kephart GM, et al. Sudden onset fatal asthma: a distinct en-

tity with few eosinophils and relatively more neutrophils in the airway submucosa. Am Rev Respir Dis 1993; 148:713–719.

32. Adcock IM, Bronnegard M, Barnes PJ. Glucocorticoid receptor mRNA localization and expression in human lung. Am Rev Respir Dis 1991; 143:A628.

33. Boschetto P, Rogers DF, Fabbri M, et al. Corticosteroid inhibition of airway microvascular leakage. Am Rev Respir Dis 1991; 143:605–609.

34. Erjefält I, Persson CGA. Pharmacologic control of plasma exudation into tracheobronchila airways. Am Rev Respir Dis 1991; 143:1008–1014.

35. Carnuccio R, Di Rosa M, Guerrasio B, et al. Vasocortin: a novel glucocorticoid-induced anti-inflammatory protein. Br J Pharmacol 1987; 90:443–445.

36. Van de Graaf EA, Out TA, Loos CM, et al. Respiratory membrane permeability and bronchial hyperreactivity in patients with stable asthma. Am Rev Respir Dis 1991; 143:362–368.

37. Kwon OJ, Au BT, Collins PD, et al. Inhibition of interleukin-8 expression in human cultured airway epithelial cells. Immunology 1994; 81:389–394.

38. Kwon OJ, Au BT, Collins PD, et al. Tumor necrosis factor-induced interleukin-8 expression in cultured human epithelial cells. Am J Physiol 1994; 11:L398–L405.

39. Kwon OJ, Jose PJ, Robbins RA, et al. Glucocorticoid inhibition of RANTES expression in human lung epithelial cells. Am J Respir Cell Mol Biol 1995; 12:488–496.

40. Sousa AR, Poston RN, Lane SJ, et al. Detection of GM-CSF in asthmatic bronchial epithelium and decrease by inhaled corticosteroids. Am Rev Respir Dis 1993; 147:1557–1561.

41. Devalia JL, Wang JH, Sapsford RJ, et al. Expression of RANTES in human bronchial epithelial cells and the effect of beclomethasone dipropionate (BDP). Eur Respir J 1994; 7(suppl 18):98S.

42. Hamid Q, Springall DR, Riveros-Moreno V, et al. Induction of nitric oxide synthase in asthma. Lancet 1993; 342:1510–1513.

43. Kharitonov SA, Yates D, Robbins RA, et al. Increased nitric oxide in exhaled air of asthmatic patients. Lancet 1994; 343:133–135.

44. Persson MG, Zetterstrom O, Argenius V, et al. Single-breath oxide measurements in asthmatic patients and smokers. Lancet 1994; 343:146–147.

45. Kharitonov SA, Yates DH, Robbins RA, et al. Corticosteroids decrease exhaled nitric oxide. Am J Respir Crit Care Med 1994; 149:A201.

46. Kharitonov SA, Yates DH, Barnes PJ. Regular inhaled budeosonide decreases nitric oxide concentration in the exhaled air of asthmatic patients. Am J Respir Crit Care Med 1995;

47. Shimura S, Sasaki T, Ikeda K, et al. Direct inhibitory action of glucocorticoid on glycoconjugate secretion from airway submucosal glands. Am Rev Respir Dis 1990; 141:1044–1099.

48. Lundgren JD, Hirata F, Marom Z, et al. Dexamethasone inhibits respiratory glycoconjugate secretion from feline airways in vitro by the induction of lipocortin (lipomodulin) synthesis. Am Rev Respir Dis 1988; 137:353–357.

49. Beato M. Gene regulation by steroid hormones. Cell 1989; 56:335-344.
50. Gronemeyer H. Control of transcription activation by steroid hormone receptors. FASEB J 1992; 6:2524-2529.
51. Miesfield RL. Molecular genetics of corticosteroid action. Am Rev Respir Dis 1990; 141:S11-S17.
52. Miner JN, Yamamoto KR. Regulatory crosstalk at composite response elements. Trends Biochem Sci 1991; 16:423-426.
53. Barnes PJ, Adcock IM. Anti-inflammatory actions of steroids: molecular mechanisms. Trends Pharmacol Sci 1993; 14:436-441.
54. Robinson DS, Durham SR, Kay AB. Cytokines in asthma. Thorax 1993; 48:845-853.
55. Barnes PJ. Cytokines as mediators of chronic asthma. Am J Respir Crit Care Med 1994; 150:S42-S49.
56. Guyre PM, Girard MT, Morganelli PM, et al. Glucocorticoid effects on the production and action of immune cytokines. J Steroid Biochem 1988; 30:89-93.
57. Ray A, Laforge KS, Sehgal PB. On the mechanisms for efficient repression of the interleukin-6 promoter by glucocorticoids: enhancer TATA box and RNA start site (1 nr motif) occlusion. Mol Cell Biol 1990; 10:5736-5746.
58. Thompson AG, Starzl TC. New immunosuppressive drugs: mechanistic insights and potential therapeutic advances. Immunol Rev 1993; 136:71-98.
59. Northrop JP, Ullman KS, Crabtree GR. Characterization of the nuclear and cytoplasmic components of the lymphoid-specific nuclear factor of activated T cells (NF-AT). J Biol Chem 1993; 268:2917-2923.
60. Paliogianni F, Raptis A, Ahuja SS, et al. Negative transcriptional regulation of human interleukin 2 (IL-2) gene by glucocorticoids through interference with nuclear transcription factors AP-1 and NF-AT. J Clin Invest 1993; 91:1481-1489.
61. Mukaido N, Morita M, Ishikawa Y, et al. Novel mechanisms of glucocorticoid-mediated gene repression: NFRB is target for glucocorticoid-mediated IL-8 gene expression. J Biol Chem 1994; 269:13289-13295.
62. Kern JA, Lamb RJ, Reed JL, et al. Dexamethasone inhibition of interleukin 1 beta production by human monocytes. Post-transcriptional mechanisms. J Clin Invest 1988; 81:237-244.
63. Shaw G, Kamen R. A conserved AV sequence from the 3' untranslated region of GM-CSF on RNA mediates selective mRNA degradation. Cell 1986; 46:659-667.
64. Grabstein K, Dower S, Gillis S, et al. Expression of interleukin 2, interferon-Y and the IL2 receptor by human peripheral blood lymphocytes. J Immunol 1986; 136:4503-4508.
65. Adcock IM, Shirasaki H, Gelder CM, et al. The effects of glucocorticoids on phorbol ester and cytokine stimulated transcription factor activation in human lung. Life Sci 1994; 55:1147-1153.
66. Crabtree GR. Contingent genetic regulatory events in T lymphocyte activation. Science 1989; 243:355-361.
67. Barnes PJ, Belvisi MG. Nitric oxide and lung disease. Thorax 1993; 48:1034-1043.
68. Barnes PJ, Liew FY. Nitric oxide and asthmatic inflammation. Immunol Today 1995; 16:128-130.

69. Di Rosa M, Radomski M, Carnuccio R, et al. Glucocorticoids inhibit the induction of nitric oxide synthase in macrophages. Biochem Biophys Res Commun 1990; 172:1246-1252.

70. Radomski MW, Palmer RMJ, Moncada S. Glucocorticoids inhibit the expression of an inducible, but not the constitute nitric oxide synthase in vascular endothelial cells. Proc Natl Acad Sci USA 1990; 87:10043-10049.

71. Robbins RA, Springall DR, Warren JB, et al. Inducible nitric oxide synthase is increased in murine lung epithelial cells by cytokine stimulation. Biochem Biophys Res Commun 1994; 198:1027-1033.

72. Robbins RA, Barnes PJ, Springall DR, et al. Expression of inducible nitric oxide synthase in human bronchial epithelial cells. Biochem Biophys Res Commun 1994; 203:209-218.

73. Lowenstein CJ, Alley EW, Raval P, et al. Macrophage nitric oxide synthase gene: two upstream regions mediate induction by interferon y and lipopolysaccharide. Proc Natl Acad Sci USA 1993; 90:9730-9734.

74. Chang KC, Morrill CG, Chair H. Impaired response to hypoxia after bilateral carotid body resection for treatment of bronchial asthma. Chest 1978; 73:667-669.

75. Xie Q-W, Kashiwarbara Y, Nathan C. Role of transcription factor NF-αB/Rel in induction of nitric oxide synthase. J Biol Chem 1994; 269:4705-4708.

76. Adcock IM, Brown CR, Kwon OJ, et al. Oxidative stress induces NF-KB DNA binding and inducible NOS mRNA in human epithelial cells. Biochem Biophys Res Commun 1994; 199:1518-1524.

77. O'Banion MK, Winn VD, Young DA. cDNA cloning and functional activity of a glucocorticoid-regulated inflammatory cyclooxygenase. Proc Natl Acad Sci USA 1992; 89:4888-4892.

78. Mitchell JA, Belvisi MG, Akarasereemom P, et al. Induction of cyclo-oxygenase-2 by cytokines in human pulmonary epithelial cells: regulation by dexamethasone. Br J Pharmacol 1994; 113:1008-1014.

79. Newton R, Adcock IM, Barnes PJ. Stimulation of COX-2 message by cytokines or phorbol ester is preceded by a massive and rapid induction of NF-kB binding activity. Am J Respir Crit Care Med 1995; 151:A165.

80. Schalkwijk C, Vervoordeldonk M, Pfeilschifter J, et al. Cytokine- and forskolin-induced synthesis of group II phospholipase A_2 and prostaglandin E_2 in rat mesangial cells is prevented by dexamethasone. Biochem Biophys Res Commun 1991; 180:46-52.

81. Goulding NJ, Godolphin JL, Sharland PR, et al. Anti-inflammatory lipocortin 1 production by peripheral leucocytes in response to hydrocortisone. Lancet 1990; 335:1416-1418.

82. Peers SH, Smillie F, Elderfield AJ, et al. Glucocorticoid and non-glucocorticoid induction of lipocortins (anrexins) 1 and 2 in rat peritoneal leucocytes in vivo. Br J Pharmacol 1993; 108:66-72.

83. Cirino G, Flower RJ, Browning JL, et al. Recombinant human lipocortin 1 inhibits thromboxane release from guinea pig isolated perfused lung. Nature 1987; 328:270-272.

84. Flower RJ. Lipocortin and the mechanisms of action of the glucocorticoids. Br J Pharmacol 1988; 94:987–1015.
85. Davidson FF, Dennis EA. Biological relevance of lipocortins and related proteins as inhibitors of phospholipase A_2. Biochem Pharmacol 1989; 38:3645–3651.
86. Brönnegard M, Andersson O, Edwall D, et al. Human calpactin II (lipocortin I) messenger ribonucleic acid is not induced by glucocorticoids. Mol Endocrinol 1988; 2:732–739.
87. Andersson SE, Zackrisson C, Hemsen S, et al. Regulation of lung endothelin content by the glucocortosteroid budesonide. Biochem Biophys Res Commun 1992; 188:1116–1121.
88. Vittori E, Marini M, Fasoli A, et al. Increased expression of endothelin in bronchial epithelial cells of asthmatic patients and effect of corticosteroids. Am Rev Respir Dis 1992; 1461:1320–1325.
89. Stankova J, Roba-Pleszczynki M. Leukotriene B_4 stimulates c-fos and c-jun gene transcription and AP-1 binding activity in human monocytes. Biochem J 1992; 282:625–629.
90. Adcock IM, Peters M, Gelder C, et al. Increased tachykinin receptor gene expression in asthmatic lung and its modulation by steroids. J Mol Endocrinol 1993; 11:1–7.
91. Collins S, Caron MG, Lefkowitz RJ. β-Adrenergic receptors in hamster smooth muscle cells are transcriptionally regulated by glucocorticoids. J Biol Chem 1988; 263:9067–9070.
92. Strader CD, Sigal IS, Dixon RAF. Structural basis of β-adrenergic receptor function. FASEB J 1989; 3:1825–1832.
93. Mak JCW, Niskikawa M, Barnes PJ. Glucocorticoids increase $β_2$-adrenoceptor transcription in human lung. Am J Physiol 1995; 12:L41–L46.
94. Nishikawa M, Shirasaki M, Mak JW, et al. Protective effects of dexamethasone on isoproterenol-induced down-regulation of pulmonary $β_2$-receptors in rat. Am Rev Respir Dis 1993; 147:A275.
95. Colotta F, Re F, Muzio M, et al. Interleukin-1 type II receptor: a decoy target for IL-1 that is regulated by IL-4. Science 1993; 261(5120):472–475.
96. Re F, Muzio M, De Rossi M, et al. The type II "receptor" as a decoy target for interleukin I in polymorphonuclear leukocytes: characterization of induction by dexamethasone and ligand binding properties of the released decoy receptor. J Exp Med 1994; 179:739–743.
97. Borson DB, Jew S, Gruenert DC. Glucocorticoids induce neutral endopeptidase in transformed human trachea epithelial cells. Am J Physiol 1991; 260:L83–89.
98. Piedimonte G, McDonald DM, Nadal JA. Glucocorticoids inhibit neurogenic plasma extravasation and prevent virus-potentiated extravasation in the rat trachea. J Clin Invest 1990; 86:1409–1415.
99. Proud D, Subauste MC, Ward RE. Glucocorticoids do not alter peptidase expression on a human bronchial epithelial cell line. Am J Respir Cell Mol Biol 1994; 11:57–65.
100. Mendelsohn FAO, Lloyd CJ, Kalhel C, et al. Induction by glucocorticoids of angiotensin converting enzyme production from bovine endothelial cells in culture and rat lung in vivo. J Clin Invest 1982; 710:684–692.

101. Owens GP, Hahn WE, Coehn JJ. Identification of mRNAs associated with programmed cell death in immature thymocytes. Mol Cell Biol 1991; 11:4177–4188.
102. Cronstein BN, Kimmel SC, Levin RI, et al. A mechanism for the antiinflammatory effects of corticosteroids: The glucocorticoid receptor regulates leukocyte adhesion to endothelial cells and expression of endothelial-leukocyte adhesion molecule 1 and intercellular adhesion molecule 1. Proc Natl Acad Sci USA 1992; 89:9991–9995.
103. Van De Stolpe A, Caldenhoven E, Raaijmakers JAM, et al. Glucocorticoid-mediated repression of intercellular adhesion molecule-1 expression in human monocytic and bronchial epithelial cell lines. Am J Respir Cell Mol Biol 1993; 8:340–347.
104. Van De Stolpe A, Caldenhoven E, Stade BG, et al. 12-0-tetradecanoyl phorbol-13-acetate and tumor necrosis factor alpha-mediated induction of intercellular adhesion molecule-1 is inhibited by dexamethasone. Functional analysis of the human intercellular adhesion molecule-1 promoter. J Biol Chem 1994; 269:6185–6192.
105. Peppel K, Vinci JM, Baglioni C. The AU-rich sequences in the 3′ untranslated region mediate the increased turnover of interferon mRNA induced by glucocorticoids. J Exp Med 1991; 173:349–355.
106. Schüle R, Evans RM. Cross-coupling of signal transduction pathways: zinc finger meet leucine zipper. Trends Genet 1991; 7:377–381.
107. Ponta H, Cato ACB, Herrlick P. Interference of specific transcription factors. Biochim Biophys Acta 1992; 1129:255–261.
108. Jonat C, Rahsdorf HJ, Park KK, et al. Anti tumor promotion and antiinflammation: down-modulation of AP-1 (fos/jun) activity by glucocorticoid hormone. Cell 1990; 62:1189–1204.
109. Schüle R, Rangarajan P, Kliewer S, et al. Functional antagonism between oncoprotein c-Jun and the glucocorticoid receptor. Cell 1990; 62:1217–1226.
110. Yang-Yen H-F, Chambard J-C, Sun Y-L, et al. Transcriptional interference between c-Jun and the glucocorticoid receptor: mutual inhibition of DNA binding due to direct protein-protein interaction. Cell 1990; 62:1205–1215.
111. Kerrpola TK, Luk D, Curran T. FOS is a preferential target of glucocorticoid receptor inhibition of AP-1 activity in vitro. Mol Cell Biol 1993; 13:3782–3790.
112. Adcock IM, Brown CR, Gelder CM, et al. The effects of glucocorticoids on transcription factor activation in human peripheral blood mononuclear cells. Am J Physiol 1995; 37:C331–C338.
113. Ray A, Prefontaine KE. Physical association and functional antagonism between the p65 subunit of transcription factor NF-κB and the glucocorticoid receptor. Proc Natl Acad Sci USA 1994 ;91:752–756.
114. Yamamoto KK, Gonzalez GA, Biggs WH, et al. Phosphorylation-induced binding and transcriptional efficacy of nuclear factor CREB. Nature 1988; 334:494–498.
115. Imai F, Minger JN, Mitchell JA, et al. Glucocorticoid receptor-cAMP response element-binding protein interaction and the response of the phosphoenolpyruvate carboxykinase gene to glucocorticoids. J Biol Chem 1993; 268:5353–5356.

116. Peters MJ, Adcock IM, Brown CR, et al. β-Agonist inhibition of steroid-receptor DNA binding activity in human lung. Am Rev Respir Dis 1993; 147:A772.
117. Stevens DA, Barnes PJ, Adcock IM. β-Agonists inhibit DNA binding of glucocorticoid receptors in human pulmonary and bronchial epithelial cells. Am J Respir Crit Care Med 1995;
118. Adcock IM, Barnes PJ. Actions of the glucocorticoid receptor on transcription factors within the cytoplasma. Am J Respir Crit Care Med 1995;
119. Szefler S. Glucocorticoid therapy for asthma: clinical pharmacology. J Allergy Clin Immunol 1991; 88:147–165.
120. Hummel S, Lehtonen L. Comparison of oral steroid sparing by high-dose and low-dose inhaled steroid in maintenance treatment of severe asthma. Lancet 1992; 340:1483–1487.
121. Pin I, Gibon PG, Kolendowicz R, et al. Use of induced sputum cell counts to investigate airway inflammation in asthma. Thorax 1992; 47:25–29.
122. Yates DH, Kharitonov SA, Robbins RA, et al. Effect of a nitric oxide synthase inhibitor and a glucocorticosteroid on exhaled nitric oxide. Am J Respir Crit Care Med 1995;
123. Okret S, Dong Y, Brönnegård M, et al. Regulationof glucocorticoid receptor expression. Biochimie 1991; 73:51–59.
124. Rosewicz S, McDonald AR, Maddux BA, et al. Mechanism of glucocorticoid receptor down-regulation by glucocorticoids. J Biol Chem 1988; 263:2581–2584.
125. Pepin M-C, Pothier F, Barden N. Impaired type II glucocorticoid-receptor function in mice bearing antisense RNA transgene. Nature 1992; 355:725–728.
126. Agertoft L, Pedersen S. Effects of long-term treatment with an inhaled corticosteroid on growth and pulmonary function in asthmatic children. Respir Med 1994; 5:369–372.
127. Haahtela T, Järvinsen M, Kava T, et al. Effects of reducing or discontinuing inhaled budesonide in patients with mild asthma. N Engl J Med 1994; 331:700–705.
128. Morell F, Orkiols R, de Gracia J, et al. Controlled trial of intravenous corticosteroids in severe acute asthma. Thorax 1992; 47:588–591.
129. Kam JC, Szefler SJ, Surs W, et al. Combination IL-2 and IL-4 reduces glucocorticoid-receptor binding affinity and T cell response to glucocorticoids. J Immunol 1993; 151:3460–3466.
130. Peters MJ, Adcock IM, Barnes PJ. High concentrations of β_2-agonists induced glucocorticoid receptor-DNA binding in rat lung. Eur J Pharmacol Mol Section 1995; 289:275–281.
131. Wong CS, Wamedna I, Pavord ID, et al. Effect of regular terbutaline and budesonide on bronchial reactivity to allergen challenge. Am J Respir Crit Care Med 1994; 15047:1268–1278.
132. Barnes PJ, Chung KF. Questions about inhaled β2-agonists in asthma. Trends Pharmacol Sci 1992; 13:20–23.
133. Spitzer WO, Suissa S, Ernst P, et al. The use of β-agonists and the rate of death and near-death from asthma. N Engl J Med 1992; 326:503–506.
134. Sears MR, Taylor DR, Print CG, et al. Regular inhaled beta-agonist treatment in bronchial asthma. Lancet 1990; 336:1391–1396.

135. Peters MJ, Yates DH, Chung KF, et al. β_2-Agonist dose reduction: strategy and early results. Thorax 1993; 48:1066.
136. Cypcar D, Busse WW. Steroid-resistant asthma. J Allergy Clin Immunol 1993; 92:362-372.
137. Lamberts SWJ, Kioper JW, de Jong FH. Familial and iatrogenic cortisol receptor resistance. J Steroid Biochem Molec Biol 1992; 43:385-388.
138. Chrousos GP, Vingrhoeds ACM, Brandon D, et al. Primary cortisol resitance in man: a glucocorticoid receptor-mediated disease. J Clin Invest 1982; 69:1261-1269.
139. Malchoff DM, Brufsky A, McDermott P, et al. A mutation of the glucocorticoid receptor in primary cortisol resistance. J Clin Invest 1993; 91:1918-1925.
140. Lane SJ, Arm JP, Staynov DZ, et al. Chemical mutational analysis of the human glucocorticoid receptor cDNA in glucocorticoid-resistant bronchial asthma. Am J Respir Cell Mol Biol 1994; 11:42-48.
141. Brown PH, Teelucksingh S, Matusiewicz SP, et al. Cutaneous vasoconstrictor responses to glucocorticoids in asthma. Lancet 1991; 337:576-580.
142. Corrigan C, Brown PH, Barnes NC, et al. Glucocorticoid resistance in chronic asthma. Am Rev Respir Dis 1991; 144:1016-1025.
143. Lane SJ, Lee TH. Glucocorticoid receptor characteristics in monocytes of patients with corticosteroid-resistant bronchial asthma. Am Rev Respir Dis 1991; 143:1020-1024.
144. Alvarez J, Surs W, Leung DY, et al. Steroid-resistant asthma: immunologic and pharmacologic features. J Allergy Clin Immunol 1992; 89:714-721.
145. Adcock IM, Lane SJ, Brown CR, et al. Differences in binding of glucocorticoid receptor to DNA in steroid-resistant asthma. J Immunol 1995; 154:3500-3505.
146. Adcock IM, Brown CR, Virdee H, et al. Transcription factor interactions in peripheral blood monocytes of steroid sensitive and resistant asthmatic patients. Am Rev Respir Dis 1993; 147:A292.
147. Adcock IM, Lane SJ, Brown CA, Lee TH, Barnes PJ. AP-1 and glucocorticoid receptor DNA binding in peripheral blood mononuclear cells from steroid-sensitive and resistant patients. J Exp Med 1995; 182:1951-1958.
148. Vathenen AS, Knox AJ, Wisniewski A, et al. Time course of change in bronchial reactivity with an inhaled corticosteroid in asthma. Am Rev Respir Dis 1991; 143:1317-1321.
149. Waalkens HJ, van Essen-Zandvliet EE, Hughes MD, et al. Cessation of long-term treatment with inhaled corticosteroids (budesonide) in children with asthma results in deterioration. Am Rev Respir Dis 1993; 148:1252-1257.
150. Selroos O, Backman R, Forsen K-O, et al. When to start treatment of asthma with inhaled steroids? Eur Resp J 1994; 7(suppl 18):151S.
151. Hoag JE, McFadden ER. Long-term effect of cromolyn sodium on nonspecific bronchial hyperresponsiveness: a review. Ann Allergy 1991; 66:53-63.
152. Thomson NC. Nedocromil sodium: an overview. Resp Med 1989; 83:269-276.
153. Bel EH, Timmers MC, Hermans JO, et al. The longer term effects of nedocromil sodium and beclomethasone dipropionate on bronchial responsiveness to

methacholine in non-atopic asthmatic subjects. Am Rev Respir Dis 1990; 141:21–28.

154. Svendsen UG, Frolund L, Madsen F, et al. A comparison of the effects of sodium cromoglycate and beclomethasone dipropionate on pulmonary function and bronchial hyperreactivity in subjects with asthma. J Allergy Clin Immunol 1987; 80:68–74.

155. Groot CAR, Lammers J-WJ, Molema J, et al. Effect of inhaled beclomethasone and nedocromil sodium on bronchial hyperresponsiveness to histamine and distilled water. Eur Respir J 1992; 5:1075–1082.

156. Bone MF, Kubik MM, Keaney NP, et al. Nedocromil sodium in adults with asthma dependent on inhaled corticosteroids in a double-blind placebo-controlled study. Thorax 1989; 44:654–659.

157. Boulet LP, Cartier A, Cockroft DW, et al. Tolerance to reduction of oral steroid dosage in severely asthmatic patients receiving nedocromil sodium. Respir Med 1990; 84:317–323.

158. Svendsen UG, Jorgensen H. Inhaled nedocromil sodium as additional treatment to high dose inhaled corticosteroids in the management of bronchial asthma. Eur Respir J 1991; 4:992–999.

159. Goldin JG, Bateman ED. Dose nedocromil sodium have a steroid sparing effect in adult asthmatic pateints requiring maintenance oral corticosteroids? Thorax 1988; 43:982–986.

160. Mullarkey MF, Blumenstein BA, Mandrade WP, et al. Methotrexate in the treatment of corticosteroid-dependent asthma. N Engl J Med 1988; 318:683–607.

161. Mullarkey MF, Lammert JK, Blumenstein BA. Long-term methotrexate treatment in corticosteroid-dependent asthma. Ann Intern Med 1990; 112:5777–581.

162. Shiner RJ, Nunn AJ, Chung KF, et al. Randomized, double-blind, placebo-controlled trial of methotrexate in steroid-dependent asthma. Lancet 1990; 336:137–140.

163. Klaustermeyer WB, Noritake DT, Kwong FK. Chrysotherapy in the treatment of corticosteroid-dependent asthma. J Allergy Clin Immunol 1987; 79:720–725.

164. Nierop G, Gijzel WP, Bel EH, et al. Auranofin in the treatment of steroid dependent asthma: a double blind study. Thorax 1992; 47:349–354.

165. Alexander AG, Barnes NC, Kay AB. Trial of cyclosporin in corticosteroid-dependent chronic severe asthma. Lancet 1992; 339:324–328.

166. Szczeklik A, Nizankoska E, Dworski R, et al. Cyclosporin for steroid-dependent asthma. Allergy 1991; 46:312–315.

167. Wright LC, Cammisuli S, Baboulene L, et al. Cyclosporin A and glucocorticoids interact synergistically in T lymphocytes: implications for asthma therapy. Am J Respir Crit Care Med 1995; 151:A675.

168. Church MK, Hiroi J. Inhibition of IgE-dependent histamine release from human dispersed lung mast cells by anti-allergic drugs and salbutamol. Br J Pharmacol 1987; 90:421–429.

169. O'Connor BJ, Aikman SL, Barnes PJ. Tolerance to the non-bronchodilator effects of inhaled β_2-agonists. N Engl J Med 1992; 327:1204–1208.

170. Roberts JA, Bradding P, Wallis AF, et al. The influence of salmeterol xinafoate on mucosal inflammation in asthma. Am Rev Respir Dis 1992; 145:A418.

171. Greening AP, Ind PW, Northfield M, et al. Added salmeterol versus higher-dose corticosteroid in asthma patients with symptoms on existing inhaled corticosteroid. Lancet 1994; 344:219–224.
172. Barnes PJ, Pauwels RA. Theophylline in asthma: time for reappraisal? Eur Respir J 1994; 7:579–591.
173. Brenner MR, Berkowitz R, Marshall N, et al. Need for theophylline in severe steroid-requiring asthmatics. Clin Allergy 1988; 18:143–150.
174. Kidney J, Dominguez M, Taylor PM, et al. Immunomodulation by theophylline in asthma: demonstration by withdrawl of therapy. Am J Respir Crit Care Med 1995; 151:1907–1914.
175. Nassif EG, Weinburger M, Thompson R, et al. The value of maintenance theophylline in steroid-dependent asthma. N Engl J Med 1981; 304:71–75.
176. Tinkelman DG, Reed CE, Nelson HS, et al. Aerosol beclomethasone dipropionate compared with theophylline as primary treatment of chronic, mild to moderately severe asthma in children. Pediatrics 1993; 92:64–77.
177. Muller M, Renkawitz R. The glucocorticoid receptor. Biochim Biophys Acta 1991; 1088:171–182.
178. Brattsand R, Axelsson B. New inhaled glucocorticosteroids. In: Barnes PJ. ed. New Drugs for Asthma. Vol 2. London: IBC Technical Services, 1992:192–207.
179. Miller-Larsson A, Lundin P, Brattsand R. Affinity for airway tissue of topical corticosteroid budesonide, but not hydrocortisone—a study in a rat tracheal model in situ. Eur Respir J 1992; 5(suppl 15):364S.
180. Ryrfeldt Å, Persson G, Nilsson E. Pulmonary deposition of the potent glucocorticoid budesonide evaluated in an isolated perfused rat lung model. Biochem Pharmacol 1989; 38:17–22.
181. Schreck R, Meier B, Männel DN, et al. Dithiocarbanates as potent inhibitors of nuclear factor-κB activation in intact cells. J Exp Med 1991; 175:1181.
182. Huang T-S, Lee S-C, Lin J-K. Suppression of cJun/AP-1 activation by an inhibitor of tumor promotion in mouse fibroblast cells. Proc Natl Acad Sci USA 1991; 88:5292–5296.
183. Barnes PJ. New drugs for asthma. Eur Respir J 1992; 5:1126–1136.
184. Israel E, Rubin P, Kemp JP, et al. The effect of inhibiton of 5-lipoxygenase by zileuton in mild-to-moderate asthma. Ann Intern Med 1993; 119:1059–1066.
185. Spector SL, Smith LJ, Glass M. Effects of 6 weeks of therapy with oral doses of ICI 204,219, a leukotriene D4 receptor antagonist in subjects with bronchial asthma. Am J Respir Crit Care Med 1994; 150:618–623.
186. O'Shaughnessy KM, Wellings R, Gillies B, et al. Differential effects of fluticasone propionate on allergen-induced bronchoconstriction and increased urinary leukotriene E4 excretion. Am Rev Respir Dis 1993; 147:1472–1476.
187. Torphy TJ, Undem RJ. Phosphodiesterase inhibitors: new opportunities for the treatment of asthma. Thorax 1991; 46:512–523.
188. Barnes PJ. Cyclic nucleotides, phosphodiesterases and airway function. Eur Respir J 1995; 8:457–462.

AUTHOR INDEX

Italic numbers give the page on which the complete reference is listed

Ullman, K. S., 40, *49*, 658, *678*
Umland, S., 289, *306*
Unanue, E. R., 209, *227*, 282, *298*,
 313, *337*
Undem, B. J., 90, *105*, 205, *225*, 244,
 256, 262, 263, 265, *273*, 654, 672,
 676, *685*
Ungar, F., 396, *430*
Unno, T., 529, *547*
Uralets, V. P., 400, *433*
Urban, J. Jr., 263, *274*
Urda, L. A., 93, *106*
Urdal, D., 212, *230*
Urdal, V., 410, *440*
Uribe, M., 409, *438*, *439*
Utz, P., 40, *49*
Utz, P. J., 111, *116*
Uwyyed, K., 558, *595*
Uyemura, K., 315, *339*

V

Vacca, A., 32, *48*, 89, *103*, 286, *303*
Vacchio, M. S., 17, *27*
Vachino, G., 290, *307*
Vadas, M. A., 210, 214, *229*, *233*,
 281, 284, 290, *298*, *301*, *307*, 325,
 345, 526, 528, *543*, *544*
Vaheri, E., 525, *542*
Vaillant, P., 653, *676*
Valent, P., 261, *272*
Valent, T., 261, *271*
Valeria, P., 389, 402, *427*
Valerius, T., 528, *546*
Valge-Archer, V. E., 40, *49*, 640, *648*
Vamvakopoulos, N., 634, *647*
van Andrian, U. H., 212, *230*
Van As, A., 534, 535, *449*, *550*
Van Bever, J. P., 558, *595*
van Boxtel, C. J., 422, *445*
Vanceri, C., 216, *234*, 285, *301*
Vancheri, C., 154, *164*, 263, *274*
Van Damme, L., 216, *235*
Van de Graaf, E. A., 167, 179, 183,
 197, 654, *677*

van den Bosch, J. M. M., 360, 363,
 378, 395, 422, *430*
van der Mark, T. W., 499, *504*, 554,
 593
van der Straeten, M., 419, *444*
Van De Stolpe, A., 661, *681*
van Essen Zandvliet, E. E., 418, *443*,
 552, 554, 555, 556, 577, 578, 579,
 591, *593*, *594*, *604*, 668, *683*
van Essen-Sandvliet, E. E. M., 627, *645*
Van Grunsven, P. M., 497, *504*
Van Herle, A. J., 565, *598*
Van Herwaarden, C. L. A., 497, *504*,
 508, *517*, 554, *593*
Vanhoutte, P. M., 276, *296*
Vanhove, B., 37, 42, *49*
van Houwelingen, H. C., 577, 578,
 579, *604*
van Leeuwen, B. H., 323, 329, *343*,
 346
Van Metre, T. E., 575, *602*
van Niekerk, C. H., 585, *605*
VanOtteren, G. M., 217, *236*
Van Otteren, J. M., 282, *299*
van Reijsen, V. C., 315, *339*
Van Riper, G., 217, *236*
Van Schayk, C. P., 497, *504*
Vanthenen, A. S., 499, *504*, 554, *593*
vanUffelen, R., 482, *492*
Van Wheel, C., 497, *504*
Vanzieleghem, M. A., 494, *503*
Vanzieleghem, M., 494, *503*
Vardimon, L., 17, *27*, 41, *51*
Varigos, Wootton, A., 89, *103*
Varkila, K., 314, *339*
Varma, N., 485, *492*
Varney, S. R., 213, *231*
Varney, V., 207, *226*, 240, *252*, 317,
 340
Varney, V. A., 213, *231*, 245, *256*,
 315, *339*, 526, 529, 530, *543*
Varnum, B. C., 54, 55, 61, 63, 66,
 78, *79*
Varsano, I., 558, 565, 566, 576, 577,
 578, *595*, *598*, *603*

SUBJECT INDEX

[Glucocorticoid receptor (GR)]
  and transcriptional interference, 31
  transcriptional transactivation domain, 5
  zinc finger, 5
Glucocorticosteroids, 173-174, 204-207, 209, 219, 393
  binding globulin, 393
  bronchoconstriction, 174
  cost–benefit of inhaled, 500
  effects on adhesion proteins, 209
  effects on cytokines, 209
  effects on gene activation, 204
  eosinophil recruitment, 219
  leukocyte inflammation, 205-206
  skin inflammation, 207
  structure, 351
    airway selectivity, 351
  transcription factors, 205
  treatment, 495-497
    asthma, 495-496
    early intervention, 496
    effect on lung function, 497
  vasoconstriction, 173
Glucose metabolism, 585
  effects of steroids, 585
Glutamine synthetase, 96
Glycosaminoglycans, 124
  extracellular matrix, 124
  basement membrane, 124
Glycyrrhetinic acid, 408
  drug interactions, 408
Goblet cell hyperplasia, 123
  epithelial changes, 123
Granulocyte macrophage–colony stimulating factor (GM-CSF), 41, 86, 115, 214, 240-241, 288, 309-310, 314, 316, 317, 318, 323, 324, 327, 329, 330, 331, 528
  allergic rhinitis, 528
  basophils, 524
    growth, 261
  and eosinophil survival, 284, 285
  epithelial cells, 527
  in the lung, 311
  pharmacodynamics, 411
  T lymphocytes, 526

Grb-2, 111
GRE(s), 4, 15, 17, 83, 99, 113, 320, 321, 330, 332
  halfsites, 83
  negative (nGRE), 15, 17
GRE_{PAL}, 83, 99
Growth, 573, 575, 590, 620
  adverse effects, 535
  age-dependency, 573
  effects of inhaled steroids, 590
  effects of intermediate steroids, 577
  effects of oral steroids, 575
  effects of short-term steroids, 575, 576
    dose-dependent effects of inhaled steroids, 576
  effects of steroids, 575
  influence of disease, 573
  inhaled steroids, 576

H

H_1-antihistamine, 523
  mast cells, 523
  perennial allergic rhinitis, 534
  seasonal allergic rhinitis, 532
Half-life, 387
  intravenous absorption, 387
  pharmacokinetics, 386
  topically active glucocorticoids, 405
Health symptom scores, 483
  oral and inhaled corticosteroids, 483
    comparison of, 483
Hemopoietic and proinflammatory cytokines, 263
Hepatic biotransformation, 364
  hepatic first-pass metabolism, 364
Hepatic blood flow, 410
Hepatic metabolism, 355, 357
  airway selectivity, 355, 357
  first-pass metabolism, 364
Herpes virus type 16 gene regulatory region, 15
High endothelial venules (HEV), 109
Histamine, 264, 528